Martin Woesler, Hans-Martin Sass (Eds.)

Medicine and Ethics in Times of Corona

Ethik in der Praxis/Practical Ethics

Studien/Studies

herausgegeben von/edited by

Ilhan Ilkilic
Universität Istanbul

Arnd T. May
Erfurt

Amir Muzur
Universität Rijeka

Hans-Martin Sass
Ruhr-Universität Bochum,
Georgetown University Washington DC

Martin Woesler
Universität Witten/Herdecke

Band/Volume 47

LIT

Medicine and Ethics in Times of Corona

edited by

Martin Woesler and Hans-Martin Sass

LIT

Cover image: Erwin J. Löhr

This book is printed on acid-free paper.

Bibliographic information published by the Deutsche Nationalbibliothek
The Deutsche Nationalbibliothek lists this publication in the Deutsche
Nationalbibliografie; detailed bibliographic data are available in the Internet at
http://dnb.dnb.de.

ISBN 978-3-643-91320-3 (pb)
ISBN 978-3-643-96320-8 (PDF)

A catalogue record for this book is available from the British Library.

© LIT VERLAG GmbH & Co. KG Wien,
Zweigniederlassung Zürich 2020
Flössergasse 10
CH-8001 Zürich
Tel. +41 (0) 76-632 84 35
E-Mail: zuerich@lit-verlag.ch   http://www.lit-verlag.ch
Distribution:
In the UK: Global Book Marketing, e-mail: mo@centralbooks.com
In North America: Independent Publishers Group, e-mail: orders@ipgbook.com
In Germany: LIT Verlag Fresnostr. 2, D-48159 Münster
Tel. +49 (0) 2 51-620 32 22, Fax +49 (0) 2 51-922 60 99, e-mail: vertrieb@lit-verlag.de

Content

Biographies

Awaya, Prof. Dr. **Tsuyoshi** B.Sc., LL.M., Ph.D., Professor of Bioethics and Medical Law, Faculty of Law, Okayama Shoka University, Okayama, Japan. (Professor Emeritus, Okayama University, Okayama, Japan). Specialization in Bioethics, Medical Law, Law and Sociology. Honors: 1. Testimony at the U.S. Congress on the Transplantation of Organs from Executed Prisoners in China, 1998, 2. Award for Promotion of Research from the Japan Association for Bioethics, 1996. *About 40 Books and Over 100 Academic Articles. F*or many years, he has been conducting fact-finding surveys, legislative researches, etc. on organ transplantation in Asian countries. Specifically, he conducted various surveys on organ trafficking in India and the Philippines, on excuted prisoners and Falun Gong transplants in China. He had a testimony and a statement on the transplantation of organs from executed prisoners in China at the International Relations Committee and the Government Reform and Oversight Committee of the United States House of Representatives on June 4, 1998: DECLARATION OF WAR ON MODERN CIVILIZATION BY THE NEW CORONAVIRUS IS A GREAT OPPORTUNITY TO REVIEW IT.

Baydar, Prof. Dr. **Tuba Erkoç** is Assistant Professor with Ibn Haldun University. She was born in Bitlis, graduated from Uludag University Faculty of Theology with a minor in Social Sciences in 2009. She completed her master's degree at the Faculty of Theology at Istanbul University in 2011 with her thesis, "Command and Prohibition in Abû Ishâq Al-Shîrâzî's Legal Thought". In 2011, her doctorate studies started at Marmara University in the field of Islamic Law and she continued to work as research assistant at the same department. In 2017, she gained the title of doctor with the thesis of "Euthanasia and Withholding Treatment: an Islamic Legal Analysis". Tuba Erkoc Baydar was born in a scholarly family and began her studies at an early age under her family. Her madrasah education continued at Bursa and at Istanbul. Meanwhile, she completed ISAM's AYP program. She has been at France, Syria and Jordan for educational purposes and in 2014, she stayed for a year at United States at Georgetown University Kennedy Institute of Ethics for conducting research and participating several courses: ISLAM'S APPROACH TO INFECTIOUS DISEASES THROUGH THE EYES OF A NINTH CENTURY MUSLIM SCHOLAR.

Beauregard, Hon. Prof. Dr. **Paul Melot de** is a partner of the international law firm of Jones Day in Dusseldorf and honorary professor of Fern University Hagen (Germany). After finishing his studies at the universities in Munich and Wurzburg with the first state exam he earned his Ph.D. under Curt-Wolfgang Hergenröder at Wurzburg University with a thesis dealing with collective bargaining agreements. After that he earned the degree of an LL.M. (labour law) at the London School of Economics (UK). He advises and publishes in regard to all matters involving German and European employment law: STRATEGIES FOR THE NEW WORLD OF WORK.

Buschmann, Dr. **Christian**, is Treasury Manager at a Frankfurt-based broker dealer, a subsidiary of one of Japan's largest banking groups. Before this he spent 11 years at a leading German Bank in several positions in Frankfurt am Main, London, and Luxembourg. He holds a diploma-degree in business administration from the Business and Information Technology School (BiTS) in Iserlohn and a MA and PhD from the Frankfurt School of Finance & Management. Since 2017 he is board member of the Allied European Financial Markets Associaton (AEFMA) and responsible for AEFMA's education programme. - cfc.buschmann@gmail.com: A SHIFT IN ECONOMIC PARADIGMS – THE NEWMALITY.

Byk, **Christian**, is Judge at the Court of Appeal in Paris, Secretary General of the International Association of Law, Ethics and Science and Chairman of the Intergovernmental Bioethics Committee of UNESCO (2017-2019). christian.byk@gmail.com: BEYOND PANDEMICS: THE REORANIZATION OF POWERS AND THE NEW FACE OF SOCIETY

Castro, Prof. Dr. **Leonardo d. de**, - Professorial Lecturer, Department of Philosophy, University of the Philippines Diliman, Quezon City. He chairs the Philippine Health Research Ethics Board and is a member of the National Ethics Committee. He has been lecturing for UNESCO's

Ethics Teacher Training Course. He has served as Senior Research Fellow at the National University of Singapore, Editor-in-Chief of the Asian Bioethics Review, Vice President of the UNESCO International Bioethics Committee, President of the Asian Bioethics Association, and Centennial Professor at the University of the Philippines. His research interests include research ethics, transplant ethics, ethics of migration, bioethics teaching and Pilosopiyang Pilipino. Decastro.bioethics@gmail.com: SUSTAINABLE COVID-19 RESPONSE MEASURES: AN ETHICAL IMPERATIVE FOR ENHANCING CORE HUMAN CAPABILITIES.

Chae, Sun Geu is Research Engineer at the Industrial Engineering Department in Hanyang University, South Korea. His research interests include data mining based on machine learning and deep learning algorithms; itwavesu@gmail.com: THE TECHNOLOGY UTILIZATION AND SOCIAL BACKGROUND THAT LED TO THE K-QUARANTINE.

Childress, Prof. em. James F. is Professor Emeritus at the University of Virginia, where he was formerly University Professor, the John Allen Hollingsworth Professor of Ethics, Professor of Religious Studies, and founding director of the Institute for Practical Ethics and Public Life. He is the author of numerous articles and several books in biomedical ethics and in other areas of ethics. His books include *Principles of Biomedical Ethics* (with Tom L. Beauchamp); the 8th edition/40th anniversary edition appeared in 2019; the book has been translated into a dozen other languages. His most recent book is *Public Bioethics: Principles and Problems* (2020). Childress has served on several national committees examining bioethics and public policy. He was vice chair of the national Task Force on Organ Transplantation, served on the Recombinant DNA Advisory Committee, and was appointed to the National Bioethics Advisory Commission by President Clinton. He is an elected member of the National Academy of Medicine: RATIONING HEALTH CARE IN THE COVID-19 PANDEMIC: IMPLEMENTING ETHICAL TRIAGE.

Dahlke, Dr. med. Eva physician in training to specialize in occupational medicine with a profound knowledge of emergency medicine and global assistance medicine. Postgraduate studies in medical ethics focusing on the interface between occupational medicine and ethics, primarily digital communication transformation concerning vulnerable groups: HOME OFFICE IN THE PANDEMIC: CURSE OR BLESSING?

DiEuliis, Dr. Diane is a Senior Research fellow at National Defense University. Her research areas focus on emerging biological technologies, biodefense, and preparedness for biothreats. Specific topic areas under this broad research portfolio include dual use life sciences research, synthetic biology, the US bioeconomy, disaster recovery, and behavioral, cognitive, and social science as it relates to important aspects of deterrence and preparedness. Dr. DiEuliis currently lectures in a variety of foundational professional military education courses across all the services: OF NEMESIS AND NARCISSUS: LESSONS COVID MAY PROVIDE FOR ENTERPRISES – AND ETHICS – OF GLOBAL HEALTH PROMOTION AND BIOSECURITY.

Donev, Prof. Dr. Dejan. Born in Skopje, North Macedonia, in 1976. He completed his studies in philosophy at the Faculty of Philosophy, Ss. Cyril and Methodius University in Skopje in 1999. He received master degree from the same University in 2005, and doctoral degree in June 2008, both in philosophy. The key research interests of prof. Donev are in Ethics, History of Ethics, especially Bioethics, Ecological Ethics and Animal Ethics. During his professional career he has published numerous scientific papers, participated in a number of referent international scientific conferences and congresses, as well as in national and regional scientific research projects. Prof. Donev is working on the Department of Philosophy at the Faculty of Philosophy,University "Sts.Cyril and Methodius", in Skopje, N. Macedonia and currently is the

Head of the Center for integrative bioethics at the same faculty. E-mail contact: donevde-jan@fzf.ukim.edu.mk: BETWEEN EGO(CENTR)ISM AND COOPERATION: WOULD PEOPLE BECOME MORALY DISENGAGED OR MORE ALTRUISTIC AFTER THE COVID-19 PANDEMIC?

Eberle, Dr. theol. Martin, studied Protestant Theology in Heidelberg, Leipzig, Berlin, Biele-feld and Madurai (India). With an interdisciplinary work on the topic "Understanding Economic Ethics. Max Weber's Studies on Ancient Judaism from a theological-ethical perspective" he received his doctorate from the Kirchliche Hochschule Wuppertal/Bethel (Germany). He is the pastor of the German Lutheran Church Washington, D.C.: HOW CAN GOD LET THIS HAPPEN? A THEOLOGICAL REFLECTION ON THE PANDEMIC.

Elisovna, Prof. Dr. Guryleva Marina doctor of medical Sciences, Professor of the Department of biomedical ethics, biomedical law with a course in the history of medicine of the Kazan state medical University. Chairman of the Local Ethics Committee for clinical research of Kazan state medical University, member of the International society of clinical bioethics. Research interests: bioethics, ethics and standards of clinical research, history of medicine, public health. E-mail: meg4478@mail.ru: BIOETHICS AND PANDEMICS IN THE MODERN WORLD: COVID-19.

Eom, Prof. Juhee is Research Professor in the Graduate School of Public Health at Yonsei University in Korea. She studied constitutional law, public law and bioethics at Yonsei University in Korea and leads an NRF-funded (National Research Foundation of Korea) project on neurolaw foundation construction in relation to emerging technology, neuroscience and ethics on legal perspectives; juheelight@gmail.com: THE TECHNOLOGY UTILIZATION AND SOCIAL BACKGROUND THAT LED TO THE K-QUARANTINE.

Fernandes, Prof. Dr. Márcia Santana - Brazil. PhD in Law (UFRGS) and Post-Doctorate in Medicine in Medical Sciences (UFRGS). Professor of the Professional Master in Clinical Research of the Hospital de Clínicas de Porto Alegre (HCPA) and Associate Researcher of the Bioethics and Ethics in Science Research Laboratory (LAPEBEC/HCPA). Collaborating Professor at PPGD-PUCRS. Professor at Feevale University. Associate and member of the board of the Institute for Cultural Studies (IEC). Fellow of the Digital Society Inititiave, University of Zurich. CV: http://lattes.cnpq.br/2132565174726788: PERSONAL DATA AND COVID-19.

Fritzhand, Prof. Dr. Ana. Born in Skopje, North Macedonia, in 1978. She completed her studies in psychology at the Faculty of Philosophy, Ss. Cyril and Methodius University in Skopje in 2001. She received master degree from the same University in 2007, and doctoral degree in May 2010, both in psychology. The key research interests of prof. Fritzhand are in Developmental psychology, Moral psychology, and the Psychology of peace and conflict. During her professional career she has published numerous scientific papers, participated in a number of referent international scientific conferences and congresses, as well as in national and regional scientific research projects. Prof. Fritzhand is currently the head of the Department of Psychology at the Faculty of Philosophy in Skopje and Vice President of the Chamber of Psychologists of North Macedonia. E-mail contact: anaf@fzf.ukim.edu.mk: BETWEEN EGO(CENTR)ISM AND COOPERATION: WOULD PEOPLE BECOME MORALY DISENGAGED OR MORE ALTRUISTIC AFTER THE COVID-19 PANDEMIC?

Gillen, Dr. theol. Erny (*1960), founder and director of Moral Factory, has taught and published on ethics in theology, medicine and organisations in Luxembourg and Freiburg i.Br. for over twenty years. As a practical ethicist, he has led Caritas in Luxembourg, was President of Caritas Europa and First Vice-President of Caritas Internationalis, and Vicar General of the

Archdiocese   of   Luxembourg   in   times   of   extensive   restructuring.-
erny.gillen@moralfactory.com: DO WE STILL NEED ETHICS?

Giordano, Prof. Dr. James, Ph.D., is Professor in the Departments of Neurology
and Biochemistry and Chief of the Neuroethics Studies Program, in the Pellegrino Center for
Clinical Bioethics, Georgetown University Medical Center, Washington DC, USA; and Senior
Research Fellow, Biosecurity, Technology and Ethics, US Naval War College, Newport RI,
USA; jg353@georgetown.edu: OF NEMESIS AND NARCISSUS: LESSONS COVID MAY
PROVIDE FOR ENTERPRISES – AND ETHICS – OF GLOBAL HEALTH PROMOTION
AND BIOSECURITY.

Goldim, Prof. Dr. José Roberto - Brazil. PhD in Medicine: Medical Clinic at the Federal University of Rio Grande do Sul (UFRGS). Master in Education (UFRGS) and Biologist. Biologist
at Hospital de Clínicas de Porto Alegre (HCPA) and head of the Bioethics Service at the Hospital. He is a Collaborating Professor at UFRGS School of Medicine, being responsible for the
disciplines of Bioethics at PPG in Medicine: Medical Sciences/UFRGS and Supervising Professor at Master's and Doctorate level at this same PPG. Associate Professor at PUCRS Medical
School, in charge of Bioethics and Gerontology discipline at PPG in Biomedical Gerontol-
ogy/PUCRS and Supervising Professor at Master's and Doctorate level. He coordinates the Bioethics Research Group - Interinstitutional Bioethics Nucleus, existing since 1998, with a line of
research on Bioethics and Complexity. He is the researcher responsible for the Bioethics and
Ethics in Science Research Laboratory of the Experimental Research Center of HCPA. In 2017
he received the Fritz Jahr International Award for Research and Promotion of European Bioethics. Fellow   of   the   Digital   Society   Inititiave,   University   of   Zurich.   CV
http://lattes.cnpq.br/0485816067416121: PERSONAL DATA AND COVID-19.

Hennig, Prof. Dr. Alicia is holding a full research position as Associate Professor of Business
Ethics at the department of philosophy at Southeast University in Nanjing, China. She obtained
her PhD in philosophy and applied ethics (business ethics) from Technical University Darmstadt, Germany with co-supervision from Thomas Pogge (Yale, CT, US). During her PhD she
worked at a leading private business school in Germany, Frankfurt School of Finance and Management, and published first working papers on China and business ethics. Her current research
focuses on Chinese philosophy and its application in organizations in the context of values, ethics and innovation. In addition to her research she also has practical working experience gained
at Chinese as well as foreign companies in China: COMMUNITARIANISM, LIBERALISM
AND CONFUCIANISM.

Hoss, Prof. em. Dr. Geni Maria holds a PhD in theology with a major in bioethics, from
Faculdade EST, Brazil. She was professor of bioethics in the courses of human sciences. Currently is an independent scholar and is also active as guest lecturer and consultant in the area of
bioethics, hospital humanization projects, health and spirituality, pastoral counseling and Christian Theology and environmental responsibility. E-Mail contact: geni.hoss@yahoo.com.br: THE
CORONAVIRUS PANDEMIC UNDER UNFAVOURABLE SOCIAL ECONOMIC CONDI-
TIONS.

Hubenko, Prof. Dr. Hanna, Ph.D., is Associate Professor in the Department of Public Health
of the Medical Institute (Sumy State University (SSU) and Founder and Head of 'Bioethics'
(NGO), hanna.hubenko@gmail.com, bioethics.ngo@gmail.com: INTEGRATIVE BIOETHICS
IN THE TIME/NOT IN THE TIME OF COVID-19: CARING, BEHAVING AND RESPON-
SIBILITIES TOWARDS FUTURE GENERATIONS.

Jurić, Prof. Dr. Hrvoje, PhD, born in 1975 in Bihać, Bosnia and Herzegovina, studied Philosophy and Croatian Culture at the University of Zagreb (University Centre for Croatian Studies), earned his PhD degree 2007 in Philosophy at the University of Zagreb (Faculty of Humanities and Social Sciences), worked since 2000 in the Department of Philosophy of the Faculty of Humanities and Social Sciences, University of Zagreb, since 2019 as Full Professor of Ethics and Bioethics. Head of the Department of Philosophy (2016-2020) and Head of Department's Chair of Ethics (since 2015). Chief Secretary of the international conferences "Days of Frane Petrić" (2002-2006) and "Lošinj Days of Bioethics" (since 2002). Since 2014 Chief Secretary of the Centre of Excellence for Integrative Bioethics, which embraces seven Croatian bioethical institutions. President of the Croatian Bioethics Society (2016-2020). Since 2017 Head of the University Centre for Integrative Bioethics of the University of Zagreb. Since 1999 Deputy Editor of the philosophical journals "Filozofska istraživanja" and "Synthesis philosophica". - hjuric@yahoo.com: PANDEMIC AS A SYMPTOM.

Kalokairinou, Prof. Eleni is Professor of Philosophy, Ethics and Bioethics, Aristotle University of Thessaloniki, E-mail: ekalo@edlit.auth.gr: AUTONOMY AND TRUST: CONCLUSIONS FROM THE GREEK MODEL OF MANAGEMENT OF THE COVID-19 PANDEMIC.

Kaluđerović, Prof. Željko (1964, Vrbas, Serbia) is employed as Full Professor at the Department of Philosophy at the Faculty of Philosophy of the University in Novi Sad, Serbia (subjects: Hellenic Philosophy, Hellenistic-Roman Philosophy, Ethics, Bioethics, Journalistic Ethics and Philosophy of Morality), and at the Department of Philosophy and Sociology at the Faculty of Philosophy of the University in Tuzla, Bosnia and Herzegovina (subjects: Ancient Greek Philosophy and Political Philosophy). Books: Aristotle and Presocratics (2004), Hellenic Concept of Justice (2010), Presocratic Understanding of Justice (2013), Philosophical Triptych (2014), Dike and Dikaiosyne (2015), Early Greek Philosophy (2017) and Stagirites (2018). He has published more than 120 papers and reviews in different science and philosophy journals in Bosnia and Herzegovina, Croatia, Germany, Greece, Hungary, Montenegro, North Macedonia, Romania, Serbia, Turkey and USA. Kaluđerović took part in around 55 international symposiums and in one international congress (9th World Congress of Bioethics). He is an editor in chief of the Journal of Philosophy *Arhe* (Novi Sad), coordinator of the Center for Bioethics at the Department of Philosophy, Faculty of Philosophy, University in Novi Sad and a member of several editorial boards of journals and proceedings, organizational, scientific and program committees of various international conferences and symposiums, E-mail contact: zeljko.kaludjerovic@ff.uns.ac.rs: SCIENCE AND ETHICS IN TIMES OF CRISIS.

Kaminsky, Prof. Dr. Carmen, PhD, is full professor for Practical Philosophy at the Faculty for Applied Social Studies at Cologne University of Applied Sciences and private lecturer at Heinrich-Heine-University-Duesseldorf, both in Germany. Her research areas of focus concern central issues of applied ethics. She published on diverse topics of medical-ethics, public health-ethics, media-ethics and ethics of social work. Her most recent works issue ethical questions of digital technologies. – carmen.kaminsky@th-koeln.de: NORMALITY "EX POST": SOCIAL CONDITIONS OF MORAL RESPONSIBILITY.

Kato, Prof. Dr. Yutaka currently holds an associate professorship in the Department of Liberal Arts at Ishikawa Prefectural Nursing University and will be a professor at Shiga University of Medical Sciences in October 2020. His main research interests include comparative study of the ethical, legal, and social dimensions of healthcare. He received a Ph.D. in medical ethics from Osaka University after completing a master's degree in religious ethics at Yale University:

CONTROVERSY IN JAPAN'S TESTING POLICY AGAINST THE NOVEL CORONAVIRUS DISEASE AND THE DIFFICULTIES SURROUNDING THE FACT.

Kegel, Hans-Peter, born on 20.04.1981 in Homburg/Saar, works as a physician in the field of occupational, social and environmental medicine since 2009. His professional experience includes the planning, implementation and evaluation of scientific studies in the field of occupational, social and environmental medicine, working in student teaching and the training and further education of medical professionals, as well as providing occupational medical care for employees at schools in the state of Rhineland-Palatinate. Previously published contributions, including book contributions, range from topics of classical occupational medicine such as occupational toxicology to questions of future trends of occupational medicine with regard to new/digital media: HOME OFFICE IN THE PANDEMIC: CURSE OR BLESSING?.

Kishore, Dr. Rishi Raj is an expert in both, Medicine and Law. He served the Ministry of Health, Government of India for nearly 35 years and was associated with the drafting of Indian Transplantation of Human Organs Act, 1994. In 1997, Dr. Kishore founded the Indian Society for Health Law and Ethics (ISHLE) of which he continues to be the President till date. In 2002, Dr. Kishore was appointed a Health Law and Bioethics Fellow in the Boston University School of Health Law, USA. He has been on the Board of Governors, World Association for Medical Law and has been the Chairman, International Committee on Organ Transplantation. He has also been a *rapporteur* for the World Health Organization. Subsequent to his retirement from the Ministry of Health in 2004, Dr. Kishore has been practicing as an advocate in the Supreme Court of India. Dr. Kishore has been working on a variety of issues in bioethics, health law and human rights such as organ transplantation, end of life, clinical trial on human subjects, assisted reproductive technologies, foetal rights, abortion, sex selection, stem cells, cloning, HIV/AIDS, DNA sampling, and human dignity. By now, he has presented nearly 100 papers in international conferences and several of his articles have appeared in leading international journals: CORONA COMBAT, HUMAN DIGNITY AND THE RIGHTS: GLOBAL REFLECTIONS AND INDIAN MILIEU - AN ETHICAL EVALUATION.

Lei, Dr. Ruipeng works at the Department of Philosophy, Centre for Bioethics, Huazhong University of Science and Technology, Wuhan, China. Contact E-Mail: lxp73615@163.com: ETHICAL AND POLICY ISSUES IN THE EPIDEMIC OF CORONAVIRUS IN CHINA. A DEFENSE FOR OFFENSIVE STRATEGY AGAINST THE SPREAD OF ZOONOSIS.

Liu, Prof. Dr. Yuli is a Professor in traditional Chinese Ethics at the Department of Philosophy, the Party School of the Central Committee of C.P.C. She graduated from Renmin University of China with Master's Degree in 1997 and got her PhD in Philosophy at the University of HULL, UK in 2002. She was a post-doctoral fellow in the National University of Singapore in 2003. She was also invited to be a visiting scholar at Yale University and the University of Trinity St. David Wales. In 2015, 2016 and 2017, she was invited to give speeches in the World Peace Convention in the UNESCO: COMMUNITARIANISM, LIBERALISM AND CONFUCIANISM.

Lolas, Dr. Fernando is Medical Doctor both at the University of Chile as well as the Central University of Chile: THE SYNDEMIC PERSPECTIVE AND THE NEED FOR HEALTH HERMENEUTICS.

Macer, Dr. Darryl, Ph.D., Hon.D., is Director, Eubios Ethics Institute, New Zealand, Japan and Thailand, Email: darryl@eubios.info: THE FOUNDATION AND FUNCTIONING OF THE WORLD EMERGENCY COVID19 PANDEMIC ETHICS COMMITTEE.

Martin, Prof. Dr. David, born 1973 in Vermont, USA, grew up in the USA, France and England. He is a pediatrician, pediatric endocrinologist, oncologist, diabetologist and hematologist. He holds the Gerhard Kienle Chair of Medical Theory, Integrative and Anthroposophic Medicine at the University of Witten/Herdecke and leads the pediatric endocrinology, diabetology and integrative pediatric oncology services in the Filderklinik, an anthroposophic hospital in Germany. He has received several prizes for his research in the field of growth, skeletal development and endocrinology and is Counselling Professor of the German National Academic Foundation. He is the founder and director of www.feverapp.org, www.warmuptofever.org, and the Clinical Foundation Course of the Eugen-Kolisko Academy www.kolisko-academy.org, faculty of www.anthroposophic-drs-training.org, scientific director of http://icihm.damid.de/en and is co-founder and co-director of www.lebens-Weise.org and www.medienfasten.org. Contact: Chair of Medical Theory, Integrative and Anthroposophic Medicine, Department of Health, University of Witten/Herdecke. David.Martin@uni-wh.de: ETHICS IN TIMES OF CORONA: SHOULD CLOSE RELATIVES OF PERSONS WITH COVID-19 BE ALLOWED TO VISIT THEIR LOVED ONES IN THE HOSPITAL?

McCullough, Prof. Dr. Laurence B., Ph.D. is Professor of Obstetrics and Gynecology in the Department of Obstetrics and Gynecology of Zucker School of Medicine at Hofstra/Northwell, Hempstead, New York, and Ethics Scholar in the Department of Obstetrics and Gynecology of Lenox Hill Hospital, New York, New York. In 2016 the President and Board of Trustees of Baylor College of Medicine (Houston, Texas) made him Distinguished Emeritus Professor in Baylor's Center for Medical Ethics and Health Policy, upon his retirement from the College after 28 years on its faculty. In 2013 he was recognized for his contribution to medical education at Baylor with the Barbara and Corbin J. Robertson, Jr., Presidential Award for Excellence in Education. He has published 590 papers in the peer-reviewed scientific, clinical, ethics, and philosophical journals, as well as 62 original chapters in scholarly books. He is the author or co-author of 8 books and editor or co-editor of 8 books. He is currently writing *Thomas Percival's Medical Ethics* and editing *Thomas Percival's Medical Jurisprudence and Medical Ethics* for the Philosophy and Medicine book series published by Springer (New York City). He lives in Austin, Texas, with his wife Linda J. Quintanilla, Ed.D., a retired community college history professor and active scholar of Mexican American history. E-Mail contact: Laurence.McCullough@bcm.edu. Contact: mctaicht@gmail.com: THE PROFESSIONAL ETHICS OF TRIAGE OF LIFE-SUSTAINING TREATMENT IN A PANDEMIC.

Miller, Irene M. celloimm@aol.com, born in Berlin, a cellist, has practiced medicine in USA, China and Africa. Now retired, she lives in New Hampshire: THE HIDDEN COST OF SOCIAL ISOLATION.

Nezhmetdinova, Prof. Dr. Farida Tansykovna, PhD of philosopher, associate Professor. Head of the Department of philosophy and law of Kazan state Agrarian University, Federal expert in the scientific and technical sphere of the Ministry of science and higher education of the Russian Federation, President of the International society of clinical bioethics, member of the Local Ethical Committee for clinical research of Kazan state medical University, Deputy Chairman of the Local Ethical Committee for clinical research of Kazan Federal University. Research interests: bioethics, social and ethical problems of modern technologies, professional education. E-mail: nadgmi@mail.ru: BIOETHICS AND PANDEMICS IN THE MODERN WORLD: COVID-19.

Omonzejele, Dr. Peter, PhD, is a philosopher and bioethicist. He trained in bioethics at the University of Witwatersrand, Johannesburg, South Africa and at the University of Central Lancashire, Preston, England. He is Professor of Cross-Cultural Bioethics in the Department of Philosophy, University of Benin, Benin-City, Nigeria. – pfomonzejele@yahoo.com: THE CORONA VIRUS PANDEMIC AND THE AL-MAJIRI SYSTEM IN NIGERIA: PROTECTING THE EXTRA VULNERABLE.

Qiu, Prof. Renzong, Professor, Institute of Philosophy, Chinese Academy of Social Sciences; Institute of Bioethics, Centre for Ethics and Moral Studies, Renmin University of China; qiurenzong@hotmail.com: A DEFENSE FOR OFFENSIVE STRATEGY AGAINST THE SPREAD OF ZOONOSIS.

Ribas, Dr. Salvador holds a PhD in Philosophy from the University of Barcelona; he is Manager for Quality Assurance in clinical trials, a Board Member of the Spanish Quality Assurance Society (SEGCIB), and also Vice-President of the International Society for Clinical Bioethics (ISCB); salvador.ribas@gmail.com: GOOD CLINICAL PRACTICE COMPLIANCE IN PANDEMIC COVID19: IT IS FEASIBLE?

Sass, Prof. em. Dr. Hans-Martin, is Professor Emeritus at Georgetown University, Washington DC and Ruhr-University, Bochum FRG, Honorary Professor at Renmin University and Peking Union Medical College in Beijing, PRC. This article is based on 2005 and 2009 lectures at Peking Union Medical College and Tsinghua University, PRC, and in hospitals in Bochum, FRG. His numerous articles and books discuss issues of bioethics, philosophy and social and political science. - sasshm@aol.com: THE CORONA VIRUS AND EMERGENCY MANAGEMENT. TRIAGE, EPIDEMICS, BIOMEDICAL TERROR AND WARFARE.

Schüz, Prof. Dr. phil. Mathias studied physics, philosophy and education at the Johannes Gutenberg University of Mainz. He was a co-initiator and long-standing member of the Executive Board of the Gerling Academy for Risk Research, Zurich, and is currently Professor of Responsible Leadership and Business Ethics at the Zurich University of Applied Sciences (ZHAW) in Winterthur, Switzerland: ETHICS APPROACHES IN DEALING WITH THE CORONA PANDEMIC.

Sean Hull is a technologist, problem solver and consultant with a 15+ year history of designing, planning and driving the delivery of strategic programs globally, primarily in the insurance domain. His track record includes work with Fortune 50 firms, Big Six Consulting, and not-for-profit organizations. Sean is a certified project manager and his academic qualifications include a Master of Business Administration (MBA) from Ashland University and a Bachelor of Arts (BA) in International Relations from the Ohio State University; sean.hull@gmail.com: POST-PANDEMIC BUSINESS PIVOT: 4 TRENDS TO WATCH.

Shim, Prof. Dr. Jiwon is Research Professor in Humanities Research Institute at Chung-Ang University in Korea. She wrote her PhD dissertations on human enhancement at Muenster University in Germany, and leads an NRF-funded (National Research Foundation of Korea) project on issues of human enhancement, artificial intelligence, and medical ethics; g1dmpkr@gmail.com: THE TECHNOLOGY UTILIZATION AND SOCIAL BACKGROUND THAT LED TO THE K-QUARANTINE.

Sun Geu Chae is Research Engineer at the Industrial Engineering Department in Hanyang University, South Korea. His research interests include data mining based on machine learning and deep learning algorithms; itwavesu@gmail.com: THE TECHNOLOGY UTILIZATION AND SOCIAL BACKGROUND THAT LED TO THE K-QUARANTINE.

Tai, Prof. Dr. Michael Cheng-tek, Chair professor of bioethics and medical humanities of the Institute of Medicine, Chungshan Medical Univeristy, Taichung, Taiwan. He earned his Ph.D. in Comparative Ethics from Concordia University in Montreal, Canada and had taught at Concordia University, Montreal, King College, Bristol, Tennessee and University of Saskatchewan, Saskatoon, Canada before his return to Taiwan in 1997. Since then he had served the dean of the College of Medical Humanities and Social Sciences and the chairman of the department of Social Medicine of the Chungshan Medical University. He was the president of International Society for Clinical Bioethics from 2006-2010 and served on the editorial board of the Journal of Medical Ethics (England), European Journal of Bioethics (Croatia), Medicine and Philosophy (China), Medical Education, Tzuchi Journal of Medicine (Taiwan) and the chief editor of Formosan Journal of Medical Humanities. He is a member of Medical Research Ethics Committee of Academia Sinica, IRB member of the National Chengchi University, Taipei, IRB member of Chungshan Medical University, Taichung and convener of the subcommittee on Education and International Relation of the Ethics Governance Committee of Taiwan National Biobank. He also sits on Medical Affairs Committee, Medical Ethics Committee and Biobank Research Committee of the Ministry of Health and Social Welfares, Taiwan. Among his monographs are *The Way of Asian Bioethics* (in English), *A Medical Ethics of Life and Death*, *The Foundation and Practice of Research Ethics*, *The Medical Humanities in the New Era* etc. and numerous scholarly papers around the world: THE QUESTION OF JUSTICE IN TREATING THE COVID-19 PATIENTS – HAS PRIORITIZING THE FITTEST TO RECEIVE THE TREATMENT BECOME THE NORM?

Wang, Prof. Dr. Robin R. is Professor of Philosophy at Loyola Marymount University, Los Angeles and The Berggruen fellow (2016-17) at The Center for Advanced Study in the Behavioral Sciences (CASBS), Stanford University. Her teaching and research center on Chinese and Comparative Philosophy, particularly on Daoist Philosophy, Women and Gender in Chinese culture and tradition. She is the author of *Yinyang: The Way of Heaven and Earth in Chinese Thought and Culture* (Cambridge University Press 2012) and editor of *Chinese Philosophy in an Era of Globalization*, (SUNY Press 2004) and *Images of Women in Chinese Thought and Culture: Writings from the Pre-Qin Period to the Song Dynasty* (Hackett 2003). She was the President of *Society for Asian and Comparative Philosophy* (2016-18). Contact: robin.wang@lmu.edu: THE MOMENT OF DAO: DESPAIR, JOY, AND RESILIENCE IN THE TIME OF GLOBAL PANDEMIC 2020.

Woesler, Prof. Dr. Martin, holds a Ph.D. in Chinese Studies and was born in 1969. He is a member of the European Academy of Sciences and Arts (Salzburg), Professor of Literature and Communication in China (Witten/Herdecke University), Xiaoxiang Scholar Distinguished Professor of Chinese Studies, Comparative Literature and Translation Studies (Hunan Normal University) and in 2020, he is appointed Jean Monnet Chair Professor. He is President of the World Association of Chinese Studies and the German China Society. His research focuses on Chinese literature, cultural comparison and social transformation processes, especially digitization, in China, including in comparison to Germany, Europe and the USA. He has received wide attention with his paper "Learning from China: Stopping the epidemic, not just slowing it down. And why 70% of Germans will not fall ill with COVID-19". *Bulletin of the German China Society* (2020.3.30)17-27, online: http://universitypress.eu/de/ 9783865152862_002.pdf: RESPONSIBILITY AND ETHICS IN TIMES OF CORONA.

Yasol-Naval, Prof. Dr. Jeanette L. - Professor at the Department of Philosophy, College of Social Sciences and Philosophy (CSSP), University of the Philippines, Diliman. She has served as the Chairperson of the Department of Philosophy and is currently the Director of the UP Padayon Public Service Office under the Office of the Vice President for Public Affairs, UP System. She has completed two Postdoctoral Research Fellowships at Kobe University, Japan where she worked in the areas Environmental Ethics and Philosophy of Food. Her current researches include emerging animal ethics in disaster and epistemological, ethical and political searches include emerging animal ethics in disaster and epistemological, ethical and political discourses in gastronomy. Contact : jlyasolnaval@up.edu.ph: SUSTAINABLE COVID-19 RESPONSE MEASURES: AN ETHICAL IMPERATIVE FOR ENHANCING CORE HUMAN CAPABILITIES.

Members, World Emergency COVID19 Pandemic Ethics (WeCope) Committee: STATEMENT ON INDIVIDUAL AUTONOMY AND SOCIAL RESPONSIBILITY WITHIN A PUBLIC HEALTH EMERGENCY

Dr. Thalia Arawi (Lebanon)
Dr. Mouna Ben Azaiz (Tunisia)
Dr. Lian Bighorse (San Carlos Apache Nation, USA)
Dr. Andrew Bosworth (Canada)
Dr. Rhyddhi Chakraborty (India, UK)
Mr. Anthony Mark Cutter (U.K.)
Dr. Mireille D'Astous (Canada)
Dr. Ayoub Abu Dayyeh (Jordan)
Dr. Nilza Maria Diniz (Brazil)
Dr. Hasan Erbay (Turkey)
Prof. Nader Ghotbi (Japan)
Prof. Abhik Gupta (India)
Prof. Soraj Hongladarom (Thailand)
Prof. Miwako Hosoda (Japan)
Prof. Dena Hsin-Chen Hsin (Taiwan)
Dr. Anower Hussain (Bangladesh)
Prof. Bang-Ook Jun (Republic of Korea)
Prof. Hassan Kaya (South Africa)
Dr. Sumaira Khowaja-Punjwani (Pakistan)
Prof. Julian Kinderlerer (South Africa)
Dr. Lana Al-Shareeda Le Blanc (Iraq)
Prof. Marlon Lofredo (the Philippines)
Dr. Manuel Lozano Rodríguez (Spain)
Prof. Darryl Macer (New Zealand)
Prof. Raffaele Mantegazza (Italy)
Dr. Aziza Menouni (Morocco)
Dr. Endreya Marie McCabe (Delaware Nation, USA)
Prof. Erick Valdés Meza (Chile, USA)
Dr. Ravichandran Moorthy (Malaysia)
Prof. Firuza Nasyrova (Tajikistan)
Dr. Suma Parahakaran (Malaysia)
Prof. Maria do Céu Patrão Neves (Portugal)
Prof. Deborah Kala Perkins (USA)
Prof. Osama Rajkhan (Saudi Arabia)
Ms. Carmela Roybal (Tewa Nation, USA)
Prof. Mariodoss Selvanayagam (India)
Prof. Mihaela Serbulea (Romania)
Dr. Jasdev Rai Singh (England)

Dr. Raquel R. Smith (USA)
Prof. Takao Takahashi (Japan)
Dr. Ananya Tritipthumrongchok (Thailand)
Dr. Lakshmi Vyas (UK)
Prof. Yanguang Wang (China)
Prof. John Weckert (Australia)
Dr. Anke Weisheit (Uganda)

Corona – A Reflection During the Pandemic

Foreword by Martin Woesler

This volume is an intellectual response of the human being to a challenge by nature, the coronavirus. The physical response by most in the world has been in the form of some kind of protectiive measures for themselves, for others, and for medical personnel working at the front-line. The microbiological response has been given by scientists to develop a vaccine.

This volume is the intellectual response of experts from disciplines such as Philosophy & Ethics, Politics, Sociology, Psychology, etc. It is a response as a result of reflection during the time when the pandemic is still soaring. Soon it will have historic value, when the vaccine is there and the pandemic persists in areas where people cannot afford the vaccination, which will be underdeveloped countries. The challenge then becomes an issue of how the world community could effectively bring the vaccination to all human beings or, at least to about two-thirds of the community, which may be sufficient for herd protection.

Although we have not invited Nobel Prize winners in their fields, we have selected through a review process papers by experts, who are often members of national or international Ethics Committees such as the official German Ethics Committee or the World Emergency COVID19 Pandemic Ethics Committee (WeCope).

Who would have expected that we would discuss Triage for civilians in 2020? This concept was developed in wartime. Although war victims are increasingly civilians, with the progress in science and technology, the world has not anticipated that hubris would bring on a natural catastrophe with more than a million deaths. Nature teaches us better. And we are well advised to listen to nature also in the even greater challenge, climate change, which may bring about a dramatic reduction of biodiversity and even more deaths in the long run. The virus may remind us that we are ultimately part of nature.

However, triage on a minor scale is everyday practice in emergency units all over the world. The doctor decides about immediate treatment (I), later treatment of severe cases (II) and of lighter cases (III) or may even decide that treatment is hopeless (IV), the latter not being covered either by the German constitution "Grundgesetz" or by the hippocratic oath.

How the world will look like after Corona is easy to answer: The same. This is what history tells us after pandemics, natural catastrophes and wars. After World War I, people swore "Never again war!", the League of Nations was founded and less than a generation later there came World War II. However, after World War II, we had the Nuremburg Trials, the United Nations and so far we have been able to avoid World War III.

Since people tend to forget how they suffered during a crisis, as soon as the crisis is over, after COVID-19 only minor changes seem feasible, but to undertake these changes is worth the effort. The human species needs to learn from mistakes to secure its survival.

When the humans changed their lives from hunters and nomads to farmers and settled in cities, diseases like leprosy, malaria, tuberculosis, influenza and smallpox spread. Two-thirds of Athenians died of typhoid fever in 430 BCE while smallpox infected the Huns, Germans and Romans 165-180 CE. Between 250-444 CE, the Cyprian plague claimed victims from Ethiopia to Britain. The Bubonic Plague between 541-650 CE killed about 50 million people, then 26% of the world's population. Leprosy grew into a pandemic in the 11th century. Spreading from Asia and arriving in Sicily in 1348, the 2nd large outbreak of the Bubonic Plague killed one third of the world's population. After the Spanish arrived in the Carribean in 1492, diseases of the Europeans like smallpox, measles and the Bubonic Plague killed about 90% of the native population in North and South America, and ended the Aztek Empire in 1520. In the 16th and 17th centuries, around 56 million native Americans fell victim to these diseases. In 1665 20% of London's inhabitants were killed by the Great Plague of London. Between 1889 and 1890 the Russian Flu killed 360,000 people worldwide. In 1918, the Spanish Flu resulted in 50 million deaths worldwide. The Asian flu in 1957-1958 caused 1.1 million deaths and was contained with a vaccine. HIV/Aids started in West Africa in the 1920s, was identified in 1981 and has killed 35 million people so far. SARS, H1N1, Ebola and Zika are the most recent diseases.[1]

COVID-19, after the Asian Flu in 1957-1958, is the second major pandemic which was not prompted just with prayers, but with a vaccine. With the outbreak, more than 150 scientific institutions worldwide immediately started to develop a vaccine.

COVID-19 will probably cost more than a million people's lives until a vaccine is found, which may stop the pandemic. Therefore, it is still a major pandemic, but in relation to the population of the world, it may affect less than 0.1 percent of the people. However, there were hotspots and villages, e.g. in Italy, and in crowded places with bad infrastructure in South America, Africa and India, where the health system collapsed. In these places, there was a higher chance to catch the disease and also a higher chance to die. Many people were suddenly confronted with the immanent death of their relatives or of themselves. Cicero declared once, there were three sorts of people, the living, the dead and those who go to sea. Not just people in quarantined cruise ships and in COVID-19 isolation stations in clinics may have felt that they belong to this third sort of people. Schroedinger has used the example of the cat, which was also in the state between life and death to describe quantum states, which are characterized by probabilities instead of a measurable status. So even if the probability to die of SARS-CoV-2 is less than 0.1 percent, it is still existential for those facing death and they deserve all the attention of the world.

This volume realizes what the governments of our world still have to learn: To stand united in times of global crisis.

Bochum, September 11, 2020

---

[1] Frederick C. Cartwright. *Disease and History*. Sutton Publishing, 2014. See also the overview article "Pandemics That Changed History". A&E Television Networks. https://www.history.com/topics/middle-ages/pandemics-timeline, accessed September 5, 2020.

Corona – A threat not just to individuals, but to social and political bodies

Foreword by Hans-Martin Sass

Medicine and Ethics share millennia of interaction in all civilizations. Sickness, epidemics, droughts, and plagues are natural events and harm or kill individuals, species, biotopes. Individuals, families, neighborhoods, cultures, businesses, and states may additionally be injured or destroyed by stealing, murdering, civil rebellion, and war. Human technologies and cultures have modified our globe and made it more livable. Fresh water supply, sanitation, healthy housing, health care systems have improved human life expectancy and happiness, - ever more rapidly during the last centuries, decades, years. The global corona pandemic, alike the global climate change, call both for long-term planning instead of short-term fixing. Science has collected a wealth of information on bacterial and viral diseases and global threats to life of biotopes, plants, animals, humans, families, villages and cities. We have a diversity of perspectives on pandemics; other viruses in our social and political bodies such as threats and malfunctions of electricity, communication, trade caused by nature, bad people or bad governments are only briefly mentioned by some authors.

We could have separated the articles into chapters such as bioethics, health care, religious or social or political studies, business, technology, management, - but each of these contribution is broader than any one discipline or activity, discussing a diversity of perspectives and interconnected issues and fears, thus becoming sources of new energy for change and encouragement. Therefore, we have just grouped the papers into larger topics. This pandemic and also the climate transformation are not routine risks, they require a new and long-term thinking by science, insurers, politicians, businesses, and last but not least by all of us and our communities. Will we need to scale back our technological, trade and political interconnections in favor of new national or even provincial stability of small communities, in narrow provincialism or solipsism? Our could new cyberspace communities including robotic companions provide new form of 'better' solidarity, love, empathy? The authors in this volume would make an ideal diverse group for a week-long conference, finding solutions and new topics for mutual enquiry and management, continuing discourses and ongoing questionings.

In world history we have significant world-changing events associated with the Chinese Yellow Emperor and Genghis Khan, Caesar, Napoleon, Washington, Lenin and other politicians. The teachings of Confucius, Laozi, Socrates, Moses, Jesus, Mohamed provided visions and values of life and culture, but some religious and philosophical doctrines at times also caused also torture and terror. Inventions and technologies such as the wheel, the steam engine and electricity have changed traffic and commerce, our houses, cars, cities, biotopes and in the present time global networks of communications and businesses. Previously, diseases have played an important role in building healthy communities with water supplies and sanitarily benefits, but the pandemic of 1917/18 with more victims than the 1914-1918 First World War did not write history the same way the war did. Will the year 2020 initiate a new significant change in ethics, lifestyle, culture, business and politics? - Today, the COVID-19 pandemic so far totals millions of infections (statistically called 'cases'!) and hundreds of thousands of deaths worldwide. Since the numbers are changing quickly with the spread in the USA, South America, and Africa, as well as with new waves coming in some parts of Europe and Asia, it is useless to give exact figures, since the book takes a few weeks to print and they will be outdated when our readers will hold this book in hands. There is no end in sight, but the hope for a vaccine within a few months. But it will not be the last virus pandemic mankind is facing.

This volume MEDICINE AND ETHICS IN TIMES OF CORONA collects 40 articles from experts and leaders in bioethics, business, philosophy, governance, medicine, religion, sociology. We present the articles in a loose order from the general to the specific and from history to the future. Given the multiplicity of challenges and topics, we have not subdivided the papers according to certain areas, which differ from traditional areas of scientific competence, since they are in flux as well. Authors work and live in 24 countries and regions: Argentina, Brazil, Chile, China, Croatia, Germany, France, Greece, India, Japan, South Korea, Luxembourg, North Macedonia, Mozambique, New Zealand, Nigeria, the Philippines, Spain, the Soviet Union, Switzerland, Taiwan, Turkey, Ukraine, and the USA. We have discussed to include national and international guidelines and regulations, but decided against, since those documents have been discussed in papers of authors here and the links are given to retrieve them from the internet, but we included three papers of the WeCope (World Emergency COVID-19 Pandemic Ethics) group of 40+ international members on issues of triage, terminology, individual autonomy and social responsibility. We also have four contributions by members or former members of the official German Ethics Council (Andreas Lob-Hüdepohl, Andreas Kruse, Kerstin Schlögl-Flierl, Jochen Taupitz).

A German publication MEDIZIN UND ETHIK IN ZEITEN VON CORONA with 16 papers includes a number of authors from this publication.

41 years ago, on July 20, 1969, the first human, Louis Armstrong, walked on the moon, 530 million on television heard him saying 'That's one small step for man, one giant leap for mankind!' Many of us remember where we were when men touched the moon. We also remember where we were on September 11, 2001 when the World Trade Center came down and changed politics and expectations. Will we remember where we were when Corona broke out in 2020? Back then, my colleague and co-editor Martin Woesler was in China, close to Wuhan, where he taught his courses as a professor with Hunan Normal University. He came back to Germany in February, to teach his courses in his second function as a professor with Witten/Herdecke University. When it became clear, that the pandemic would be life-threatening, he paused all his duties, became a volunteer, took a loan from the bank and imported 60,000 masks from China to Germany. That was at a time in March, when there were almost no masks available in Germany and the German government claimed masks were of no use. He delivered them day by day as donations by foot, bike and car to Corona Ambulances, to hospitals and clinics, to old people's homes, to the German Red Cross, old neighbors etc. He informed the German public in a widely read paper[1] about measures how to contain the virus, asked in TV interviews not to stigmatize infected people and not to discriminate against Asian people in Germany who were (wrongly) suspected to carry the virus. He simply dedicated his life to save other people's lives, as millions of volunteers did all over the world.

As the global press and in particular the ongoing civil unrest and demonstrations in the USA document most clearly, the Corona virus itself is not the single one contamination of our times, we see a multitude of social and political infections most visibly in the deadly choke hold of over 8 minutes by a white US policeman murdering a black man - George Floyd. His last words were: 'I cannot breathe!' When authors here say 'let us breathe again'; they don't discuss just the corona virus, but these new dimensions of living, community, solidarity, - of staying healthy, of becoming healthier, of enjoying new and stable connections in living together in our political, social, and cultural bodies.

Will 2020 mark a historical change of peoples and cultures? Will our political and social bodies change and become more resilient and stronger or will they face new infections and need to transform themselves? A special section of the papers is also dedicated to an outlook.

Washington, September 11, 2020

---

[1] Martin Woesler. "What we can learn from China – To stop the pandemic, not just to flatten the curve. And why not 70% of Germans will fall ill with Corona." *Bulletin of the German China Association*, Bochum (2020.3.29):17-27, online: http://universitypress.eu/de/9783865152862_002.pdf.

Rationing Health Care in the COVID-19 Pandemic: Implementing Ethical Triage

James F. Childress, University of Virginia, USA

Abstract

This paper critically examines current debates in the U.S. about rationing scarce medical resources in the COVID-19 pandemic to address current and anticipated shortages of ventilators, medications, vaccines, etc., in light of several ethical principles, including medical utility, social utility (e.g., ensuring essential social functions), equal regard (e.g., random selection), and justice/fairness. Given the disproportionate impact of COVID-19 on disadvantaged people in the U.S., this essay considers how rationing criteria and procedures should attend to health disparities resulting from structural injustice.

Key Words

Rationing; justice/fairness; medical utility; narrow social utility; health inequities; tragic choices

1. Introduction: Just Rationing in an Unjust System

Having recently co-taught a course for three hundred medical students on Confronting Epidemics: Perspectives from History, Ethics, and the Arts, I can safely say that societies learn and act on very few lessons from previous epidemics or pandemics—they tend to respond badly in each new outbreak. Societies also suffer "amnesia" about past—even recent past—ethical wisdom on such matters as rationing health care in a public health crisis. (Wikler 2020) As a result, important, thoughtful, and carefully crafted guidance developed by government bodies, ethics committees, professional associations, the World Health Organization, and the like over the last twenty years or so in preparation for a possible influenza pandemic has been poorly mined even though much of it is relevant to the current coronavirus pandemic. While this coronavirus is novel, the ethical issues and dilemmas it generates are not new, even if they manifest differently for various reasons.

However, lessons and ethical guidance from the past, even if recalled, would not be sufficient because each pandemic has its own distinctive features, including the particular biological agent involved, its modes and ease of transmission, the range of biological responses to infection, the groups it most often targets, its responsivity to different interventions, and the development and availability of different preventive and therapeutic interventions.

I analyze several ethical issues that the COVID-19/SARS-CoV-2 pandemic raises for rationing, triage, or allocation of scarce medical and public health interventions that could benefit particular individuals and the community. I use the terms "rationing," "triage," and "allocation" more or less interchangeably, while being attentive to the distinctive rhetorical features and elements of decision making each highlights. As two policy analysts note, the language of "allocation" suggests manageable and largely pragmatic, even if hard, choices, while "rationing" and "triage" suggest harsher choices in emergency and war or war-like circumstances—as reflected in the common language of war against the SARS-CoV-2 virus. (Rettig and Lohr 1981)

Our question is what constitutes just and fair rationing of preventive and therapeutic measures in this public health crisis. An answer requires determining what is due individuals and groups in these circumstances, under altered standards of care. Formally, justice mandates treating similar cases in a similar way and dissimilar cases dissimilarly. But it is not always clear which similarities and dissimilarities are morally relevant. The material criteria of justice identify characteristics that constitute relevant similarities and differences among people in the distribution of health care in a public health crisis, including urgency of need, level of risk, probability of a successful intervention, probability of societal contribution, etc. (Beauchamp and

Childress, 2019: chap. 7)

In the U.S., the overall health care system is blatantly unjust, especially because it fails to provide funds to ensure that everyone has timely access to an adequate level of health care. Obtaining medical treatment often presupposes the ability to pay out of pocket or to have insurance pay. This arrangement contributes to significant health inequities, including severe morbidity and mortality among people of color who bear the brunt of the pandemic. There is a general consensus that insurance status should not affect decisions about the hospitalization of persons with COVID-19. In actuality, many infected people seek medical attention later than they should because of their lack of insurance, thereby continuing to expose others and to delay discovery of clusters of infection. Moreover, those with insurance may still have to pay for testing if they can get it. A connected problem is the legacy of systemic or structural injustice experienced particularly, but not only, by African Americans and Native Americans and others who now have higher rates of hospitalization and death from COVID-19. Below I consider how corrective or reparative justice should figure into rationing in this pandemic.

Among the different levels of allocation, macroallocation decisions determine how much of a good—say, a resource such as personal protective equipment (PPE) or ventilators—is available during a pandemic. These macroallocation decisions, which in the U.S. are set through a mix of public and private institutions and mechanisms, determine the extent of scarcity and hence the severity of decisions of microallocation, rationing, or triage, which in turn determine who will receive a particular scarce resource. The notoriety of ethical dilemmas in microallocation may lead to revisions in macroalloction decisions—in the U.S. dramatic public controversies about patient selection for dialysis helped to create an exceptional federal program in 1973 to (largely) cover the costs of dialysis and transplantation for end-stage kidney disease.

Two sets of criteria are needed in microcallocation: for exclusion/inclusion and for prioritization/selection from eligible candidates. In debates about rationing ICU beds and ventilators in the current pandemic, I concur with those who argue that we should use looser exclusion/inclusion criteria—focused on need and probable benefit—rather than categorically excluding large groups, even though this will increase the burden of prioritization/selection, and that these exclusion/inclusion criteria for ICU beds and ventilators should be applied to all patients needing intensive care and ventilators, not only to patients with COVID-19. (White and Lo 2020) I will first turn to two clusters of moral considerations captured by the principles of utility and of equal regard and their implications for rationing across a variety of potentially scarce medical and public health interventions.

2. The Principle of Utility: Medical Utility

The principle of utility—of doing the greatest good or maximizing welfare—has been and remains prominent in allocation decisions. But it is also controversial in part because some wrongly assume that it entails a commitment to utilitarianism and thus to making the principle of utility the sole or ultimate source of moral judgment. However, properly interpreted, this principle is simply one prima facie principle along with others—in particular cases it can override other principles or yield to them depending on the circumstances. (Beauchamp and Childress 2020: 217, 243) Moreover, the principle of utility needs to be specified, as well as balanced against other principles.

Decisions about rationing usually focus on individuals' needs and probable outcomes with and without certain resources. As a form of rationing, triage is designed to produce the greatest good under conditions of scarcity, often, as noted, in extreme emergencies and wartime circumstances. Hence, it is consequentialist and generally utilitarian in the sense of seeking to produce the greatest good (within the limits noted above and without adopting traditional utilitarian values).

The distinction between medical utility and social utility in important in specifying the principle of utility. Rationing according to medical utility seeks to maximize the welfare of persons suffering from or at risk for disease. Judgments of medical utility incorporate several factors, including medical need (e.g., degree of urgency), probability of a successful outcome, and amount of resources required. And these must be balanced because, for example, the severity of medical need may reduce the likelihood of successful treatment. At a minimum, there must be a need for the medical intervention being considered, such as the likelihood of dying without a ventilator. But then, in a triage context, the probability of a successful outcome, as determined by clinical judgment and prognosis, becomes critical.

Saving the most lives has generally been the primary goal of rationing or triage of ICUs and ventilators in a pandemic, but it is not uncontroversial or unproblematic. To start, there are debates about the algorithms for predicting death without the intervention and survival with the intervention. These debates are beyond the scope of this essay other than to say that they need constant scrutiny to reduce bias. Instead, I will focus on other ethical issues in developing point systems.

The widely accepted aim of saving the most lives is not clear cut. Should this be survival to discharge, or for a year, or for five years, etc.? One reason for favoring the modest goal of survival to discharge is that the longer-range predictions focus heavily on co-morbidities, which frequently burden people of color who are dying at such high rates from COVID-19. In principle, their chances of receiving a ventilator in case of need would increase if the goal were short-term survival, such as to discharge, rather than, say, five-year survival.

Some argue that the proper end or aim of triage, the value to be maximized, should be "life years" or even "quality-adjusted life years" (QALYs) rather than individual lives. However, it would be a moral mistake not to consider how life years are distributed among patients and not to include efforts to reduce the number of individual deaths even while attempting to increase the number of life years. Moreover, rationing based on anticipated life years would reduce priority for patients with co-morbidities that would have little or no impact on their survival to discharge or even for one year or perhaps five years but could later shorten the length of their lives.

Another major counterargument is practical: the health care team has limited time and information to acquire such precision. In a crisis, it would be time consuming and, even then, would require information that is very hard to obtain. Moreover, these longer-range predictions would be quite uncertain. This counterargument applies even more strongly against proposals to focus on QALYs, which would also be problematic for other reasons, particularly because their use tends to neglect other issues of justice, including the needs of people with disabilities.

Rationing according to patients' anticipated life years has been a secondary goal in this pandemic in some contexts (for instance, in Italy). And it could be a legitimate "tie-breaker" between two patients who otherwise have identical point scores in terms of probable survival. It also overlaps with another secondary or supplementary criterion: life cycle. Younger people are sometimes included in the category of the "worst off" because they stand to lose the most years of life, since they are not as far along in the life cycle as older people also needing intensive care. Priority to younger patients based on anticipated life years can legitimately function as a tie breaker where judgments of medical utility are otherwise roughly equal.

This is different from using age as an exclusion criterion in a pandemic in which the elderly are at higher risk, with or without co-morbidities. Philosopher Franklin Miller (2020) defends age as a cut-off for access to ICUs and ventilators. He suggests starting with age 80, which is just above the average life expectancy in the U.S.; such patients arguably have already had their "fair innings." In the COVID-19 pandemic, elders also stay longer in the ICU and die at higher rates even when placed on ventilators. If the demand for ICU beds and ventilators increases, Miller would lower the cut-off age to 70 with and then without co-morbidities to meet the demand.

Several responses to Miller's proposed age limit are in order. First, underlying medical conditions may be more important than biological age even at 80. (Segal 2020) As White and Lo (2020) argue, we need to avoid broad group exclusion criteria in part because of individual variations, such as the presence of other medical conditions. In addition, Miller's proposal would set a bad precedent in support of "ageism" and "ageist" policies and practices. For this reason, many medical institutions' policies during this pandemic rightly rule out discrimination against patients on the basis of age, as well as on the basis of many other irrelevant factors. But, again, age can still legitimately function as a tie-breaker in favor of a younger patient when comparative needs and prognoses are equal.

3. Supplementing Medical Utility with Narrow Social Utility

The object of judgments of utility may be societal welfare rather than medical welfare (though obviously the latter may contribute to the former). This is one source of opposition to invoking utility in rationing health care—it seems to go in the direction of social value or social worth thus violating the principle of equal regard, to be discussed below. However, it is important to distinguish broad social utility from narrow social utility. Broad social utility is rightly rejected as a basis for rationing health care by virtually all secular and religious perspectives. Nevertheless, narrow social utility, also called instrumental value, can be employed, and it applies, albeit in complicated ways, in this pandemic.

Many proposals recognize and emphasize the moral legitimacy of giving some priority for some interventions to health care workers (HCWs) and others who fill essential social roles and discharge essential social functions. (White and Lo 2020; Emanuel et al. 2020) A major reason is to ensure that crucial medical and social responsibilities will be met in the pandemic. Philosopher Daniel Wikler insists that essential caregivers "must be protected, both to induce all to pitch in and to keep them in the action; and they must be treated when ill, both to restore them to the front lines and as a further incentive to keep going." (Wikler 2020) Much depends on the particular intervention being rationed. For instance, in discussions about rationing ventilators, which have perhaps too often been taken as the paradigm case, questions have been raised about whether HCWs and other essential workers experiencing such a severe case of COVID-19 as to require a ventilator can be expected to return to work anytime soon if they survive.

Some bioethicists note that calls for giving priority to HCWs needing ventilators in a pandemic have increased substantially from discussions 10 to 15 years ago about rationing in a possible influenza pandemic; they reasonably surmise that this increase stems in part from the failure in the U.S. in the current pandemic to provide HCWs with the PPE they need. (Chen, Marshall, and Shepherd 2020) They further argue that there are ethically preferable ways to recognize HCWs' assumption of risk and to make up for not equipping them adequately.

Facing the possible lack or significant delay of future instrumental value because of HCWs' and others' limited prospects of returning to work anytime soon after ventilator support, some bioethicists resort to retrospective reciprocity to support priority for those who have assumed risk in their essential work or other important related activities. (Emanuel et al 2020) Such claims can even support provisions for one-time contributors, such as subjects or participants in pandemic-related research. (Emanuel et al. 2020) Consider a person who volunteers for a challenge study during the development of a successful vaccine for SARS-CoV-2 but receives a placebo in the process. (Elliott 2020) Arguably, reciprocity would require that he or she receive a vaccine when successfully developed or, in the absence of a successful vaccine, receive points toward another needed resource, such as an anti-viral drug.

Instead of assigning priority for medical treatments based on narrow social utility, other possibilities include using narrow social utility as a tie-breaker or incorporating it into a "weighted lottery," as we will consider below. Moreover, the strength of arguments for or against prioritization for HCWs, first responders, and others on grounds of their instrumental value depends in part on what is being distributed. As we have seen, it is harder to justify priority for ventilators than priority for preventive measures, such as PPE and vaccines or even for anti-viral treatments such as remdesivir.

In any event, debates about who counts or should count as an essential worker direct our attention to the important role of the community in setting allocation criteria. Not only should allocation criteria be transparent, and explained and justified to the community, but they should actually be developed with public input and engagement. Such public involvement, a matter of participatory justice, is essential for the community's trust and cooperation, both indispensable in a public health crisis.

4. The Principle of Equal Regard

Another cluster of ethical concerns falls under the egalitarian principle of equal regard, which requires treating everyone as an equal, according to fair procedures, in the distribution of goods and burdens. It does not require that everyone receive the same resource. Instead, it permits rationing according to fair procedures. One fundamental question is whether this principle of equal regard is compatible with the principle of utility, as I have defined and specified it in terms of medical utility and broad and narrow social utility.

In contrast to some interpretations, medical utility does not infringe the principle of equal regard for individual persons and their lives. Instead, medical utility insists on counting each individual as an individual. My claim is that counting numbers of individual lives is compatible with a principle of equal regard.

By contrast to medical utility, judgments of social utility do infringe the principle of equal regard. But we need to distinguish narrow from broad conceptions of social utility. Judgments based on broad social utility focus on the differential overall social value of people's lives including but extending well beyond their various roles and functions. By contrast, judgments of narrow social utility consider only the differential value of specific social roles and functions and assign some priority to individuals who fill those roles and discharge those functions. Following the principle of equal regard, it is unjustifiable to use judgments of broad social utility as a basis for rationing in public health crises, but it is ethically justifiable, under some circumstances, to incorporate judgments of narrow social utility into rationing, when narrowly focused on specific and urgent functions and essential services.

If we accept judgments of both medical utility and narrow social utility in triage in the current pandemic, while rejecting broad social utility, there are still ways to express equal regard within and beyond these judgments. Equal regard supports approaches that recognize the transcendence of persons over their social roles and functions and that provide fair equality of opportunity. Hence, proponents of equal regard often argue for a mechanism, such as random selection or a lottery, which can embody and express these values. For instance, random selection or a lottery can serve as a tie-breaker when patients have identical points in medical utility. (Emanuel, et al. 2020) Random selection has often been employed when new medical resources are extremely scarce; over time, this has occurred for several new drugs, including HIV/AIDS drugs, before supplies became plentiful.

A "weighted lottery" can also express equal regard even when judgments of narrow social utility are employed. It is important to ensure that enough individuals survive who can effectively discharge essential social functions. However, it may not be necessary to save all individuals who hold essential social roles. Instead, it may be fair to put essential workers at some risk through a weighted lottery. In such a lottery, individuals in essential social roles would receive additional weights in order to ensure that enough of them will be saved to meet definite social needs, including but not limited to providing health care, fighting fires, delivering food, etc. In this weighted lottery, some persons in essential social roles may not receive treatments. (Childress 2020: Chap. 12; Elster 1989: 47-48, 113-115)

Random selection or a lottery is often joined with "first come, first served" or queuing as an expression of equal regard. "First come, first served" is generally acceptable for hospital admissions and for obtaining and continuing treatments. In addition, interpreted as time on the waiting list, it generates some priority points for candidates for a kidney transplant. However, in the COVID-19 pandemic, under circumstances of extreme scarcity with life and death at stake, "first come, first served" is indefensible as an allocation criterion. One important reason is that background societal injustice may result in people being inadequately aware of and informed about their symptoms, not seeking or receiving medical advice and care early enough, and thus being slow in being treated. In short, unjust background conditions may delay a person's arrival for treatment. Moreover, as we will see later, "first come...." creates special problems in reallocation.

5. Mitigating Health Inequities

The disproportionately high number of COVID-19-related hospitalizations and deaths among African Americans, Native Americans, and other racial/ethnic minorities in the U.S. dramatically highlights the country's health inequities. When we examine the detrimental social determinants of health rooted in systemic or structural injustice (Powers and Faden 2019), racism is certainly a primary example. Outcomes of racism overlap in part, though not entirely, with the effects of lower socio-economic status. Hence, it is not surprising that residents of low-income areas have greater chances of being hospitalized for COVID-19. (Price-Haywood 2020) Accordingly, some ethical frameworks have proposed using metrics such as the Area Deprivation Index (ADI) to identify patients from disadvantaged communities in order to increase their chances of receiving scarce treatments in a weighted lottery. (Pennsylvania Department of Health 2020)

The "Ethical Allocation Framework for Emerging Treatments of COVID-19," prepared by the Pennsylvania Department of Health and other state departments and agencies, represents an important and promising effort to reduce the potential impact of health disparities, such as co-morbidities, on what I have called judgments of medical utility or what it views as "allocating scarce treatments to maximize community benefit." (Pennsylvania Department of Health 2020) This framework focuses primarily on remdesivir, an anti-viral treatment which at this time is available in only limited supply after receiving an Emergency Authorization Approval from the U.S. Food and Drug Administration, but it is designed to apply to other emerging treatments as well. It avoids exclusion of individuals based on various irrelevant characteristics, such as race, religion, ethnicity, age, gender, etc., and it emphasizes individualized assessments. Most importantly for this essay, it seeks to provide meaningful access to all and, at the same time, "to proactively mitigate health disparities in COVID-19 outcomes." (Pennsylvania Department of Health 2020) Its rationale is that of equal respect, what I have called equal regard.

The document's instructions for a weighted lottery allocation among patients who meet the current clinical eligibility criteria emphasize heightened priority for individuals who live in disadvantaged areas, as indicated by an ADI score of 8-10 (these scores fall between 1 and 10, with 10 being the worst). (This ethical framework also gives heightened priority to essential workers in a weighted lottery.) Even patients who are not expected to live more than a year because of chronic, end-stage conditions are included in the lottery but are assigned lower weights.

This ethical framework attempts to incorporate corrective or reparative justice in response to health inequities, and acute care facilities in Pennsylvania are expected to develop ethical treatment policies and protocols consistent with it. While this ethical framework is promising and significant, particularly as a symbolic commitment to reducing health inequities, difficult questions remain. One is whether the ADI accurately and reliably applies at the individual patient level; this is important because the ethical framework stresses an individualized assessment. Another question is whether the ethical framework, formulated for "emerging treatments," can and should be applied across the entire range of possible scarce public health and medical interventions. For instance, the public health rationale that this framework uses may not extend easily to rationing intensive care and ventilators. Application of the ADI to such decisions may raise charges of unfairness in life/death decisions, perhaps especially if used in a point system rather than in a weighted lottery or as a tie-breaker. And this may damage public trust.

Just public health requires more upstream interventions, especially to prevent or reduce some of the health conditions that cause severe morbidity and increased mortality among patients with COVID-19. But in the midst of a pandemic, it may only be possible to try to reduce the impact of these conditions on patients' health and survival and to prevent these conditions from disadvantaging patients in an allocation framework that also emphasizes medical utility or community benefit.

Preventive interventions such as PPE and vaccines (if and when a safe and effective vaccine is developed) are important. A shortage of PPE has made it difficult for many people to take steps to protect themselves and others, but protection has also faltered because some living conditions (e.g., overcrowding) and some work environments (e.g., essential work that requires physical presence in close quarters) make social distancing difficult if not impossible. Still priority distribution of PPE, such as masks and sanitizers, to disadvantaged communities can help. If a safe and effective vaccine is developed and available, prioritization in distribution can also be justified because of the risks both of infection and of bad outcomes among African Americans and other racial/ethnic minorities. But vaccine acceptance may be limited in part because of widespread distrust of government-sponsored, encouraged, or mandated vaccinations among African Americans and others. (Jamison, Quinn, and Freimuth 2019)

Tragic Choices: Reallocation of ICU Beds and Ventilators

Many bioethicists argue that there is no moral difference between withholding (not starting) and withdrawing (stopping) life-saving interventions, however significant the psychological differences between these actions may be. (Beauchamp and Childress, 2020: 161-165) The psychological differences are often quite weighty—withdrawing treatment, such as ceasing intensive care or stopping a ventilator, seems to many clinicians to be closer to killing a patient than does withholding such interventions. However, not only is the distinction between withholding and withdrawing conceptually flawed, and not only can it lead to overtreatment, but, perhaps less obviously, it can actually lead to undertreatment because clinicians may be reluctant to start treatments they fear being locked into continuing. And yet it is often important to start treatments in order to gauge a patient's response or determine more accurately a person's prognosis; hence, decisions to withdraw treatments can often be ethically superior to decisions to withhold treatments because they can be better informed. However, any decision to remove a patient from intensive care or to withdraw a ventilator in order to make room for another patient on the grounds that the latter has a better prognosis creates serious ethical as well as psychological conflicts.

Reallocation of intensive care and ventilators in this pandemic has received wide, but by no means universal, support in the ethics literature (Emanuel, et al. 2020; White and Lo 2020; Truog, Mitchell, and Daley 2020). In my judgment, it can be ethically justifiable under certain conditions. Earlier I noted that while "first come, first served" is often viewed as an expression of equal regard, just as random selection is, it is problematic in part because unjust background circumstances may affect when patients seek and receive care. Nevertheless, in considering reallocation even in a pandemic that necessitates rationing, treatment should be continued for patient X in the ICU or on the ventilator unless there is strong evidence that X will not survive even with that treatment coupled with strong evidence that patient Y, in need of the ICU bed or ventilator, has a significant probability of surviving. A slight difference in probable benefit between the two patients is not enough. Moreover, importantly, withdrawal of a treatment is not tantamount to abandonment, that is, cessation of care. Care should continue, particularly in the form of palliative care. Just care under altered standards in a public health crisis is still care, even if not every possible intervention can be provided or continued.

Writing in the New York Times, Jennifer Senior (2020) stresses that this pandemic has thrust upon clinicians "a devil's kit of choices no healer should ever have to make." In Italy, doctors were reported "weeping in the hospital hallways because of the choices they were going to have to make." (quoted in Truog, Mitchell, and Daley 2020) Tragic choices often create moral distress, injury, and trauma, even when agents believe they made the right choices. This may occur because of the tension between physicians' training and commitments to prioritize the care of the most ill patients on the one hand and the demands of saving the most lives through triage on the other. Many institutions have developed ethical criteria and procedures to mitigate the individual clinician's burden, for example, in ventilator reallocation, but these measures, including role separation through the use of a triage committee, may not be sufficient to eliminate the clinician's moral distress.

In conclusion, rationing or triage in a public health crisis poses wrenching ethical questions. In confronting such tragic choices—where fundamental social-cultural-ethical values are at stake—societies must "attempt to make allocations in ways that preserve the moral foundations of social collaboration." (Calabresi and Bobbitt 1978: 18) What we decide and how we decide it are vitally important. The choices we make in this pandemic not only signal who we are now (e.g., a

society committed to saving lives, to equal regard, to justice/fairness, to correcting health inequities, and so forth—or not); they also communicate who we are becoming. The ethical burden is ours: our choices can either shore up or undermine the foundation for current and future public trust.[1]

Acknowledgements
I thank my colleagues at the Center for Health Humanities and Ethics, School of Medicine, University of Virginia, and the Ethics Committee, UVA Health, for rich and illuminating discussions of many of these topics.

References

Beauchamp and Childress 2019. Beauchamp, Tom L. and James F. Childress. Principles of Biomedical Ethics. New York: Oxford University Press, 2019 8th edition

Calabresi and Bobbitt 1978. Calabresi, Guido, and Philip Bobbitt, Tragic Choices. New York: W.W. Norton & Company, 1978.

Chen, Marshall, and Shepherd, 2020. Chen, Donna T., Mary Faith Marshall, Lois Shepherd. Prioritize Health Care Workers for Ventilators? Not So Fast. Bioethics Forum, June 8, 2020 [URL: https://www.thehastingscenter.org/prioritize-health-care-workers-for-ventilators-not-so-fast/ Visited June 13]

Childress 2020. Childress, James F. Public Bioethics: Principles and Problems. New York: Oxford University Press 2020, Chap. 12, "Triage in a Public Health Crisis"

Elliott 2020. Elliott, Carl. An Ethical Path to a Covid Vaccine. New York Review of Books, July 2, 2020

Elster 1989. Elster, Jon. Solomonic Judgements. Cambridge: Cambridge University Press, 1989.

Emanuel, Persad, Upshur, et al. 2020. Emanuel, Ezekiel J., Govind Persad, Ross Upshur, et al. Fair Allocation of Scarce Medical Resources in the Time of COVID-19. The New England Journal of Medicine 382 (2020): 2049-2055

Jamison, Quinn, and Freimuth 2019. Jamison, Amelia M., Sandra Crouse Quinn, and Vicki S. Freimuth. 'You don't trust a government vaccine': Narratives of institutional trust and influenza vaccination among African American and white adults. Social Science and Medicine 221 (2019): 87-94

Miller 2020. Miller, Franklin G. Why I Support Age-Related Rationing of Ventilators for COVID-19 Patients. Hastings Bioethics Forum, April 9, 2020 [URL: https://www.thehastingscenter.org/why-i-support-age-related-rationing-of-ventilators-for-covid-19-patients/ Visited June 15, 2020]

Pennsylvania Department of Health, et al. 2020. Pennsylvania Department of Health, Pennsylvania Emergency Management Agency, Pennsylvania Department of Human Resources. Ethical Allocation Framework for Emerging Treatments of COVID-19 (2020)2020 [URL: https://www.health.pa.gov/topics/disease/coronavirus/Pages/Guidance/Ethical-Allocation-Framework.aspx, visited June 15, 2020]

Powers and Faden 2019. Powers, Madison and Ruth Faden. Structural Injustice: Power, Advantage, and Human Rights. New York: Oxford University Press 2019

Price-Haywood, Burton, Fort, et al. 2020. Price-Haywood, Eboni, Jeffrey Burton, Daniel Fort, and Leonardo Seoane. Hospitalization and Mortality among Black Patients and White Patients with COVID-19. New England Journal of Medicine. May 27th, 2020.

Rettig and Lohr 1981. Rettig, Richard and Kathleen Lohr. Ethical Dimensions of Allocating Scarce Resources in Medicine: A Cross-National Study of End-Stage Renal Disease. Unpublished manuscript, 1981

Segal 2020. Segal, J. Bradley. Why I Don't Support Age-Related Rationing during the Covid Pandemic. Hastings Bioethics Forum, May 18, 2020 [URL: https://www.thehastingscenter.org/why-i-dont-support-age-related-rationing-in-treating-covid-19/ Visited June 15, 2020]

Senior 2020. Senior, Jennifer. The Psychological Trauma that Awaits Our Doctors and Nurses, The New York Times, March 29, 2020

Truog 2020. Truog, Robert D., Christine Mitchell, and George Q. Daley. The Toughest Triage—Allocating Ventilators in a Pandemic. New England Journal of Medicine 382 (May 21, 2020) 21: 1973-1975.

White and Lo 2020. White, Douglas B. and Bernard Lo. A framework for rationing ventilators and critical care beds during the COVID-19 pandemic. JAMA 323 (2020) 18: 1773-1774

Wikler 2020. Wikler, Daniel. Here are rules doctors can follow when they decide who gets care and who dies. The Washington Post, April 1, 2020

James F. Childress is Professor Emeritus at the University of Virginia, where he was formerly University Professor, the John Allen Hollingsworth Professor of Ethics, Professor of Religious Studies, and founding director of the Institute for Practical Ethics and Public Life. He is the author of numerous articles and several books in biomedical ethics and in other areas of ethics. His books include *Principles of Biomedical Ethics* (with Tom L. Beauchamp); the 8th edition/40th anniversary edition appeared in 2019; the book has been translated into a dozen other languages. His most recent book is *Public Bioethics: Principles and Problems* (2020). Childress has served on several national committees examining bioethics and public policy. He was vice chair of the national Task Force on Organ Transplantation, served on the Recombinant DNA Advisory Committee, and was appointed to the National Bioethics Advisory Commission by President Clinton. He is an elected member of the National Academy of Medicine.

The Professional Ethics of Triage of Life-Sustaining Treatment in a Pandemic

Laurence B. McCullough, Zucker School of Medicine at Hofstra/Northwell, USA

Abstract

In a pandemic emergency that overwhelms the capacity to provide life-sustaining treatment, the concept of medically reasonable applies to an at-risk population of patients and creates the *prima facie* ethical obligation of physicians to reduce mortality and morbidity in this population by preventing unacceptable opportunity costs. This is the professional ethics of triage. This paper identifies the implications of the professional ethics of triage for the development and deployment of triage of life-sustaining treatment in a hospital when resources become overwhelmed by a pandemic.

Key Words

ethical principle of beneficence, ethical principle of respect for autonomy. professional ethics in medicine, professional ethics of triage, professional virtue of integrity, triage, unacceptable opportunity cost

1. Introduction[1]

Pandemics, including the highly infectious disease COVID-19 and other that will follow it in the future, can become so large in scale that affected individuals and their clinical needs can overwhelm available medical resources. This outcome can also occur with mass casualty events, such as a terrorist attack using weaponized biological agents or large-scale, multiple shootings. Planning for such events places a priority on coordinating and managing resources so that healthcare delivery organizations are not overwhelmed and can meet the needs of everyone who presents for care and thereby becomes a patient. This is easier to accomplish in countries with national systems of healthcare or high levels of effective cooperation among healthcare organizations.

In the United States, there is no national system of health care. Instead, the United States has a complex combination of public and private healthcare organizations. Among private healthcare organizations, there are not-for-profit or voluntary and for-profit healthcare organizations. Some voluntary healthcare organizations are sectarian, sponsored by faith communities, including Baptist, Jewish, Methodist, Roman Catholic, and Seventh Day Adventist healthcare organizations. Other private healthcare organizations are secular. There are large public payers such as Medicare (federal program for those 65 years of age and older) and Medicaid (state-federal program for the medically indigent). There are also large health publicly held insurance companies such as United Health Care and Aetna. No one payer is in charge, making coordination among healthcare organizations a challenge, compounded by intensive competition among healthcare organizations and groups of healthcare organizations.

There will be circumstances in which efforts to manage the very high volume of patients in a pandemic or mass casualty event fail to prevent healthcare organizations from being overwhelmed. In clinical circumstances in which not every patient's needs can be met, priorities must be set in triage policies (McCullough 2020). This will especially be the case for life-sustaining treatment and other critical care medicine resources. The response to the clinical reality of overwhelmed healthcare resources is the professional ethics of triage, applied to provision of life-sustaining treatment. Triage of life-sustaining treatment is especially challenging in the COVID-19 pandemic because this disease can cause life-threatening multi-organ disease

---

[1] Portions of this paper have been adapted, with permission, from McCullough 2020.

resulting for some patients in rapid pulmonary decompensation. As a consequence, individuals with symptoms of serious COVID-19 have a risk of mortality in the absence of rapid access to life-sustaining treatment in a hospital.

2. Professional Ethics in Medicine

Two physician-ethicists, John Gregory (1724-1773) of Scotland and Thomas Percival (1740-1804) of England, invented professional ethics in medicine (McCullough 1998; McCullough, Coverdale, Chervenak 2020). They deliberately framed it as secular so that it could be transreligious transcultural, and transnational, as it must be to guide clinical practice in the pluralistic societies of their time and ours. Two ethical principles and one professional virtue are pertinent to the professional ethics of triage.

2.1 Ethical Principle of Beneficence

The ethical principle of beneficence creates the *prima facie* ethical obligation to identify and provide clinical management that, in deliberative (evidence-based, rigorous, transparent, and accountable) clinical judgment is predicted to result in net clinical benefit. Such clinical management is medically reasonable (McCullough, Coverdale, Chervenak 2020).

2.2. Professional Virtue of Integrity

The professional virtue of integrity creates the *prima facie* ethical obligation to practice medicine to standards of intellectual and moral excellence. Intellectual excellence is achieved by habitual adherence to the discipline of deliberative clinical judgment. Moral excellence is achieved by making the protection and promotion of the health-related interests of the patient the physician's primary concern and motivation, keeping self-interest systematically secondary (McCullough, Coverdale, Chervenak 2020).

2.3. Ethical Principle of Respect for Autonomy

The ethical principle of respect for autonomy creates the *prima facie* ethical obligation of the physician to empower the patient to make an informed and voluntary decision about whether to authorize clinical management that has been offered or recommended (McCullough, Coverdale, Chervenak 2020). The first step is to identify the medically reasonable alternatives for the clinical management of the patient's condition or diagnosis. The second step is to provide the patient with clinically salient information about the nature of the clinical management and its clinical benefits and risks. The third step is to support the patient to come to an adequate understanding of this information, to identify his or her relevant values and beliefs, and to assess the medically reasonable alternatives on this basis. The final step is to ensure that the patient's decision-making process is voluntary, i.e., free of internal and external controlling influences (Beauchamp and Childress 2013).

3. Professional Ethics of Critical Care Medicine

Life-sustaining treatment takes the forms of medication and machines that supplement or supplant vital organ function, including oxygenation (mechanical ventilation, extra-corporeal membrane oxygenation), circulation (cardiopulmonary resuscitation, blood-pressure medications, implantable mechanical circulation devices, intraventricular pumps), and removing toxins from blood (renal dialysis).

3.1. Beneficence-Based Outcomes of Life-Sustaining Treatment

Life-sustaining treatment has both short-term and long-term goals, both beneficence-based.

The short-term goal of life-sustaining treatment is prevention of imminent death. The long-term goal of life-sustaining treatment is survival with at least some interactive capacity. This long-term goal rejects vitalism, the view that there is an absolute or unlimited beneficence-based ethical obligation of physicians to preserve life until the patient is actively dying (death is imminent) or death occurs. In the global history of medical ethics, there is no professional ethics in medicine that has embraced vitalism (Baker and McCullough 2009). Some faith communities, including some schools of Islam and of Judaism, have embraced vitalism (Baker and McCullough 2009; McCullough, Coverdale, Chervenak 2020).

3.2. Initiating and Discontinuing Life-Sustaining Treatment

Critical care management should be recommended when in deliberative clinical judgment it is predicted to achieve *both* the short-term and long-term goals of life-sustaining treatment. When in deliberative clinical judgment life-sustaining treatment is predicted not to achieve the short-term goal or the long-term goal, it is not medically reasonable. If life-sustaining treatment has been initiated, it should be discontinued when in deliberative clinical judgment it is no longer medically reasonable. The physician should make a clear recommendation that life-sustaining treatment should be discontinued. If life-sustaining treatment has not been initiated when, in deliberative clinical judgment, it is not medically reasonable, it should not be initiated. The physician should make a clear recommendation that life-sustaining treatment should not be initiated (McCullough 2020).

3.3. Response to Requests for Life-Sustaining Treatment that is not Medically Reasonable

When life-sustaining treatment that is not medically reasonable is requested to be continued or to be initiated, this request should not be implemented. The ethical principle of beneficence creates a *prima facie* ethical obligation only to provide medically reasonable clinical management, an ethical obligation reinforced by the professional virtue of integrity.

4. Professional Ethics of Triage

4.1. The Professional Ethics of Triage and the Professional Ethics of Medicine

The professional ethics of triage brings the professional ethics of medicine to bear on the responsible management of life-sustaining treatment when clinical need overwhelms the number of critical care beds, including those that can be rapidly created and staffed. This was the response of many hospitals in COVID-19 "hot-spots" in the United States, especially New York City.

4.2. Two Necessary Conditions for any Adequate Triage Policy

In the triage literature, two necessary conditions for any adequate triage policy have been identified. The first is that "Triage systems must be simple, easy to remember, and amenable to quck memory aids" (American Academy of Pediatrics et al. 2011, 125). The second is that triage criteria must be "objective" in the specific sense that bias has been eliminated or, failing that, minimized to the greatest degree feasible. This means that "[e]thnic origin, race, sex, social status, sexual preference, or financial status should never be considered in triage decisions" (Nates et al. 2016, 1567).

4.3. Critical Care Management and its Limitations

The provision of critical care should be understood as a trial of management, with ethically justified, beneficence-based criteria for its initiation and discontinuation, as explained above (Consensus statement of the Society of Critical Care Medicine's Ethics Committee regarding futile and other possibly inadvisable treatment. 1997; Kon et al. 2016). Life-sustaining treatment should be initiated when, in deliberative clinical judgment, it is reliably predicted to result in reducing the risk of mortality and preserving at least some interactive capacity, i.e., when its two goals can be achieved. Life-sustaining treatment should continue until it is no longer medically reasonable (the patient is well enough to be discharged to a lower level of clinical management, the patient is too sick to benefit from critical care management and should be transferred to palliative and hospice care, or the patient dies). When the test of medical reasonableness fails, life-sustaining treatment should not be started or should be discontinued (Brett and McCullough 1986, 2012; Blackhall 1987). Violations of this ethical obligation violate the ethical principle of beneficence and the professional virtue of integrity.

4.4. Prevention of Unacceptable Opportunity Costs

In conditions of severe scarcity, the focus simply shifts from beneficence-based ethical obligations to an individual patient to beneficence-based ethical obligations to a population of patients. There is a beneficence-based and integrity-based ethical obligation to provide medically reasonable clinical management to a specified population of patients. The means to fulfill this beneficence-based and integrity-based ethical obligation is the prevention of unacceptable opportunity cost: the use of life-sustaining treatment for a patient for whom in deliberative clinical judgment that use is not medically reasonable and that use blocks access to life-sustaining treatment for a patient for whom it is medically reasonable to initiate critical care management. To prevent unacceptable opportunity costs and thereby to prevent unacceptable clinical harm to other patients, life-sustaining treatment should not be initiated and should be discontinued when it is not medically reasonable. Inasmuch as intubation is time sensitive, decision making must be rapid, to end the unacceptable opportunity cost rapidly. Unacceptable opportunity costs with respect to life-sustaining treatment are neither clinically nor ethically benign. Effective prevention of unacceptable opportunity does not require coordination among hospitals. The non-system of healthcare in the United States therefore does not pose any obstacle to the implementation of professional ethics in triage.

Permitting unacceptable opportunity costs to occur violates the harm principle, the beneficence-based ethical obligation to prevent harm to innocent others, especially when those others lack the capacity to consent to being exposed to risk of harm (Beauchamp and Childress 2013). It is well understood in all ethical theories that no one has the right willfully harm others, with well-known exceptions such as self-defense, defense of others, or in just war.

4.5. Beneficence-Based Ethical Obligation to Reduce Mortality While Preserving At Least Some Interactive Capacity

In the professional ethics of triage, clinical criteria are beneficence-based and integrity-based. Their focus is on the beneficence-based ethical obligation to achieve the short-term and long-term goals of life-sustaining treatment, by reducing mortality while preserving at least some interactive capacity in a population of patients, the clinical needs of which outstrip available resources.

Criteria for triage management in statements from professional organizations appeal solely to these beneficence-based goals (using Glasgow Coma Scale [https://www.glasgowcomascale.org/]) (Consensus statement of the Society of Critical Care Medicine's Ethics Committee regarding futile and other possibly inadvisable treatments 1997; Consensus statement on the triage of critically ill patients 1994; Guidelines for intensive care unit admission, discharge, and triage 1999; Nates et al. 2016). Such criteria meet an important clinical practice test: "Triage systems must be simple, easy to remember, and amenable to quick memory aids" (American Academy of Pediatrics et al. 2011, 125).

Because triage criteria focus on reduction of mortality and preservation of at least some interactive capacity, they are biologically reductionist by design (Engel 1977). Biological reductionism eliminates what George Engel (1913-1999) called the psychosocial dimensions of health and disease and therefore eliminates these sources of bias. This becomes a powerful asset in triage management because biological reductionism ensures that "[e]thnic origin, race, sex, social status, sexual preference, or financial status should never be considered in triage decisions" (Nates et al. 2016, 1567).

In addition, from the perspective of biomedically reductionist clinical judgment, other considerations are ruled out as irrelevant to deliberative clinical judgment about initiating or discontinuing life-sustaining treatment. The chronological age of the patient by itself is irrelevant to the physiologically based prediction of outcomes because chronological age cannot be equated with physiologic age. Discontinuing medically reasonable critical care management of an older patient in favor of a younger patient and prioritizing patients based on age *simpliciter* are therefore ethically impermissible. Quality of life, engaging in valued life tasks and deriving satisfaction from doing so, is an autonomy-based concept. Quality-of-life judgments are matters for each individual with at least some interactive capacity to determine for himself or herself. This includes the quality of life of those with disabilities. Achieving the goal of survival with at least some interactive capacity rules out as ethically impermissible any judgment by others that a patient has such a low or unacceptable quality of life that life-sustaining treatment should not be initiated or should be discontinued.

4.6. Organizational Policy

When life-sustaining resources become overwhelmed and the biomedically reductionist criterion of survival with at least some interactive capacity has been applied, every critical care bed will be occupied by patients under the condition of medical reasonableness. Other patients for whom, in deliberative clinical judgment, a trial of critical care management is medically reasonable should be informed that access to life-sustaining treatment will not be offered and that the team will attempt transfer. If transfer is not feasible, the team will do their best to provide for a dignified, respectful dying process. Within resource constraints, clinical management for these patients should aim to provide palliative and hospice care to accepted standards. The outcome for some patients of acceptable opportunity costs will be ethically justified deaths. This is not a new clinical ethical category. The already existing clinical ethical category of justified deaths includes deaths subsequent to ethically permissible discontinuation of life-sustaining treatment. The professional ethics of triage simply expands this clinical ethical category.

Healthcare organizations should develop and implement triage policies that apply the professional ethics of triage to conditions of severe scarcity. In their internal and external communications healthcare organizations should explicate their triage policies, to prevent misinformation and misunderstanding of them. These policies should acknowledge that patients' deaths may justifiably occur when the policies are applied in conditions of extreme scarcity. Ethically justified deaths resulting from triage should be disaggregated from overall mortality statistics, to prevent unjustifiably distorting the mortality statistics of individual physicians and healthcare organizations.

These communications should make clear that the healthcare organization is fully committed to use its resources to defend the professional staff of the organization in response to professional liability claims of wrongful death, negligence, and other torts for the simple reason that the professional staff have fulfilled their professional responsibility to provide life-sustaining treatment on the basis of an ethically justified clinical standard of triage. Every healthcare organization has the ethical obligation to sustain the professional integrity of its physicians, nurses, and other healthcare professionals. Failure to fulfill this ethical obligation will undermine an organizational culture of professionalism (Chervenak and McCullough 2005). This ethical obligation has a crucial implication: All litigants should be informed that the organization will respond vigorously to all complaints and will not settle out of court when organizational triage policy has been implemented without medical errors. Countries with national health systems should have appropriate policies to this effect.

4.7. Triage Process

The beneficence-based criterion of survival with at least some interactive capacity requires only deliberative clinical judgment for its clinical application. This means that the triage process should be led by physicians with the requisite training and experience to make deliberative clinical judgments about the medical reasonableness of initiating and discontinuing life-sustaining treatment. These physicians should be held in the highest professional regard by their colleagues, to promote confidence and trust in the organization's triage policy and its implementation.

There is no role for others. Specifically, there is no role for clinical ethicists because, qua ethicists, they do not have the fund of knowledge or skillset to make deliberative clinical judgments of any kind. The role of clinical ethicists is restricted to contributing to the professionally responsible adaptation of existing triage guidelines into organizational triage policy. Such policy should state that clinical ethics consultations in individual cases are unnecessary.

Triage officers have the integrity-based ethical obligation to the population of patients, to their professional colleagues, and to the organization to document their decisions in patients' records. Triage officers will experience a potentially jarring frameshift. To discharge the responsibility to apply triage criteria, these physicians will need to shift their focus of concern and judgment away from the needs of an individual patient in a physician-patient relationship to the needs of a population of patients in a physician-population relationship (Chervenak et al. 2020). Organizational leaders should not underestimate the need for full support of the professional integrity of triage officers who are charged with making and documenting decisions about the medical reasonableness of life-sustaining treatment. This support should include periodic retrospective review of the triage officers' decisions. A well-designed, communicated, and implemented triage policy will obviate the need for appeals of triage decisions by professional staff. Appeals by clinicians therefore should not be permitted.

The same holds true for appeals from patients, their surrogate decision makers, family members, and friends. This includes patients or family members with social and political influence in the community. The justification for a policy of no appeals from these parties is simple: The ethical principle of respect for autonomy plays no role in the formation of the concepts of medical reasonableness and an unacceptable opportunity cost and their clinical application by triage officers. Permitting patients or those claiming to speak for them to override the decisions of a triage office creates the risk unnecessary and therefore impermissible unacceptable opportunity costs, an egregious violation of the harm principle compounded by the amount of time required to file and adjudicate an appeal.

Consent plays no role in the professional ethics of triage. When the beneficence-based criterion of survival with at least some interactive capacity is not satisfied, patients or their surrogates should be informed by the triage officer that life-sustaining treatment will not be initiated or discontinued, as explained above. Psychosocial support for patients and their families should be provided, remotely if necessary

5. The Appeal to Justice Has No Place in the Professional Ethics of Triage

The professional ethics of triage makes no appeal to "public-focused duties to promote equality of persons and equity in distribution of risks and benefits in society" (Hastings Center 2020). There is a serious philosophical problem with appeals to the ethical principle of justice in proposed triage policies.

In the history of Western philosophy, the classic source for the general formulation of this ethical principle is Aristotle, who held that like cases should be treated alike. This formulation is so abstract that it lacks practical application. We need to know in what respect cases are alike.

Articulating an applicable principle of justice requires specification (Richardson 1990). As H. Tristram Engelhardt, Jr. (1996), persuasively showed, the various specifications of justice, including utilitarianism in its various forms founder in the context of a pluralistic society. Specifications of justice that appeal variously to equality, equity, fairness, and equal or equitable distribution of resources (Hastings Center 2020) are unavoidably contentious, because there is no authoritative philosophical specification of the ethical principle of justice (Engelhardt 1996; Chervenak and McCullough 2015). .

Perhaps the most influential justice-based approach to triage has been proposed by Douglas White and colleagues (White et al. 2009; White and Lo 2020). White and colleagues specify justice as utilitarian and procedural justice. They appeal to the work of Norman Daniels, which is deeply influenced by the modified utilitarianism of John Rawls (1921-2002). They also specify criteria that procedural justice should meet: "public engagement, transparency in decision making, appeals to rationales and principles that all can accept as relevant, oversight by a legitimate institution, and procedures for appealing and revising individual decisions in light of challenges to them" (White et al. 2009: 137) White and colleagues claim that this specification of justice supports a multi-principle bioethical framework for triage: "saving the most lives, maximizing the number of "life-years" saved, and prioritizing those who have had the least chance to live through life's stages" (White et al. 2009: 132). No argument is made to support their Rawlsian specification of utilitarian justice. Engelhardt's critique is not even acknowledged.

The ethical principle of justice in Aristotle's formulation and its multiple specifications is invoked to prevent bias. It is therefore at least ironic that the clinical application of White's framework results in the introduction of bias in its use of the criterion of five-year survival (University of Pittsburgh April 15, 2020). Critical care physicians understand well that social determinants of disease and injury influence who become their patients. Triage criteria based on survival with at least some interactive capacity assume that social determinants play no role in the provision of critical care from admission to discharge, because the critical care team is solely and completely in control of the processes of patient care. Nor do social determinants or nonclinical factors play a role in the physiological profiles and their measures incorporated into triage policies.

The processes that result in five-year survival are not solely and completely under the control of the critical care team. Indeed, no healthcare professional has this kind of control over these processes and therefore over their outcomes post-discharge. It is well recognized that social determinants of health and disease, including ethnic origin, race, sex, social status, sexual preference, and financial status, influence post-discharge mortality. The justice-based appeal to "saving the most lives, maximizing the number of "life-years" saved, and prioritizing those who have had the least chance to live through life's stages" (White et al. 2009: 132), far from eliminating bias in triage decisions, introduces bias.

This critique applies to all triage criteria based on post-discharge survival and supports another critique of White's approach (University of Pittsburgh 2020). White's proposed policy explicitly calls for eliminating the influence of social determinants of health and disease and then implicitly includes them in the five-year survival criterion. This is a straightforward violation of the principle of non-contradiction

6. Conclusion

The professional ethics of triage is elegantly simple, requiring appeal only to the ethical principle of beneficence and its complementary professional virtue of integrity that generate the key clinical ethical concepts of an unacceptable opportunity cost and the anti-vitalist ethical concept of survival with at least some interactive capacity. The result is triage policy that is easy to remember, rapidly clinically applicable, and free of bias. Triage policies that propose to add justice-based considerations are challenging to remember (which specification of justice is invoked and why), not rapidly clinically applicable (two prognostic judgments must be made and then integrated(University of Pittsburgh 2020)), and riddled with bias that reinforces, and does not even minimize, the ethically impermissible influence of deleterious social determinants of health and disease on the outcome of life-sustaining treatment and other forms of critical care management in a pandemic that overwhelms the resources of healthcare organizations.

References

American Academy of Pediatrics; American College of Emergency Physicians; American College of Surgeons - Committee on Trauma. 2011. American Academy of Pediatrics; American College of Emergency Physicians; American College of Surgeons - Committee on Trauma. Model uniform core criteria for mass casualty triage. Disaster Medicine and Public Health Preparedness 5 (2011):125–128.

Baker and McCullough 2009. Baker RB, McCullough LB, eds. The Cambridge World History of Medical Ethics. Cambridge: Cambridge University Press 2009.

Beauchamp and Childress 2013. Beauchamp TL, Childress JF. 2013. Principles of Biomedical Ethics. New York: Oxford University Press 2013, 7th ed.

Blackhall 1987. Blackhall L. Must we always use CPR? New England Journal of Medicine 317(1987): 1281-1285.

Brett and McCullough 1986. Brett AS, McCullough LB. When patients request specific interventions: Defining the limits of the physician's obligation. New England Journal of Medicine 315 (1986): 1347-1351.

Brett and McCullough 2012. Brett AS, McCullough LB. Addressing requests by patients for nonbeneficial interventions. Journal of the American Medical Association 307 (2012): 149-150.

Chervenak and McCullough 2005. Chervenak FA, McCullough LB. The diagnosis and management of progressive dysfunction of health care organizations. Obstetrics and Gynecology 105 (2005): 882-887.

Chervenak and McCullough 2015. Chervenak FA, McCullough LB. Ethics in perinatal medicine: A global perspective. Seminars in Fetal and Neonatal Medicine 20 (2015): 364–367.

Chervenak et al. 2020. Chervenak FA, Grünebaum A, Bornstein E, et al. Expanding the concept of the professional integrity of obstetrics during a public health emergency [published online ahead of print, 2020 May 6]. Journal of Perinatal Medicine 2020;/j/jpme.ahead-of-print/jpm-2020-0174/jpm-2020-0174.xml.

Consensus statement of the Society of Critical Care Medicine's Ethics Committee regarding futile and other possibly inadvisable treatments. 1997. Consensus statement of the Society of Critical Care Medicine's Ethics Committee regarding futile and other possibly inadvisable treatments. *Critical Care Medicine* 25 (1997): 887–891.

Consensus statement on the triage of critically ill patients. Society of Critical Care Medicine Ethics Committee. 1994. Consensus statement on the triage of critically ill patients. Society of Critical Care Medicine Ethics Committee. Journal of the American Medical Association 271 (1994): 1200–1203.

Engel 1977. Engel GL. The need for a new medical model: a challenge for biomedicine. Science 196 (1977): 129-136.

Engelhardt 1996. Engelhardt, Jr., H. Tristram. The Foundations of Bioethics. New York: Oxford University Press 1996, 2nd ed.

Guidelines for intensive care unit admission, discharge, and triage. Task Force of the American College of Critical Care Medicine, Society of Critical Care Medicine. Guidelines for intensive care unit admission, discharge, and triage. Task Force of the American College of Critical Care Medicine, Society of Critical Care Medicine. Critical Care Medicine 27 (1999): 633–638.

Hastings 2020. Hastings Center. Ethical Framework for Health Care Institutions and Guidelines for Institutional Ethics Services Responding to the Novel Coronavirus Pandemic. March 16, 2020. Available at https://www.thehastingscenter.org/ethicalframeworkcovid19/, accessed June 2, 2020.

Kon et al. 2016. Kon AA, Shepard EK, Sederstrom NO, et al. Defining futile and potentially inappropriate interventions: a policy statement from the Society of Critical Care Medicine Ethics Committee. Critical Care Medicine 44 (2016): 1769–1774.

McCullough 1998. McCullough LB. John Gregory and the Invention of Professional Medical Ethics and the Profession of Medicine. Dordrecht, The Netherlands: Kluwer Academic Publishers (now Springer), 1998.

McCullough 2020. McCullough LB. In Response to COVID-19 Pandemic Physicians Already Know What to Do. [published online ahead of print, 2020 Apr 23]. American Journal of Bioethics 2020; 1-4.

McCullough, Coverdale, Chervenak 2020.McCullough LB, Coverdale JH, Chervenak FA. Professional Ethics in Obstetrics and Gynecology. Cambridge and New York: Cambridge University Press 2020.

Nates et al. 2016. Nates JL, Nunnally M, Kleinpell R, et al. ICU Admission, Discharge, and Triage Guidelines: A Framework to Enhance Clinical Operations, Development of Institutional Policies, and Further Research. Critical Care Medicine 44 (2016): 1553–1602.

Richardson 1990. Richardson HS. Specifying norms as a way to resolve concrete ethical problems. Philosophy and Public Affairs 19 (1990): 270-310.

University of Pittsburgh 2020. University of Pittsburgh. 2020. Department of Critical Care Medicine. Allocation of scarce critical care resources during a public health emergency.

April   15,   2020.
https://ccm.pitt.edu/sites/default/files/UnivPittsburgh_ModelHospitalResourcePolicy_2020
_04_15.pdf, accessed June 2, 2020.

White et al. 2009. White DB, Katz MH, Luce JM, Lo B. Who should receive life support during
a public health emergency? Using ethical principles to improve allocation decisions. An-
nals of Internal Medicine 150 (2009): 132-138.

White and Lo 2020. White DB, Lo B. A Framework for Rationing Ventilators and Critical Care
Beds During the COVID-19 Pandemic [published online ahead of print, 2020 Mar 27].
Journal of the American Medical Association 2020;10.1001/jama.2020.5046.

Laurence B. McCullough, Ph.D. is Professor of Obstetrics and Gynecology in the Department
of Obstetrics and Gynecology of Zucker School of Medicine at Hofstra/Northwell, Hempstead,
New York, and Ethics Scholar in the Department of Obstetrics and Gynecology of Lenox Hill
Hospital, New York, New York. In 2016 the President and Board of Trustees of Baylor College
of Medicine (Houston, Texas) made him Distinguished Emeritus Professor in Baylor's Center
for Medical Ethics and Health Policy, upon his retirement from the College after 28 years on its
faculty. In 2013 he was recognized for his contribution to medical education at Baylor with the
Barbara and Corbin J. Robertson, Jr., Presidential Award for Excellence in Education. He has
published 590 papers in the peer-reviewed scientific, clinical, ethics, and philosophical journals,
as well as 62 original chapters in scholarly books. He is the author or co-author of 8 books and
editor or co-editor of 8 books. He is currently writing *Thomas Percival's Medical Ethics* and
editing *Thomas Percival's Medical Jurisprudence and Medical Ethics* for the Philosophy and
Medicine book series published by Springer (New York City). He lives in Austin, Texas, with
his wife Linda J. Quintanilla, Ed.D., a retired community college history professor and active
scholar of Mexican American history. E-Mail contact: Laurence.McCullough@bcm.edu.

The Corona Virus and Emergency Management
Triage, Epidemics, Biomedical Terror and Warfare

Hans-Martin Sass, Georgetown University Washington, USA

Abstract

Our cultures and states have moral and legal rules of what do in normal situations. But in situations of war, terror, famine and triage, we face emergencies which require extraordinary actions and means; the actual Corona Pandemic is such a situation. We have to ask ourselves and our institutions and governments what to if 'mother nature' or 'bad people' cause extraordinary dangerous and deadly situation for ourselves and for our communities. I use case-studies to discuss ethical and political solutions and remaining uncertainties.

Key words

emergency, epidemic, extraordinary situations, normal situations, pandemic, situational ethics, terror, triage, responsibility, warfare

> *You govern a kingdom by normal rules; you fight a war by exceptional moves; but you win the world by letting alone[1]*

1. Normal and extraordinary situations

Life has normal and abnormal times; this is true for individuals, families, and also communities and states. There are certain technical and moral norms which guide our behavior, make us successful and reliable in everyday life and in professional life. These guides govern our behavior and the expectations of others. The rule 'love you neighbor', known as the golden rule in all cultures. We define good people in contrast to bad people as to be those who act of an attitude of compassion, who care for others, in particular for those who are close to them: parents, family, neighborhood, but not excluding strangers. The concept of compassion is valid for everyone, for personal and for professional activities. Businessmen should not exploit or steal or otherwise hurt their customers. Generals have to fight the enemy, not their own government or the people of their country; homebuilders have to build stable and reliable houses. For emergency and extraordinary situation such as pandemic events 'playbooks', are available for leaders, most of them not at the public domain.[2] The medical profession, physicians and nurses, have their own code of ethics, more clearly defined in medical ethics: a great physician has to combine expertise and ethics, professional knowledge and human compassion. He should not make difference between his patients and treat everyone fairly and just; he should treat everyone professionally and morally as if he were his own father or mother. As famous Confucian doctor Sun Simiao in his book 'On the Absolute Sincerity of Great Physicians' wrote: 'A Great Physician should not pay attention to status, wealth or age; neither should he question whether the particular person is attractive or unattractive, whether he is an enemy or fried, whether he is a Chinese or a foreigner, or finally, whether he is uneducated or educated. He should meet everyone on equal grounds. He should always act as if he were thinking of his close relatives. (Sun Simiao: On the Absolute Sincerity of Great Physicians) In the Western world Hippocrates, who

---

[1]   Lao Tzu 1989. Lao Tzu. *Tao The Ching*, transl. Wu J CH, London, Shambala.

[2]   Executive Office of the President of the United States. *Playbook for early Response to high-consequence emerging infections disease Threats and biological Infections (Not for Public Distribution)*, [google]; But the 'handbook' Schweizerische Eidgenossenschaft. Bundesrat fuer Gesundheit, 2019 [3.ed] Pandemieplan. Handbuch fuer die betriebliche Vorbereitung. Betriebe aufrechtungerhalten. Mitarbeiter schuetzen, was and is intentionentially public.

is called the father of Western medicine, expressed the same ethics by means of an oath to be sworn by physicians: 'Into whatever houses I go, I will do so only for the benefit of the sick, avoiding all willful injustice and harm'.[3]

In modern times, we have certain requirements for the ethics of a good physician[4]. These requirements are based in the tradition, are taught in medical ethics classes, but above all by role model and behavior of clinicians, doctors and nurses who are exemplary teachers of their students and rightly called masters of the arts and sciences of healing, i.e. combining expertise and ethics, professionalism and compassion. The requirements for a trust-based communication and cooperation with the patient and the family include the following norms and standards: (1) the care for the individual patient who is your first obligation; only thereafter come obligations to the family, the hospital, society; (2) every intervention requires the information and the consent of the patient [or his family] out of respect for the dignity of individual values and personal choice; (3) do not treat without informed consent; (4) treat everyone fair and equal, e.g. do not make a difference between the poor and the rich, men or women, or people of so-called social worth such as public officials or dignitaries; (5) treat those who need the help most, first. It is the usual practice that emergency care is given priority over routine treatment in hospital wards; doctors are called to the emergency room and other patients and non-emergency procedures have to wait.

2. Triage in disaster, catastrophe and in war

The case: A bus accident has happened on the road. All 30 people are hurt, some very severely and might die if not helped immediately; among the passengers is a nurse who could help, but she is also hurt. A local ambulance with one doctor and two nurses with some emergency equipment happens to come by. The doctor recognizes his mother to be among the more severely hurt. How would you set priorities, if you were the physician, would you treat your mother first, or those who might die if not helped immediately? Would you give the nurse a priority treatment in order to get one more trained nurse to help?

The bus accident case presents a situation of triage. Triage occurs in natural or man-made catastrophes, in severe epidemics or endemics, after acts of terrorism and in war. There are established rules of professional conduct and ethics of triage; for medical as well as ethical reasons these rules are different. The general rule is: safe as many lives as possible in the shortest possible time or in the time available. Such a triage ethics is reverse to what is professionally and ethically mandated in normal situations. Triage ethics include: (1) give preferential care to of medical or management worth, who can assist you; (2) care for those first, who are least hurt; (3) allow those, who are hurt most, to die; (4) provide treatment, if necessary, without consent.

Of course, there will be a professional and very personal conflict for the doctor in postponing the treatment of his own mother, actually putting her into the sequence of a treatment list, which contains the easiest cases first and the most complicated cases last, i.e. violating the principle of 'filial love' [xiao] for the benefit of 'neighborly and patriotic love' [zhong]. The ethical reasoning give for the triage situation is the reverse commitment of the physician and the health care system to safe life: save as many lives as possible and don't safe those lives, which need it most. Giving the nurse a preferential treatment contradicts the principle of fair and just health care directly, but it helps indirectly to increase the quantity of care given to everyone on the list

---

[3] Sass, Hans-Martin. Medizin und Ethik, Stuttgart, Reclam 1989, 351f.
[4] Qiu Renzong. The Art of Humanness, in: *J Medicine Philosophy* 13(1988)3:277-300.

of a sliding scale people needing less help and more help and very much help.

NATO instruction in a handbook on 'Emergency War Surgery'[5] differentiates between ordinary and extraordinary triage: 'Ordinary triage classifies the wounded so all will receive optimum care, while mass casualty triage treats the injured according to salvage value when the injured overwhelm available medical facilities and not all can be treated'. In making triage decisions, pressure of time to treat certain cases earlier than others complicates medical and ethical decisions even further. In traditional virtue theory, this would mean that 'neighborly and patriotic love [zhong] in those extreme situations becomes a more urgent virtue that 'filial love' [xiao] and that 'colleagues' as potential partners become preferential treatment.

3. Fighting Epidemics

Case Study: Two dozen family members and friends attend the marriage of Mr. and Mrs. Schmidt. They come from different provinces, some even from abroad. During the festivities they got infected with a highly lethal virus, such as the SARS virus, Ebola or a pathogen similar to the actual Corona virus. Twenty die; only four survive. By using high-tech and low-tech modes of transportation, they spread this highly contagious virus around many provinces and around the globe, causing one billion people to die. - The case of the Schmidt family spreading a highly lethal virus around the globe results from the easiness, safety, and affordability of global travel. Global travel is a high achievement made possible by a combination of high-tech developments in hardware and software and skilled businesses and good governance; it is definitely a contribution to global enterprise, communication and cooperation, not at least to better understanding each other. But global travel can spread dangerous viruses and other dangerous material more easily around the globe than before. Countries are fixed to their respective geographic place, people, viruses, materials are not. Two different scenarios describe the destructive potentials of the high-tech context for human health, human life, and human culture: (1) the 'natural' spread of global diseases, and (2) the terrorist, aggressive, or criminal use of pathogens to kill or to terrorize. For scenarios, ordinary citizens and public officials must translate classical theories of 'just war' into the high-tech context of biomedical terror and warfare.

Global mobility causes global spread of infectious diseases: We don't have to wait for terrorists, criminals or foreign countries to use biomedical devices for killing, terror or warfare. High-mobility of people, made possible by integrated global travel, and global networks of trade and commerce make the spreading infectious diseases easy and dangerous. To fight these side-effects of the high-tech context of the modern globalized world, high-tech interventions are necessary. First among those high-tech defenses are (a) a high-tech research capacity, including the education and continuing education of epidemiologists and other experts, (b) a high-tech infrastructure of informing and communicating with experts and, even more important with citizens. Of particular importance is the full, clear and easy to understand information and advice to all citizens about the dangers, about self-protection, and about shelters or facilities for help. If full and easy to understand information is not given, then public authorities will lose trust and people might not follow advice and instructions. Of secondary nature, but unavoidable and probably less effective if not supported by well informed and trusting citizens is the control of travel.

To prevent the spread of the disease, ways of spreading have to be blocked rigorously; this might include the total stop of mobility for people and some merchandise. Of course, a few or many civil and human rights will have to be restricted. Following the minimax principle, such

---

[5] NATO Handbook Emergency War Surgery, 2011.

restrictions on travel and mobility need to be balanced against the lethal and contagious character of a particular disease and the extent of such a temporary restraint needs to be communicated fully and openly. Also, the establishment of an independent governance and monitoring committee would be highly advised for two purposes: to control actual restrictions and make those who are in control aware that they are monitored, and to keep and preserve the trust of the people, who suffer under those restrictions, and later report in public on their findings. Unfortunate, as these destructive side-effects of a high-tech world and highly mobile people are, they are just a side-effect, not a dilemma which would call to reduce global travel and mobility. People and viruses can travel geographically, countries cannot; therefore, countries are obligated to restrict the movements of people and viruses. This includes unfortunate actions such as quarantine facilities, mandatory inoculation, restriction of movements, and other burdens on individual lives and lifestyles.

4. Public Health Ethics and Acts of Terror and War

Here is a slightly different case: Not the nice people of the Schmidt family, but a handful of neurotic or fundamentalist extremists, ready to commit terror and killing via their own suicide deliberately infect themselves with a highly contagious and lethal virus. They 'distribute' the deadly virus not accidentally as the Schmidt people did, but deliberately. They strategically infect many other people who then will infect many more on a global scale: in buses or subways leading to airports, in movie theaters or sports events, in planes and trains. Many pathogens in military or research arsenals or new strains of pathogens or deliberately modified and even more deadly strains can be used for that purpose. .Human history is full of deliberate poisoning of water; in 1000 BC the Hettites used plague bacteria in Northern China and Siberia; in 1346 AD the Mongols through infected corpses over the walls of Jaffa in Crimea; in the Second World War the Japanese through Bubonic bazillions into the Chinese town of Ningbo[6]. Biomedical terrorism and biomedical killing will be a powerful side-effect of the modern world of global integration. The already mentioned instruments of high level of research, readiness to test, to inform, to advise and to react by immunization, restriction of mobility, and quarantine need to be used for the protection of innocent citizens and of humankind. But levels of uncertainty and risk are higher than in naturally occurring situations of medical triage or endemic infection catastrophes, because of the deliberate strategic destructive powers of evil-doers.[7]

There is a variety of scenarios of modern high-tech biomedical destruction, terror, and war: Evil-doers might work alone or with a few friends, might have support networks, get help or encouragement even from governments, or governments themselves might use biomedical warfare.

(1) In cases of biomedical terrorism, only a few might be killed because of poor planning by terrorists or swift reaction by public authorities. As one purpose of terrorism is killing and the other purpose to terrorize the survivors and to breed scare and fear, it is very important that authorities and experts give the lay citizen all necessary information of how to protect herself or himself and how the pathogen lives and becomes distributed; only then will the citizen feel some sort of power over the terrorist, the attack, the terror and the angst and fear.-

(2) When and if terrorists work alone in small cells, the best defense and prevention against all forms terrorism and radical discontent in society is to support healthy cultural and ethical

---

[6] Sass HM 2020 Health and Happiness of Political Bodies, Lit: Zürich 2020: 31f.

[7] Henderson DA 1999 Smallpox as a biological Weapon; medical and public Health Management, in: J American Medical Association 281(22)2127-2137.

environments, inform and educate the people to be risk competent and vigilant and responsible citizens. Global high-tech networks of communication and travel allow good-doers as well as evil-doers to work successfully in reaching their goals. We may call the situation a dilemma; being strongly in support of technology as a tool to cultivate raw nature and uncivilized societies, I rather call it a side-effect we need to be aware of and protect ourselves against. -

(3) Terrorists most likely will have direct or indirect support from international groups, even from governments, alike the sea pirates always had. If this is the case, then those groups and governments need to share the blame and punishment and be exposed publicly. -

(4) If biomedical killing is one of the options seriously contemplated by governments, the best defense against those dangerous weapons for killing masses of innocent people are a high level of research and preparedness and, unfortunately, a policy of threatening to retaliate similarly. During the times of the Cold War this was called the strategy of 'mutual assured destruction (MAD). The acronym MAD, when not read as acronym, means mad, irate, imprudent, senseless, i.e. it makes the calculation to win for a potential aggressor too uncertain and also the probability of losing one's own population and power. For an intellectual and academic ethicist without real responsibility and power in those situations, it is futile and irresponsible to even evaluate the arguments pro and contra in analytical and ethical terminology; it will be the very personal responsibility of those in public office to make such decisions, which are beyond human capacities to calculate, and to live with those decisions for the rest of her life and in history.

(5) It has been mentioned that protection of certain high-tech biomedical research from patenting and public knowledge would be necessary to curb dual-use or abuse of knowledge for terrorism or other immoral use, in particular methods used to modify microbes to make them resistant to drugs. As secrecy this might be a means to slow the distribution of knowledge, centuries of technology development have shown that firewalls against double-use or spin-off rarely work in the long run. But certain principles of governance to prevent potential abuse of biomedical knowledge definitely is warranted, also in scientific publication and patenting. Bu then, potential terrorists and mass killers do not need to develop their own, potentially more deadly biomedical weapons, as the arsenals of biomedical research are full of deadly pathogens. Also, pathogens such as dangerous forms of flu or other viruses will develop naturally and evil-doers, in particular suicidal killers, will find ways to infect themselves and infect as many people as possible before they might die.

5. Does Crisis Ethics Justify Exceptional Ethical Moves

Is the fight against biomedical terrorists and killers of any kind a war and thus allows using methods and means, which are ethically accepted in wartime? Furthermore: does the same apply to situations of emergency caused by natural disasters or man-made catastrophes? Is the possible destruction of large numbers of people and culture so eminent, that extraordinary means are justified? European military theory and ethics, similar to Chinese military theory and ethics, has as set of principles which need to be recognized to fight a just war. There are five requirements to justify a war as a means of last resort: use of power must legitimate; it must be a just cause; it must have the right intentions; it must the mean of last resort; it must be an obligation (potestas legitima, causa justa, recto intention, ultima ratio, modus debitus).

(1) The person or institution using power must be legitimate. This definitely was and is the case for elected government which has the obligation to protect its people. But in modern times, international corporations such as Amazon, Tencent, Google, having an annual budget of more than most nations wield a tremendous power and professional organizations in the high-tech

context such as those of engineers, physicians, internet experts have a legitimate power to advise governments and to be partners or executors of powers in the protection of the people. But they can do otherwise, such as treating people who would be high value because of their skills, with preferential treatment, because they will be valuable assets to fight epidemics or situations of triage. Not only generals and high public officials are essential assets in fighting catastrophes, whether natural or man-made. Actually, nurses or doctors are of higher immediate value than high bureaucrats who do not bring any special skill to situations of triage and great danger to a high number of people.

(2) The cause must be just, i.e. it must serve the purpose of protecting innocent people and the population for which the government is responsible, in modern times even responsible for the survival and health of the global population. In the case of biomedical destruction, but causes would justify the exercise of warlike powers. It is under discussion, whether or not preventive war is justified as the fight against microbes, once spread, is extremely difficult in biomedical and epidemiological terms, but also in terms of protecting civil and human rights. Saving people's life always has been and always must be the highest order of every compassionate and civilized person, especially of physicians and health care expert and of high public officials.

(3) The use of war or warlike powers has to come from the right intentions, i.e. the argument that one wants to protect the people must be serious; it would unethical and unjust to use that argument only to build a stronger power base for oneself. A means to check this requirement is to check whether the means used, are precisely appropriate for the purpose. Temporary restrictions of civil liberties never are allowed for the purpose of gaining more power or hurting other parties or persons in the process of politics and business, or for enriching oneself.

(4) War and warlike situations need to be the means of last resort, after all other means to protect the health and life of the people have been exhausted. In combination with other principles such as highest levels of information, civil ethics and public preparedness, citizens will understand and support the measures taken on their behalf. Restriction of civil liberties, such as quarantine and treatment or immunization against a person's will, must only be used as means of last resort. Other public health activities such as information campaigns requiring mandatory attendance are of lower impact on civil liberties.

(5) Finally, the exercise of warlike power needs to be an obligation, a duty of those who resort to these interventions and acts as a last resort. For public officials the highest duty is the protection of the people, their lives and livelihood; this is a common-sense duty, but also supported by all religions, and by Confucian and socialist reasoning. It is important that everything be done to avoid situations of high emergency and danger to high numbers of people, i.e. prevention of catastrophes by means of vigilance, safety regulations, education of experts and people, and quick responses, which might keep the proportions of disasters as small as possible.

Thus, natural and man-made disasters do, indeed, justify using the model of just war under the condition, that these five specific requirements are met. It would be advisable that ethicists and strategists in public office and in professional organizations develop more detailed lists of principles for monitoring the exceptional powers given to or taken by those who act in warlike situations in the high-tech context.

A personal word: It is extremely unpleasant and uncomfortable for an ethicist to argue in favor of restricting civil rights and liberties and in favor of abandoning people in severely pain and suffering and helping those who are less sick or hurt. My moral and intellectual background comes from childhood experiences of the 2nd World War in Europe and the student and intellectual revolution of 1968. I have seen some of the immoralities and atrocities associated with times of war and after-war. I also cherish the civil rights of free and open modern societies. I hate war and I hate everyone who takes away civil rights from people without an extremely strong and persuasive justification. However, the dangers of high-tech biomedical attacks and destruction are so threatening, that I strongly feel that the just war theory and ethics must be employed in evaluating and in guiding the situation those responsible in public office, experts in their specific fields, and above all educated and responsible citizens find themselves in the context of high-tech biomedical risks and options. Unfortunately, it cannot be excluded that sooner or later a natural disaster such as a new bird virus or any other pathogen might develop to which humankind is not immune. In the global situation of high mobility of merchandise and people, such a contagious pathogen can spread rapidly around the globe, not only within one country, and cause hundreds of millions, of not billions, of fellow humans to die.

6. Prevention and Preparedness is Essential in Public Health!

There is a number of medical and ethical issues which need to be discussed in detail as means of prevention and preparedness. Traditional measures in public health already have caused controversy among bioethicists and suspicion in certain populations. Polio vaccination in Nigeria has met resistance by strong forces in traditional culture and was introduced by poor government education programs. But vaccination programs as a means of prevention for diphtheria, tetanus, whooping cough, meningitis, flu, measles, mumps, rubella, hepatitis A, and flu immunization is a service to the individual as well as to the community. Education in how to prevent the spread of disease or to reduce the risk of occupational or lifestyle related accidents also are important features in the protection of health for the individual as well as the community.[8]

Preparedness for biomedical disasters of mass proportions includes not only training of health care professionals; cooperation with other local experts and public authorities is essential. Material has to be pre-positioned, facilities other than hospitals have to be determined as shelters or for quarantine. Health care workers and other disaster relief personnel have to be immunized preventively, if and when a specific bacterial or viral pathogen infection or attack cannot be excluded. Such immunization programs are costly and also might have side-effects on the health of those immunized. Ethical and professional issues associated with mandatory preventive immunization programs need to be addressed prior to immunization. Some health care workers will be quarantined together with patients; those who for a variety of personal or family reasons rather should or would not be quarantined need to be identified long before and formal quality criteria for selection need to be developed and publicly and professionally discussed prior to implementation.

Prevention, whenever and wherever possible, is important to reduce dangers, once they cannot be avoided or averted. Prevention methods include immunization programs, education of citizens to be vigilant and alert, to follow safety recommendations and instructions. Another means to reduce the severity of a catastrophe is appropriate training and rehearsal, in particular, when many parties on the local level are involved. The chain of command needs to be established in such realistic training programs. Also, material needs to be ready and pre-positioned, so that it is readily available where it is needed.

Additional to natural catastrophes, the same measures of prevention and preparedness need to be applied to the possibility of man-made disasters, those by accident and in particular those

---

[8]   Moreno J ed., 2003, In the Wake of Terror: Medicine and Morality in a Time of Crisis, Cambridge MA, MIT.

caused intentionally. Given the immoral and criminal intentions of a few determined criminals to kill innocent civilians, it also cannot be excluded that they will find neurotic or criminal expert to help them to specifically engineer deadly pathogens just for the purpose of killing fellow humans. It has been discussed to, in particular, to limit information and scientific publication on molecular research knowledge of manipulating pathogens, as such knowledge can be used by criminals to construct even more deadly viruses or bacteria. While the dissemination of knowledge rarely can be suppressed for longer periods of time, patents cannot be granted and further research will be hampered, including research on developing vaccines and antibodies for rapidly changing pathogens, as the recent H5N1 flu virus seems to be.

As disaster management is service to the people under extraordinary circumstances, public officials and health care providers need to prepare themselves during normal times for extraordinary times. Therefore, rehearsals and planning and implementation exercises are extremely important. It is essential to determine the chain of command, to have more than one means of communication, to preposition materials and goods, also to include the private market sector.

Private market businesses such as supermarkets, hardware stores, hotels offer special routine service to the people; they are profit oriented and have experience to change services and goods depending on demand. The profit motivation and the skills of private business should not be underestimated in contributing to manage big and unexpected crises and disasters. In particular, when natural disasters can be foreseen, private business will preposition goods and services and might be quicker in a response to mass calamities, as has been shown in relief efforts for hurricane victims. It would be prudent for public officials in control of disaster relief to not also micro-manage the private sector, rather encourage the private sector to cooperate in relief efforts, whenever possible. The Daoist saying 'you win the world by letting alone' can be translated into the emergency situation when not everything can be done by public officials and should not be done by public officials and response teams. There is a certain prudence in the market and in people who know their skills and who are compassionate, that they as citizens and as professionals will help where they feel help is needed and can be provided by them. Thus, the encouragement of civil ethics, i.e. the ethics of citizenship and neighborly love, is one of the most important tasks of public officials and of public discourse and culture. Civil war like protests and riots after the murder of George Floyd, a citizen of black color by policemen caught on camera, and non-sensitive stupid and arrogant twitter remarks by the US President, show that medical diseases of great social impact can translate into the disease of the entire political and social body.[9]

7. Hard Conflicts in Great Danger

There are some 'hard cases' which had been discussed in the bioethics literature and unfortunately are occurring again and again. I mention just three: (1) Investigational torture of terrorists in order to gain information which could save hundreds, thousands or millions from attack and death; (2) killing out of compassion and mercy; (3) saving the life of an enemy in situations of limited resources.

(1) Investigational torture. The case: A terrorist was captured who very likely has information on the whereabouts of other members of his team, his superiors and of plans of immanent attacks on I high number of people. The captors ask you to assist and consult as medical expert

---

[9] Cf Sass HM 2020 Health and Happiness of the Political Body, Zürich, Lit; Sass HM 2009 Ethische Risiken und Prioritaeten bei Pandemien, Bochum: ZME; Sass HM 2007 Bioethics and Biopolitics. Beijing Lectures[chin, engl], Xian, fmmu.press.

in proceedings of torture as a means of last resort to save very many innocent people in immediate danger. What would you do? Possible benefits are evident and include the saving of highest numbers of innocent people, work as a disincentive for potential criminals and could lead to capture of other criminals. The World Medical Organization in 1982, and again in 2004, passed a resolution that 'medical ethics during armed conflict are identical to those in peacetime'.

(2) Merci-killing. The case: After a car accident, a triage situation develops and the most severely hurt cannot be treated; they scream in extreme pain and agony; some ask to be killed. They know and everyone else knows that they cannot be saved and that all of them will die a painful death. Would you active kill those who plea for that, would you also kill the others who are in similar agony but only scream? Situations like this have been reported from the battle fields of the past when wounded soldiers were screaming between enemy lines with no hope to salvage them. In some cases, their soldier friends shot them, in other cases they listened to the screams of their comrades for hours and hours. Merci-killing is an issue which does not occur only in warlike situations; it is an everyday issue in treating terminal patients who are in pain and suffering. Professional codes of conduct in Western as well as in Chinese medicine refuse vehemently the active killing of a fellow human as contrary to the rules of ethics and nature, and the obligations of physicians; but there are situations where compassionate health care professionals and family members have resorted to killing patients or their loved ones out of merci and compassion.

(3) Costly health care for an enemy. The case: United States Special Forces capture a combatant in Eastern Afghanistan, only to find out that he needs dialysis treatment. The prisoner refuses the treatment, saying he would rather be dead than in the hands of the enemy. Doctors are reluctant to treat without informed consent. Two days later, the US Secretary of Defense orders dialysis treatment, arguing that the prisoner might have valuable information on other terrorists and on planned attacks. What would you have done? [10] The Geneva Convention on treating prisoners of war requires equal and fair treatment to all, prohibits medical experiments on prisoners if those are against the prisoner's interests, and requests informed consent.

There are more than these three cases to which an answer is not easily found and in regard to which bioethicists, health care professionals, public officials, and each and every one of us might have different opinions. Research literature in bioethics documents and reflects these different opinions. Hard cases rarely can be solved in the classroom and should not be solved in the classroom by giving instructions, such as you would give instruction in a cookbook or for standard treatment in medical care following quality norms. These are cases of a very personal matter where ethical and medical analysis is not enough to make decisions or to criticize decisions. The moral agent to make those decisions, beyond the capability of moral calculation, is the person in the actual situation. Only in an actual situation, the interaction and combination of expertise and ethics can be the final test for professional and compassionate behavior based in personal responsibility. Decisions might be right or might be wrong; one might regret to have made a certain decision at a later date. One might regret not to have involved oneself in interrogational torture because it became evident that 1000 or even more lives could have saved, if one had not refused.

8. Disaster Ethics is Partnership Ethics: Serve the People

There are many other sources of social and political disaster[11]. Extraordinary situations of

---

[10] Zupan et al., 2004 Dialysis for a Prisoner of War, in: Hastings Center Report 34(6)11f.

[11] Fukuyama F 2014 The Sources of pollical Dysfunction, in: Foreign Affairs, Sept/Oct 2014;5-26.

challenge to physician's and health care expert's need to focus on professionalism and compassion. But there might be no clear-cut answers, pointing to different roles and obligations and duties for health care professionals: Some in the field of public health, some in consulting or treating the individual patient, some in consulting on prevention, some in accompanying and comforting the frail and dement, some in consulting public officials, some in being elected to a public office based on skills and knowledge as an expert in the care for health. High-tech cultures depend essentially on skills and compassion of experts, individual citizens and communities. Physicians and other health care workers play many roles in modern society: treating patients in acute and in chronic situations, consulting and advising citizens in regard to lifestyle, nutrition, occupational and environmental health, researching and improving family and clinical medicine and epidemiology, advising government and corporations in regard to safety and reduction of risk to health, preparing, advising and cooperating in the management of natural disaster, endemics, biomedical terror and warfare. Dr. Research, Dr. Acute, Dr Consult, Dr Care, Dr. Manage, Dr Prepare, Dr Govern, Dr Teach, Dr Partner, Dr Special, Dr Example, they all display special skills in their craft.

Whether treating patients in the family medicine or in high-tech medicine, in disasters, endemics, or in war, physicians need to cooperate with others, with people who organize emergency logistics, who understand radiation, pathogens or earthquakes, who can coordinate and manage. But above all, it will depend on the compassion and team spirit, all these people bring together with their skills. Real situations are different from simulated situations. But anticipatory simulation and preparedness allows for better managing extreme situations. Discussing the extreme challenges of crisis ethics, triage, endemics, and biomedical terror and warfare in the classroom or in preparation meetings results not in a protocol that produces moral solutions, but those discussions and actions 'enhance awareness of the many moral aspects of the daily practice in which professionals operate'. What the classroom discussion in medical ethics, in public health ethics and in the ethics of emergency care cannot do, is to prescribe a list of 'to do' and 'do not'. But case studies and analytical evaluation of medical and moral options can help to develop what has been called 'moral competence': 'the ability to see what is morally relevant in a situation, knowing the points of view from which one sees it, understanding that others may see it differently, and then, with others, responding well to what one sees'[12]. Classroom teaching is easy; life is not easy; making ethical decisions in exceptional situations is not easy; easy to understand is the obligation to safe life, to alleviate pain and to professionally consult in matters of a healthy lifestyle and the enhancement of life; difficult is the implementation of all of this.

Extreme situations require extreme, sometimes very unpleasant and very extraordinary means of protecting individual lives, families, neighborhoods and communities. Those extraordinary means need to be guided by principle and prudence, strategically coordinated, and executed with skill and compassion. Surviving disasters makes individuals, communities, institutions and corporations stronger.

Conclusion

'The 'heart has its own reasons, which reason cannot argue with', as Blaise Pascal once said. Acting in extraordinary situations must guarantee that basic and proven rules of behavior in protecting people and people's lives and that normal rules will not be violated without cause. But there are limits to logical moral argumentation based on rules, principles, regulations; we

---

[12] Verkerk M, Lindemann H, Maeckelberghe E et al. 2004 Enhancing Reflection. An interpersonal exercise in ethics education, in: Hastings Center Report 34(6)31-38.

often work just on intuitions of caring for loved ones and the community. The recent video-taped murder of George Floyd, a colored US citizen in an over 8-minute choke grips by a racial white police officer caused - additional to the over Covic-19 150.000 US deaths by the end of July 2020, and arrogant and stupid comments by the US President - civil-war-like protests and demonstrations in many US cities for weeks. Situational emotion and protest have led to hate and hardship of the entire political body. In normal situations and even more so in extraordinary situations the individual conscience is the highest justice in applying norms and principles, but the individual conscience is not slavishly bound to those normal rules till 'we can breathe normally again'.

References

Executive Office of the President of the United States. *Playbook for early Response to high-consequence emerging infections disease Threats and biological Infections (Not for Public Distribution)*, [google]

Fukuyama F 2014. "The Sources of pollical Dysfunction" *Foreign Affairs*, Sept/Oct 2014;5-26

'handbook' Schweizerische Eidgenossenschaft. Bundesrat fuer Gesundheit, 2019 [3.ed] Pandemieplan. Handbuch fuer die betriebliche Vorbereitung. Betriebe aufrechtungerhalten. Mitarbeiter schuetzen

Henderson, DA 1999. "Smallpox as a biological Weapon; medical and public Health Management" *J American Medical Association* 281(1999)22:2127-2137

Lao Tzu 1989. *Tao The Ching*. Transl. Wu J CH, London, Shambala 1989

Moreno J ed., 2003, "In the Wake of Terror: Medicine and Morality in a Time of Crisis", Cambridge MA, MIT

NATO Handbook Emergency War Surgery, 2011

Qiu, Renzong 1988. "The Art of Humanness", *J Medicine Philosophy* 13(1988)3:277-300

Sass, Hans-Martin 1989. *Medizin und Ethik*, Stuttgart: Reclam 1989

Sass, Hans-Martin 2007. *Bioethics and Biopolitics*. Beijing Lectures [chin., engl.], Xian, fmmu.press

Sass, Hans-Martin 2009. *Ethische Risiken und Prioritäten bei Pandemien*, Bochum: ZME 2009

Sass, Hans-Martin 2020. *Health and Happiness of Political Bodies*, Lit: Zürich 2020

Verkerk M, Lindemann H, Maeckelberghe E et al. 2004. "Enhancing Reflection. An interpersonal exercise in ethics education" *Hastings Center Report* 34(2004)6:31-38

Zupan et al., 2004. "Dialysis for a Prisoner of War" *Hastings Center Report* 34(2004)6:11f

Hans-Martin Sass, PhD, is Professor Emeritus at Georgetown University, Washington DC and Ruhr-University, Bochum FRG, Honorary Professor at Renmin University and Peking Union Medical College in Beijing, PRC. This article is based on 2005 and 2009 lectures at Peking Union Medical College and Tsinghua University, PRC, and in hospitals in Bochum, FRG. His numerous articles and books discuss issues of bioethics, philosophy and social and political science. - sasshm@aol.com.

The Question of Justice
in Treating the COVID-19 Patients
-- has prioritizing the fittest to receive the treatment become the norm?

Michael Cheng-tek Tai, Chungshan Medical University, Taiwan

Abstract

The development of medical technology in the 21 century has been most remarkable as medical scientists are generally able to dissect the mystery of illness that people suffer. But the novel onset disease we call Covid 19 of 2020 has been spreading rapidly without signing of respite and has already caused the death of close to ninety hundred thousand people worldwide by the end of August. The health professionals working day and night to save patients' lives have been in a dilemma for the ventilator that is needed to treat and save life has been in dire short supply. A poignant bioethical dilemma has confronted the clinicians and eventually some health professionals passed the ventilator from the older patients to the younger ones on the basis of the survival of the fittest in order to save more lives. This article attempts to argue that this practice of selecting who lives and who dies violates the principle of medical ethics and the world must find a way to solve it.

Key words

COVID-19, ventilator, survival of the fittest, justice, respect of life

1. Introduction

COVID 19 has turned the world upside down. The whole world is devastated by this coronavirus that has killed more than three hundred and fifty thousand people so far worldwide. In treating its infected patients, health professionals found that the needed ventilator to save life is in dire short supply posing a dilemma of how to distribute this scare medical equipment.

2. Ventilator, a tool to save life when a patient develops breathing problem

When a patient cannot breathe properly, ventilator can take over by forcing air into the lungs at certain intervals to prevent immediate death from occurrence therefore gaining time to treat the patient. There are two types of ventilation: mechanical and non-invasive. Non-invasive ventilation involves a face mask fitted over the mouth and nose with no tube required to establish the airway. But when someone needs a longer-term help to breathe, a mechanical ventilator is required. A mechanical ventilator is connected to a tube inserting into the patient's windpipe through nose or mouth. The COVID 19 pandemic which strikes the world in early 2020 found humankind being ill-prepared to meet the challenge because the ventilator that is needed to treat the patient has been depleted. Not only ventilator is in short supply, the mask to prevent the infection is also extremely lacking. As a result some elderly patients have been denied of this last life-saving tool for the reason that younger patients may have better chances of recovery therefore the elderly has been denied its access. News report has this: "hospitals in Italy are no longer intubating patients over the age of 60, with some doctors being forced to make agonizing decisions about who lives and who dies in the face of the ongoing coronavirus pandemic, according to shocking eyewitness reports from healthcare professionals." (McGrath 2020).

3. Justice, a principle of medical ethics advocating fairness to all

Justice is the one of the major principles of medical ethics upholding that "requires us to treat every patient as equal and provide equivalent treatment for everyone with the same problem" (Parsons 1992:15). Robert Veatch of Kennedy Institute of Ethics said that " people in simi-lar situation should be treated equally" (Veatch 2000:122). Beauchamp and Childress, the au-thors of the *Principles of Medical Ethics* wrote: " no person should be treated unequally despite all difference with other persons" (Beauchamp 1983:187). In medical school teaching, students are taught to treat every patient equally. In other words, no gender, color, creed, social status of patient should stand on the way to affect how a patient is cared for. A patient is a patient, no difference in age, gender, color… that all deserve the best possible care and treatment he or she needs regardless of anything. Hippocrates' oath that every medical student studies and also takes before starting clinical training is vividly visible in all medical school. They vow that they will not violate their role as healers and swear that they will observe the solemn oath of non-maleficence, beneficence, respecting autonomy and upholding justice in clinical practice. H. M Sass, former director of European Ethics Section of the Kennedy Institute of Ethics put it this way: "a great physician has to combine expertise and ethics, professional knowledge and human compassion…he should not make difference between his patients and treat everyone fairly and just" (Sass 2007:383).

The principle of justice has been described as the moral obligation to act on the basis of fair arbitration. It is linked to fairness, entitlement and equality. In health care ethics, this can be subdivided into three categories: fair distribution of scarce resources (distributive justice), re-spect for people's rights (rights based justice) and respect for morally acceptable laws (legal justice) (Gillon 1994). The terms fairness, desert, and entitlement have been used by philoso-phers to explain the idea of justice, while equitability and appropriateness of treatment are used in interpretations.

At the time when medical supplies of any kind are inadequate and limited, can a physician be allowed to play the role of God deciding who lives and who dies? Beauchamp and Childress have indicated "… until it has been shown that there is a difference between their relevant to the treatment at stake" (Beauchamp 1983:187), can some other measures be considered. Here we found that there are two different types of justice, the formal justice and material justice. (Beauchamp 1983:186) Formal justice can be understood as the treatment that is given at 'the first come first served" basis. In this sense, everyone receives the equal chance without any dif-ference. If the elderly patient is the first to be admitted to hospital, he or she will have the privi-lege to receive a ventilator when needed, the younger patient coming later would have to wait till another ventilator is available. Formal justice is not comparative while material justice is comparative to be determined by the degree of emergency or recoverability or otherwise. When medical resources are limit, Tom Beauchamp and James Childress mentioned " justice is com-parative when one person deserves can be determined only by balancing the competing claims of others persons against his or her claims. Justice is non-comparative by contrast when desert is judged by a standard independent of the claims of others, e.g. by the rule that an innocent person never deserves punishment." (Beauchamp 1983:185).

In daily practice, quite often we notice the material justice is applied that each patient is served according to individual need. This pandemic experience gives us a great lesson that hos-pital should be prepared to meet all kind of challenge at all time, therefore all needed medical equipment should be in place and stored especially for the medical center that is expected to be capable of dealing with all problems in all situation.

Justice in medical ethics can be complicated and complex as everyone's concept of fairness tends to be different. The Medical Portal of the Royal Society of Medicine in UK has suggested four aspects to consider when confronting the troubling decision-making dilemma:

1. Is this action legal?

2. Does this action unfairly contradict someone's human rights?

3. Does this action prioritize one group over another?

4. If it does prioritize one group over another, can that prioritization be justified in terms of overall net benefit to society or agree moral conventions? (Portal n.d.)

This fourth aspect seems to justify the act of denying elderly patient to ventilator while giving it to the younger one. It argues that the younger patients have better chances of recovery therefore, this act therefore is justifiable. Though this argument is based on utilitarian ground, it is a violation of the principle of justice to "treat every patient as equal and provide equivalent treatment for everyone with the same problem" (Parsons 1992:15). Therefore in order to avoid any situation like this from arising, medical institutes should be prepared anytime to meet the challenge of the unpredictable outbreak of contagious diseases. In other words, hospital must always be ready to provide needed medical services with ample storage of medical supplies and devices.

4. Respect to the elderly as an expression of filial piety in Confucianism

The practice of bypassing the elderly to give the needed ventilator to the younger patients of COVID-19 can be deemed as un-filial in Confucianism. The center of Confucian teaching is based on compassion and its implementation is fulfilled through filial piety which is to respect one's own parents and then extended it to other elderly. Parents have sacrificed themselves in nursing, raising and supporting children when children were little. This act of kindness must be reciprocated by children when parents grow old.

The Chinese character for filial piety is Hsiao(xiao) which is composed of two letters, the top is old (lao), the bottom is son (er/chu). The character itself depicts son as supporting and carrying the old. As parents become senile no longer able to take care of themselves, the children have the obligation to support and care of them.

This reciprocity is an act of filial piety but to love one's own parents is not enough, this obligation and respect must be extended to other elderly as well in society. Mencius, the second greatest sage of Confucianism said: "Treat the aged in your family as they should be treated and extend this treatment to the aged of other people's families. Treat the young in your family as they should be treated and extended this treatment to the young of other people's families" (Mencius 1a.7). Fung Yu-lan, one of the most important Chinese philosophers of modern time interpreted it in this way: "to extend the love for one's family so as to include persons outside ... is nothing forced in any of these practices because the original natures of all men have in them a feeling of commiseration which makes it impossible for them to bear to see the suffering of others." (Fung 1948:72). According to Fung, filial piety is an inborn nature of humankind and once it is cultivated, the whole community will be benefitted, none of the sick has to suffer the pain of being left out in time of need because in order to fulfil the expectation of filial piety, people should be aware and prepared to meet the challenge of urgent call.

Confucian teaching always upholds benevolence or compassion. This virtue needs to be cultivated so that the whole society can be harmonious and prosperous. In book of Great Learning it says when one's inner character is cultivated, the family life can be regulated. When the family life is regulated, the nation can be rightly governed. When the nation is rightly governed, the whole world peace will prevail. [Legge 1971:1.5]

Therefore filial piety is the foundation of world peace and universal harmony. Any activity that falls short of respect toward the elderly on the base of filial piety cannot be regarded as good and just. Thus justice in the Confucian tradition is not understood as fairness but as right-eousness and ought-ness of a situation (Tai 1997:60). Using filial piety as an example, the elders deserve the right to have the first share in time of destitution. It is not about fair or not, but about a question of a respect toward the elderly. The western concept of fairness and equality are missing in Confucian society. (Tai 2009:123) In most of East Asian countries the elderly are given free entrance to some public facilities such as museum or exhibition center that the rest of people need to buy a ticket to get in. In train and bus, some seats are reserved only for the eld-erly. All these are the expressions of filial piety because justice is not understood as fairness rather it has the implication of respect and is known as righteousness to do the right thing and the right thing to do (Tai 2019:89-92). The pre-eminence of filial duty is clearly demonstrated by the following Chinese saying: Of all virtues, filial piety is the first. In general, filial piety requires children to offer love, support, and deference to their parents and other elders in society such as teachers, professional superiors, or anyone who is older in age.

As the westernization takes shape in the Orient, the virtue of this respect toward the elderly has been blurred. The most serious challenge to the bedrock of filial piety came in the early dec-ades of the 20th century. Lu Xun (1881–1936), China's acclaimed and influential writer, criti-cized filial piety and argued that the hierarchical principle favoring elders over youth prevents the young adults from growing to adulthood. Mao Tse-tung also attempted to ride of this Con-fucian virtue during the Cultural Revolution but he failed. This tenet remains important to Con-fucian society this day.

In modern Chinese, filial piety is rendered with the words Xiao xun, meaning 'respect and obedience'. While China has always had a diversity of religious beliefs, filial piety has been common to almost all of them; historian Hugh D.R. Baker calls respect for the family the only element common to almost all Chinese people. (Baker 1979:98)

In Korean culture, filial piety is also of crucial importance. (Yim 1998:163-186) In Taiwan, filial piety is considered one of eight important virtues, among which filial piety is considered supreme. It is "central in all thinking about human behavior". (Jordan 1998:267-284) The Viet-namese common man is expected to show respect to people who are senior to him in age, status, or position. At home, he should show respect to his parents, older siblings, and older relatives. This is expressed by obedience in words and action. Respect is part of the concept of filial piety.

From Confucian tradition, denying elder's need for a ventilator to treat the infected disease is regarded as disrespectful of the sacrifice and contribution of these older people to the younger generation and to the society as a whole. It does not mean that the younger patients should re-treat a step behind and yield everything to the elderly. Parents are willing to do anything for their children by giving in of themselves for the benefit and growth of the young. The idea of reciprocity of the human relationship for caring for one another when able not only between children and parents but also including all people in community is an realization of compassion and righteousness. Besides looking after one's own parents, Mo-tzu, another thinker of a differ-ent branch of Confucianism proposed an universal love to advocate that all should be cared for in the same way including other peoples' parents, families and countries just like one's own.

5. Should the fittest be selected to give ventilator?

The concept of "the Survival of the Fittest" is borrowed here to describe what happened in some places which might have deprived the right of the elderly to use respirator due to shortage of supplies. What happened in Italy of passing the elderly patient their use of ventilator to younger patient appears to be contradictory to the professional teaching in medical school. At this COVID 19 pandemic, we noticed that some elderly patients have been let die without giving them respirator to offer them chances of recovery simply because the older the patients, the more likely they will perish while the younger patients will have better chances of healing.

"Survival of the fittest" is a phrase that originated from Darwinian evolutionary theory as a way to describe the mechanism of natural selection. The biological concept of fitness is defined as reproductive success. The phrase can also be interpreted to express a theory or hypothesis that "fit" as opposed to "unfit" (https://en.wikipedia.org/wiki/Survival_of_the_fittest). Some of the elderly patients have been regarded as "unfit" for their chance of recovery is slim. This situation can occur and it is indeed unfortunate and pitiful. We must be reminded that "people must not attempt to impose their own 'truth' on others", as wrote H.M.Sass. (Sass 2016:111)

In late March this year, nearly 1,400 of the most prominent bioethicists and health leaders in USA signed an urgent letter to Congress and the White House, imploring the U.S. government to immediately use its federal power and funds to respond to the COVID-19 pandemic as a matter of moral imperative. Among the five requests it posted, "ensure the manufacture and distribution of needed supplies" came first. It also asked to protect the vulnerable. (Hastings 2020).

This petition clearly indicates that every patient needs to be cared for and protected as it is a solemn duty of health professionals. Refusing to give ventilator to elder patient when they need it is a serious violation of medical ethics although it can be due to the compromise made in a situation where medical resources are scarce. Patients with better chances of survival thus are given the ventilator for the sake of saving more lives.

American medical ethicists and medical leaders who signed the letter stressed in their appeal that no one's life is more valuable than the life of another. Sun Simiao, the father of Chinese medical ethics, put it in 6th century: "Life is precious, heavier than thousand pounds of gold." ... "Whenever a great physician treats diseases.....he should commit himself firmly to the willingness to take the effort to save every living creature." (Tai 2011:25). H.M.Sass put it this way: "a great physician has to combine expertise and ethics, professional knowledge and human compassion... he should not make difference between his patients and treat everyone fairly and just" (Sass 2007:383). When a physician sees a patient, what he sees in front of him should only be a person needing help without distinguishing between the white and the black, the rich and the poor, nor should there be a difference between the young and the old. Skin color, wealth, gender or social privilege should not stand on the way of treating the sick. Sass interpreted this way: " a great physician should not pay attention to status, wealth or age; neither should he question whether the particular person is attractive or unattractive, whether he is an enemy or friend, whether he is a Chinese or a foreigner, or finally, whether he is uneducated or educated. He should meet everyone on equal grounds. He should always act as if he were thinking of his close relatives" (Sass 2005:15).

The unfortunate situation of lacking medical resources may occur at times and bioethicist may be forced to adopt some consequential approach to choose who to live and who to die. But medical professionals must bear in mind that every life is worthy and weights the same and deserves to be treated in the best way they can. It is health professionals' duty to be well prepared to meet any kind of emergence. The survival of the fittest violates the sacred profession of health care. Facing the threat of COVID-19 pandemic, medical professional should uphold the dignity of humankind, follow ethical guidelines and guarantee everyone's access to medical assistance and respect her/his right to healing.

6. Be prepared – Taiwan as an example

Taiwan's remarkable experience in containing COVID-19 in 2020 proves that justice is not only about equality, it also calls for readiness to meet the challenge so that everyone can be treated fairly. The ethical dilemma happened in Italy never took place in Taiwan.

When the outbreak of COVID 19 first started in January, 2020, some experts predicted that Taiwan would have the highest number of cases outside of China because it sits only 180 kilometers away from the coast of China and also has frequent air flights between two countries with close commercial connection. While China has had over 80,000 COVID-19 cases to date, Taiwan has kept its number of confirmed cases just around 400 and only 7 death. Some international health experts credit this to Taiwan's quick preparation and early intervention.

Although Taiwan has high-quality universal health care, its success lies in its preparedness, speed, central command and rigorous contact tracing. Anticipating the high demand for masks in late January, the Taiwanese government right away purchased the manufactory machine to produce needed mask immediately. Taiwanese citizens can go to designated drug stores across the country to buy a specific number of masks on a weekly basis. (Dewan 2020) Ventilator, swap and hospital isolation ward/room …have never run insufficient.

H.M Sass prophetically stated: "global mobility causes spread of infectious diseases: we don't have to wait for terrorists, criminals or foreign countries to use biomedical devices for killing, terror or warfare, high mobility of people, made possible by integrated global travel and global networks of trade and commerce make the spreading infectious diseases easy and dangerous" (Sass 2007:389) and voiced for early precaution and preparation.

Be prepared, get ready to meet any challenge is the lesson Taiwan learned from the SASR epidemic in 2003 where Taiwan paid a heavy price. Now, they are ready. Justice is not only about equality and fairness, it is also about readiness and preparation to act quickly.

7. Conclusion

Medical principles remind us to be dutiful in serving the medical needs of the sick. All of these principles have something to do with attitude and awareness. But without being well prepared, good intention to serve is not enough. COVID 19 should teach all the world a new lesson that we must be prepared, be ready to meet the challenge of next wave of unexpected new contagious disease.

Many elderly patients have died because they never got the chance to have ventilator to help breathe at the critical time. Even if they received the respirator, some of them might still die but at least they were cared for equally, same as other younger patients. If we can learn the lesson, their death will not be in vain. Human society should be a community of love and mutual respect where every life is worthwhile to live and to save.

References

Anon. n.d. https://en.wikipedia.org/wiki/Survival_of_the_fittest

Baker 1979. Baker, Hugh D. R. (1979), Chinese Family and Kinship, New York, Columbia University Press

Beauchamp 1983. Beauchamp T, Childress J: Principles of Medical Ethics. New York, Oxford University Press, Second edition. 1983

Dewan 2020. By Angela Dewan, Henrik Petterson and Natalie Croker, CNN April 16, 2020--
https://www.cnn.com/2020/04/16/world/coronavirus-response-lessons-learned-int

Fung 1948. Fung YL: A Short History of Chinese Philosophy. New York, The Free Press1948

Gillon 1994. Gillon R: Medical ethics: four principles plus attention to scope in BMJ, 1994 Jul
16; 309(6948): 184–188. https://doi.org/10.1136/bmj.291.6490.266

Hastings 2020. Hastings Center News, COVID-19, Ethics, Health and Health Care, Public
Health. Published on: March 24, 2020

Jordan 1998. Jordan, D.K: Filial Piety in Taiwanese Popular Thought, in Slote, Walter H; Vos,
George A. De (eds.), Confucianism and the Family, SUNY Press,1998: 267-284

Legge 1971. Legge, James (trans.) Confucius: Confucian Analects, The Great Learning and The
Doctrine of the Mean. New York: Dover 1971 "Things being investigated, knowledge became complete. Their knowledge being complete, their thoughts were sincere. Their
thoughts being sincere, their hearts were then rectified. Their hearts being rectified, their
persons were cultivated. Their persons being cultivated, their families were regulated.
Their families being regulated, their States were rightly governed. Their States being
rightly governed, the whole kingdom was made tranquil and happy."

McGrath 2020. McGrath Ciaran: Italian hospital makes heartbreaking decision not to intubate
anyone over the age of 60: Friday, Mar 20, 2020,
https://www.express.co.uk/news/world/1257852/Italy-coronavirus-intubating-elderly

Mencius 1a.7

Parsons 1992. Parsons AH, Parsons PH: Health Care Ethics. Toronto, Wall & Emerson Inc.
1992

Portal n.d. The Medical Portal on Medical Ethics Explained : Justice
https://www.themedicportal.com/blog/medical-ethics-explained-justice Hasting

Sass 2005. Sass HM: "Emergency Management in Public Health Ethics: Triage, Epidemics,
Biomedical Terror and Warfare" *Eubios Journal of Asian and International Bioethics*.
2005

Sass 2007. Sass HM: Bioethics and Biopolitics. Sian, China: Fourth Military University of
Medicine Publishing Press 2007

Sass 2016. Sass HM: Cultures in Bioethics. Zurich Lit Verl.AG GmbH & Co. 2016

Tai 1997. Tai MC: Principles of medical Ethics and Confucius' Philosophy of Relationship in
Religious Studies and Theology, University of Saskatchewan, Canada, Vol 16, No.2, 1997.

Tai 2009. Tai MC: The Way of Asian Bioethics. Taipei: Princeton International Publishing Co.
2009

Tai 2011. Tai MC: An Asian Perspective of Western or Easter Principles in a Globalized Bioethics in Asian Bioethics Review March 2011, Vol 3.(1)

Tai 2019. Tai MC: Eubios Journal of Asian and International Bioethics 2019. Vol 29 (3):89-92

Veatch 2000. Veatch RM: The basics of Bioethics. Upper Saddle River, New Jersey, Prentice
Hall. 2000

Yim 1998. Yim, D: Psychocultural Features of Ancestor Worship, in Slote, Walter H.; Vos,
George A. De (eds.), Confucianism and the Family, SUNY Press, 1998:163-186

Michael Cheng-tek Tai, Ph.D., Chair professor of bioethics and medical humanities of the Institute of Medicine, Chungshan Medical Univeristy, Taichung, Taiwan. He earned his Ph.D. in Comparative Ethics from Concordia University in Montreal, Canada and had taught at Concordia University, Montreal, King College, Bristol, Tennessee and University of Saskatchewan, Saskatoon, Canada before his return to Taiwan in 1997. Since then he had served the dean of the College of Medical Humanities and Social Sciences and the chairman of the department of Social Medicine of the Chungshan Medical University. He was the president of International Society for Clinical Bioethics from 2006-2010 and served on the editorial board of the Journal of Medical Ethics (England), European Journal of Bioethics (Croatia), Medicine and Philosophy (China), Medical Education, Tzuchi Journal of Medicine (Taiwan) and the chief editor of Formosan Journal of Medical Humanities. He is a member of Medical Research Ethics Committee of Academia Sinica, IRB member of the National Chengchi University, Taipei, IRB member of Chungshan Medical University, Taichung and convener of the subcommittee on Education and International Relation of the Ethics Governance Committee of Taiwan National Biobank. He also sits on Medical Affairs Committee, Medical Ethics Committee and Biobank Research Committee of the Ministry of Health and Social Welfares, Taiwan. Among his monographs are *The Way of Asian Bioethics* (in English), *A Medical Ethics of Life and Death*, *The Foundation and Practice of Research Ethics*, *The Medical Humanities in the New Era* etc. and numerous scholarly papers around the world.

Responsibility and Ethics in Times of Corona

Martin Woesler, Hunan Normal University, Changsha, P. R. China

Abstract

How far can the self-responsibility of the individual (e.g. the policy in Sweden) master situations, in which mass compliance is required? Should fundamental rights be restricted? What responsibility should scientists have who encourage 'herd immunity' and populist leaders who deny the threat? Are authoritarian societies better prepared to fight the virus than liberal ones? Given the various ways COVID-19 can be transmitted due to the different national measures of precaution and prevention: Are "nations" the right category in a globalized world? Does the fight against a virus justify the rise of non-virus related deaths among patients, the unemployed, for instance? What consequences do triage, isolated dying, restrictions of contacts/religious practices and face masking have? Are they justified?

Key words

Legal responsibility, scientists, politicians, herd immunity, dictators, populists, Triage, deaths, International Criminal Court, masks

1. Normativity

Ethics are normative, they depend on basic assumptions and values (such as that human life is worth protecting), they are subjective (why shouldn't the life of e.g. bacteria be worth protecting instead), they depends on time, culture, region, values and beliefs. From a non-normative point of view, there is no reason why human life should be worth protecting (and not, for example, the life of many other living creatures whose lives are threatened by humans, such as bacteria on the meso-level). In this understanding, the cognitivism of meta-ethics is rejected, i.e. that it is always only about relative values (e.g. good or bad from a human perspective) and never about true or untrue. Let us therefore remain in normative ethics. From the basic assumption that human life is worthy of protection, assumptions can be derived, such as that biodiversity must be preserved to enable the survival of the human species. From this, in turn, it can be deduced that climate change must be mitigated, the environment protected and the economy made more sustainable.

There are also more weakened forms in which it is not about life, but about life worth living, about dignity, freedom and the satisfaction of needs with maxims such as that freedom finds its limits in the freedom of others.

However, there is no coercive logic for applied ethics, such as which measure would be preferable, especially since acting with ethical motives can have unethical consequences.

Now there are choices that, each with its own probability, can save a different number of lives. Classical questions are the "lesser of two evils" or whether a mass murderer should be killed (e.g. Hitler by assassination), when this might save a large number of people.

2. Ethics

From an ethical point of view, even the murder of the mass murderer would be reprehensible, among other things, because one does not know for sure whether the mass murderer would actually have killed more people if he was not murdered. However, negative utilitarian grounds are often cited when a dictator is assisinated. If one executes a mass murderer out of "revenge" or "atonement" for murders committed in the past, this is unethical at first, since it is neither clear whether the murderer would have continued to murder, nor whether the execution would have a deterrent effect on copycats. What appears ethically justifiable may be different from different perspectives. It is therefore to be argued at most with probabilities or one can seek for compromises, like to arrest a dictator to prevent him from doing further harm. However, the legal system also provides for punishment for injustice committed without this punishment being ethically justifiable. According to Foucault, in most regions of the world we have overcome the centralist disciplinary society and in most societies we find ourselves in decentralised control societies.

If one were to base one's actions purely mathematically on the number of human lives to be saved, then every person in developed countries like Germany, the USA etc. would have to take his or her money to save as many people as possible in Africa who are threatened by starvation. In practice, this would hardly be possible, as the national economies then might collapse and a redistribution and migration of peoples would take place, which in turn would result in hunger and suffering. Also it would rob the top performers of their means.

In practice, there are also decisions about which one of two lives is the preferred one to be saved. Here there are triage principles like in seafaring, that "women and children" go off the ship first and the captain last, a selective practice which is not endorsed by many constitutions (also not by the German Basic Law).

3. Ethical Decisions in Times of Corona

The Corona pandemic brings us a special situation: Where only limited medical capacities (intensive care beds, ventilators/respirators, qualified personnel) are available, a triage decision is made.

| 34.7 USA[1] (about 177,000 ventilators)[2] |
| 29.2 Germany (about 25,000 ventilators)[3] |
| 12.5 Italy |
| 11.6 France |
| 9.7 Spain |

Table 1: Number of intensive care beds per 100,000 inhabitants in 2017, selected countries, partly with number of ventilators.[4]

In fact, however, the triage decision only affects a comparatively small fraction of the infected people, as only about 15% become seriously ill and about 5% require artificial respiration (figures from practice, in which usually only persons with symptoms were tested, so that there is a high number of unreported cases of untested ill persons). In Germany, for example, such triage decisions probably did not occur, partly because of additional capacities. This is also a classic triage decision, which has led to a further deterioration in many clinical pictures and de facto to more deaths.

By far the biggest triage decision is made by politicians and experts with the lockdown. An early lockdown can keep the number of infected persons (and thus also the number of deaths) many times lower, the lesser evil in this case being deaths and suffering through job loss (in-

---

[1] https://www.sccm.org/Communications/Critical-Care-Statistics, visited March 29, 2020.

[2] *New York Times.* https://www.nytimes.com/2020/ 03/18/business/coronavirus-ventilator-shortage.html, visited March 29, 2020.

[3] *New York Times* 2020.

[4] Rhodes 2020.

cluding suicides), domestic violence, etc.

4. The Responsibility of Experts and Politicians

This paper looks at the triage decisions of the experts and politicians who are more or less responsible for hundreds of thousands of deaths by deciding on a lockdown.

The focus here is on those among the experts who, for example, have refused protection measures to the population on the argument of "full protection". They have accepted up to 5% expected deaths of their respective populations. Not even - and this comparison is misleading in many respects - doctors experimenting on population groups in the service of totalitarian regimes are responsible for such high death rates.

The motives of these experts are base: craving for recognition, irresponsible transfer of experiments from the computer or laboratory to the environment, etc. If in retrospect these experts want to justify themselves by saying that they thought about full protection but not about the deaths it would cost, this is unbelievable and the claimed fact is untrue.

Another focus is on those populists and dictators among the politicians who have abused their political power to deliberately and intentionally sacrifice hundreds of thousand lives of their compatriots. To prevent a lockdown or at least delay it until one's own re-election is in jeopardy, requires considerable criminal energy and coordinated effort. Not only did a narrative have to be found which, similar to warmongering, would lead the masses to their doom.

Their motives are also base: It was about retaining power and personal gain. However, once their actions are exposed, these goals are also called into question.

Ethics is certainly the supreme discipline of the sciences. Every other discipline must find out for itself where the limits of ethical and unethical actions are.

What is the question of quantitative rescue in times of Corona? Who are the decision-makers? What responsibility do they have?

Here it is striking that there are different mortality rates in different countries. Thus, political decisions have a direct influence on death rates. To what extent do the decision-makers actually bear responsibility for the dead who would not have died if they had made a different decision? Contrary to the avoidance effect (With this I mean the effect that effective vaccinations appear to be unnecessary in retrospect because the feared wave of disease has not materialized - but among other things because of the vaccination!), death rates can be read concretely. However, a moral judgement of the decisions presupposes that these decisions were made in an informed manner.

It is considered how informed the decisions were made. Right at the beginning of the epidemic it was difficult to estimate the reproductive factor of the virus and mortality. However, after a complete national course was observed in China, the reproductive factor was assumed with 3.

Virus/ Syndrome	Start	Cases	Deaths	Mortality	Countries
Ebola	1976	33,577	13,562	40.4%	9
Nipah	1998	513	398	77.6%	2
SARS	2002	8,096	774	9.6%	29
MERS	2012	2,494	858	34.4%	28
SARS-CoV-2*	2019	25,079,330	843,842	3.9%	188

*State: July 30, 2020. Figures: Johns Hopkins University.

Table 2: Comparison of different epidemics. Sources: CDC, WHO, New England Journal of Pathology. Status: MERS November 2019, Ebola January 24, 2020, quoted by *Business Insider*.

Even during earlier epidemics that were stopped without full protection (Ebola, bird flu, SARS etc.), similarly strong contact restrictions were actually imposed in the (albeit not global) region vulnerable to infection.

There are indeed a few epidemics where we are now protected by full protection of the population. For more than a century, however, this has never been achieved through intentional infection of the population with a disease, but rather through comprehensive vaccination (full protection for measles, mumps, rubella is achieved at a vaccination rate of about 95% according to the formula 1-(1/R)).[5]

Even during the Spanish flu of 1918-1920, when protective measures were complicated by the chaos of war, only about a quarter of the people in the world were infected.

So when SARS CoV-2 broke out in China, the outbreak was brought under control locally or regionally relatively quickly, for example by immediately suspending domestic flights and quarantining Wuhan.[6] Any conspiracy theory of a US soldier having brought the virus to China or the virus being artificially developed in a lab in Wuhan do not become true[7] even if repeated by populists and dictators for political reasons.

However, the Chinese government has made a decision that also deserves international investigation: for a certain period of time, it was no longer possible to fly from Wuhan domestically, but it was possible to fly to other countries. That means that infected people could fly abroad unhindered and in fact this was how the virus spread. This decision turned the epidemic into a pandemic.

Lauren Gardner from Johns Hopkins University provided an interactive map[8] as early as January 2020, which outlined the scenario of a US-wide and worldwide distribution.

In addition to observing the national outbreak in China, policy makers relied on the as-

---

[5] Robert Koch Institute „Nationales Referenzzentrum für Masern, Mumps, Röteln". https://www.rki. de/DE/Content/Infekt/NRZ/MMR/mmr_node.html, visited March 29, 2020.

[6] „Fallzahlen aus China. Jetzt 26 Tote durch Coronavirus". *Tagesschau* (January 24, 2020), visited July 30, 2020: https://www.tagesschau.de/ausland/corona-china-103.html.

[7] An accidental transmission either in the food market or the nearby lab seems more reasonable, since accidents with SARS infected bats were reported at the lab several times before 2020. However, the possibility of an individual terrorist attack even with such biological weapons becomes more likely in the future. See Sass 2020. Hans-Martin Sass. Health and Happiness of Political Bodies, Zürich: Lit Verlag 2020.

[8] https://coronavirus.jhu.edu/map.html. Further interactive maps: https://news.google.com/covid19/map, https://interaktiv.morgenpost.de/corona-virus-karte-infektionen-deutschland-weltweit/.

sessment of experts. Thus, the role of the experts must be considered first. In Germany, Christian Drosten, virologist at the Charité and chief virologist at the Robert Koch Institute, explained that even if the spread of COVID-19 were to be slowed down, "60-70% of Germans" would fall ill "anyway" with COVID-19 in the next "two years or even longer" until full protection was achieved.[9] He repeated this several times until April 2020 in the Grimme Prize-awarded "Corona-Updates" on public NDR broadcasting station. With a mortality rate of 3.94% for example, Drosten's words implied almost 2.2 million deaths. In fact, even with much more infectious and deadly diseases in human history, full protection often has not been achieved. In most cases, outbreaks remained regionally limited or, if they spread globally, the infection rate usually did not exceed 10% of the total population. This is also due to the fact that the reproduction factor, which for Corona is often given as R=3, only describes the unchecked spread that hardly occurs in practice, so it should be called R_{max}=3 or R≤3. Human fear alone, which instinctively keeps people at a distance, reduces this factor.

The following experts, to whom governments referred, have advocated the fastest possible spread, with the aim of achieving full protection, thereby risking millions of lives: Christian Drosten (Germany), Klaus Püschel (Germany),[10] Karin Mölling (Switzerland, March 14, 2020),[11] Anders Tegnell (Sweden), (Great Britain)[12], Jaap van Dissel (Netherlands, "The idea is: we want to allow the virus to spread in a controlled way among those who have little problem with it").[13] Anders Tegnell (June 4, 2020),[14] and Karin Mölling (March 24, 2020) admitted their mistakes.

A herd immunity/full protection was also propagated by virologists and politicians in Brazil.[15]

When the approval ratings of the following dictators and populists among the population dropped, thus endangering their re-election, the following ones rowed back: Donald Trump (wore a mask for the first time on July 11, 2020), Boris Johnson (on March 12, 2020 he set out to achieve herd immunity as quickly as possible, on March 15, 2020, after King's College published the expected high death figures, he rowed back).[16]

Dutch Prime Minister Mark Rutte, who on March 16, 2020 in a television address had called for herd immunity: "We can slow down the spread of the virus and at the same time build

---

[9] Ibid.

[10] Coroners on Corona: „Wir können Infektionen nicht verhindern". https://www.n-tv.de/wissen/Wir-koennen-Infektionen-nicht-verhindern-article21702978.html, n-tv Wissen, April 8, 2020.

[11] Radio program of rbb with statements by Professor Karin Mölling: https://www.radioeins.de/programm/sendungen/die_profis/archivierte_sendungen/beitraege/corona-virus-kein-killervirus.html.

[12] Gareth Davies. „What is herd immunity and will it stop coronavirus in the UK?" The Telegraph (March 21, 2020), visited July 30, 2020: https://www.telegraph.co.uk/news/2020/03/15/what-herd-immunity-mean-will-stop-coronavirus-uk/.

[13] Michael Hammerl. Herdenimmunität erreichen? Niederlande rudern zurück. Kurier (March 18, 2020), visited July 30, 2020: https://kurier.at/politik/ausland/herdenimmunitaet-erreichen-niederlande-rudern-zurueck/400785917.

[14] „Epidemiologe Anders Tegnell räumt Fehler bei Corona-Kurs ein". SWP (June 4, 2020), visited July 30, 2020: https://www.swp.de/panorama/corona-schweden-raeumt-fehler-ein-epidemiologe-anders-tegnell-virologe-46794203.html.

[15] Katherine Funke. Uns bleibt nur, auf die Impfung zu warten, Süddeutsche Zeitung (May 29, 2020), visited July 30, 2020: https://www.sueddeutsche.de/kultur/welt-im-fieber-brasilien-katherine-funke-serie-gastbeitrag-1.4923746.

[16] Sebastian Borger. Mit Herdenimmunität gegen das Coronavirus. Johnson verzichtet auf die harte Tour. Tagesspiegel (March 15, 2020), visited July 30, 2020: https://www.tagesspiegel.de/politik/mit-herdenimmunitaet-gegen-das-coronavirus-johnson-verzichtet-auf-die-harte-tour/25646150.html.

up a controlled group immunity", rowed back in parliament on March 18, 2020: His government did not aim for "group immunity" after all, he said in parliament. In the long term, however, it could be the consequence of the pandemic.[17]

At the beginning of the pandemic, when hardly any masks were available in Germany, the Robert Koch Institute had spoken out against masks on the grounds that they were almost ineffective. This was in line with the WHO's statement. When it became clear that they had been mistaken, the Robert Koch Institute continued to declare that it had not revised its assessment of masks. Nevertheless, homemade masks were suddenly recommended which "did not protect the wearer, but others". Indeed, each barrier protects both sides and special masks (FFP-2, FFP-3) also protect the wearer substantially, may even allow immunization.[18] Better would have been (as is quite naturally done in China) an indication that the dust protection masks with valve, worn in many places, allow unhindered exhalation and are therefore not suitable.[19]

In fact, the only true logic became known early on, namely that the curve must be flattened by taking hard measures as early as possible ("flatten the curve" movement), in order to avoid overloading the health system on the one hand and to survive the time until the vaccine would arrive with as few deaths as possible.[20]

Another strategy was to trivialize the situation. This included statements such as those made by Brazil's President Jair Bolsonaro that it was a "mild flu".[21] Bolsonaro himself ignored the opinions of his health minister and leading experts, and with statements such as "we all have to die sometime" he deliberately showed himself to be combative.[22]

The Brazilian president also recommended the ineffective drug chloroquine and hydrochloroquine, just like his counterpart Donald Trump.[23]

Recommendations such as that of the Belarusian autocrat Alexander Lukashenko to fight the virus with vodka were also playing down the danger.[24]

---

[17] Michael Hammerl. Herdenimmunität erreichen? Niederlande rudern zurück. Kurier (March 18, 2020), visited July 30, 2020: https://kurier.at/politik/ausland/herdenimmunitaet-erreichen-niederlande-rudern-zurueck/400785917.

[18] Gandhi, Monica, and George W. Rutherford. "Facial Masking for COVID-19 – Potential for 'Variolation' as We Await a Vaccine". *New England Journal of Medicine* (2020.9.8), https://www.nejm.org/doi/full/10.1056/NEJMp2026913

[19] Alexandra Leistner. "Warum Träger von FFP2/3-Masken mit Ventil eigentlich Egoisten sind". Euronews (June 8, 2020), visited July 30, 2020: https://de.euronews.com/2020/06/08/warum-trager-von-ffp2-3-masken-mit-ventil-eigentlich-egoisten-sind.

[20] Inga Barthels. "Entwicklung einer Pandemie. Eine Grafik zeigt, warum die Verlangsamung der Coronavirus-Epidemie so wichtig ist". Tagesspiegel (March 12, 2020), visited July 30, 2020: https://www.tagesspiegel.de/wissen/entwicklung-einer-pandemie-eine-grafik-zeigt-warum-die-verlangsamung-der-coronavirus-epidemie-so-wichtig-ist/25636718.html.

[21] Marian Blasberg, Jens Glüsing. "Das Virus seines Hasses" Spiegel (May 1, 2020), visited July 29, 2020: https://www.spiegel.de/politik/ausland/jair-bolsonaro-und-die-corona-krise-in-brasilien-das-virus-des-hasses-a-6bfeb692-4ed5-404d-acbc-2c49e2cc2429.

[22] Christoph Gurk. "Wir alle müssen irgendwann sterben" Süddeutsche Zeitung (March 30, 2020), visited July 30, 2020: https://www.sueddeutsche.de/politik/brasilien-wir-alle-muessen-irgendwann-sterben-1.4862370.

[23] Marian Blasberg, Jens Glüsing und Ralf Neukirch. "Umstrittenes Mittel gegen Corona in Brasilien und den USA. Kokain der Rechtsradikalen". Spiegel (25.05.2020), visited 30.07.2020, https://www.spiegel.de/politik/ausland/warum-sich-jair-bolsonaro-und-donald-trump-fuer-chloroquin-zur-coronabekaempfung-einsetzen-a-e3fefafd-5240-4d02-9826-785e0430f65b.

[24] "Lukaschenko empfiehlt Wodka und Traktor gegen Coronavirus", n-tv (17.05.2020), visited 30.07.2020 https://www.n-tv.de/der_tag/Lukaschenko-empfiehlt-Wodka-und-Traktor-gegen-Coronavirus-article21649790.html.

Tragic in this context is the demonstrative appearance of an Italian mayor in a café without a mask, stating he did not see the virus: He died of Corona a short time later. This is somewhat reminiscent of John Major's demonstration in front of running cameras when he ate a British beef steak during the BSE scandal. However, it is not known whether he subsequently contracted Kreutzfeld-Jakob disease.

Seemingly trivializing, but actually worsening and at least grossly negligent was Trump's advice to inject a disinfectant or cleaning agent.[25]

According to Bob Woodward, on January 28, National Security Adviser Robert O'Brien warned Trump: "This *will* be the biggest national security threat you face in *your presidency*."[26] Trump was very early well informed and well aware of the deathly danger. On February 7, 2020, he told Bob Woodward coronavirus was dangerous, highly contagious, airborne and "deadly." Trump went on to say that coronavirus was maybe five times "more deadly" than the flu. "This is more deadly. This is five per- you know, this is five percent versus one percent and less than one percent. You know? So, this is deadly stuff." Despite knowing better, he decided to play down the threat, as he told Bob Woodward on March 19, 2020: "I wanted to always play it down. […] I still like playing it down, because I don't want to create a panic."[27]

And Trump denied, belittled and played down the virus like no one else.[28] He railed vehemently against protective masks and strictly rejected a nationwide mask obligation. He also regularly expressed the desire to bring public life back up to speed. In recent months, the US president has been conspicuous for the way he downplayed the risks of the pandemic - only to emphasize just a few days later how bad the situation was. Here are a few quotes by Donald Trump:[29]

Jan. 22: On whether he was worried about a pandemic: "No, we're not at all. And we have it totally under control. It's one person coming in from China."

Jan. 24: "It will all work out well."

Jan. 29: "Just received a briefing on the Coronavirus in China from all of our GREAT agencies, who are also working closely with China. We will continue to monitor the ongoing developments. We have the best experts anywhere in the world, and they are on top of it 24/7!"

Jan. 30: "We think we have it very well under control. We have very little problem in this country at this moment — five. And those people are all recuperating successfully. But we're working very closely with China and other countries, and we think it's going to have a very good ending for it. So that I can assure you."

Feb. 2, eight cases; 0 deaths: "Well, we pretty much shut it down coming in from China. … We can't have thousands of people coming in who may have this problem, the coronavirus. So we're gonna see what happens, but we did shut it down, yes."

[25] Wulf Rohwedder. "Trump zu Corona-Maßnahmen Sommer, Sonne - und Spritzen?", Tagesschau Faktenfinder (April 24, 2020), visited July 30, 2020, https://www.tagesschau.de/faktenfinder/trump-corona-desinfektionsmittel-101.html.

[26] Robert Costa, Philipp Rucker. „Woodward Book" . *Washington Post*. (Sep 9, 2020, 11:55 am EDT). URL https://www.washingtonpost.com/politics/bob-woodward-rage-book-trump/2020/09/09/0368fe3c-efd2-11ea-b4bc-3a2098fc73d4_story.html.

[27] Mike Hayes, Meg Wagner and Veronica Rocha. Tapes of Trump's conversations released. CNN (Sep 9, 2020, 8:05 p.m. ET). URL https://edition.cnn.com/politics/live-news/trump-woodward-book-09-09-2020/h_5bb44945ec0cf0eba9cdd92ab28fde3c, visited on Sep 11, 2020..

[28] The following quotes have been listed in: Trumps Irrungen in der Corona-Krise „Das Virus wird keine Chance gegen uns haben", July 22, 2020, 21:16 Uhr, https://www.tagesspiegel.de/politik/trumps-irrungen-in-der-corona-krise-das-virus-wird-keine-chance-gegen-uns-haben/26026870.html.

[29] The following quotes were mostly collected by the *Washington Post* on March 12 and constantly updated on their website (the author of this chapter added a few from Trump's official Twitter account). Accessed on September 8: https://www.washingtonpost.com/politics/2020/03/12/trump-coronavirus-timeline/ cf. BBC: https://www.bbc.com/news/world-us-canada-52775216.

Feb. 7: "Nothing is easy, but [Chinese President Xi Jinping] … will be successful, especially as the weather starts to warm & the virus hopefully becomes weaker, and then gone."

Feb. 10: "I think the virus is going to be — it's going to be fine."

Feb. 14: "We have a very small number of people in the country, right now, with it. It's like around 12. Many of them are getting better. Some are fully recovered already. So we're in very good shape."

Feb. 19: "I think it's going to work out fine. I think when we get into April, in the warmer weather, that has a very negative effect on that and that type of a virus. So let's see what happens, but I think it's going to work out fine."

Feb. 24: "The Coronavirus is very much under control in the USA. … Stock Market starting to look very good to me!"

Feb. 25: "You may ask about the coronavirus, which is very well under control in our country. We have very few people with it, and the people that have it are … getting better. They're all getting better. … As far as what we're doing with the new virus, I think that we're doing a great job."

Feb. 25: "CDC and my Administration are doing a GREAT job of handling Coronavirus, including the very early closing of our borders to certain areas of the world."

Feb. 25: "I think that's a problem that's going to go away."

Feb. 26 - 15 cases; 0 deaths: "Because of all we've done, the risk to the American people remains very low. … When you have 15 people, and the 15 within a couple of days is going to be down to close to zero. That's a pretty good job we've done."

Feb. 26: Q: This is spreading — or is going to spread, maybe, within communities. That's the expectation.

A: It may. It may.

Q: Does that worry you?

A: No. ... No, because we're ready for it. It is what it is. We're ready for it. We're really prepared. ... We hope it doesn't spread. There's a chance that it won't spread too, and there's a chance that it will, and then it's a question of at what level.

Feb. 27: "Only a very small number in U.S., & China numbers look to be going down. All countries working well together!"

Feb. 27: "It's going to disappear. One day, it's like a miracle, it will disappear."

Feb. 28: "We are working on cures and we're getting some very good results."

Feb. 28: "I think it's really going well. We did something very fortunate: we closed up to certain areas of the world very, very early — far earlier than we were supposed to. I took a lot of heat for doing it. It turned out to be the right move, and we only have 15 people and they are getting better, and hopefully they're all better. There's one who is quite sick, but maybe he's gonna be fine. … We're prepared for the worst, but we think we're going to be very fortunate."

Feb. 28: "Now the Democrats are politicizing the coronavirus. ... And this is their new hoax."

Feb. 29: "We're the number one travel destination anywhere in the world, yet we have far fewer cases of the disease than even countries with much less travel or a much smaller population."

March 2: "On average, you lose from 26,000-70,000 or so and even some cases more from the flu. ... So far, we have six [coronavirus deaths] here."

March 4: "Some people will have this at a very light level and won't even go to a doctor or hospital, and they'll get better. There are many people like that."

March 5: "With approximately 100,000 CoronaVirus cases worldwide, and 3,280 deaths, the United States, because of quick action on closing our borders, has, as of now, only 129 cases (40 Americans brought in) and 11 deaths."

March 6: "We did an interview on Fox last night, a town hall. I think it was very good. And I said: 'Calm. You have to be calm. It'll go away.' "

March 7: "It came out of China, and we heard about it. And made a good move: We closed it down; we stopped it. Otherwise — the head of CDC said last night that you would have thousands of more problems if we didn't shut it down very early. That was a very early shutdown, which is something we got right."

March 7: "We're doing very well and we've done a fantastic job."

March 8: Retweets a story about Surgeon General Jerome Adams playing down the risk of coronavirus for Trump personally.

March 9: "The Fake News Media and their partner, the Democrat Party, is doing everything within its semi-considerable power (it used to be greater!) to inflame the CoronaVirus situation, far beyond what the facts would warrant. Surgeon General, 'The risk is low to the average American.' "

March 9: "So last year 37,000 Americans died from the common Flu. It averages between 27,000 and 70,000 per year. Nothing is shut down, life & the economy go on. At this moment there are 546 confirmed cases of CoronaVirus, with 22 deaths. Think about that!"

March 10: "As you know, it's about 600 cases, it's about 26 deaths, within our country. And had we not acted quickly, that number would have been substantially more."

March 10: "And it hit the world. And we're prepared, and we're doing a great job with it. And it will go away. Just stay calm. It will go away."

March 11 - 1100 cases; 0 deaths: "I think we're going to get through it very well."

March 12: "It's going to go away. ... The United States, because of what I did and what the administration did with China, we have 32 deaths at this point ... when you look at the kind of numbers that you're seeing coming out of other countries, it's pretty amazing when you think of it."

March 13: Says the Food and Drug Administration "will bring, additionally, 1.4 million tests on board next week and 5 million within a month. I doubt we'll need anywhere near that."

March 14: "We're using the full power of the federal government to defeat the virus, and that's what we've been doing." Also retweeted supporter Candace Owens, who cited "good news" on the coronavirus, including that "Italy is hit hard, experts say, because they have the oldest population in Europe (average age of those that have died is 81)."

March 15: "This is a very contagious virus. It's incredible. But it's something that we have tremendous control over."

March 16: "If you're talking about the virus, no, that's not under control for any place in the world. ... I was talking about what we're doing is under control, but I'm not talking about the virus."

March 17: "We're going to win. And I think we're going to win faster than people think — I hope."

March 23: "America will again and soon be open for business. ... Parts of our country are very lightly affected."

March 24 - 52,700 cases; 913 dead: "You're going to lose a number of people to the flu. But you're going to lose more people by putting a country into a massive recession or depression."

On seeking to reopen portions of the American economy by April 12: "It's such an important day for other reasons, but I'll make it an important day for this, too. ... I would love to have the country opened up and just raring to go by Easter."

March 25: "There are large sections of our country — probably can go back to work much sooner than other sections. ... It's hard not to be happy with the job we're doing, that I can tell you."

March 26: "They have to go back to work; our country has to go back. Our country is based on that, and I think it's going to happen pretty quickly."

March 29: "So you're talking about [worst-case scenarios of] 2.2 million deaths, 2.2 million people from this. And so if we could hold that down, as we're saying, to 100,000 — it's a horrible number, maybe even less — but to 100,000. So we have between 100 and 200,000, and we altogether have done a very good job."

March 30: "New York is really in trouble, but I think it's going to end up being fine. We're loading it up, we're stocking it up. ... And then by a little short of June, maybe June 1, we think the — you know, it's a terrible thing to say, but — we think the deaths will be at a very low number. It'll be brought down to a very low number from right now, from where it's getting to reach its peak."

March 30: "Stay calm, it will go away. You know it is going away."

March 31: "It's going to go away, hopefully at the end of the month and if not, it hopefully will be soon after that."

April 2: "Our states, generally speaking, it's like lots of different countries all over. We have -- many of those countries are doing a phenomenal job. They're really flat."

April 3: "The CDC is advising the use of nonmedical cloth face covering as an additional voluntary public health measure. So it's voluntary; you don't have to do it."

April 7: "It did -- it will go away."

April 8 - 423,100 cases; 18,100 dead: "I'd love to open with a big bang, a beautiful country, and just open."

April 9: "There are certain sections in the country that are in phenomenal shape already. Other sections are coming online; other sections are going down."

April 10: "Hard to believe that if you had 60,000 [deaths] -- you could never be happy, but that's a lot fewer than we were originally told and thinking."

April 22: "It may not come back at all [in the fall/winter]."

April 28: "This is going to go away. And whether it comes back in a modified form in the fall, we'll be able to handle it."

April 29: "It's going to go. It's going to leave. It's going to be gone. It's going to be eradicated."

May 5: "Will some people be affected? Yes. Will some people be affected badly? Yes. But we have to get our country open."

May 5: "With or without a vaccine, it's going to pass."

May 6: "This virus is going to disappear. It's a question of when."

May 8 - 1.3 million cases; 71,300 deaths: "This is going to go away without a vaccine."

May 11: "We have met the moment, and we have prevailed. ... We've prevailed on testing, is what I'm referring to."

May 14: "If we didn't do any testing, we would have very few cases."

May 15: "It'll go away — at some point, it'll go away."

May 19: "Many of these people aren't very sick, but they still go down as a case."

June 15: "Even without [widespread testing], you know, at some point this stuff goes away and it's going away. Our numbers are much lower now."

June 15: "If we stopped testing right now, we'd have very few cases, if any."

June 16: "I always say, even without it [a vaccine], it goes away."

June 17: "The numbers are very minuscule compared to what it was. It's dying out."

June 17: "It's going to fade away. But having a vaccine would be really nice. And that's going to happen."

June 18: "America is better supplied and more prepared to [reopen] than, I would say, just about any other place."

June 18: "It is dying out. The numbers are starting to get very good."

June 20 - 2.2 million cases; 113,500 dead: "Many call it a virus, which it is. Many call it a flu, what difference?"

June 21: "Our Coronavirus testing is so much greater (25 million tests) and so much more advanced, that it makes us look like we have more cases, especially proportionally, than other countries."

June 23: "You know, people get sick from the other also. It's not just from the virus. They get sick from all of the other things that happen. You know what I mean."

June 23: "Cases are going up in the U.S. because we are testing far more than any other country, and ever expanding. With smaller testing we would show fewer cases!"

June 25: "If we didn't want to test, or if we didn't test, we wouldn't have cases. But we have cases because we test."

June 25: "So when you do 30 million, you're going to have a kid with the sniffles, and they'll say it's coronavirus — whatever you want to call it. ... In some cases, it's people that didn't even know they were sick. Maybe they weren't. But it shows up in a test."

June 25: "Our Economy is roaring back and will NOT be shut down. 'Embers' or flare ups will be put out, as necessary!"

July 1: "I think we are going to be very good with the coronavirus. I think that, at some point, that's going to sort of just disappear, I hope."

July 2: "There is a rise in Coronavirus cases because our testing is so massive and so good, far bigger and better than any other country."

July 3 - 2.8 million cases; 123,200 deaths: "I think, and this is important, anyone who needs a test yesterday or needs one today gets a test. They are here, they have tests, and the tests are beautiful. Anyone who needs a test gets a test."

July 4: "By so [so much testing], we show cases — 99 percent of which are totally harmless — results that no other country can show because no other country has testing that we have, not in terms of the numbers or in terms of the quality."

July 5: "New China Virus Cases up (because of massive testing), deaths are down, 'low and steady'. The Fake News Media should report this and also, that new job numbers are setting records!"

July 6: "Deaths from the China Virus are down 39%, while our great testing program continues to lead the World, by FAR! Why isn't the Fake News reporting that Deaths are way down? It is only because they are, indeed, FAKE NEWS!"

July 9: "So we have tests; other countries don't do tests like we do. So we show cases; other countries don't show cases."

July 9: "We have cases all over the place. Most of those cases immediately get better. They get — people — they're young people. They have sniffles, and two days later, they are fine."

July 9 - 3.1 million cases; 126,700 deaths: "For the hundredth time, the reason we show so many Cases, compared to other countries that haven't done nearly as well as we have, is that our TESTING is much bigger and better. We have tested 40,000,000 people. If we did 20,000,000 instead, Cases would be half, etc. NOT REPORTED!"

July 14: "No other country tests like us. In fact, I could say it's working too much. It's working too well. We're doing testing and we're finding thousands and thousands of cases. If it's a young guy who's got sniffles, who's you know 10 years old, gets tested, all of a sudden he's a case and he's gonna be better tomorrow."

July 19: "It's going to disappear and I'll be right."

July 21: "It will disappear."

July 21: "You will never hear this on the Fake News concerning the China Virus, but by comparison to most other countries, who are suffering greatly, we are doing very well - and we have done things that few other countries could have done!"

July 22: "I say, 'It's going to disappear.' And they say, 'Oh, that's terrible.' ... Well, it's true. I mean, it's going to disappear."

July 31: "We have more Cases because we do more Testing. It's Lamestream Media Gold!"

Aug. 1: "If we tested less, there would be less cases."

Aug. 3: "It's under control as much as you can control it."

Aug. 3: "Cases up because of BIG Testing! Much of our Country is doing very well. Open the Schools!"

Aug. 5: "It will go away like things go away and my view is that schools should be open."

Aug. 5: "No question in my mind, it will go away."

Aug. 6: "So because we have the tests, we give them cases. Other countries that don't do this testing, they don't have cases."

Aug. 7: "It's going to disappear."

Aug. 10: "It's very interesting because we're so far ahead of testing, we have more cases. If we had much smaller testing, would have fewer, but we feel that having testing is a very important thing."

Aug. 11: "Many people get it and they have — like kids, they get it, they have the sniffles — young kids, almost none have a serious problem with it."

Aug. 12: "When you do as much testing as us, however, as you understand, you develop more cases."

Aug. 13: "It's going to be going away."

Aug. 17: "It's going away, but we're also going to have vaccines very soon."

Aug. 17: "The China plague will fade."

Aug. 24: "It's all coming back so fast that you'll see it, and the pandemic goes away. The vaccines are going to be, I believe, announced very soon."

Aug. 31: "Once you get to a certain number, you know, we use the word 'herd,' right? Once you get to a certain number, it's going to go away."

The tobacco industry, chemical industry, pharmaceutical industry and the automotive industry were all sentenced to high compensations for playing down risks.

Even if historical comparisons are (always) misleading, the role of experts, who are responsible for numerous deaths, must be critically reviewed in the future, as well as the role of doctors working in dictatorships, who are responsible for the loss of human life, for example.

What responsibility do political decision-makers generally bear? Do the victims of war also go on the accounts of these decision-makers? What is the situation with defensive wars? What national goals justify fighting "to the last man", "wanting total war", "not taking prisoners"? What goals justify taking up arms in the event of a warlike attack? Wouldn't the saving of human lives always be more important than the resistance associated with victims?

After the development of the epidemic in China was known, and the first cases occurred in Europe, later in the United States, South America and Africa, each state leader was responsible, due to the information situation, to immediately carry out a lockdown of about one month according to the Chinese model, with mask recommendation, distance rules, contact restrictions and especially no more large events in closed rooms.

Most countries in the world implemented these measures and survived the pandemic with a manageable number of infected and dead before the vaccine was expected to be available at the turn of 2020/2021.

Of course, there were also countries where, despite countermeasures, cramped accommodation led to a rapid spread; even in Germany, which survived the pandemic well, there were further local outbreaks in the meat processing industry with ventilation systems without sufficient fresh air supply. As predicted in my paper of the end of March 2020,[30] the worst spread took place in slums in South America, Africa and India.[31]

But there were also deliberately induced mass deaths: populists and dictators placed their hoped-for popularity and retention of power above the lives of their people and continued to base this existential decision on moods captured by the analytical instruments of social media. Accordingly, they unanimously claimed that the pandemic did not exist or was harmless, they claimed that the population had to infect themselves as quickly as possible in order to achieve full protection, they used their function as role models and appeared without a mask or social distancing. They mobilized followers, which led to a division of society into virus-warners and deniers, so that in case of conflicts, the masks of people who protected themselves were torn down. These populists and dictators argued with economic reasons. This narrative was dramatic in its consequence: there were numerous higher death figures than the global average (and even much higher than in countries where the lockdown was carried out early).

History will show how many deaths the populists and dictators are responsible for. This snapshot from July 29, 2020 may give a first insight:

Country/Region	Leader	In-fected him-self	Deaths	Deaths excee-ding global average	Deaths in promille / population	Mortality rate among infec-ted
World			660,593	0	0.0844961	3.94%
USA	Donald Trump	?	152,042	126,825	0.5094485	3.43%
Brazil	Jair Bolsonaro	Ja	88,792	72,900	0.47210125	3.57%
Russia off.*	Vladimir Putin	?	13,673	4,243	0.12251068	1.65%
Russia est.*	Vladimir Putin	?	32,662	23,232	0.29265479	3.94%
Belarus off.*	Alexander Lukaschenko	Ja	543	-258	0.05724829	0.81%
Belarus est.*	Alexander Lukaschenko	Ja	2,654	1,853	0.27983346	3.94%
Great Britain	Boris Johnson	Ja	45,961	40,840	0.75831722	15.21%
Sweden			5,730	4,866	0.5601173	7,18%

Table 3: To go over dead bodies for survey results. Dictators and populists and their blood toll.

*off./est.: The death figures officially reported by Russia and Belarus appear incorrect due to the resulting untypical

---

[30] Martin Woesler. "What we can learn from China – To stop the pandemic, not just to flatten the curve. And why not 70% of Germans will fall ill with Corona." *Bulletin of the German China Association*, Bochum (2020.3.29):17-27, online: http://universitypress.eu/de/9783865152862_002.pdf.

[31] Christian Wolf. „Corona in Schlachtbetrieben: ‚Deprimierende Zustände'". WDR.de (09.05.2020), visited July 30, 2020: https://www1.wdr.de/nachrichten/themen/coronavirus/corona-schlachtbetriebe-fleischindustrie-100.html.

lethality for the virus. Based on experience with officially reported figures and their erratic developments due to changes in the counting methods in countries with autocrats and populists, the official figures (off.) are compared here with a figure estimated (est.) by the author, which is based on the global average (3.94%) instead of the obviously embellished lethality rate (0.81% and 1.65% respectively).

Another way to count the death victims of a single person's vanity is to calculate how many deaths could have been avoided if the lockdown had come one or two weeks earlier. Since the death toll is still on the rise, this is again just a random snapshot as of September 11, 2020:

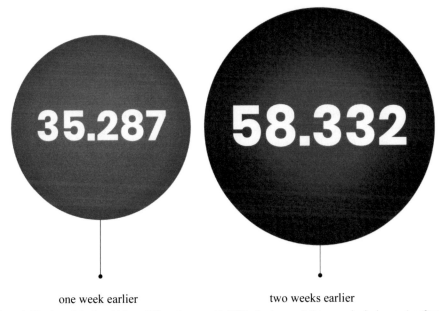

one week earlier two weeks earlier

Figure 1: Number of deaths which could have been avoided if the hygiene and distance rules had come 1 or 2 weeks earlier. Source: *Columbia University*. Published by *ThePioneer* and *statista*.

While war decisions are often based on a misconception that one is superior to the opponent (even if deaths were accepted and therefore any war decision is unethical), the populist measures of dictators and populists have been based solely on the interest of maintaining their personal power. Right at the beginning of the national outbreaks, it was clear that this political decision would lead to high death rates. At the latest after the first hundreds or thousands of deaths, this knowledge could no longer be denied. These deaths were therefore knowingly and unethically accepted. Whether or not this is a base motive and 1st degree murder only a court could judge.

Therefore, similar to war criminals, these populists and dictators must be brought before an international court. The number of US civilian victims of COVID-19 soon surpassed the number of US servicemen and women killed in Korea, Vietnam, Iraq and Afghanistan over an aggregate 44 years of fighting.[32]

---

[32] Cf. https://www.bbc.com/news/world-us-canada-52775216: Korean War (1950-1953): 36,500, Vietnam War (1961-1975): 58,000, Iraq War (2003-2011): 4,500, Afghanistan (2001-today): 2,000.

When Trump turned out to be a lying, divisive, polarizing president with racist, chauvinist, misogynistic views, who harasses and fires his staff, always looking for scapegoats and praising himself, his opponents could not have come up with a better scenario for the demise of this populist than that Trump, through wrong political decisions, could become personally responsible for hundreds of thousand civilian deaths at home. Now this scenario has come true and the approval ratings for Trump have dropped to 41.5% (cf. Biden: 49.5%, Source: realclearpolitics.com August 30, 2020) by August 30, 2020. Irrespective of whether this voter attitude continues until election day or whether Trump succeeds in jeopardizing the United States Post Service with the aim of voiding the postal vote or if he may stay in office on November 3, 2020 through voter manipulation via social media as he did in his election in 2016, the question of responsibility for and consequences of political action is asked in this paper.

It remains to be seen how the mass murder of civilians will be legally dealt with. One can expect complaints from individual relatives for failure to provide assistance, for example, to those who have lost their parent through COVID-19, and who may document, for example, missing hygiene measures (such as masks, disinfectants, rules on spacing and visits) a refused transfer from the old people's home to a hospital or similar.

Trump has clearly violated his Oath of Office: "I do solemnly swear that I will faithfully execute the Office of President of the United States, and will to the best of my Ability, preserve, protect and defend the Constitution of the United States." Trump added like all presidents since George Washington: "So help me God."

5. Using the means of justice to hold those responsible to account

The International Criminal Court in The Hague, which started operating in 2002, has also been targeting incumbent presidents since around 2012.

Here I quote from a newspaper description of the Court's Work:

"The court shall prosecute the most serious crimes such as genocide, crimes against humanity and war crimes. In doing so, it is to judge those primarily responsible if no prosecution takes place in the country where the crimes take place. But this is only so if the country in question has acceded to the Rome Statute, the founding document of the ICC, and is a member state. In most cases, the countries concerned themselves request that the investigations be opened. In other cases, such as the Western Sudanese crisis region of Darfur or Libya, the UN Security Council has referred the cases to the ICC."[33]

"The situation became really dramatic, however, after the charges were brought against six Kenyans who were initially held responsible for the murders, mutilations, rapes and expulsions following the controversial presidential election at the end of 2007. Three defendants remain: Uhuru Kenyatta, president of Kenya since March 2013, William Ruto, his vice-president, and Joshua arap Sang, who had worked for a hate radio and has been on trial with Ruto since September 2013, because both are accused of being responsible, among other things, for the fact that more than 100 Kikuyus were burned alive in a church in the Rift Valley. The victims were mostly women and children who had wanted to escape the violence and seek a "safe" place to live. The trial against Kenyatta has not yet been called after several planned opening dates, because the chief prosecutor has lost all relevant witnesses over the years. They have withdrawn their statements, have gone into hiding, and some may even have been murdered.

---

[33] Source: https://www.tagesspiegel.de/politik/internationaler-strafgerichtshof-moerder-und-praesidenten/10284198.html.

Kenya has threatened to withdraw from the ICC. The African Union is demanding that acting presidents be exempted from prosecution in the future."[34]

The case of Donald Trump is comparable: He too, through his untrue statements and hatred, including on Twitter, contributed to both COVID-19 deaths and race riots. In fact, the USA does not recognise the International Criminal Court. Nevertheless, the Court does investigate American citizens, for example, possible war crimes committed by soldiers and CIA agents in Afghanistan. The USA revoked Chief Prosecutor Bensouda's entry visa in 2019 and in June 2020 defended themselves against investigations into possible war crimes in Afghanistan. A charge against dictators for mass murder would be possible, even against populists like Trump for mass murder of US civilians and nationals of other countries in the USA would be legally possible, even if it was only of a symbolic nature. A sentence of imprisonment would in all probability not be enforceable, since Trump would not recognize the jurisdiction of the court and probably would not have to fear extradition when visiting one of the approximately 127 states that are members of the court (60% of all states).

6. Final Remarks

In the USA, there are already lawsuits with large compensation sums in the event of health damage, such as in the tobacco industry, the diesel and glyphosate scandals. In such cases, even responsible company managers receive prison sentences. This case involves a historically unprecedentedly high number of civilian victims. The president was able to escape an impeachment trial for him blackmailing the Ukrainian president and combining state office and election assistance, by his Republican majority in the Senate. However, an indictment of Donald Trump and other populist rulers and dictators, even after the end of their terms of office, for mass murder appears to be urgently necessary from the point of view of justice, regardless of the outcome, be that the possibility of imprisonment or the actual start of punishment.[35]

References

Anon. 2020a. „Epidemiologe Anders Tegnell räumt Fehler bei Corona-Kurs ein". SWP (04.06.2020), besucht am 30.07.2020: https://www.swp.de/panorama/corona-schweden-raeumt-fehler-ein-epidemiologe-anders-tegnell-virologe-46794203.html.

Anon. 2020b. „Trumps Irrungen in der Corona-Krise ‚Das Virus wird keine Chance gegen uns haben'" *Tagesspiegel* (22.07.2020) 21:16 Uhr, https://www.tagesspiegel.de/politik/trumps-irrungen-in-der-corona-krise-das-virus-wird-keine-chance-gegen-uns-haben/26026870.html.

Anon. 2020c. *Rechtsmediziner über Corona: „ Wir können Infektionen nicht verhindern".* https://www.n-tv.de/wissen/Wir-koennen-Infektionen-nicht-verhindern-article21702978.html, n-tv Wissen, 8. April 2020.

Anon. 2020d. https://www.sccm.org/Communications/Critical-Care-Statistics, besucht am 29.3.2020.

---

[34] Source: https://www.tagesspiegel.de/politik/internationaler-strafgerichtshof-moerder-und-praesidenten/10284198.html.

[35] "US-Tabakkonzern zu Milliarden-Schadensersatz verurteilt". Welt.de (July 20, 2014), visited July 30, 2020: https://www.welt.de/newsticker/news1/article130355478/US-Tabakkonzern-zu-Milliarden-Schadensersatz-verurteilt.html; Roland Nelles und Marc Pitzke: "Freispruch für Trump. Sechs Lehren aus dem Impeachment-Debakel." Spiegel (February 6, 2020), visited July 30, 2020: https://www.spiegel.de/politik/ausland/trump-impeachment-sechs-lehren-aus-dem-debakel-a-cfbde9a5-cc80-4a86-8808-18e7114b25d7.

Anon. 2020e. Interaktive Karten: https://coronavirus.jhu.edu/map.html,
    https://news.google.com/covid19/map, https://interaktiv.morgenpost.de/corona-virus-karte-
    infektionen-deutschland-weltweit/.

Anon. 2020f. "Fallzahlen aus China. Jetzt 26 Tote durch Coronavirus". Tagesschau
    (24.01.2020), visited 30.07.2020: https://www.tagesschau.de/ausland/corona-china-103.html.

Anon. 2020g. "Lukaschenko empfiehlt Wodka und Traktor gegen Coronavirus", n-tv
    (17.05.2020), visited 30.07.2020 https://www.n-tv.de/der_tag/Lukaschenko-empfiehlt-
    Wodka-und-Traktor-gegen-Coronavirus-article21649790.html.

Anon. 2020h. "US-Tabakkonzern zu Milliarden-Schadensersatz verurteilt". Welt.de
    (20.07.2014), visited 30.07.2020:
    https://www.welt.de/newsticker/news1/article130355478/US-Tabakkonzern-zu-Milliarden-
    Schadensersatz-verurteilt.html.

Barthels 2020. Barthels, Inga. "Entwicklung einer Pandemie. Eine Grafik zeigt, warum die Ver-
    langsamung der Coronavirus-Epidemie so wichtig ist". Tagesspiegel (12.03.2020), visited
    30.07.2020: https://www.tagesspiegel.de/wissen/entwicklung-einer-pandemie-eine-grafik-
    zeigt-warum-die-verlangsamung-der-coronavirus-epidemie-so-wichtig-ist/25636718.html.

Blasberg et al. 2020a. Blasberg, Marian und Jens Glüsing. "Das Virus seines Hasses" Spiegel
    (01.05.2020), visited 29.7.2020: https://www.spiegel.de/politik/ausland/jair-bolsonaro-und-
    die-corona-krise-in-brasilien-das-virus-des-hasses-a-6bfeb692-4ed5-404d-acbc-
    2c49e2cc2429.

Blasberg et al. 2020b. Blasberg, Marian, Jens Glüsing und Ralf Neukirch. "Umstrittenes Mittel
    gegen Corona in Brasilien und den USA. Kokain der Rechtsradikalen". Spiegel (25.05.2020),
    visited 30.07.2020, https://www.spiegel.de/politik/ausland/warum-sich-jair-bolsonaro-und-
    donald-trump-fuer-chloroquin-zur-coronabekaempfung-einsetzen-a-e3fefafd-5240-4d02-
    9826-785e0430f65b.

Borger 2020. Borger, Sebastian. „Mit Herdenimmunität gegen das Coronavirus. Johnson ver-
    zichtet auf die harte Tour" Tagesspiegel (15.03.2020), besucht am 30.07.2020:
    https://www.tagesspiegel.de/politik/mit-herdenimmunitaet-gegen-das-coronavirus-johnson-
    verzichtet-auf-die-harte-tour/25646150.html.

Davies 2020. Davies, Gareth. „What is herd immunity and will it stop coronavirus in the UK?"
    The Telegraph (21.03.2020), online besucht 30.07.2020:
    https://www.telegraph.co.uk/news/2020/03/15/what-herd-immunity-mean-will-stop-
    coronavirus-uk/

Funke 2020. Funke, Katherine. „Uns bleibt nur, auf die Impfung zu warten" Süddeutsche Zei-
    tung (29.05.2020), besucht am 30.07.2020: https://www.sueddeutsche.de/kultur/welt-im-
    fieber-brasilien-katherine-funke-serie-gastbeitrag-1.4923746.

Gurk 2020. Gurk, Christoph. "Wir alle müssen irgendwann sterben" Süddeutsche Zeitung
    (30.03.2020), visited 30.07.2020: https://www.sueddeutsche.de/politik/brasilien-wir-alle-
    muessen-irgendwann-sterben-1.4862370.

Hammerl 2020. Hammerl, Michael. „Herdenimmunität erreichen? Niederlande rudern zurück".
    Kurier (18.03.2020), online besucht 30.07.2020:
    https://kurier.at/politik/ausland/herdenimmunitaet-erreichen-niederlande-rudern-
    zurueck/400785917.

Leistner 2020. Leistner, Alexandra. "Warum Träger von FFP2/3-Masken mit Ventil eigentlich

Egoisten sind". *Euronews* (08.06.2020), visited 30.07.2020: https://de.euronews.com/2020/06/08/warum-trager-von-ffp2-3-masken-mit-ventil-eigentlich-egoisten-sind.

Nelles et al. 2020. Nelles, Roland und Marc Pitzke. "Freispruch für Trump. Sechs Lehren aus dem Impeachment-Debakel." *Spiegel* (06.02.2020), visited 30.07.2020: https://www.spiegel.de/politik/ausland/trump-impeachment-sechs-lehren-aus-dem-debakel-a-cfbde9a5-cc80-4a86-8808-18e7114b25d7.

New York Times 2020. https://www.nytimes.com/2020/03/18/business/coronavirus-ventilator-shortage.html, besucht am 29.3.2020, im Folgenden: *New York Times* 2020.

rbb 2020. Radioprogramm des rbb mit Aussagen von Prof. Dr. Karin Mölling: https://www.radioeins.de/programm/sendungen/die_profis/archivierte_sendungen/beitraege/corona-virus-kein-killervirus.html.

Robert Koch-Institut 2020. „Nationales Referenz-zentrum für Masern, Mumps, Röteln". https://www.rki.de/DE/Content/Infekt/NRZ/MMR/mmr_node.html, besucht am 29.3.2020.

Rohwedder 2020. Rohwedder, Wulf. "Trump zu Corona-Maßnahmen Sommer, Sonne - und Spritzen?", Tagesschau Faktenfinder (24.04.2020), visited 30.07.2020, https://www.tagesschau.de/faktenfinder/trump-corona-desinfektionsmittel-101.html.

Sass 2020. Hans-Martin Sass. Health and Happiness of Political Bodies, Zürich: Lit Verlag 2020.

Wolf 2020. Wolf, Christian. „Corona in Schlachtbetrieben: ‚Deprimierende Zustände'". *WDR.de* (09.05.2020), visited 30.07.2020: https://www1.wdr.de/nachrichten/themen/coronavirus/corona-schlachtbetriebe-fleischindustrie-100.html.

Appendix: Table with full figures as basis for table 3 above.

Country/ Region	Leader	Infec- ted himself	Deaths	Num- ber of deaths excee- ding global average	Deaths pro- mille/ popu- lation	Population	Infected	Morta- lity rate among infec- ted
World			660,593	0	0.0844961	7,818,029,847	16,810,315	3.94%
USA	Donald Trump	?	152,042	126,825	0.5094485	298,444,300	4,461,216	3.43%
Brazil	Jair Bolsonaro	Yes	88,792	72,900	0.47210125	188,078,300	2,498,668	3.57%
Russia off.*	Vladimir Putin	?	13,673	4,243	0.12251068	111,606,600	828,990	1.65%
Russia est.*	Vladimir Putin	?	32,662	23,232	0.29265479	111,606,600	828,990	3.94%
Belarus off.*	Alexander Lukaschenko	Yes	543	-258	0.05724829	9,485,000	67,366	0.81%
Belarus est.*	Alexander Lukaschenko	Yes	2,654	1,853	0.27983346	9,485,000	67,366	3.94%
Great Britain	Boris Johnson	Yes	45,961	40,840	0.75831722	60,609,200	301,455	15.21%
Sweden			5,730	4,866	0.5601173	10,230,000	79,782	7.18%

Martin Woesler is a Chinese Studies scholar, born in 1969. He is a member of the European Academy of Sciences and Arts (Salzburg), Professor of Literature and Communication in China (Witten/Herdecke University), Xiaoxiang Scholar Distinguished Professor of Chinese Studies, Comparative Literature and Translation Studies (Hunan Normal University) and in 2020, he is appointed Jean Monnet Chair Professor. He is President of the World Association of Chinese Studies and the German China Society. His research focuses on Chinese literature, cultural comparison and social transformation processes, especially digitization, in China, including in comparison to Germany, Europe and the USA. He has received wide attention with his paper "Learning from China: Stopping the epidemic, not just slowing it down. And why 70% of Germans will not fall ill with COVID-19". *Bulletin of the German China Society* (2020.3.30)17-27, online: http://universitypress.eu/de/9783865152862_002.pdf.

Normality "ex post":
social conditions of moral responsibility

Carmen Kaminsky, Cologne University of Applied Sciences, Germany

Abstract

In countries that successfully "flattened the curve", people now rightfully demand restoration of their rights to self-determination. Nevertheless, the pandemic is not over yet and we cannot simply go back to an "ex ante" way of living. A new normality "ex post" will at least demand individual actors to keep responsible space to others. We are, hence, held to stress the moral responsibility that belongs to our fundamental understanding of individual self-determination. However, if we demand self-determined individuals to act morally, we collectively have to strive for conditions that enable them to do so. What do we collectively have to change, if we want to enable individuals to realize their interests responsibly?

Key words

COVID-19; social impacts; exit strategies; moral responsibility; distance keeping

Introduction

Merely half a year ago most Europeans hadn't thought that social life could change that quickly. Relying on the stability of the social structures we live in, we were rather making plans for spring and summer; some planning to celebrate their wedding with all their beloved ones in May, others looking forward to travelling abroad and yet others anticipating their businesses to overcome the doldrums of wintertime. Whatever the individual prospects and plans were in January 2020, they were abruptly thwarted by restrictive measures that followed the public health threat posed by the Corona-virus.

To a surprisingly comprehensive extent the German public confirmed the quickly launched new rules, putting up with all the disappointments, troubles, sorrows and distress that this caused individually. Be it for reasons of personal fear or thorough insight into collective necessity, the individual willingness to refrain from the safeguards of accustomed interactive practices, proved unprecedented. Admittedly there are more complex linkages to the individual motivation that finally led to the success the stout-hearted political decisions and restrictive measures achieved, namely the "flattening of the curve". It must not be overseen, though, that the majority of individuals accepted to temporarily waive their personal interests for the benefits of the common good, i.e. public health and public health service. The German Chancellor Angela Merkel therefore rightfully and repeatedly marked this as a noble gesture.

Now, as in Germany the curve is flattened and public health service is acutely not at stake anymore, the public is getting increasingly impatient. While still wearing masks and still keeping appropriate distance to others, many people demand to immediately abrogate the state of emergency and to restore the living conditions they were used to before the pandemic. "Let's go back to normal" is the slogan that fits this demand. Anyhow, the pandemic is not over yet and, hence, the demand to furthermore restrict the "ex ante" practices and force people to continue to conform with new rules, is just as strongly expressed. Especially those who worry about getting infected and sick demand patience and protection.

Yet, no matter how the rapidly developed „new normality" may personally be judged, it's permeating, extremely negative effects on all interconnected dimensions of social life provides reason enough to refrain from lock-down measures as soon as possible.

Political decision-makers are therefore under pressure to quickly design change and develop respective strategies for a normality "ex post" the state of emergency. The challenge is yet sophisticated, one of the first critical endeavors being the determination and moral justification of aims and milestones in the regulatory process. In this context the most recent German discourse prevails consensus on the foremost aim to prevent the risk of a backdrop. However, as the German Ethics Council pointed out, any measures to reach this aim are subject to thorough justification:

„Against this backdrop, the question arises as to how long the measures to slow the course of the pandemic and, more particularly, the ones designed to reduce physical contact, are justified. The justification of these lockdown measures necessitates an extremely complex balancing of goods under conditions of uncertainty from their introduction and throughout their entire duration." (German Ethics Council 2000:4 f)

Nevertheless, whatever goods need to be balanced in the further process, it should not be overseen that the most effective means to prevent a "second wave", is and remains to have people keeping a reasonable physical distance to each other. *The responsible and moral behavior of individuals thus becomes the crucial aspect of the next regulatory steps to be taken.* Therefore, any withdrawal or prolongation of restrictive measurements is firstly to be related to the individuals' own capacities to, in terms of close proximity to others, realize appropriate precautious and protective decisions. As we are commonly dependent on the individual actor's decisions and our mutual considerateness, we have to make sure not to overstrain given capacities. In preparing for a normality "ex post" we are thus held to turn towards conditions that impede or else foster reasonable physical distance to be kept while participating in social life. In how far can we rely on the individual actors' responsibility and how can we avoid overstraining conditions?

In this paper I am concerned with social conditions of the responsible individual actor's decision-making in terms of physical contact to others. In particular I am concerned with potential overstrains that occur in the interrelation between individual decisions and respective social practices. In the following, at first, three different, yet interconnected overstraining aspects will be outlined. At this point beforehand, it can be stated that we are to concede that in explicable respects we indeed overstrain individuals, if – again in terms of keeping reasonable physical to others – we demand them to act precautious and protectively. On this ground it is not only justified but demanded to take further regulative action. However, as will be argued in the second paragraph, respective regulations should not follow a rather epidemiologically founded taxonomic strategy, but rather a socially integrative strategy that is founded in the demands of a liberal, democratic society. The third paragraph, eventually, comprises tentative propositions to direct policy making in striving for a normality "ex post".

I. Personal Space in Social Interaction

When critically considering the individual actors' intention to act responsible and morally in regard to keeping physical distance to others, we have to take a closer look at the factual social surroundings in that respective acts are to be realized. While actors might be willing and personally competent to perform precautious and protectively, they may still be hindered to perform appropriately. Due to customized structures of social interaction actors can in some cases, for reasons that they cannot fully overlook, regularly fail to realize their intentions. It is these cases that potentially overstrain the individual actors' capacity to manage the risk to infect or be infected with COVID-19.

Communication and nonverbal understanding

As a matter of fact the *physical space we personally keep to others is not subject to our own, solely individual decision-making.* Rather it is the result of more or less outspoken mutual negotiation and mediation. In terms of inches we intend to keep to others, we are thus dependent on the other's vigilant awareness and willingness to peacefully bargain, balance and respect each individual's according needs.

The general necessity and procedural complexity of these trials is not easy to assess; it was however humorously brought to the point by no other than Arthur Schopenhauer. In §396 of his Parerga and Paralipomena[1] Schopenhauer presents a fable, telling about the awkward state of affairs in a society of porcupines. Being naturally endowed with spikes and yet being essentially vulnerable, the porcupines perennially have to negotiate the closeness and distance to be kept, to provide each other the needed warmth without injuring or getting injured.

Doubtlessly our human social interactions generally parallel with the fable's society of porcupines: Neither can we overcome the interrelation of demands and threats of intimacy nor can we once and for all determine the length of appropriate space. In fact, mutual negotiations of getting close and staying away are situationally inevitable to meet our individual needs in social interaction. The fact that COVID-19 has rapidly let grown the "spikes" of a yet unknown number of individuals, does not at all facilitate respective mutual negotiations. To the contrary, the currently quite distinctly emerging claim for mutual considerateness touches sore points of often incompetent, sometimes even reckless, in any case inappropriate social behavior. The limited individual actors' opportunities to situationally engage successfully in respective negotiations was, for instance, made subject to discussion in the "me-too"-debate. It is however not only the others' refusal to negotiate that limits the individual actors' successful precautious and protective performance.

In addition we have to consider the fact that in human social interaction we do not only negotiate *about* the physical distance we want and have to keep to others, but also communicate *with* the physical distance we keep. In keeping a certain space between each other, we nonverbally communicate e.g. our relational attitudes, feelings, expectations, intentions and social positions. *Thus, the physical distance we maintain in social interactions, clearly is itself a communicative act.* Although usually unconsciously performed, it is packed with contents we need to interpret correctly to gain a stable foundation for our more abstract, verbal communications and relating cooperative interests. When the non-verbal communication fails, because the other physically gets too close or stays too far away, we feel discomfort and are far too much concerned to engage in an openminded conversation.

To avoid such discomfort, irritation and failure of communication, we are thus prompted to take a closer look on the meaning that keeping a certain physical distance has in human interaction. Social cooperation does not only rely on more or less meticulously worded conversation, but also on mutual comprehension of the meanings contained in habitually shown nonverbal, i.e. physical expressions. The fact that during the "emergency-state" most people were willing to refrain from such habits showed what efforts it takes to fulfil daily routines without relying on customized physical expressions. Obviously people took the efforts and coped. This fortunate

---

[1] "A number of porcupines huddled together for warmth on a cold day in winter; but, as they began to prick one another with their quills, they were obliged to disperse. However the cold drove them together again, when just the same thing happened. At last, after many turns of huddling and dispersing, they discovered that they would be best off by remaining at a little distance from one another. In the same way the need of society drives the human porcupines together, only to be mutually repelled by the many prickly and disagreeable qualities of their nature. The moderate distance which they at last discover to be the only tolerable condition of intercourse, is the code of politeness and fine manners; and those who transgress it are roughly told—in the English phrase—to keep their distance. By this arrangement the mutual need of warmth is only very moderately satisfied; but then people do not get pricked. A man who has some heat in himself prefers to remain outside, where he will neither prick other people nor get pricked himself." (Arthur Schopenhauer 1881: § 396)

experience should, however, not mislead our anticipations of the mid- and long-term future.

We should rather take into account that framing "state of emergency"-narratives and not least the prospect of the measures to be limited in time, contributed a lot to the interactive discipline we luckily experienced. In particular we shouldn't overlook that the disciplined behaviors were burdened with a leap of faith in the stability of relations habitually expressed and maintained by nonverbal signs, e.g. gestures and physical closeness. Wherever such faith proved unfounded, for instance in communication with little children or people, who for reasons of cognitive limitation did not have access to understand the framings of behavioral change, emotionally devastating situations occurred.

Although at this point further considerable empirical aspects cannot be discussed[2], it should be noted that by situationally realizing a certain space to others, individuals – more or less consciously – make use of well-established, meaningful nonverbal signs. To demand of individuals making a minimum distance of 60 inch their new default, thus compares to demanding of them to speak without knowing the meanings of words. In this respect we must acknowledge that with suggesting and even demanding from individuals to keep more space to others, we strongly interfere in – and most probably harm – customary practices and behavioral patterns that are extremely important for peaceful and successful social interactions.

Taking into account the *structural importance of established nonverbal communication*, the expectation that individuals could and would without further ado confirm to keep the suggested distance to others, thus seems a kind of window dressing. As single persons can in their social interactions not individually decide on the distance they keep to others, their reasonable and responsible performance remains highly dependent on their situational agreements with others. And the less the contractual parties can rely on the validity of the non-verbal subtext established in the sphere they are negotiating in, the more conversation is needed to situationally avoid harsh conflicts and even the destruction of bearing relationships.

Self-exclusion from social life

Provided that it is true for actors that in the given state of social communication they cannot rely on their untroubled performance of precautious and protective distance keeping, at least some will be prone to rather withdraw from social encounters. Indeed it is at least consistent with the precautious intentions of those, whose "skin thinned" as well as with the protective intentions of those, whose "spikes grew" due to the pandemic, to stay at home and avoid mixing with the inconsiderate crowd. At least, for both groups it is reasonable to stay clear of situations in that they could be harmed or harm others. However, again we have to consider and question the factual opportunities to act accordingly.

Let alone at this point that most actors don't even know about their infectious position, we

---

[2] With his 1966 published work (Hall (1966): The Hidden Dimension) Hall founded the interdisciplinary research area of Proxemic that empirically investigates and describes signals that individuals exchange by taking a certain position in physical space. Proxemic has since become an established field of research in Psychology as well as in Communication studies. - It is especially owed to Edward T. Halls works that we could learn more about the basic structures and mutually accepted patterns of the non-verbal "language" our social interaction relies on. According to his findings and by now rather commonly known is that by the physical distance we keep, we define, mark out and respect the intimate, personal, private, social and public spheres of interaction. Depending on our cultural upbringing, gender and social status, there are empirically verifiable and in terms of inches measurable differences in the distance we expect and claim to be respected. Within our community we nevertheless all rely on the sturdy signals of spheres in that we intend to interact. Any deviation from the communities' defaults of distance keeping thus leads to at least embarrassing, more often irritating and sometimes painful communicative and eventually cooperative failure.

must acknowledge that individuals can, for diverse reasons, in fact not refrain from physical interactions. Depending on the respective actors' surrounding social conditions – including living conditions such as dwellings, housemates, reliability of supply, professional life – the individual is dependent on physical contact to others. Withdrawal from physical social interaction might therefore result in existential risks that are to be balanced with the risks of imposing or being imposed to risks of a COVID-19 infection. As a matter of fact, in worst cases they even by far outweigh the risks of COVID-19.

It is thus to be conceded at this point that for some individual actors voluntary self-quarantine or reluctant participation in social encounters is indeed a reasonable means to realize their precautious and protective intentions. On the other hand, depending on their concrete living conditions, many individuals are factually overstrained to proceed accordingly. Without reliable, vigorous support to compensate the harms combined to their terminated exclusion, they will factually not be able to realize their considerate intentions.

Structurally forced misconduct

Social life consists of people getting together to participate, co-operate, and, at times, to just enjoy their mutual presence. Of course, for functional necessity and sometimes for more dispensable reasons, getting physically close is therewith combined. Nevertheless, togetherness and especially physical closeness is not always wanted and yet not always avoidable. As a matter of fact, while taking part in social life individuals do not always have the opportunity to voluntarily decide on their physical closeness to others. Even though they might at times want to prevent close proximity, they will still find themselves in situations that inevitably thwart their plans. For many physical closeness to others is, for instance, a condition of their dwellings, for others an inevitable part of their profession and yet others unexpectedly end up in jam-packed public transport or stodged places. Lock-down measures highlighted respective structures and settings.

Hence, no matter how factually preconditioned, inevitable or unexpected situations of non-voluntary closeness to others may be, we have to acknowledge that they structurally undermine the individuals' responsible decisions. It is by conditions of social life that individuals fail to realize precautious and protective acts. They might even be structurally forced to misconduct.

In this respect we have to be aware that concerning non-voluntary close proximity, individuals adopt relevantly different positions. For example do service-givers take a quite different position from service-takers. While the former e.g. are constantly dependent on close proximity to their customers the latter in most cases can chose as to when and to whom they want to get close. And furthermore generally, the opportunity to avoid non-voluntary physical closeness is, as is known, dependent on decent income. Poor income does thus not only correlate with health-related inequalities but also with inequalities in chances to act responsibly and morally. The currently often mentioned phrase of us "all sitting in one boat" serves thus untrue when it comes to the individual's chance to manage personal corona risks.

To summarize in short: reflecting on the individual actors' opportunities to – in terms of physical distance to others – practically execute precautious and protective intentions, revealed massive obstacles. Overcoming such obstacles does for namable reasons obviously not lie in the hands of individual actors. As a matter of fact we are thus to concede that taking back restrictive measures and therewith leave precautious and protective actions to individual decisions, does indeed overstrain individual actors. We therefore cannot renounce the task to, with legitimate power of policy making, intervene in existing structures of social life. On this assessment, however, the question arises, what strategic concept could and should guide policy making and therewith our common normality "ex post".

II. Taxonomic vs. integrative strategies of policy-making

Taking into account that due to the pandemic's dynamic – to stick with the metaphor – the individual's spikes grew in different, as yet individually unknown lengths, we might consider to guide our regulations by flanking taxonomic concepts. One promising approach obviously being the idea to differentiate according to the threat potentials and vulnerabilities individuals have to manage in social interactions. Intensified testing and respective classification of individuals (into groups according to their relative risk and threat potential), currently thus seems to provide strategies worth considering (see e.g. Gertner; quoted by Milano 2020).

The considerable idea behind this being to identify a hopefully rapidly growing number of people who can, without any further normative attention, get close to each other, because their immunity status provides them – to again stick with the metaphor – with a "thicker skin". At the same time, so the presumed taxonomic concept, paying special normative attention to those, whose skin due to corona thinned down and those whose spikes evidently grew strongly.

It is however obvious, that testing and classifying the population into groups does not at all provide us from difficult decisions and their painful effects (see Romero quoted by Friedersdorf 2020). To the contrary, it may well be, that by realizing the concept, we may evoke new and even stronger unjust inequities.

"Given the uncertainty around the scientific facts concerning immunity as well as the reliability of serology tests, careful consideration must be given to the ethical issues underlying decisions to issue immunity passports. In addition to potentially prolonging the spread of COVID-19, it may be that, in our efforts to benefit society and our economies, we create yet another type of inequity. This could arise from the limited availability of tests, which disadvantaged people, who are most in need of work, may not be able to access, especially if they have no one to advocate for them. (Xafis et al. 2020)

Let alone at this point the indicated problematic side-effects of the taxonomic concept, the concept itself must be questioned as a guiding scope for policy-making. At first and overall the concept is to be criticized for its narrowed foundation in epidemiological thinking. However understandable it is in this time, to lapse into epidemiological categories, we have to acknowledge that, given the emergency-state of public health service is overcome, policy making is by constitution foremost bound to other values than public health. The policy-making perspective decisively has to take a point of view that stresses the needed social cohesion of a population. Seen from this point of view, policy making is prompted to design regulations that serve an unobstructed, well-functioning *integrative* concept of social participation. To deliberately distinguish and therewith separate and exclude groups of people from the commonalities of (physical) social interactions does, in fact, serve as counteract to democratic societies' *quest for integrative and inclusive structures of participation.* Following the taxonomic strategy thus completely misses the key problem to be solved by policy-making.[3] Thus, not at all ignoring, but rather acknowledging the immunological differences of individual states, public policy-making in the context of deliberative democracy is summoned and urged to not only design acceptable living conditions but also, with equal importance, participative chances for *all*. The foremost task be-

---

[3] It is to be stressed at this point, that exclusion strategies that might be appropriate for epidemiological endeavors and emergencies must to an extend generally be ruled out for policy making. As we learned from most atrocious practices in history, policy-making must not be guided by the idea of in- and out-grouping individuals from the community.

ing that individuals independent from their respective immunological state, may freely and safely take part in social life.

To meet this participative aim we are held to generally confess uncertainty in regard to the other's vulnerability and infectious state.[4] Nonetheless, given that in cases certain immunological states of individuals are known, we still have to deal with the as yet unsolved problem arising. It does consist in finding practical ways to integrate and stay close to those whose skin thinned as well as to those whose spikes might have grown a lot. *The key question for policy-making therefore is, how we must and are allowed to change our interactive commonalities, if we want them to suit for the participation of all members of our community.* Therewith combined is the foremost task, to guide and enable individual actors to realize their precautious and protective intentions in their mutual physical encounters.

As an intermediate result it can at this point be concluded that in regard to mid- and long-term governance of the pandemic, there is no alternative as to address the conditions that support or demotivate and even defeat the individuals' responsible social interaction in all its situational spheres. Instead of concentrating on the immunological status of individuals, our attention should therefore be drawn to the communicative situations in that persons are to negotiate and manage their (immunological) diversity and corresponding needs.

III. Designing social interaction "ex post"

Regarding mid- and long-term perspectives, we want for everybody (not only some) to freely and safely take part in the whole range of social interactions (not only some) that do include physical encounters with others. With only acceptable risk-taking and risk-posing it must in predictable time be possible for everyone to meet family and friends, go to work, go shopping, take part in or attend cultural events, go clubbing, engage in organizations, travel or else, to make a long list short, to participate in all the joys and burdens that social life involves.

To meet this aim, the crucial task for policy-making is to appropriately design the communicative surroundings in which reasonable and responsible individual acts can be realized. The appropriateness of respective regulations albeit underlying the demands of an *integrative concept* that needs to suit individuals most irrespective of their immunological state. In this regard it may at this point be more than a marginal note to indicate that this demand is not to be spared, once a vaccine is developed. Although the whole world is desperately waiting for a vaccine rapidly to be developed and although we are obliged to have vaccination available to anyone who wants it, we for constitutional reasons prima facie still mustn't force nor, with the threat of exclusion, press individuals to be vaccinated.

Pursuing this line of thought, however, leads to the question, as to what aspects of social life are more precisely to be looked at and how they can and should be addressed by policy-making.

To gain a first approach it is worthwhile turning towards the obstacles and conditions that in the beginning were identified to defeat individual actors' chances to realize their precautious and protective intentions. On this ground it can tentatively be proposed that policy-making should concentrate on three different aspects:

---

[4] This is not to say that testing and knowing about the populations and one's own individual infection-state is irrelevant. To the contrary, governments, collective bodies as well as individuals do have a crucial interest and right to know about the distribution of health-related threats. And as we can presuppose that individuals' neither want to harm nor want to be harmed by others, they need access to their personal infectious state.

(1) Supporting understanding and negotiation competences in public communication

Subject to studied confirmation it must be assumed that the less we commonly insist in physical distance being kept, the more individuals will lapse back to their "ex ante" established practices. This expectable relapse into personal habits and their respective conventional patterns, is not, at least not only, due to the individuals' erroneous assessment of the persisting corona risks. It seems to be more likely that problematic behavioral relapses occur for other very simple, pragmatic and psychological reasons.[5] Especially in situations of crowdedness, "ex ante" behavior tends to become default practice again. To avoid this trend and therewith to avoid once more increasing infections and to eventually having to reset restrictive measures, suitable efforts should be undertaken. For this it seems worthwhile to thoroughly investigate the communicative factors that contributed to the disciplined common acceptance of "keep distance"-recommendations during the "emergency-state".

As, for instance, the impact of framings on social communication is beyond doubt (see Ekman Reese et al.: 2020), the particular words and narratives, that framed the "emergency-state" should be payed particular attention. First analytic remarks (see: eurolanguage 2020) on the wordings that were e.g. used to translate "lockdown" to the German public, reveal that in the broader public the used words fostered the common perception of measures being rightfully undertaken and clearly terminated. On this perceptive basis they eventually contributed to the mutual understanding and acceptance of demanded distance-keeping.

As the "emergency-state" fortunately is over, the framings[6] that constituted current "new normality", however, cannot prepare for normality "ex post". To found and stabilize an appropriate normality for the mid- and long-term perspective, it will therefore be important to find and use new wordings and narratives that support the integrative aims to be met in the normality "ex post". In social communications such framings must suffice to offer opportunities to individually claim and correspondingly ease the willingness to keep physical distance. It seems obvious that such wordings and narratives should definitely not to be founded in codes of anxiety and fear but rather – as Schopenhauer had already recommended for the society of porcupines – in codes of politeness and fine manners.[7]

---

[5] So it was, for instance, most recently reported of German flight passengers, who initially strictly followed the new normality's rules until their plane landed and, to fetch luggage from the overhead-compartments, the whole crowd didn't care for appropriate distance to be kept anymore. However, in judging individual behavior, we have to regard, that, firstly, there are just no alternatives available that with equal common comprehensibility could replace gestures and other meaningful distance related patterns of physical expressions. More than that, secondly, people seem to goad each other into behaviors that are oblivious to all else in the moment, including the pandemic risks. (Television program „Hart aber fair" (ARD, June 15th 2020). The report referring to the first tourists going to Mallorca/Spain after the pandemic lock-down measures.)

[6] „Framing essentially involves *selection* and *salience*. To frame is to *select some aspects of a perceived reality and make them more salient in a communicating text, in such a way as to promote a particular problem definition, causal interpretation, moral evaluation, and/or treatment recommendation* for the item described. (...) Frames, then, *define problems* – determine what a causal agent is doing with what costs and benefits, usually measured in terms of common cultural values; *diagnose causes* – identify the forces creating the problem; *make moral judgments* – evaluate causal agents and their effects; and *suggest remedies* – offer and justify treatments for the problems and predict their likely effects." (Entman 1993:52)

[7] In this respect preparations for a normality "ex post" should additionally include suggestions to replace "ex ante" habitually practiced gestures with others that under the given conditions proof appropriate. To collectively watch models presenting patterns of alternative gestures can help to define a normality "ex post" and obviously, a good deal of humor can help to commonly cope with the upcoming changes. So it is as yet neither watched nor done without a certain comic effect, when German Foreign Minister Heiko Maas in recent case instead of shaking hands, softly knocked elbows with his Israeli interlocutor, Gabi Ashkenasi. The mutually performed gesture worked well

All in all the importance of measures that support and guide social communication in the common transfer to a normality "ex post" should not be underestimated. It doubtlessly lies in a liberal society's common interest, to initiate and fund respective initiatives and projects. In other respects more official regulations are desirable.

(2) Implementing norms and establishing assistive services

To enable individual actors to fully realize their precautious and protective intentions, supporting official regulations and the establishment of assistive services, proves highly desirable. As discussed above, in regular cases individual actors are overstrained to meet the challenges combined with foreseeable side-effects of their prospective precautious and protective acts. Such overstrains burden not only, but particularly those, who for their known infectious state, reasonably want to temporarily relinquish their physical participation. Not only do they have to fear about their regular income and job security. They also need to organize being supplied for their daily needs and services and furthermore, not least, need to organize temporary replacement in all the manifold social obligations they usually fulfil. In striving to act responsible and morally, actors are thus highly dependent on a well-functioning supportive social surrounding.

Without further ado it is, however, not to assume for actors, to regularly dispose of accordingly competent and reliable contacts. Experiences in the "new normality" rather suggest that the less actors can rely on the supportive functionality of their personal social surrounding, the less they will be able to manage the challenges imposed by side-effects of their intended actions. Eventually, so must be presumed, actors will rather waive their precautious and protective plans.

Consequences that follow from the individual actors' overstrain in regard to management of side-effects of their precautious and protective intentions must, however, in any case not simply be accepted. To the contrary. Primarily out of respect for the actor's autonomy, and furthermore for reasons social cohesion and mutual dependency, we are collectively compelled to ease and support the individual's ability to manage burdening side-effects of her moral actions. In the given pandemic situation tangible interests to reduce infectious risks, add to the concept.

To enable successful management and therewith foster responsible and moral self-determined actions, the regulatory implementation of suitable supportive means is thus of enhanced common interest.

In this context official regulations should address two different aspects. On the one hand regulations should be designed to *reduce the scope of challenging side-effects*. In this respect suitable regulations will presumably mainly consist of individual rights of claims. For instance legal entitlements to financial support, security of workplace and income. On the other hand regulations should provide *support for the individuals practical management*. These regulations will basically consist in the implementation of institutionalized assistive services, e.g. services for child-care and further services that can temporarily surrogate the individual's social engagement.

(3) Changing structural settings

Last but not at all least, for reasons of justice, and even more in regard to civil liberties, policy makers are compelled to take a closer look at settings that undermine or substantially reduce the individual's chances to responsible and moral decision-making. Being aware of the differences in personal risks, the challenge consist in critically restructuring certain settings of interaction in social life. Admittedly, the challenge is not easy to be met. It is yet unclear what

---

to show that their diplomatic negotiations had gone peacefully. And yet both commented their new gestural performance with an amused smiling.

settings and what structures are to be addressed and how, i.e. by what means and to what ends they should be restructured. Obviously, due to the complexities of social life and it's manifold settings of encounters, there are no sweeping answers. Hence, we have to take effort and proceed systematically.

Roughly speaking the necessary approach must consist of a 3-step proceeding.

- The *first* step consisting in *analyzing* and differentiating social encounters according to their constituent potential for (too) close proximity.

In this step a differentiated view on critical social encounters is to be achieved. Whereby critical encounters are to be understood as social settings that do not without waiving participation allow individuals to perform their precautious and protective acts, i.e. to realize their responsible and moral intentions. Presumably in this step attention is drawn for instance to conditioned closeness (i.e. in dwellings), created closeness in crowds (i.e. intentional jam-packing), functional closeness (i.e. in person-related services) and further relevant situations.

- The *second* step requires respective *evaluation* in regard to the individual's chances to predict and to avoid being exposed to social encounters that do not allow precautious and protective acts. The manifold social events that by their organizers on purpose are designed to be jam-packed might serve as an example at this point. And the professional person-related services – ranging from child-care, hair-dressing, assistance, taxi-driving to medical services – might serve as yet another.

Where thorough evaluations reveal settings that individuals cannot escape without self-exclusion from common practices of social life, the next step should be commenced.

- This *third* and crucial step is concerned with the *change* of settings that in the analytic and evaluative process proved problematic.

Change in this context means to identify, design and implement strategies that result in preventing individuals from unavoidably being exposed to risks or inevitably pressed to impose risks to others while participating in common practices of social life.

Depending on the particular case, considerable strategies might require not more than measures to make people line up instead of having them in a throng. In other cases digital options, e.g. Apps that inform about the crowdedness of places, might be worth considering. In many cases, however, it will turn out that suitable strategies will strongly affect customized social practices and especially those that constitute economic security of many.

Thus, in striving for a normality "ex post" we must be aware that what is at stake, is not only important foundations of public communication and therewith individual opportunities to realize responsible acts. The functionality of as yet sustainable businesses, even economic branches and respective social practices is at stake, too. For this reason, all in all the challenge is to find balance in keeping social life in function and at the same time expand and broaden participative opportunities for those whose "spikes have grown" as well as those whose "skin thinned". Predictably, however, this challenge will result in tough controversies and even conflicts, when it comes to decisions about what measures to implement. Whatever strategies will be suitable in the particular case, is, of course, subject to conscientious studies, transparent communication, public discourse and not least the willingness and stout-hearted use of legitimate power to indeed induce change of critical settings.

From a moral point of view it is nevertheless to be stressed that the maintenance of businesses and customized practices can hardly outweigh the values, represented by the society's fundamental promotion of the individual's responsible and moral participation. Owed to our constitution the right to participative self-determination weighs heavier than the security of particular businesses and their practices. It is thus to consent the assessment that George Annas had years ago put in words:

„Sacrificing human rights under the rubric of national security is almost always unnecessary and counterproductive in a free society." (Annas 2007:1093)

Concluding remarks

In liberal societies the functioning of social life is and remains highly dependent on the individuals' responsible and moral self-determination. In the end it is the individuals' decisiveness to follow their own interests with considerate precautious and protective intentions that maintains trouble-free, well-functioning interactions, social cohesion and finally the functioning of social-life.

On the other side, the individuals' limited options and opportunities to proceed correspondingly, became more than obvious in dealing with the corona-pandemic. It became clear that no matter how willing and decided individual actors may be, to keep reasonable physical distance to others, the conditions under which they are acting, in many respects regularly thwart their plans. This, of course, must not be simply accepted as a matter of fact.

We are collectively compelled to take the critical detections as an occasion and thoroughly scrutinize the conditions under which we expect individuals to strive for self-fulfillment in a responsible and moral way. Our aim must be to eliminate any obstacles to mutual respect and considerateness in social life. Accomplishing the aim clearly requires a sophisticated and far-sighted willingness to change conditions correspondingly and therewith constitute a social normality "ex post". To master this admittedly difficult task, the liberal societies' constitution provides the compulsory and reliably guiding basis. A normality "ex post" should offer safe and sound participation for all and demand of any participating person – to close with Schopenhauer's words – to follow the "code of politeness and fine manners".

References

Annas, George J. (2007): Your liberty or your life. Talking Point on public health versus civil liberties, EMBO reports VOL 8 | NO 12 | 2007, p. 1093-1098.

Entman, Robert M. (1993): Framing: Toward clarification of a fractured paradigm. Journal of Communication; 43, 4; p.51-58.

Eurolanguage (2020): Sprachkulturelle Vielfalt in Zeiten von Corona – wie sprechen wir über Corona? Blog, 04.05.2020, URL: https://www.eurolanguage-translations.com/wie-sprechen-wir-ueber-corona/ (accessed 16.06.2020)

Friedersdorf, Conor (2020): How to Protect Civil Liberties in a Pandemic. There are much bigger worries than temporary stay-at-home orders. The Atlantic, 24 April 2020; URL: https://www.theatlantic.com/ideas/archive/2020/04/civil-libertarians-coronavirus/610624/ (accessed June 5th 2020)

German Ethics Council (2020): Solidarity and Responsibility during the Corona Virus Crisis. Ad Hoc Recommendation. Berlin (published 27.03.2020)

Milano, Brett (2020): Restricting civil liberties amid COVID-19 pandemic. Harvard Law School faculty Charles Fried and Nancy Gertner discuss new restrictions on individual freedoms. The Harvard Gazette, March 25th 2020; URL: https://news.harvard.edu/gazette/story/2020/03/new-restrictions-on-civil-liberties-during-coronavirus/ (accessed June 5th 2020)

Reese, Stephen D.; Gandy, Oscar H. Jr.; Grant, August E. (eds.) (2001): Framing Public Life. Perspectives on Media and Our Understanding of the Social World. Mahwah, NJ: Lawrence Erlbaum Assoc.

Schopenhauer, Arthur (1851/1986): Sämtliche Werke in fünf Bänden: Band V: Parerga und Paralipomena II. Frankfurt am Main: Suhrkamp, § 396. (english translation: anonymous)

Xafis ,Vicki; Schaefer, G. Owen; Labude, Markus K.; Zhu, Yuji; Hsu, Li Yan (2020): The Perfect Moral Storm: Diverse Ethical Considerations in the COVID-19 Pandemic, Singapore: National University of Singapore and Springer Nature Singapore (online 28 May 2020)

Carmen Kaminsky, PhD, is full professor for Practical Philosophy at the Faculty for Applied Social Studies at Cologne University of Applied Sciences and private lecturer at Heinrich-Heine-University-Duesseldorf, both in Germany. Her research areas of focus concern central issues of applied ethics. She published on diverse topics of medical-ethics, public health-ethics, media-ethics and ethics of social work. Her most recent works issue ethical questions of digital technologies. – carmen.kaminsky@th-koeln.de.

Ethics Approaches
in Dealing with the Corona Pandemic

Mathias Schüz, Zurich University of Applied Sciences, Switzerland

Abstract

In times of crisis, ethical leadership is necessary. This can be seen in decisions that reflect the three basic ethical approaches in dialogue with all those affected and take into account all available expert knowledge, resources and capabilities to the best of our knowledge and belief. An ethical manager should be credible and trustworthy towards his followers through virtues such as fairness, honesty and be a role model for them. He should also be critical of himself with regard to prejudices and biases against the facts as presented by various experts. He should admit his mistakes and be willing to correct them. They should be more concerned with the common good than with their own, i.e. have an altruistic attitude. Under time pressure, the three test questions mentioned above can at least give them a rough idea of the ethical content of their planned decisions. Consider (1) the reciprocity test, which asks about fairness for all affected persons, respect (2) the daylight test, which asks about the public acceptance of a decision, and conduct (3) the empathy test, which implies a role reversal of the decision maker with those of the affected persons.

Key words

Ethical Leadership

Introduction

The COVID 19 pandemic has turned the world economy upside down. Millions of people - like countless day labourers in India - lost their jobs and thus their livelihoods with the close-down ordered by political leaders. Countless companies worldwide have already had to file for bankruptcy. The survival of millions of small and medium-sized companies, but also of large corporations, is at stake. Their survival can hardly be secured with tried and tested patterns of leadership.

Irreversible consequences have already occurred with the worldwide spread of the pandemic. The disruptions in the interplay between supply and demand along global supply chains are particularly far-reaching. Examples of this are the gastronomy, the aviation industry and global tourism. The cruise ship industry alone employed more than one million people worldwide, who contributed to a global added value of $ 150 billion annually (CLIA, 2019). With the closure of the cruise industry they have lost most of their jobs. In view of the threat of infection by the corona virus and the necessary protective measures, it will hardly be possible to provide services that cover costs. However, the forced lock-down in industries such as these may also have the positive side-effect of a break in recovery for the massive disturbances to the balance of nature.

The global crisis of the COVID-19 pandemic forced and still forces rapid decisions and accordingly challenges leaders in politics and business. In view of the unprecedented health and economic consequences, they had to rethink their decision-making processes - more or less consciously - also from an ethical point of view. Particularly in exceptional times of crisis, it has always been clear that many years of experience and tried and tested guidelines are hardly sufficient to protect the population, companies and organisations from the negative consequences in a responsible manner. Ethical responsibility is therefore particularly in demand in politics and business. This article would like to outline some basic principles in this regard.

Does ethics now offer decision-makers in politics and business guidance to solve the global problem of the pandemic? To what extent can it contribute to responsible action in crises such as the one currently triggered by the COVID-19 pandemic? The article shows that two different approaches to ethics compete for the sovereignty of interpretation, namely in the polar comparison of *ethics of utility* and *ethics of duty*. The current crisis makes it abundantly clear that there is a risk of ethics in such a definition of the approaches. Only the dialectical abolition of the supposed opposites via the third typical approach of ethics, the *ethics of virtue*, breaks up the rigid fronts.

The three approaches then prove to be *complementary*. As in the separation of powers in democratic political systems, they ensure that no one gets out of hand. Instead, they open up new spaces for creative solutions to difficult problems. However, the degrees of freedom gained have their price: responsible action can no longer claim to be absolute. It is proving to be an *art* whose form of expression must prove itself and face competing solutions.

The contribution is structured as follows: First, the conflict potential of different perceptions and interests to which decision makers are exposed is analysed. In the second step, a theory of ethical responsibility is presented as well as the complementary approaches of ethics associated with it. In the third step, the model will then be applied to the problems associated with the pandemic in order to identify patterns of solution. In the fourth step, recommendations for ethical leadership will be summerized.

1. Decision makers in conflict with different perceptions and interests

To cope with the COVID-19 pandemic, the responsible politicians in each country are challenged to make decisions on how to best protect the population from the risks involved. It is the hour of health ministers who listened to the advice of experts in epidemiology and virology to influence government decisions. These in turn are also based on the influence of ministers of the interior, foreign affairs, finance and economics. Each of them represents different interests, such as public security, community of states, economy. In order to make the right decision, i.e. to choose the right means to achieve the desired goal of overcoming the pandemic, different interests and the values behind them must be taken into account.

As Max Weber has already stated, "the unintended versus the intended consequences" of a decision must be weighed up. The question is "what will it *cost to* achieve the intended purpose in the form of a likely violation of *other* values? (Weber, 1968, p. 5, transl. by the author) This makes it clear that every decision makes a selection from a bundle of different possibilities, and thus blocks a number of paths:

Bringing a "weighing up to a decision is ... *no* longer a possible task of science [and its experts], but of the willing human being [here: the politician]: he weighs and chooses according to his own conscience and his personal world view between the values in question. Science can help him to become *aware that all* action, and of course, depending on the circumstances, *non-action*, means in its consequences *taking sides in* favour of certain values, and thus - something that is so often misunderstood today - regularly *against others*. (Weber, 1968, p. 5, transl. by the author; cf. Schüz, 1999, p. 36 f)

Hence, the politicians must shoulder the responsibility for their decisions. The advising (scientific) experts, who, as Weber makes clear, are themselves constantly bringing their "personal world views" to the field of empirical science, are never able to teach what they should, but what they can and, at best, want to do within the bounds of possibility. (Weber, 1968, p. 6)

This early insight by Weber has deepened in the sociology of science. As Ulrich Beck points out: "The unambiguousness of scientific [expert] statements has given way to the insight into their decision making, method dependence, context dependence." (Beck, 1991, p. 141, transl. by the author) In times of crisis, responsible politicians cannot alone rely on the findings of the supposedly exact sciences. In their tunnel vision, they may well grasp important connections, but at the same time they fade out others. Therefore, the responsible politician will never be able to rely on them completely.

2. A theory of ethical responsibility

This clarifies the framework within which responsible decisions can be taken. As Georg Picht (1969, p. 323) has already pointed out, responsible action means that an acting subject has to answer *for* the *consequences of* his actions towards *authorities*. Depending on the answer to the question "What have you done?" or "What are you doing now?" or "What do you plan to do?", the respective authority will make its judgement. Responsibility in this sense is thus a "three-digit predicate" (Nida-Rümlin, 2011, p. 23) or a "three-digit relation" (Zimmerli, 2014, p. 22) between the acting subject S, the consequences C and authority A. Accordingly, a politician, *for* example, has to answer *to the* various interest groups, for example his voters, *for* the consequences of his decisions. It can be represented as follows:

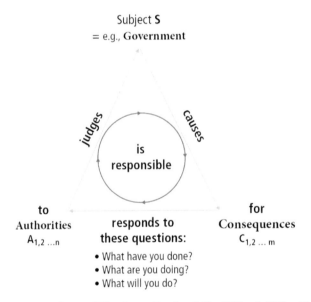

Figure 1: The three-digit relation of responsibility. Source: Based on Schüz, 2012, p. 9; 2019, p. 56.

No matter what decision a government makes in the event of a pandemic, it will trigger a multitude of intended and unintended consequences and will have to answer for them before a multitude of different interest-groups. The consequences of a close-down of public life are manifold. The side effects, repercussions and remote effects are hardly manageable. On the one hand, it protects against infection with the virus, and on the other it forces many commercial enterprises to cease their activities - with consequences that in some cases cannot be ignored. Depending on the interests of these groups, the consequences will be assessed differently, even controversially. Some will welcome a close-down of the economy, while others will criticise it.

The acting subject can only be held responsible for what he or she could decide independently and freely. Responsible action thus presupposes a certain degree of freedom. There is only room for manoeuvre where alternatives open up. There are almost always possibilities to act in this or another way. Where this scope is no longer given, the behaviour is determined.

The scope for responsible action is limited or opened up by the respective *situation*, the available *resources* and the *abilities* or *degrees of freedom of* the actors. For example, the close-down of public life can be relaxed if the reproduction rate R of the virus is less than 1. Otherwise it should rather be maintained. If sufficient financial resources are available, commercial enterprises can be kept alive more easily with bridging money. And the intellectual capacity and flexibility of the decision-makers allows for a more differentiated consideration of the different values of the interest groups. The latter should therefore be an important competence of a leader in politics and business, so that they can exercise their position responsibly. However, limited resources can also restrict the degree of freedom, for example if there are strong dependencies on powerful interest groups and they consider certain measures to be unacceptable.

Viewed holistically, every responsibility refers beyond the fulfilment of a function, compliance with laws or consideration of interest groups. Since every action, as the physicist and philosopher Heinz v. Foerster once expressed it, has consequences that interact with the universe, it is also subject to "universal responsibility" (Picht, 1969, p. 338; cf. Schüz, 2019, p. 65):

"When I ask myself 'Am I part of the universe?' and answer 'Yes, I am!', I decide here that whenever I act, not only I change, but the universe changes as well. Something, it's not just me that changes, but the universe, too. . . . This position [. . .] ties my actions inseparably to my responsibility" (Foerster, 1991, p. 66)

It is obvious that the finite consciousness of man will never be able to overlook the causal networks that his actions trigger in the whole. Nevertheless, he should be aware of his entanglement with the universe and at the same time give up any fantasies of omnipotence. The ideal can never be achieved. Nevertheless, the striving for it should never be abandoned. The idea of universal responsibility is at the same time the call to achieve the best possible results in cooperation with all other responsible persons. The recourse to insights of ethics is indispensable in this context.

3. Complementary ethical approaches as a basis for decision-making

According to which standards should the decision makers now make their choices? Ethics has a special role to play here. For it ensures that all those affected by a decision get along well (cf. Schüz 1999:156). In connection with responsibility, it must answer three questions: (1) What consequences do I want to strive for in order to get along well with as many affected persons as possible? (2) What duties should I respect in order to ensure a good livelihood with all those affected? (3) What capabilities should I develop to get along well with as many people as possible? In short: What do I want, what should I do and what can I contribute? These questions are of great importance for the ethical management of the Corona crisis. They refer to the three different approaches of ethics: the ethics of utility (utilitarian ethics), duty (deontological ethics) and virtue (aretological ethics).

According to the principle of "greatest good of the greatest number", the *utility ethics* examines the consequences of a decision or action, whether it causes more benefit than harm for the majority of those affected. It is not concerned with maximizing self-interest, as is often said of business life, but at least with fair bartering relationships with all stakeholders along the entire value chain. Political decisions such as the close-down ordered to contain the COVID-19 pandemic should also be based on fair relations with as many affected parties as possible. If, for example, companies lose their customers because of the measures adopted, the government should make resources available to compensate financially for the losses and - above all - justify the measures. For each restriction imposed, the persons affected should be able to see an equivalent benefit, such as the preservation of their health.

The decision that guarantees a fair exchange ratio for those affected is useful. With every restriction imposed by politics, an equivalent benefit should be evident in return. The test question of whether the decision guarantees a fair exchange relationship for those affected (*reciprocity test*) can be seen as an important contribution to the ethics of utility.

The *ethics of duty* as a judging authority sets standards for action and demands, for example, the observance of human rights or the protection of the dignity of all creatures. The basic value of the former clearly demands the protection of the freedom or the right of self-determination (autonomy) of all those affected by a decision. In principle, therefore, the restriction of the freedom of movement of the citizens concerned should in no way be at issue.

Whether or not I am in compliance with such duties must be examined separately. The *daylight test* checks whether a decision or action was actually taken in accordance with rules accepted or required by the company. It reads: "Would you accept it if tomorrow your decision or action became public?" However, this presupposes freedom of speech and freedom of the press.

And the *ethics of virtue* appeals to the actor to develop good behaviour such as mindfulness, courage and empathy. Those who are mindful avoid risky tunnel vision, those who are courageous can also point out dangerous consequences to their superiors or in front of supervisory bodies or even to the public, and those who are empathic are able to put themselves in the position of those affected emotionally. Here the *empathy test* is relevant, which asks: "How would you feel if you were affected by your own decision or action? (Cf. Schüz, 2020, 239 f).

We now have the necessary tools together to apply them to the Corona crisis.

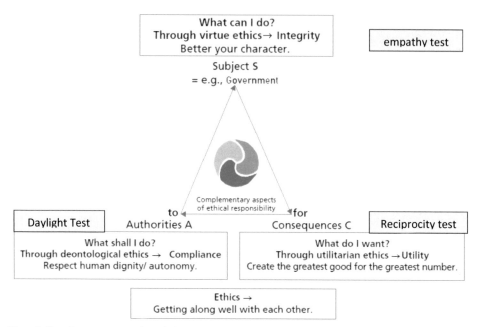

Figure 2: Complementary approaches of ethical responsibility. Source: Based on Schüz 2019:246.

4. Ethical Responsibility applied to the Corona-Crisis

In the Corona Crisis, the two camps of utilitarian and deontological ethicists were and are primarily opposed to each other. The former have the well-being of the majority in mind. The *utility ethicists* (utilitarians) demand that the well-being of the majority must be ensured. It would therefore be absurd to make the majority suffer at the expense of a minority of mainly old people or people with poor health. They favoured the solution of "herd immunity" - according to the motto: "Let the coronavirus run free, then a small minority of the old and sick might die, but the majority of humanity - the young and the healthy - will survive, now immune to the virus, and the economy will suffer even smaller losses on top of that". Public life will be preserved. Although a majority of people will then be infected by the virus, they will acquire the necessary antibodies if the symptoms are mild. They also argue with the freedom rule that prohibits curfews. Ethical action is taken when the short and long-term consequences are weighed against each other. Countries such as Sweden, initially also the USA and UK, favoured this approach.

The *ethicists of duty* (deontologists) advocate the opposite. The adherents of this ethics approach demand the protection of the minority who, due to their age or other predispositions, have to reckon with massive damage to their health, possibly even pay with their lives. For them there is the red line of human rights, according to which all people have the same inviolable dignity - whether young, old, weak or sick. Everything must be done to preserve their lives, no one must be favoured and sacrificed for the benefit of others. Every person has the same right to the best possible assistance to protect his or her health integrity. In case of doubt, the economy must step back in favour of an optimally effective health system. They therefore recommend isolating as many people as possible in order to minimize the risk of infection for the elderly and sick. They also argue with the principle of freedom, according to which freedom ends at the limit of the freedom of the other person when the latter thereby gets in trouble. Those act ethically who do everything in their power to save human lives. Therefore, their call for a close-down seems to be ethically justified. The fact that they herewith simultaneously restrict human rights in turn seems paradoxical, but corresponds to the typical problem of a conflict of goods or a conflict of duties, which deontologists often have to face.

With the global shutdown, most countries have followed this path. The politicians responsible for it justified their decision by referring to human rights. This is welcome, considering how, in recent history, the murder of minorities or dissidents was justified by the common good. In order to protect the lives of endangered persons, major restrictions were imposed on everyday and economic life. This had and has very strong economic and social effects, the final extent of which cannot yet be accurately estimated. In any case, billions of people have had to accept drastic consequences, even threatening their very existence.

The dialectic of good and evil

Obviously, both paths are associated with risks and opportunities. The close-down had unexpected consequences. While social risks increased considerably, the natural environment was able to breathe a sigh of relief. (Fulterer et al. 2020:7) For decision-makers in politics they represent a dilemma. On closer inspection, the arguments of both camps have both fundamental strengths and weaknesses.

The *ethicists of duty* run the risk, in good faith, of saving the lives of particularly endangered people in the short term, but in the long term they risk putting other people's lives at risk by closing down. In India, for example, the imposed curfew had led to mass migration. Millions of people lost their income as day labourers and could no longer afford the expensive agglomerations. They therefore returned to their home villages with lower living costs. In overcrowded buses, they now threatened to spread the coronavirus even more. Or they hoped for donations from private organizations in order to be able to physically survive at all.

The *utility ethicists,* on the other hand, protect the economy and thus the lives of the majority in the short term. They disregard the avoidable suffering of minorities by pointing out that the number of deaths caused by the corona virus is much lower compared to that caused by the close-down. In addition, the lives of thousands of people are at risk with the close-down due to untreated diseases. By leaving minorities unprotected, they threaten fundamental achievements of modern enlightenment.

The triage problem

The dilemma of the two ethical approaches is also evident in the so-called triage problem. As a result, only one ventilator is available - as has happened in Italian, French or Spanish hospitals - for the treatment of two patients seriously ill with coronavirus. To whom should the life-saving measures be given? (Cf. Mandry 2020)

Some utilitarians explicitly recommend giving preference to younger patients. The ethicists of duty reject such preferences as age-discriminatory, since no person has a higher intrinsic value than another. (Cf. Fateh-Moghadam/Gutmann 2020)

This principle formulated in the human rights is already rooted in the ethics of the modern Enlightenment as irrevocably formulated and justified by Immanuel Kant in his categorical imperative: A human being must never be misused merely as a means to this or that end, but must always be respected in his dignity, that is: in his right to self-determination. (Cf. Kant, 1994, p. 36) Thus, according to the Swiss Society of Intensive Care Medicine, no decisions may be made based on "age, sex, place of residence, nationality, religious affiliation, social status, insurance status or chronic disability". (Scheidegger et al. 2020)

In the polar opposite of the two approaches, they claim the good way for themselves and consider the other to be evil. As a way out the third approach of virtue ethics offers itself.

The third way - dialectics of ethical approaches

Is the conflict between the contradictory ethical approaches solvable? Yes, because there is still a third approach: The virtue ethics (Aretologie) could, as a tip on the scales, to a certain extent bring about a separation of powers in the weighing of ethical dilemmas. In the sense of Aristotle, who elaborated virtue ethics in a very differentiated way following his teacher Plato, it examines the respective situation, the existing resources and abilities of the actors in order to solve a given problem. (Cf. e.g. Aristotle 2009:1106a-b).

For example, the mentioned Society for Intensive Care Medicine, despite its basic deontological attitude, recommends taking the patients' chances of survival - i.e. a utilitarian point of view - into account when resources are scarce for the triage problem. Accordingly, the treating physician should refer to both ethical approaches. What might this look like in concrete terms?

The attending physician can only make a decision on the use of a ventilator in favour of one or the other seriously ill patient to the best of his knowledge and belief. In order for this to succeed, he should have virtues such as life experience, intuition and empathy for the person concerned. However, there is no guarantee that his decision will actually be the right one. Perhaps his final decision will benefit both patients after all. But it may just as well be wrong for both. As practice shows, in the latter case the attending doctors have to live with the bad outcome and work through their feelings of guilt. With the acceptance that human action can fail in principle, the courage to face such borderline situations in life again and again may grow.

The current situation is also a test of strength for individual states or even the world community, in which they have to weigh up different positions and interests. The highly complex situation of the Corona crisis requires virtues such as mindfulness, empathy, but also courage and self-control. The fact that individual states have arrived at different, sometimes even contradictory solutions in the process is shown precisely by the situation-related openness of virtue-ethical considerations. Decisions must never be taken alone, but should always be discussed with representatives of different interest groups. It is important that contrary expert opinions are considered equally and transparently and that the decision-making process is communicated accordingly.

From the point of view of virtue ethics it is therefore understandable why each state has chosen its own solution. For everyone is in a unique situation and has different resources and capabilities. Countries that have sufficient financial resources can, for example, finance short-time work by the state. This considerably cushions the economic fall through the close-down. However, considerable differences have also emerged between such financially strong countries. While in Switzerland, government guarantees allowed banks to grant larger loans to companies in need within a few days, Austria demanded that companies advance short-time work compensation for three months. Many companies there had to file for insolvency as a result. In the USA, which does not even know about short-time work benefits, companies were forced to release their employees immediately. This led to a real explosion in the number of unemployed to 40 million nationwide.

The role of the impartial observer

The great ethicist and founder of modern economics, Adam Smith, referred to the important role of the "impartial spectator" in ethical decisions (cf. Smith 2014:69, 81, 94 f). The latter also makes his recommendations contrary to his own interests in order to resolve an ethical conflict on the basis of its "universel benevolence" (Smith 2014:207) for the benefit of all those affected, also in the long term. This can be done on an individual basis, with the responsible actors self-critically questioning their own position and responding attentively to that of the other participants. In this way, the impartial observer takes on the role of the individual conscience or, in Kant's ethics, resembles the "inner judge" who presides over the "inner court of justice" in order to judge his or her own actions as to whether or not they meet ethical duties. (Cf. Kant 1994:§13) In order to strengthen the power of judgement, however, virtues such as the *courage* to look at one's own dark sides and hidden interests neutrally (cf. Schüz 2019:319 f), *mindfulness* (cf. Ruedy/Schweitzer 2010) and *deliberation* on the basis of knowledge of ethical duties and consequences (cf. Zhong 2011) are required.

But this can also be done collectively, as Smith calls for neutral countries to assume a mediating role and make recommendations (Smith 2014:135). In the Corona crisis, this function could perhaps be assumed by the UN or neutral countries such as Switzerland. After all, according to evaluations by the London Deep Knowledge Group, Switzerland regularly receives top marks for its handling of the COVID-19 pandemic. (DVK 2020) Their experience could serve as a role model for other countries.

Certainly, the time pressure of a sudden pandemic hardly allows for lengthy discourses. These should have been conducted prophylactically as balanced proposals for a crisis scenario before the outbreak of the current pandemic. After the experience of the first SARS corona epidemic in 2002, a number of countries have learned their lesson and at least developed risk analyses and coping strategies. Taiwan, Singapore and South Korea have prepared their health care systems for this on the basis of such forward-looking studies. The German Bundestag also had a year 2012 to prepare a detailed risk study on an impending pandemic caused by a SARS corona virus (Deutscher Bundestag 2013:5 f) Thus the German government, like many other countries, is unlikely to have been unprepared.

It would now have to be examined to what extent the manifold approaches to solving the Corona crisis were actually based on a transparent weighing process worldwide within the individual nations. Furthermore, whether this process was executed in the sense of the three ethical approaches, or how far hidden interests of individual groups were the decisive factor for one or the other solution. Particularly in view of the recent lifting of the lockdown in Europe and the feared second wave of infection by the corona virus, such a weighing should therefore also be carried out on an inter-, if not transdisciplinary basis.

In particular, there is a need for a wide range of perspectives on the opportunities and risks of the strategies used to overcome the corona crisis. Strategies such as the planned use of various tracking apps, the compulsory vaccination with electronically retrievable markers as an immunity card considered in some places, the requirement for proof of corona virus antibodies, etc. Even a one-sided understanding of physical health, which is based unilaterally on the findings of orthodox medicine and excludes alternative medicine, could miss opportunities for crisis management. In any case, the virtuous-ethical approach is open to a variety of solutions and integrates impact considerations as well as respect for recognised ethical obligations. The perception of ethical responsibility is more than just observing existing rules. It is an art which, especially in times of uncertainty and global problems, is challenged to avoid one-sidedness and instead develop innovative solutions.

5. Basic insights of ethical leadership

To sum up, in times of crisis, ethical leadership is necessary. This can be seen in decisions that reflect the three basic ethical approaches in dialogue with all those affected and take into account all available expert knowledge, resources and capabilities to the best of our knowledge and belief. An ethical manager should be credible and trustworthy towards his followers through virtues such as fairness, honesty and be a role model for them. (cf. Brown/Trevino 2006) They should also be critical of themselves with regard to prejudices and biases against the facts as presented by the various experts. They should admit their mistakes and be willing to correct them. They should be more concerned with the common good than with their own, i.e. have an altruistic attitude (cf. Morris 2019).

Under time pressure, the three test questions mentioned above can at least give them a rough idea of the ethical content of their planned decisions. Consider (1) the reciprocity test, which asks about fairness for all affected persons, respect (2) the daylight test, which asks about the public acceptance of a decision, and conduct (3) the empathy test, which implies a role reversal of the decision maker with those of the affected persons.

References

Aristotle 2009. Aristotle. *Nicomachean Ethics*, translated by David Ross, New York: Oxford University Press. Available at: https://socialsciences.mcmaster.ca/econ/ugcm/3ll3/aristotle/Ethics.pdf, retrieved on: 9 January 2019.

Beck 1991. Beck, Ulrich. «Wissenschaft und Sicherheit», in: *Politik in der Risikogesellschaft* (hrsg. v. Ulrich Beck). Frankfurt a. M.: Suhrkamp.

Brown/Treviño 2006. Brown, Michael E./ Treviño, Linda K. «Ethical Leadership: A review and future directions», in: *The Leadership Quarterly*, 17, pp. 595-616.

CLIA 2019. CLIA – Cruise Lines International Association: *Cruise Industry Outlook Report*. Available at: https://cruising.org/en/news-and-research/press-room/2019/december/clia-releases-2020-state-of-the-cruise-industry-outlook-report, retrieved on 10 June 2020.

Deutscher Bundestag 2013. Deutscher Bundestag. *Unterrichtung durch die Bundesregierung: Bericht zur Risikoanalyse im Bevölkerungsschutz 2012*. Deutscher Bundestag Drucksache 17/12051 vom 3.01.2013. Available at: https://dipbt.bundestag.de/dip21/btd/17/120/1712051.pdf, retrieved on 30 June 2020.

DKV 2020. DKV – Deep Knowledge Group. *COVID-19 Regional Safety Assessment (200 Region)*. Available at: https://www.dkv.global/covid-safety-assesment-200-regions, retrieved on 30 June 2020.

Fateh-Moghadam/Gutmann 2020. Fateh-Moghadam, Bijan/ Gutmann, Thomas. «COVID-19 und Intensivmedizin: 'Wir brauchen eine öffentliche Diskussion über die gerechte Verteilung von lebensrettenden Ressourcen'», in: *Universität Basel*. Available at: https://www.unibas.ch/de/Aktuell/News/Uni-Research/COVID-19-und-Intensivmedizin-Wir-brauchen-eine-oeffentliche-Diskussion-ueber-die-gerechte-Verteilung-von-lebensrettenden-Ressourcen.html, retrieved on: 30 June 2020.

Foerster 1991. Foerster, Heinz v. «Through the Eyes of the Other», in: *Research and Reflexivity* (ed. by F. Steier). London: Sage Publications, pp. 63–75. Available at: http://cepa.info/1729, retrieved on: 30 June 2020.

Fulterer 2020. Fulterer, Ruth et al. „Zehn unerwartete Folgen der Pandemie" *Neue Zürcher Zeitung* (NZZ) (7. Mai 2020)7.

Kant 1994a. Kant, Immanuel. '*The Metaphysical Principles of Virtue* [1797]', Book II, in: *Ethical Philosophy* (translated by James W. Ellington). Indianapolis: Hackett (2nd ed.), pp. 1–161.

Kant 1994b. Kant, Immanuel: *Grounding for the Metaphysics of Morals* [1785], Book I, in: Ethical Philosophy (translated by James W. Ellington). Indianapolis: Hackett (2nd ed.), pp. 1–69.

Mandry 2020. Mandry, Christof"Lernen aus der Corona-Krise. Triage, Ethik und politische Theologie», in: *feinschwarz.net* vom 20. April 2020. Available at: https://www.feinschwarz.net/corona-krise-triage-ethik-politik/, retrieved on: 3 June 2020.

Morris 2019. Morris, Lancey. «7 Characteristics of Ethical Leadership and Why the matter – A Checklist for ethical and mindful leadership», available at: https://www.thegrowthfaculty.com/blog/ethicalleadershipwilldriveresultsin2020, retrieved on 10 July 2020.

Nida-Rümelin 2011. Nida-Rümelin, Julian: *Verantwortung*. Stuttgart: Reclam.

Picht 1969. Picht, Georg. «Der Begriff der Verantwortung», in: *Wahrheit – Vernunft – Verantwortung – Philosophische Studien*. Stuttgart: Klett, pp. 318-372.

Ruedy/Schweitzer 2010. Ruedy, Nicole E./ Schweitzer, Maurice E. «In the Moment: The Effect of Mindfulness on Ethical Decision Making», in: *Journal of Business Ethics*, vol. 95, pp. 73-87.

Scheidegger 2020. Scheidegger, Daniel et al. COVID-19-Pandemie: *Triage von intensivmedizinischen Behandlungen bei Ressourcenknappheit*, in: Schweizerische Gesellschaft für Intensivmedizin (SGI), available at: https://www.sgi-ssmi.ch/de/news-detail/items/422.html, retrieved on: 30 June 2020.

Schüz 1999. Schüz, Mathias. Werte – Risiko – Verantwortung. Dimensionen des Value Managements. München: Gerling Akademie Verlag.

Schüz 2012. Schüz, Mathias. "Sustainable Corporate Responsibility – The Foundation of Successful Business in the New Millenium", in: Central European Business Review, No 2, Prague: VSE, p. 7-15. Available at: http://cebr.vse.cz/cebr/article/view/34, retrieved on 10 June 2020.

Schüz 2019. Schüz, Mathias. *Applied Business Ethics – Foundations for Study and Daily Practice*. Singapore/ New Jersey/ London: World Scientific.

Schüz 2020. Schüz, Mathias. «Ethische Verantwortung von Führungskräften in Unternehmen», in: *HR-Wissen kompakt – 10 Insights von führenden Experten*, Personal Schweiz – Das Buch 2020. Zürich/ Kissing/ Paris/ Wien: Weka Business Media AG, pp. 237-241.

Smith 2014. Smith, Adam. *The Theory of Moral Sentiments* [1759]. Los Angeles: Enhanced Media Publishing.

Weber 1968. Weber, Max. «Die Objektivität sozialwissenschaftlicher und sozialpolitischer Erkenntnisse», in: *Methodologische Schriften*. Frankfurt a. M.: S. Fischer, pp. 1-64.

Zhong 2011. Zhong, C.-B. The Ethical Dangers of Deliberative Decision Making. *Administrative Science Quarterly*, 56 (1), pp. 1–25. Available at: https://doi.org/10.2189/asqu.2011.56.1.001.

Zimmerli 2014. Zimmerli, Walther. «Verantwortung kennen oder Verantwortung übernehmen? – Theoretische Technikbewertung und angewandte Ingenieurethik», in: *Verantwortung von Ingenieurinnen und Ingenieuren* (hrsg. v. L. Hieber, Hans-Ullrich Kammeyer). Wiesbaden: Springer, pp. 15-24.

Prof. Dr. phil. **Mathias Schüz** studied physics, philosophy and education at the Johannes Gutenberg University of Mainz. He was a co-initiator and long-standing member of the Executive Board of the Gerling Academy for Risk Research, Zurich, and is currently Professor of Responsible Leadership and Business Ethics at the Zurich University of Applied Sciences (ZHAW) in Winterthur, Switzerland.

Integrative bioethics in the time/ not in the time of COVID-19:

Caring, Behaving and Responsibilities towards Future Generations

Hanna Hubenko, Sumy State University, USA

Abstract

As a bioethicist, I observe society integrally (among the responsibilities of which obligatory are help and caring for *Vulnerable Groups* of the population), using the transdisciplinary methodologies of the postmodern paradigm. The importance of such view / position can be reasoned by the recent experience of quarantine: if a certain population group is not included in the COVID-19 protection plan, then the whole society is at risk. As a teacher, I see/approve a solution through education – my stakes are on the *New Generation* – more responsible and conscious. As a bioethicist, the solution is also presented through the creation of a new methodology on the Platform – a stake on *Integrative Bioethics*. I suggest an 'InplatBio'– an integrative bioethics platform. InplatBio and its transdisciplinary methodologies give us the opportunity to cross the borders of the contemporary culture into responsibilities towards future generations.

Key words

Bioethics, Contemporary Culture, Caring, Civil Liberty, Education, Integrative Bioethics Platform (InplantBio), Vulnerability

1. How do we make decisions in a condition of an 'existential vacuum'?

During the COVID-19 period, there is a need for tools that would help unprotected / vulnerable population groups. In areas such as education and public health, these can be coverage of practices and recommendations when making difficult decisions. The mechanism for creating these tools is based on transdisciplinarity, which helps uniting into teams and increases the level of trust in society. Will these recommendations only be a screen for decision-making? It is especially possible, when speaking about post-Soviet countries, deprived of justice and legal order. All the above mentioned affects the understanding of right and wrong. I think this requires, first of all, feedback - as the potential for support (primarily psychological) and publicity - as the opportunity of inclusion in society. In the text, we will also consider several uniting bioethical practices from different parts of the world, get acquainted with the Integrative Bioethics Platform. As one of the opportunities to collect successful and failed cases from the pre- and post-Covid life of different countries, so that as many people as possible get acquainted with their experience of changing behavior and finding the right resources for making decisions in vital moments.

2. Integrative Bioethics and its Platform

Let us examine the blocks in more details: integrative bioethics and its platform; the theory of generations and human behaviour. Is bioethics relevant in 21st century? This issue became especially clear during the COVID-19 epidemic, when questions about ethics, equality, and injustice unfolded around us every day. I want to underline, that we get the answer in accordance with the level of understanding that injustice penetrated / was in social systems long before the pandemic. Why were state systems not ready, why didn't bioethics do more to anticipate these problems and mitigate them? It is difficult to find the answer, but here / in this article, I want to pause / speak my thoughts about young people, the theory of generations. I am talking about generations that live now; generations that are involved in the history of the formation of today's reality and the future. I would like to note that my view will illuminate an attempt to look at the problem from a triangular perspective, as a bioethicist, scientist and teacher.

It is time for the bioethicists to ally in the global meaning of this word. This is why my suggestion, to create an InplatBio– Integrative Bioethics Platform is on the table. InplatBio and its transdisciplinary Methodology – is an opportunity to cross the borders of the «own» culture, in the time/not in the time of COVID-19. The methods, that are used on the InplatBio: cases; author-made cartoons; documentaries; comics; «helpful humor»; storytelling; narrations of professionals, that are already occupied in the hybrid professions – increase the speed and the direction of the social changes. In the text it is possible to apply such types of behavioural science and bioethics: **Overcoming Fear (Laziness) Of Changes** decrease the effort and increase the reward; **Using Creative Interactive** change the worldview; **«Happiness Nudges»** build a conscious way to yourself; **Realising Your Actions** create a feedback – communication. This pandemic has shown us, that the world is intertwined, and we are as strong as our «weakest unit». It is time to change the modern discourse: to talk more about the «economics of caring», move to the equality discourse, solidarity, caring and human safety.

Among all concepts of bioethics, «*Integration*» is an attempt to establish a discourse between various points of view and a perspective in the interaction of bioethical issues in order to provide direction within a certain discussion. By providing different positions, integrative bioethics can direct people who are faced with ethical / bioethical issues. Therefore, in integrative bioethics, the idea of accepting various points of view as serious, without any form of hierarchy, but without falling into ethical relativism, is active. Another important aspect is the fact that the discussion of these issues creates a society's sensitivity to them (Hubenko 2016: 206-207). Such transition requires a paradigm shift, the ability to make the «invisible visible», and also solidary seek real economic solutions. In my opinion, *integrative bioethics*[1] fulfils an individual claim, since it is a methodological attempt to find out **how** we can speak not only about bioethical, but also other complex topics and **what** should be done in crisis situations. This basis of discourse has not been completed to this day, we are not ready to speak on topics that do not offer a certain result, for example, one accepted for a minority.

I would like to note the idea that each society in the quarantine period projects «accustomed» response skills, and in situations dealing with the vulnerable groups, these skills and experience are new, the ability to react correctly becomes dull, as invisible aspects of society's life show themselves. At the same time, the attitude towards vulnerable groups is the litmus test of the society's ethics and the well-being of all citizens' life. Undoubtedly, Ukraine is changing its post-Soviet views, a small number of projects (Suka Zhizn[2]; «Put a life into a suitcase[3]»; «Solidarity»[4], etc.) run by the huge organizations and volunteers occupy first places in terms of public trust. This shows that Ukrainians support such movements and, perhaps, in this sense, become more moral, thanks to mutual help. However, in Ukraine, there are still echoes of the past: below I would like to outline a few cases showing weaknesses during quarantine, while in reality, hiding behind declarative laws and regulations, far from life and understanding of the problem of existence in an invisible zone.

---

[1]   The integrative bioethics platform is based on the methodology of integrative bioethics. The questions of integrative bioethics and its methodology are outlined in the following articles: Rinčić I., Sodeke St. Ol., Muzur A. (2016); Hoffmann Th. S. (2018); Sass H.-M., Muzur A. (2017).

[2]   Media project about Homeless People in Ukraine: Suka Zhizn [https://bzh.life/ua/lyudi/suka-zhizn-kak-kievlyanin-sozdal-proekt-pomoshchi-bezdomnym-blagodarya-postam-v-instagram - accessed: June 20, 2020].

[3]   The exhibition-installation «Put your life in a suitcase» the purpose of which «through emotions and feelings» is to draw attention to the problems of internally displaced persons in Ukraine – https://www.ukrinform.ru/rubric-kyiv/2697357-vmesti-svou-zizn-v-cemodan-otkrylas-vystavkainstallacia-o-zizni-pereselencev.html – accessed: June 20, 2020].

[4]   The site «Solidarity» was created to help Ukrainians through the coronavirus epidemic – [https://v2020.org.ua/] .

3. Special Cases

Case 1. Quarantine without shelter: At the beginning of March 2020, about 50,000 children were sent home - from boarding schools, children's homes (orphanages) and social and psychological rehabilitation centres. Some children met their parents for the first time. In fact, boarding schools were closed in one day, and it was necessary to urgently return children to their families. Nobody checked whether the children are expected at home and whether there is room for them? If no one came for the child, the boarding school workers transported the fosterlings themselves. The fact is that in Ukraine boarding schools are subordinate to the Ministry of Education and Science, and social services - to the Ministry of Social Policy[5]. The communication bridge, as we can see, could not be built between the services. In 2017, Ukraine began to introduce a boarding school reform, the ultimate goal of which was to eliminate boarding schools, substituting them with family-type orphanages and foster homes, and failed to be implemented.

Case 2. Silent problems: Due to quarantine the severely ill patients are discharged from the palliative departments of Kiev hospitals. We are talking about people at high risk who are in the last stage of life. Despite the fact that hospices really declare the presence of mobile services in reality, we face following: while long-term health facilities hospitalize patients from all over Kiev, their on-site services provide medical support in certain areas only and, according to experts, have limited human and material resources. There are some patients who have lost access to essential medical care, and there are also patients who have nowhere to be discharged and who cannot be taken care of at home[6]. At the same time, the Ministry of Health never actually approved the order, which defines what a mobile palliative care service is, which functions is it supposed to pursue.

Case 3. Pandemic inside a pandemic: The number of calls to the domestic violence prevention hotline during quarantine is recorded every day: in March, 1,600 calls were received (in comparison, the largest number of calls was recorded during the New Year's holidays - 1,100 times). According to Yekaterina Khanyovo[7], coordinator of the prevention and counteraction of gender-based domestic violence direction: «the number of appeals to the «Slavic Heart» charity fund, that operates in Donbass, has doubled since the beginning of quarantine. Now the risk of domestic violence in the frontline zone also grows because of the economic instability caused by the quarantine. In areas near the demarcation line, jobs were often associated with services for residents of uncontrolled territories.

Case 4. Excessive cargo: It took teachers who really tried to maintain the quality of the educational process during the quarantine, much longer to prepare for online classes than before. At the same time, there were those who transferred communication with students into a written form – through giving them a lot of written assignments and refusing to actually teach

---

[5] Read the details of an independent publication on social and cultural trends in the post-Soviet countries of Eastern Europe, an article by Alena Vishnitsky «Quarantine without a bed» [https://zaborona.com/karantin-bez-lizhka/ - accessed: June 1, 2020].

[6] See article by Margarita Tulup, coordinator of the project «Pravosyllia», that is devoted to the rights violations in Correctional Facilities. Co-grounder of the palliative support centre «La Vita» - https://www.slidstvo.info/news/deyaki-kyyivski-likarni-vypysuyut-nevylikovno-hvoryh-patsiyentiv-dodomu/ (2 of April 2020).

[7] See also: Aliona Kryvuliak, coordinator of hotline directions of the social organization «La Strada»; Oksana Rasulova «Pandemic inside of a pandemic». The influence of the quarantine on the domestic violence – [https://hromadske.ua/posts/pandemiya-vseredini-pandemiyi-yak-karantin-v-ukrayini-vplivaye-na-domashnye-nasilstvo].

classes. There were those, who generally barely got in touch with students. Moreover, the degree of involvement of teachers in distance learning does not affect their salaries. This situation once again actualized the issue of a fair level of salaries in higher education institutions and the *question of the quality of knowledge*. Modern universities are tied to a wage scale and cannot set salaries based on the individual performance of teachers.

I think these four cases can help the reader to feel the underdevelopment of Ukrainian society in understanding the sensitivity of the decision-making[8] needs for all, including vulnerable groups of society. In my educational practice, I often use cases like this, in the solution of which students show a high level of empathy and inclusion. I am sure that Generation Z («Zetas») can fundamentally change our society. These changes will be more significant than those that previous generations succeeded in. Another question is that the post-Soviet space is a space that «fractures» individuals, and even those who are now 40 years old grew up and were brought up in a poor state riddled with corruption and nepotism. What youth grew up on has become for it a natural and integral part of life, or a social norm. Thereby, it delays the development by irredundant prejudices. As a result, most of the of the Ukrainian population believes that «strong leaders can do more for the country than all the laws and discussions».[9] Unfortunately they are *non-responsible* for their actions, *non-obligations* and concern for future generations. Given the fact that future generations are in a constant state of dependence on the actions of modern people, this is exactly the relational structure that is important to nurture and implement as a motivational one. It's about this kind of *caring* – visible and important, I wrote above, and it's precisely it that can provide a reliable theory of commitment: where people in the present can provide the conditions necessary to maintain the peace for future generations, which allow friendly and happy relationships[10] to flourish.

4. The Integrative Bioethics Platform

Transdisciplinarity. The Transdisciplinarity Of Integrative Bioethics includes the following elements in its description: Acquiring a complex of knowledge / integrative bioethics; Application of knowledge in the life process; Creating new / transdisciplinary spaces: a) introduction of bioethical education for the new generation, b) awareness of the role of bioethical knowledge, c) to enlighten scientific, social and political decisions / bioethical vision to solve global problems in the modern world (Hubenko 2020: 177).

Inclusion. Inclusion is a social ideal of humanism and tolerance, which is impossible without conscious acceptance of «Otherness» as a chance for mutual beneficiation. Also, this concept - is a great, tireless scripter of switching-on (Hubenko 2020: 174). Inclusion includes the following elements in the description: Access of all residents of the city to the blessings and everyday life; Publicity and openness (discussion of ideas in public spaces, public hearings; Actions of public organizations, etc.) Accessibility and switching-on (accessibility of flannel; recognition of moral democracy and human rights; framing a broad social movement, that is able to

---

[8] I want to gather cases and solutions from various countries. In this way we will be able to save transnational experience for help and support of all those in need. Gathering of all the international data on the InPlatBio could have a therapeutic meaning – as the acknowledgment that this problem is visible.

[9] See Irina Bekeshkina research: Are the people the engine of reforms or the brake? - [https://www.youtube.com/watch?v=Q6ScKt5kTOc&fbclid=IwAR0iBaYAeclXQy54eKD_tW6SEGHxyN2Gl6A1 npG9KWZ050HDRarBEXTTnDE; also see studies of Deloitte in CIS- https://www2.deloitte.com/ru/ru/pages/about-deloitte/articles/millennialsurvey.html - accessed: June 30, 2020].

[10] Studies of Richard Davidson, Willejanur Ramanchandrani and Sean Aco. Now it is especially important not to concentrate on the universe economy, but on making people happy.

fulfill its liberty). **Intersubjectivity** and perception of «Otherness» (the right to the city - is the right to change ourselves by changing the city; the interaction of grass-root initiatives and city authorities) (Hubenko 2020: 175).

Integrative bioethics showed the importance of mixing for me. In light of these characteristics, we can work out mechanisms for operating with vulnerable groups of the population – as markers of readiness to newly formed skills of interaction and care. It is very important to embed this insight into society. Do you understand what else is important? It is important to understand a certain **center** of life support. Then, for example, in the community, not only leader as the source of all decisions and commitments, will be important, but the whole team. For example, in the case of Covid - it became clear to many people that unpredictability is fraught with challenges and crises as well as opportunities. But for them to appear, the environments «inside» and «outside» must be structurally similar. An element of uncertainty should be implanted in the corporate / team environment.

Several examples of bioethical practices from around the globe and based on these considerations, we propose to speculation and creation of an ***Integrative Bioethics Platform*** – InPlat-Bio, that is online and offline present. The integrative bioethics platform is a structure that integrates knowledge of all areas of bioethics/bioethical knowledge integration platform, providing open scientific information to the wider audience. Examples of such offline platforms in any field are bioethicist-specialists production (courses, trainings, experience sharing). Society has been in need of a qualitatively new mental paradigm for both professionals and citizens in general for quite a long time. It enhances the relevance of integrative bioethics' programs, defines philosophical and methodological foundations of bioethics, as well as the content of training guides, programs and methodological recommendations aimed at their implementation into the process of both - training of bioethics professionals and retraining of specialists in other fields (Hubenko 2014: 80).

Our main idea on the online-platform InplatBio is to highlight scientific, social, and political decisions/approaches to the ethical problems in the modern world (these may be ethical codices, bioethical standards, civil involvement projects, art initiatives, etc.). On this platform, we also want to highlight new hybrid professions in the areas, which were not possible to combine before (for example, through project programs). We suggest using the experience of bioethicists as a mechanism in well-established rules of connecting, a «glueing a humanities person to a science person». Such hybrids may be new professions as new interests or hobbies for one to feel like a happy citizen and form positive social factors for the development of a «new personality» and society in general (Hubenko 2020: 181-182)[11].

---

[11] We have first introduced the idea of hybrid professions, with bioethicists as an example, with a colleague from Spain, Salvador Ribas, at the I International bioethics conference: Teaching and learning in bioethics, January 24-25, 2019.

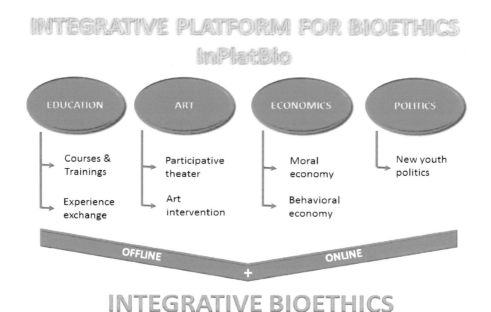

Figure 1 – Scheme of Integrative bioethical platform (authors report materials «Bioethics Workshop: Urban-Cultural Project» from the International conference «The 21st Rijeka Days of Bioethics. Urban *Bioethics: From Smart to Living Cities. Bioethical Debate, Reflections and Standards», Rijeka/Croatia,* 17–18 of May 2019)[12]

The platform contains *interactive methods* (cartoons; comics; narratives from specialists who already work in the field of hybrid professions - bioethicists); a new youth policy will be created on the platform - a career portal - a mentoring commission of specialists from different parts of Europe (*taking into account the statistics of youth opinion*), etc. (Hubenko 2020).

4. Human behavior and culture of society[13]

During the pandemic, I started lessons with questions about how students feel during isolation, what would they like to change, and how do they see the future? Sometimes the answers sounded quite unusual - the students were confused by the inability to imagine their further future, but later at the end of the course, many of them thanked for these questions and emotional support. In fact, these reactions were therapeutic for us. They gave the opportunity to think about the meaning of life and how to create a better future, being at home.

Social norms and the behavior of the people around us affect how we live and how we make decisions. This pandemic has shown us that it is important to unite. This showed us that

---

[12] The scheme is also disclosed in the article: Hubenko, Hanna (2019) *Urban Bioethics Plan: Studies for the Conscious Citizen*, Filosofiya Osvity. Philosophy of Education, *24*(1), 236.

[13] The material for the section «Human behavior and culture of society» was also used in the German-language collection «Medizin und Ethik in Zeiten von Corona» in the section «How has the pandemic changed our societies?», Hubenko H(2020), *New bioethics: how we make decisions in a condition of «existential vacuum»*.

there is strength in collective action. Compared to pre-COVID life, where more attention was paid to the culture of «*me*», has now shifted to «**we**» and the understanding that people still need support, empathy and interaction. We also understand that the motivation to changing human behavior does not depend on age, gender, culture etc., but primarily depends on the psychological state of the person.

In this paper, I combine the studies of Cass Sunstein[14], BJ Fogg[15], Dan Arieli[16], Lori Santos[17], Chiara Varazzani[18], Dilip Soman[19], as well as the materials of the online Nudgstock festival[20], for my own understanding of the issue that has been tormenting me for a long time - why people do not change their behavior, being aware that it is dangerous to the health, own life and the life of the Planet as a whole? It's very difficult to make a decision, and if the series of critical questions does not end, then it also drains psychologically. I am trying to relate together the research of world scientists to adapt the author's mechanism in the field of education and in the public debate field[21].

There are different ways to apply behavioral science: overcoming fear (laziness) of changes: *reduce effort and increase reward* (and we're not talking about cash reward, but about empathy and care). In this way, we can reduce the panic of uncertainty and make it easier to accept changes (or accept the Other). Bri Williams[22] presented the equation of *effort versus reward*: for many people, if the efforts are greater than the received rewards, it is much more difficult to convince the person/himself to change his behavior. Thus, we can try to simplify the mechanism of doing the right things and complicate the mechanism of the wrong ones. I like this example during COVID-19: Lush's '30-Second Soap', which is designed to dissolve after 30 seconds of usage, makes it easier to understand just how long it takes to wash your hands thoroughly[23].

Here is another example: I am currently/at the moment taking the course «Allies: Solidarity School with LGBT +» from Freedom House[24], the motivation for passing which was prejudice and fear towards representatives of LGBTI Communities in Ukraine, both in the field of education and in society as a whole. I began to include cases of discrimination in my courses, and I

---

[14] See also: Nudge: Improving Decisions about Health, Wealth, and Happiness (with Richard H. Thaler, 2008).

[15] BJ Fogg (2019) *Tiny Habits: The Small Changes That Change Everything,* Houghton Mifflin Harcourt, 320 pp.

[16] On the website you can familiarize yourself with the work of Dan Ariely - http://danariely.com/.

[17] Lori Santos. The Happiness Lab, Podcast - https://www.happinesslab.fm/.

[18] Chiara Varazzani, Behavioral Science Needs More Neuroscience, Podcast – [https://behavioralgrooves.com/episode/chiara-varazzani-behavioral-science-needs-more-neuroscience/ visited June 2, 2020].

[19] Dilip Soman (2015). *The Last Mile: Creating Social and Economic Value from Behavioral Insights,* Rotman-UTP Publishing, 296 pp.

[20] Nudgestock 2020 - the World's Leading Festival of Behavioural Science and Creativity – [https://nudgestock.co.uk/about-nudgestock-2020/ - visited 12 June, 2020].

[21] The material is also used in the German-language collection «Medizin und Ethik in Zeiten von Corona», Hubenko H., *2020.*

[22] Bri Williams is an expert in behavioral influence – how to apply behavioral economics to decision-making so you delete hesitation and maximize every interaction. Watch Talk: Lazy, scared, and overwhelmed [https://www.youtube.com/watch?v=ObFrZImxYeI&t=4383s - visited 12 June, 2020].

[23] Research carried out by health authorities has found that people fail to wash their hands effectively 97% of the time. To help them get into the habit, Lush has released a soap that dissolves after 30 seconds, showing how brands can nudge people into hygienic and healthy behaviours [https://www.canvas8.com/signals/2020/06/16/lush-soap.html - visited June, 2020].

[24] The course aims to support and development LGBTI + allies in the human rights movement in Ukraine.

conducted a survey on the attitude of students to the LGBTI Community – the answers before and after the courses changed significantly - negative/aggressive attitude was transformed and, basically, earlier they were built on nescience. Such practices help to accept *the Other* much easier. We, as teachers, greatly facilitate the student's efforts to accept the *new/unknown*. This, of course, is a difficult example to consider this method, but is very deep, since includes the timeliness of knowledge, didactic knowledge and methods that improve the qualifications of the highest level of the teacher (see *Case*. ***Exorbitant burden*** above).

Also, we must use our creative Interactivity: *to change your worldview (more interesting)*: think like comedians; as art critic, etc. I am very impressed with the method that I often use in the classroom - humor, satire as *«Helpful Humor»*[25]. I really believe that humor can be a power-ful tool when used correctly[26]. I want to give extraordinary examples of art usage[27], stand-up performances at discussing very difficult topics: gender stereotypes, discrimination and vio-lence. For example, Iliza Vie Shlesinger is a stand-up comedian, who jokes about the «typical» behavior of men and women. Her audience hardly intersects with those who have already taken feminism into their hearts, freed themselves from imposed stereotypes, and know what intersec-tionality is. Daniel Sloss is a stand-up comedian, the best part of this stand-up comedy is that our prejudices and stereotypes do not disappear automatically, but at the cost of active cognitive efforts, as well as systematic sexual violence - at the cost of active intervention, including legal one[28]. This forces the listener/viewer to face violence and discrimination, explaining that, actu-ally, there is no joke that can neutralize such an experience.

«happiness Nudges» [29] . *to build a conscious path to yourself*. Many people think that more money can make them happy, but studies show that it is not true. Being happy at work and at home, showing concern and empathy for *«Otherness»* and the *Other* – this can be a good skill for both present and future generations.

The existential vacuum during COVID-19 exposed the problems of societies, especially the realities of vulnerable groups. The modern situation with Covid, expressing V. Frankl's teach-ing (Frankl 2006), transferred people into an atmosphere of *existential vacuum* and showed that the lack of knowledge about the meaning of modern human existence causes fear and neuroses. That's what, filling this gap through awareness, contains preventive, quick methodological step in education[30]. Basically, all it really takes is **just to be/remain a Human**; realizing actions: *to*

---

[25] Watch and read Peter McGraw is a professor of marketing and psychology at the University of Colorado Boulder and a global expert in the scientific study of humor; Watch Talk: Shtick to Innovation: Serious lessons in creativity and execution from comedy's rebels – [https://www.youtube.com/watch?v=Zjse4E8iqnk&t=10317s - visited 12 June, 2020].

[26] Ibid.

[27] The UnLonely Project has created a community through its Stuck At Home Together initiative. You can watch a short film, then participate in an online conversation. You can view others' art or share your own. And for motiva-tion to get started, the group has designed creative challenges, like crafting a self-portrait from objects around the house - https://www.artandhealing.org/.

[28] See the article: «You will be very uncomfortable»: 5 stand-ups for those who are tired of sexist jokes – [https://povaha.org.ua/vam-bude-duzhe-nezruchno-5-stendapiv-dlya-tyh-hto-vtomyvsya-vid-seksystskyh-zhartiv/ visited 30 June, 2020].

[29] I use the term « Nudge » in the context of the book: Thaler, R., & Sunstein, C. (2008). Nudge: Improving decisions about health, wealth and happiness, New Haven, CT: Yale University Press, 293 pp; as well as on the basis of fes-tival reports Nudgestock 2020 - the World's Leading Festival of Behavioural Science and Creativity – [https://nudgestock.co.uk/about-nudgestock-2020/ - visited 12 June, 2020].

[30] The material for the «existential vacuum » was also used in the German-language collection "Medizin und Ethik in Zeiten von Corona" in the section « Interaktive, lebensnahe Instrumente und Maßnahmen », Hubenko (2020*), New bioethics: how we make decisions in a condition of «existential vacuum».*

create a feedback - communication. In this context, I want to note an interesting fact, as a teacher, of sometimes falling into the trap of «overestimating the final result». I think we tend to underestimate the complexity of the issue or problem, especially if the experience of mastering knowledge is new, in the case of quarantine, which carries a danger to life. And this remains a significant point for people who find/develop solutions, because you can immerse yourself in the problem and lose touch with reality. Therefore, it is so important to communicate in trans-disciplinary platforms and listen/hear feedbacks. It is very important not to fall into the trap of **knowledge bias** and look at the information through the eyes of a student, listener, any *Other* and/or culture of the society where this information is announced. On the other hand, we are looking for difficult solutions when, in fact, the most basic human needs in difficult times - support, care, openness/honesty - are on the surface[31].

5. Future Prospects

I think that it's time for bioethics to unite in the global sense of the word. I think it's time for Others to hear what specific practices exist in different social conditions. Therefore, it is so important to communicate on transdisciplinary platforms and listen/hear feedbacks. InplatBio and its transdisciplinary methodology - is an opportunity to go beyond the culture. Methods that InplatBio uses: cases; author cartoons; documentary films, comics; storytelling; narratives from experts who are already working in the field of hybrid professions increase the speed and direction of social changes. Examples include the impact of art and pop culture on social changes; helpful humor.

It is important to organize a special section on the ***InplatBio*** platform in the future, which deals with the processes of implementing measures of necessary protection against possible power abuse in connection with the expansion of restrictive measures by government bodies. And such a policy should first ensure that any restrictions are appropriate and proportionate. Activists and human rights defenders should continue to work to monitor, document and report human rights violations, and advocate for societal changes to better protect all people rights.

An equally ambitious form of cooperation is that we can provide a platform - the Institute (School) of Bioethics - for exchange of ideas, methods of teaching bioethics and improving bioethics education in general. Moreover, there is a shortage of bioethicists, and the method of qualification directly through individual research and initiatives is not enough. Teacher communication networks provide environment conducive to teacher learning. Thus, for essential communication skills, both networks and the development of relationships with various organizations and associations are important.

Another way to collaborate is creation of transdisciplinary bioethics course designed for both, students and teachers. The courses are multidisciplinary. Subjects should include aspects of ethics, law, architecture, cognitive science, pedagogy and sociology. Trainees from different countries could choose teachers-bioethicists courses, which represent various fields. Since there is still no center or organization where courses could be organized / listened to, the teaching team might be organized so that the course is taught in different universities. Usage of online courses, webinars – is a modern source of information about the development of bioethics in Ukraine and European countries. Participation in international workshops is also the starting point for building international networks (Hubenko 2016).

---

[31] The material was also used in the German-language collection "Medizin und Ethik in Zeiten von Corona" in the section «What does the new training program look like?», Hubenko (2020), *New bioethics: how we make decisions in a condition of «existential vacuum».*

Conclusion

This pandemic showed us that our world is interconnected, and we are as strong as our «weak link» is. When we are going through this and any other crisis, we have to remember that people should be in the center of attention. Each of us can spread kindness, listen to others, show support and solidarity, and speak out against discrimination. The emergence of global ethical thinking in this context is important not only because the global nature of the world's problems and their causes are becoming more and more clear, but also for the providing of social support (including lifestyle changes). That is why, when asking the question - is bioethics relevant, the correct answer remains its relevance, which lies both in its assignment and in its significance for future generations. The described characteristics of integrative bioethics - transdisciplinary, inclusiveness – help to be / dress «in someone else's skin» - which means, that you understand the problem much broadly and more sensitive.

And although questions of leadership and team remained on the surface of reasoning; care economics, ways to apply behavioral science, etc. - they all have deep-sea subtext - the need of changing approaches to work and life – *to build trust, long-term relationships and visibility. To change the modern discourse: to speak more and reasonably about the «economy of care», to move away from the militarized discourse of «fighting the virus» and «war», and go to the discourse of equality, solidarity, care and human security* (Potapova 2020). I want to emphasize the main thesis, all that is really required during and outside the crisis – is just to be / remain human for yourself, for the *Other,* for *new generations* and for *all live.*

References

Fogg, BJ (2019), Tiny Habits: The Small Changes That Change Everything, *Houghton Mifflin Harcourt*, 320 pp.

Frankl, Viktor E. (2006), Man's Search for Meaning, *Beacon Press*, 184 pp.

Hoffmann, Thomas Sören (2018), The origins and basic approaches of the emergence of a new bioethics and the program «Integrative Bioethics». Part 1 (translation from German by Hanna Hubenko), *Philosophy of Education*, 1 (22), 211-223.

Hubenko, Hanna (2014), Integrative pedagogical bioethics as a new direction of training specialists, *Higher Education of Ukraine*, 3, 75-81.

Hubenko, Hanna (2016), Models Integrative Bioethics in Different Countries, *Filosofiya Osvity. Philosophy of Education*, 19(2), 206-217

Hubenko, Hanna (2019), Urban Bioethics Plan: Studies for the Conscious Citizen, *Filosofiya Osvity. Philosophy of Education*, 24(1), 231-241

Hubenko, Hanna (2020), Urban Bioethics – The Architect of a Healthy City, *JAHR*, 21, 171-188.

Soman, Dilip (2015), The Last Mile: Creating Social and Economic Value from Behavioral Insights, *Rotman-UTP Publishing*, 296 pp.

Sisk, Bryan A., Mozersky, Jessica, Antes, Alison L. and DuBois, James M. (2020), The «ought-is» problem: An implementation science framework for translating ethical norms into practice, *American Journal of Bioethics*, 20(4): 69.

Sass, Hans-Martin and Muzur, Amir (2017), 1926-2016 Fritz Jahr's Bioethics: A global Discourse, Wiem: *LIT Verlag*, 242.

Schalatek, Liane (2020), COVID-19 uniquely affects women. Here are many of the ways it does. - https://ua.boell.org/en/2020/06/11/covid-19-uniquely-affects-women-here-are-many-ways-it-does

Soman, Dilip (2015), The Last Mile: Creating Social and Economic Value from Behavioral Insights, *Rotman-UTP Publishing*, 296 pp.

Potapova, Oksana (2020), The Economics of Care: How Quarantine and the COVID-19 Pandemic Change Communities, NGO Practices, and Government Policies – https://genderindetail.org.ua/library/ukraina/ekonomika-turboti-yak-karantin-i-pandemiya-covid-19-zminyuyut-spilnoti-praktiku-gromadskih-organizatsiy-ta-derzhavni-politiki

Thaler, R., & Sunstein, C. (2008), Nudge: Improving decisions about health, wealth and happiness, New Haven, CT: *Yale University Press*, 293 pp.

Rinčić, Iva, Sodeke, Stephen Olufemi and Muzur, Amir (2016), From integrative bioethics to integrative bioethics: European and American perspectives, *Journal international de bioéthique et d'éthique des sciences*, 4 (27), 105-117.

Hubenko, Hanna, Ph.D., is Associate Professor in the Department of Public Health of the Medical Institute (Sumy State University (SSU) and Founder and Head of 'Bioethics' (NGO), hanna.hubenko@gmail.com, bioethics.ngo@gmail.com.

Do we still need Ethics?

Morals hold the direction between opposite poles

Erny Gillen, Moral Factory, Germany

Abstract

The Corona crisis has created a collective situation worldwide for which many people were not prepared to subordinate their love for freedom, their ideas of self-realisation and their individual needs to social ethical requirements. This article shows which forms of ethics help to make productive use of existing moral reservoirs with their inner tensions for the future, before biological, climatological or technical constraints increasingly will reduce or even close down free choices. A supple and fluid morality, which aims at what is good, right, just and healthy, can learn from the way medicine deals with life crises.

Key words

freedom, health, medicine, morality, Moral Factory, self-realisation,

What morals are back?

Will the crisis triggered by the coronavirus also change our morals and ethics in the long term? It is already clear that we as a species are capable of changing our behaviour and actions very quickly and purposefully in the face of potential and real threats. For a long time, this evolutionary advantage, to which humanity owes its present cultures, was no longer as tangible and observable as it has been since the beginning of 2020.

When the severe COVID-19 disease broke out, there was a lack of proven therapies and the risk of over-stretching our health care systems was real. Slowly but surely, a unique and new collective situation emerged that infiltrated the consciousness of people around the world. The invisible virus could potentially affect anyone and it makes no difference. It came from the realm of nature, leaping from animals to humans as hosts and back again.

How would less scientifically developed cultures have reacted to this invisible and creeping phenomenon? Would they also have hidden and locked themselves away from the incomprehensible? Would they have protected themselves with prayers and expelled the virus and all those visibly affected by it with exorcisms? Would they also have washed their hands and protected their airways in the open street? Or would they have excluded particularly affected areas or groups from their societies? Narratives and images about plague, cholera, malaria or the so-called Spanish flu suggest that the current behavioural patterns are archaically deeply rooted in human beings, as not yet fixed animal (Nietzsche 1954: No. 61). The movement data freely provided by Apple and Google (Yogeshwar) even show that most people did not wait for the policy of lockdown at all, but had already consistently withdrawn from circulation days before the respective nationally declared crisis situations. Here it becomes clear that it was not politics that set the pace, but the actions of citizens and their expectations of politics.

The dictum "First the eating, then the morality" could have been well documented by extraterrestrial observers as well. The hamster purchases and police operations in shopping malls will be remembered as lasting images, as will the struggle for the last roll of toilet paper, condoms, or bottles of red wine in the otherwise busy temples of consumption in the Western world with their contemplative display cases and flaneurs. What the roll of toilet paper, the condom, or the bottle of red wine meant for individuals was the masks for the states that were not afraid to mobilise their also military means and forces for pirate shopping on the black market and to set up blockades in the open trading area. The observers from outer space could have documented another archaic reaction, namely the protection of territory. The sovereignty reflex of grown groups (Han) led to border closures in the European Union, for example, which are difficult to explain from an epidemiological point of view, and the largest ever worldwide return flights of the own population.

The external observers would probably have written in their logbooks: "As far as we can tell, an unseen phenomenon seems to provoke a largely orderly retreat into the safety of their own nests and groups. Within a few days and weeks it became quiet on planet Earth. The view to the highest mountains and into the depths of the oceans has improved considerably. The pristine nature spreads again to the cities and settlements. From this distance there is not (anymore) much of the reported human superiority to be seen. Whether and when the inhabitants will come out of their hiding places again cannot be predicted at the beginning of April 2020, according to the calendar applicable on planet Earth. "

What could not be seen from this great distance are the high moral achievements on the new front of the disease. Many people have not been idle in their initial shock. The will to live and survive made not only the individual but also the human species resilient and creative in dealing with the new enemy. Doctors and nurses, salesmen and transporters, producers of food and hygiene products were recognised as systemically relevant to this situation and received organised applause from the hiding places. A new public sphere, new forms of private, commercial and political communication emerged thanks to cables and virtual networks laid earlier, which made it possible to connect people who were otherwise physically close to each other and among decision-makers from the protected spaces. Despite all the self-isolation, people have found ways to communicate and to organise themselves locally, regionally and even globally, away from the increasingly better understood sources of danger. Their language and their ability to cooperate strategically under new conditions has also confirmed humanity as the crown of creation to the new viral contender called Corona. The love of freedom that otherwise isolates the individual, his exclusive ideas of self-realisation and individual needs had recognised and accepted the needs of the community as a current priority. We will come back to the different motives for this abrupt change in the behaviour of many.

At the time of writing this paper in June 2020, people still face their most difficult challenge. How should they organise their social and economic activities under the new conditions of the Corona crisis? The cyber-specialists from extraterrestrial space heard a hullabaloo in countless video conferences and telephone calls, as is typical for new beginnings. They were unable to determine the exact meaning because they lacked the code for the human language system. But the increase in the intensity of the conversations and several repetitive sounds such as 'benefit', 'state', 'or', 'ruin', 'vaccine', 'therapy' and 'COVID19' 'and' 'politics' alone suggested that at least three large clusters dominated the lively exchange.

The will to live and survive is also in the foreground in this phase, in which everyone slowly comes to the surface again, and with it the second nature of man, his morality. Non-governmental organisations and critical parties are openly raising the questions: in which directions society, public health and joint economic activity should evolve? How should the three public goods of 'public health', 'social life' and 'economic activity' be better balanced? The balance to be achieved must respect human rights as much as the natural environment, which must also provide future generations with its resources.

The United Nations and companies that are concerned about sustainability and justice join this discourse about people's morality for the future. On the other hand those questions face a wall of silence or open resistance. Behind this wall stand united those who are convinced that the Corona story was just a serious accident. After the accident sites have been cleared up and the victims have been compensated, everything should continue as it was before the tragic event. It is to be feared that the old rifts between the one and the other, the good and the bad, the value conservatives and the open liberals will once again dominate the discussions. The either-or logic is back. And with it the big moral questions: What is good? What is right?

Using opposite polarities productively

It is precisely here at the interface of morality that it is worth pausing for a moment. Are we on a helpful track when we approach the questions of morality with exclusive answers? Does good exclude evil? Or are we dealing with a living polarity (Guardini)? If the not-good does not simply coincide with evil as its negation, but represents its opposite polarity, then both can be thought of together. What would apply to moral intentions should also apply to the determination of factual logic with its counter-concepts of 'right' and 'wrong'. If we dare to leave behind the exclusive dualism in order to allow productive polarities, we take a step into another way of understanding morals and ethics.

For this unusual understanding of morals and ethics as a continuous process between the polarities that determine them, we can learn a lot from practical medicine and nursing. This also moves between polarities, namely between 'healthy' and 'sick'. The one pole can only be understood in the tension with the other. Patients, nurses and doctors know what is going on in a person who experiences his body as healthy or sick for the first time. What happens to him opens up new dimensions that have always been present but were not consciously perceived. It is similar with moral bipolarity: it comes to the surface and into consciousness together with a dilemma.

Did the toilet paper hunters act right or wrong at the beginning of the crisis? Or perhaps they acted right and wrong? As a first step, I would like to argue that good and bad intentions determine us in a mixed and unseparated way, as well as our right and wrong actions. The next step will be to show how the respective opposites kinetically interact as polarities of a living tension. Before that, it will be clarified in more detail what a bipolar tension is in relation to a contradiction or an excluding dualism.

The problem addressed is as old as the history of philosophy. Well-known and controversial are above all the last great attempts of dialectic, with which Hegel and many others tried to resolve such tensions. In this process, the tension between polarities, such as rich and poor, those without rights and the powerful, is lifted to a third level in a tour de force of reason, on which the polar opposites dissolve and reconcile within the same people. Communism or socialism did not succeed to effectively reconcile the opposites in a given society. Rather, they have created or allowed new antagonisms and injustices to arise. Also Christianity in the discipleship of Jesus of Nazareth has not succeeded in opening a third way, but oscillates indecisively between opposite positions. At the same time, the One made its Founder did not want to abolish the law, but to fulfil it with his Sermon on the Mount.

Is the short phase of the collective situation of consciousness, created by the corona virus, of being one vulnerable human family enough to respond to dualisms and constraints with a philosophy of the living-concrete? Today's science and medicine could be our guide with their approach of trial and error on the trail of a renewed understanding of morality and ethics. Their approach owes its success, among other things, to Karl Popper's recipe, which reversed the logic of power through proof by the logic of falsification. In an open society, one can and should happily experiment. As long as society is willing to learn from mistakes, it remains in a logic of research. What is good and right, evil and wrong is not determined in advance, but is tested and openly evaluated with determination.

Nobody simply knows and there is no secret knowledge that is only accessible to a few. The search for therapies and vaccines to challenge the uninvited virus shows how science works. Interim results and hypotheses are controversially and respectfully examined and rejected, written and rewritten among experts. Science is the skillful handling of knowledge and ignorance.

Politics, too, has had to come out before the people as a power that navigates from point to point between knowledge and ignorance, between certainty and uncertainty. Between acting too quickly and intervening too hesitantly, the crisis managers in the respective countries had to explain themselves almost daily on the basis of new findings and other arguments. As long as the plausibility and in some cases also the authenticity of the decision-makers was given, the majority of people followed what they understood and accepted.

In the first hot phase around COVID-19, the majority of us as humanity have proven that our morality is very quickly adaptable and changeable when we are individually and socially challenged. The observer from outside can easily prove this with the photographs of deserted places and streets, groups keeping their distance and the many masks that have become fashionable. The people on the outside behave differently before the crisis than during and after it. But why do they do this? Out of a moral conviction that they do not want to harm themselves or others? Out of selfish fear of being infected themselves? Out of pure fashion?

The danger of dualism lurks behind the answers, especially when one motive is qualified as good and the other as bad. Should we now focus on the reasons, i.e. the real moral question, the good and bad behaviour or the right and wrong doing? After the Second World War, now the penultimate collective experience of large parts of the world, common normative sentences were agreed upon in the constitution of human rights without giving reasons for them, because otherwise the signatories would not have found agreement (Kühnlein-Wils). Even today we all pay the price of this compromise of the powerful. Can our tolerance of ambiguity today withstand the fact that normative sentences are understood and justified in this way by the one and in another?

The direction within the polarities makes the difference

In order to decisively put a stop to the appearance and the real danger of arbitrariness or relativism, it is time to come to the productivity criterion of the theory of polarities[1]. It inscribes itself in a philosophy of life, in dissociation from a philosophy of being or technology. Life as an expression of entropy develops along the fuzziness of the immovable. Where the blurs leave the subject free to choose, he or she is free to choose and to realise his or her decision as an individual. Where the subject does not leave its choice to chance, but submits it to its will, it acts morally and ties its expectation of the future to this decision.

Again, the constitutive contrast between 'sick' and 'healthy' from medicine can help us as an analogy. It all depends on the direction our actions take. The sick person can let go in his illness and surrender to it. But he can also struggle and fight for his dwindling health together with his doctors and nurses. In both cases one will avoid the extremes and try to keep the leading direction "health" in mind.

But are we even able to determine a direction? Many individual decisions, which are perceived as free, can today be calculated statistically and in part down to the individual person from their previous behaviour, that is to say: their choices can be foreseen (Zuboff). Yesterday's

---

[1] I am here adopting the formal principle developed by Romano Guardini in his main work in the 1920s, (Der Gegensatz), however, without his idiosyncratic content. He formulated his theory at a similarly uncertain time as the one we are currently experiencing between latent and acute crises and uncertainties. The call for clarity, unambiguity and power was as great then as it is today. Between the great ideologies and narratives of liberalism, socialism or communism, he wanted to use his own doctrine of polar oppositions to clear a specific path for humane development that was not exclusive but inclusive.

economy before the corona break, which some are striving for again, can be described as a de-centralised and interconnected planned economy in more or less open systems of competing and cooperating interests. With the 'just in time' or 'on demand' functions, production and distribution chains were created in the large data centres of the economy, which served the customer and his sometimes individualised product more and more efficiently, even into personalised medicine. The energy consumption for the virtual machine of our global economy is enormous and is constantly increasing. Some people see this form of satisfying their needs as having no alternative. They have built their lifestyle on the smooth running of this invisible market.

Since the price is paid in money and the costs to others and to nature are kept behind the curtain of not-knowing, the economic machine driven by money and profit can determine the rhythm of life of the payers as well as that of its maintenance staff. Incidentally, from the machine's point of view it does not matter who it serves or whether it stutters because of supply or demand. The bigger it is and the faster it turns, the more unimportant are the occasional local failures, whether on the input or output side.

This economy was massively slowed down and partly stopped by the lockdown for the sake of people's lives and survival. The hygienic conditions under which the economic machine can be restarted were quickly worked out and are already largely in place among the people. But even among the business lobbyists, the TINA representatives (There Is No Alternative) are making themselves scarce. The money-makers in the central banks and political leaders more and more link the holding of vast sums of money to moral conditions such as the renunciation of dividends or bonus payments, but also to more climate-friendly growth. Less audible are the voices demanding more justice for this 'reset' of the economy.

But who is to shape this bumpy and step by step new start with money borrowed from the future? Does money finally reveal itself in this reset as a narrative without any ties to services or products? To whom is the newly printed money entrusted? The customers, the producers or service providers? How do we finance the systemically relevant social and health centres? What role should the state play? What role is left to the decision-makers in the economic centres?

These questions and many more are open to free choices. The current blurs and acute uncertainties are a wide doorway for our freedom. Here and now, it must be enough to mention some alternatives and options, such as an unconditional basic income or low-emission or emission-free production. Again, it is not about playing off the right or the good against the wrong or the evil. Otherwise we would be back in the scheme of dualism. In this tense polarity, however, it is morally important to give a direction to one's choices and actions. Good intentions are better than bad ones, and right action is preferable to wrong.

The Corona situation has shown that we are able to reorganise ourselves quickly and purposefully as human beings if we recognise the situation, understand the reasons and accept them. In this still ongoing situation, will it be possible to develop a narrative for a good and just coexistence of all people worldwide in order to become more crisis-resistant and resilient to future threats to our species? Do we develop an open-ended moral language that unites us and uses the spectrum of polarities to make statements of direction that serve different interests?

In concrete terms, this would mean enriching the private and public discourse with questions of moral direction and justification. We are "back again from our hiding places" with our silent, tested and adaptable morals. We just have learned that life is not just routine, but remains open for beautiful and ugly surprises. In that vein we should now also be able to deal with our own anthropodicy in a relaxed and calm way: we can act good and bad, just and unjust. The Corona crisis has produced enough positive and negative situations and experiences that cannot be divided up again dualistically, but sometimes flowed into each other unseparated and mixed up. In this field of tension, from which we cannot escape if we want to develop, it is important to give priority to the good and the right. And that, in turn, can only be done in discourse and action. We should no longer hide from our reasons and motives. In this explicit work on our morals, professional ethicists can, where desired and helpful, step in as moderators.

Professional ethics, which itself does not represent an moral point of view of its own, cultivates the philosophical craft of right argumentation and knows the pitfalls of naturalistic fallacy, for example, when a direct conclusion is drawn from is to ought. Medicine, military and slowly also the economic sciences have already partially integrated these competencies for their own humane development and use comprehensible moral arguments in dealing with their counterparts. These differ from biological, climatological or technical arguments. The latter do not automatically guide action, but provide data from the nature of things, which are to be incorporated into political and moral calculations. It is about goals and not about methods, as the nationally differing distance rules or multiple, hygienic and fashionable mouth and nose protection utensils show. Morality dies a slow death where it is replaced by practical constraint instead of being understood as a creative way to shape our freedom.

Test and evaluate freedom!

Which pairs of polarities can help us to shape the future in freedom and responsibility? As I have already explained, my thesis here is that moral thought and action is a matter of development that cannot be separated from the polarities of good and evil, right and wrong. Even from our wrong, evil or unjust actions we can learn how and what we can do better if we have the courage to attribute the negative to ourselves. None other than Pope Francis writes a remarkable sentence about this in Evangelii gaudium, his declaration of government for the further development of the Catholic Church: *"Even people who can be considered dubious on account of their errors have something to offer which must not be overlooked" (n. 236).*

Develop ideas for reality

We remain learners if we keep the polarity between reality and ideas permanently in mind and evaluate it. Which realities determine our lives, and which ideas? Especially the novel corona virus has shown us and still shows us that we have not yet fully grasped it with our readymade ideas. Whether vaccines will ever be able to combat it is as open as the search for a drug. Whether business trips will ever regain their familiar and symbolic meaning is just as questionable as permanent home schooling. In any case, our wealth of ideas and the courage to implement them effectively has experienced an undreamed-of heyday with the crisis. What was introduced as a substitute solution may also partly survive beyond the Corona period, such as working from home.

But the reality that we create anew with our decisions is constantly changing. This reality must be examined with the primordial question of morality: Should we do that? We are back at the reasons and motives why we act in this or another way. These give life our identity and take it away from the rule of the nobody, as Hannah Arendt put it in a nutshell. Reality does not have to be as it is. Where it is fragile or blurred, we can work alone and together to change it. For this we need ideas that can be tested as hypotheses until they are discarded or sufficiently improved. In this way we give reality a first place and make it the benchmark for our ideas. Perhaps it is precisely our mass society that is about to breaking up into many new real segments, which will make it harder for future pathogens than the current monoculture.

Open existing spaces for time

A second polarity that can help us in the moral evaluation of meaningful next steps is the constitutive tension of space and time. We have first outwitted the virus with our understanding of space and time. By buying time by retreating into safe spaces, we have tactically deprived it of its breeding ground. The same tactic is used with the countless bridge loans. The self-invented time has often helped man to cunningly dig a pit for the stronger ones as they ascend from the realm of primeval nature. With time, we have been able to create ever new and larger spaces, which we have designed with our own cultures. As people who are at home on the go, we need spaces that change with us and our situations; not fortresses for eternity. Our fictional external observers from extraterrestrial space will easily recognise the traces of the new pathogen in the architecture and urbanism of the future, as well as we are able to follow the traces of the cholera epidemic along the underground sewers and wide boulevards in Paris and many other cities.

Learning Transfer

How we should use the time in the race against the impending climate catastrophe is another question to our morality, which we cannot avoid further in our current directly or indirectly threatened spaces. Whether we have enough time to work out technical solutions is uncertain. Just as uncertain is whether a few will manage to escape to Mars, while planet Earth is slowly becoming uninhabitable for most. With the polarity of space and time, time should be used to point the way for the design of our changing habitats. Together with our creative power to create effective and symbolic realities, the binomial space and time provides us with an excellent toolbox for shaping the future. Whether our lifelong and survival skills are sufficient to technically master the artificially intelligent and partly autonomous systems we desire is another major question for our morality and future. Since these systems do not share our sense of time, the risk is all the greater that we are in the process of outwitting ourselves with this last invention of mankind.

What ethical structures (Gillen (a)) should now be created in order to approach the questions of the future under the impulse of the corona crisis in an open, but cheerful discourse about our morals? Ethical advisory bodies have proven their worth, especially during the acute threat. Moral movements such as "Fridays for Future" or "Black Lives Matter" unite millions of people to denounce the bloody and dirty wounds of our future-blind economy and ruthless coexistence. The unmistakable calls for more justice among people and with nature need honest forums that test and evaluate changes in terms of hypotheses before they become radicalised, because no progress can be seen. Ethics as an applied philosophy should be further integrated into all areas of academic teaching and research. Decisive for the future will also be small-scale moral experiments by courageous citizens who, over time, will create alternative spaces and realities and thus effectively exemplify which other possibilities are realistic. Only lived morality is convincing. The Corona situation has also confirmed this in an exemplary manner.

Man has the resources to shape his life differently. If he orients himself again and again to the good, the right, the just and the healthy, he will find points of application as an individual and as a member of his species to shape himself and his environment in such a way (Gillen (b)) that the freedom of all of us will also in future become larger and not smaller. Freedom is the vehicle for our morality and responsibility. For them it is worth the effort!

12.6.2020

References

Nietzsche 1954. Nietzsche, Friedrich, Jenseits von Gut und Böse, in: Works in three volumes, Munich 1954, Volume 2.

Yogeshwar 2020. Yogeshwar, Ranga, phase two. First, citizens, politics and science were in harmony in the Corona Crisis. That is changing rapidly and that is dangerous, in: Frankfurter Allgemeine Zeitung, Saturday, May 2, 2020, No. 102, page 9.

Han 2020. Han, Byung-Chul, La emergencia viral y el mundo de mañana, in: El Pais, 22 March 2020: https://elpais.com/ideas/2020-03-21/la-emergencia-viral-y-el-mundo-de-manana-byung-chul-han-el-filosofo-surcoreano-que-piensa-desde-berlin.html, accessed 9 June 2020.

Guardini 1985, Guardini, Romano, The Contrast. Attempts at a philosophy of the living-concrete, Mainz: Mathias Grünewald-Verlag, 1985, 3rd edition.

Popper 1935. Popper, Karl, Logic of Research. On the epistemology of modern science, Vienna: Springer-Verlag, 1935.

Kühnlein-Wils 2019. Kühnlein, Michael; Wils, Jean-Pierre, The West and Human Rights. In interdisciplinary discussion with Hans Joas, Baden-Baden: Nomos Publishing Company, 2019.

Zuboff 2019. Zuboff, Shoshona, The Age of Surveillance Capitalism. The Fight for A Human Future at The New Frontier of Power, New York: Hachette Book Group, 2019.

Arendt 2016. Arendt, Hannah, Vita activa oder vom tätigen Leben, Munich: Piper, 2016 (18th edition), p. 51.

Gillen 2005 (a). Gillen, Erny, promote and demand so-called 'ethical committees' ethical competence?", in: European Research Society for Ethics. (Ed.). Societas Ethica. Annual Report 2005, 2005, ISSN: 1814-8204, 2005.

Gillen 1989 (b). Gillen, Erny, How Christians act and think ethically. On the debate about the autonomy of morality in the context of Catholic theology, Würzburg: Echter, 1989.

Francis 2020. Francis, Pope, Evangelii gaudium: http://www.vatican.va/content/francesco/de/apost_exhortations/documents/papa-francesco_esortazione-ap_20131124_evangelii-gaudium.html, accessed 9 June 2020.

Dr. theol. Erny Gillen (*1960), founder and director of Moral Factory, has taught and published on ethics in theology, medicine and organisations in Luxembourg and Freiburg i.Br. for over twenty years. As a practical ethicist, he has led Caritas in Luxembourg, was President of Caritas Europa and First Vice-President of Caritas Internationalis, and Vicar General of the Archdiocese of Luxembourg in times of extensive restructuring.- erny.gillen@moralfactory.com

The Pandemic Crisis and what it reveals about Western and Eastern Ethics

Alicia Hennig, Southeast University, P.R. China

Abstract

Eastern ethics, specifically Confucian ethics, stresses the value of social relations, the individual as embedded in society. In Confucianism, a human being is not considered as 'human' per se merely on the basis of her biological and physical features that are different from animals. Western ethics, on the other hand emphasizes the value of the individual, freedom, and the idea of inherent human dignity *qua* being 'biologically' human. What are the implications of these very different perspectives regarding human dignity and the role of the individual in society? Is it possible to combine these two perspectives and thereby advancing our understanding of ethics and what makes a good human being?

Key words

Eastern ethics, Confucian ethics, human, dignity, individual, society, good and evil

1. Introduction

Most characteristic of Chinese philosophy in general is its pragmatic nature and 'this-world concerns', which are expressed in its orientation towards every-day life and related problems (Chan 1967; Fung 1958; Moore 1967). It concentrated on studying human affairs more broadly and made character cultivation a major tenet in order to maintain social order. In the context of character cultivation, constant learning and self-improvement are particularly emphasized in Classical Confucianism.

Through Confucius (Chinese: *Kongzi* 孔子, 551–479 BC, Chan 1969) born in the mid fifth century BC in the state of Lu in today's Shandong province in China (Slingerland 2003), emerged the most prominent way of thinking associated with *ru* 儒. Originally presenting a class of scholar-officials specializing in transmitting and preserving the ideological legacy of the previous Zhou dynasty (1111 to 249 BC, Chan, 1969), *ru* became synonymous for the Confucian way of thinking (Slingerland 2009). *Ru* in that way is a "philosophy of social organization" and of daily life (Fung 1958:22), combining the preserved Zhou traditions with a more 'egalitarian' approach, enabling anyone regardless of social rank to become morally *good* if willing and committed.

Being almost unimpeded[1] for over more than two millennia, Confucianism and later Neo-Confucianism as the dominant state doctrine and religion had a significant and long lasting influence on the way of Chinese thinking (Chan 1967). Nevertheless, it is important to keep in mind that Confucius's own 'philosophy' is only a part of what is subsumed under the label Confucianism or in Chinese *ru jia* 儒家.

2. Confucian Ethics

Confucian ethics largely rests on three core concepts derived from Confucius' philosophy. These are *li* 禮, ritual, which is embedded in a hierarchical system of social relations; *yi* 義, appropriateness (Yu, 2006; Slingerland, 2009), and *ren* 仁, translated with benevolence (Chan

---

[1] Confucianism as state doctrine ended with the downfall of the Qing Empire in 1912 (Chan 1969) and further declined through the revolution and the introduction of Communism in 1949 (ibid.), where under Mao's reign it was deemed 'reactionist' and was consequently banned. Yet, a steady come back of Confucian thought, and Chinese traditional culture more broadly can be observed since Mao's death (Wren 1984; The Economist 2007).

1969), humaneness (Allan 1997), or humanity (Ivanhoe 2000). The latter, *ren,* is the capacity that makes the human being an exemplary human being and hence a role model, *junzi* 君子.

The Zhou li 禮

The most important – and inherently practical – element Confucius took from the foregone Zhou traditions was *li*. Confucius was very fond of what he recognized as praiseworthy traditions in Zhou dynasty conveying virtue and wisdom (Slingerland 2003), which he perceived as being significantly distorted during his lifetime.

In the past, *li* may have referred to mainly religious ritual, but by the time of Zhou dynasty it already prescribed objectively proper behavior in a broader sense, referring to rite, ceremony, and general manners (Schwartz 1985; Lai 2006). Through ritual, the human realm and the realm of the spirits were bound together. *Li* also reflected hierarchical relations, as what was regarded as proper behavior was highly dependent on one's status in society. As Schwartz (1985:67) puts it: "[…] what makes *li* the cement of the entire normative socio-political order is that it largely involves the behavior of persons related to each other in terms of role, status, rank, and position within a structured society". Thus, *li* in its entirety stands for the "foundation of human society" (Schwartz 1985:71).

To master *li* one had to undergo intensive training in the sense of learning the classics and music, which requires a "personal investment in the performance of actions and quality of character" (Sim 2007:57). Through this training and investment, the way of perfect ritual practice could be internalized. Hence, *li* fulfilled two functions: to "reshape[ing] one's innate endowment" and to have "a kind of behavioral language" (Slingerland 2009:118) available, which allows one to become a good human being. *Li*, however, was not about blindly following rules and mechanically performing ritual. As noted above, already in Zhou dynasty, sincerity was seen as a requirement for truthfully following *li*. Accordingly, *li* requires "emotional commitment, combined with a refined sensibility, on the part of the practitioner" (Slingerland 2009:122; cf. *LY*[2] 3.12, 3.26, 17.11, and 19.1).

Yi 義 Appropriateness

Yi implies the capacity of having the 'right' sense regarding one's behavior (Yu 2006; Slingerland 2009) and feelings (Yu 2007). It requires a deeper understanding and internalization of what is 'proper' or 'right'. Having *yi* signals a more profound understanding of morality beyond compliance with formal rules and moral codes (Slingerland 2009). Only this allows for the necessary flexibility to respond to a variety of situations (ibid.; cf. *LY* 4.10, 15.37). As Lai (2006:80) puts it: "Moral reasoning is characterized by flexibility. There is attention to the relevant details of each situation (Analects 1:8; 18:8) and this includes consideration of the particular circumstances and disposition of individuals". Hence, what is *yi* (appropriate) in each situation will vary (Sim 2007). Essentially, *yi* is "a sense of how to apply[ing] the rites in a given circumstance" (Sim 2007:167; cf. Lai 2006). *Yi* thereby enables the capacity of proper ethical judgment, which prevents following rules, like *li*, blindly.

According to Yu (2007), however, there are actually two dimensions to *yi*. On the one hand, *yi* can be seen as a quality or characteristic of ethical action. This quality implies that the action taken is in accordance with the values of the actor's socio-cultural environment. This is the "outer" *yi* represented by "what is appropriate to do" (Yu 2007:144). On the other hand,

---

[2] If not indicated otherwise, the translation used here for Confucius's *Analects/Lunyu* (*LY*) is Slingerland's (2003).

there is the "inner" *yi*, which is more of an intellectual capacity, representing a quality of an ethical agent, that is, "the virtue of judging and doing what is appropriate" (ibid.). Similar to Aristotle, *yi* enables a person not just to comply with formal rules or to follow a role model, but to judge for herself autonomously.

Ren仁Humanity

Ren originally referred to an aristocratic and martial, and hence physical, ideal. However, Confucius transformed *ren* into an ethical ideal (Slingerland 2009), thereby also emphasizing the relational, deeply social aspect in this notion. *Ren* cannot be learned in solitude but only be cultivated in human relations since it does not present an intellectual quality or a kind of scientific knowledge (Lin 1974).

Although often translated as "benevolence" or "humanness"/"humanity"[3], *ren* is more than just a single virtue. Sinologists usually differentiate between *ren* presenting a particular virtue (narrow sense) and *ren* presenting an "all-encompassing ethical ideal" (broader sense) (Shun, 2002:53; cf. Slingerland 2009; Sim 2007). Regarding the first interpretation, *ren* is considered a virtue amongst other Confucian virtues, which is linked with wisdom, *zhi* 智, ritual, *li* 禮 and learning, *xue* 學 (Sim 2007). The second interpretation considers *ren* as the "goal of all cultural practices" (Slingerland 2009:121; cf. Lin 1974), and is seen as being "linked up with virtually all other basic Confucian concepts" (Tu 1985:87; cf. Sim 2007). Thereby, *ren* symbolizes a kind of 'overarching virtue' of Goodness (Slingerland 2003, 2009), a "manifestation of humanity on its commonest and highest state of perfection" (Sim 2007: 25). According to Slingerland (2009; cf. Shun 2002), *ren* in the Analects is more often used in this latter, general sense.

There appears to be an interdependent, symbiotic relation between *ren* and *li* (Hennig 2016). Without *ren*, a person is unable to observe *li* properly (*LY* 3.3) and can only follow it in a mechanistic, blind way, thereby reducing abiding by *li* to a mere formality to maintain face or reputation (Lin 1974). Only having *ren* enables a person to follow *li* by heart and by what is natural (ibid.). On the other hand, being able to properly observe *li* only makes a person being *ren* (*LY* 12.1).

Both Confucius and Mencius (Chinese: *Mengzi* 孟子, 371–289 BC, Chan 1969) see human nature as inherently good and as being an inborn capacity (Schwartz 1985; Lai 2006). Yet, Mencius, in contrast to Confucius, emphasizes four particular virtues[4]: *ren*, *yi*, *li*, and in addition *zhi* 智 (wisdom) (Yu 2007). The virtues can be realized through four predispositions or 'sprouts', *si duan* 四端, residing in each person's *xin* 心 (literally translated as "heart", but meaning 'heart-mind'[5]), which are compassion, respect, shame, and a sense of right and wrong (Chong 2009; Allan 1997; cf. *Mencius* 2A6[6]). *Xin* has "affective, cognitive, and volitional elements" (Ivanhoe, 2009, p. xii), helping us to exercise (self-)reflection as to eventually making us

---

[3] However, according to Sim (2007), *ren* as humanity does not imply a kind of love, which is supposed to be extended beyond one's relatives. It is not comparable to Mozi's idea of universal love'. Rather, *ren* "is applied in decreasing intensity within concentric circles around the individual" (Niedenführ and Hennig 2020; cf. Yan 2001).

[4] The term 'virtue' (*de* 德) in Chinese philosophy, however, is different to the ancient Greek concept, where it presents "acquired moral habits" (Zhang 2016:19). It stands for potency or capacity and thus virtues in Chinese philosophy do not present primary faculties but "only secondary faculties enabling actions (e.g. the quality of justice as propensity to act justly)" (ibid.).

[5] That *xin* is translated with "heart-mind" instead of literally only "heart" also indicates that for Mengzi reason and emotion are going together (Chong 2009).

[6] If not indicated otherwise, the translation for the *Mencius*/*Mengzi* used here is Bloom's (2009).

realize the joy in moral action. The predispositions emerging out of *xin* are a person's "native endowment", *cai* 才 (Chong 2009:XX) or "ability" (Robinson 2016:183), for being good[7]. Although having *cai*, the sprouts can only flourish and develop further into virtues and thereby fully actualize *xing*, human nature, if these are nurtured (through reflection and learning), and are provided with the right environmental conditions (Chong 2009; cf. *Mencius* 6A8; Ivanhoe 2000; Schwartz 1985). However, although all people generally dispose of sufficient *cai*, the concrete 'level' of it may vary (Allan 1997). Similarly, although human beings have these sprouts, which theoretically guarantee human goodness, not every human being is actually good (Van Norden 2005).

Same as Confucius, Mencius believed in the importance of *li*, and that these need to be learned, as the *li* are "ultimately the external expressions of a capacity for 'humanity [*ren*] and righteousness [*yi*]'" (Schwartz 1986:264). *Yi* in the *Mengzi*, however, is seen as an "innate moral sensitivity to moral righteousness" (Lai 2006:75), which is not an innate quality and thus needs to be cultivated (Yu 2007). *Ren* is interpreted as a feeling of compassion and expressing humaneness, similar to Confucius. It is "to be human in the fullest sense, the state that people reach when their shoots which sprout in their hearts have been nurtured to attain their greatest glory" (Allan 1997:110). Humaneness is the highest virtue in early Confucian thinking, as only this quality makes a human truly human and separates us from animals: "To be "humane" [*ren*] is to be the most perfectly developed example of the human species" (ibid.). Mengzi believes that everyone principally can become a sage since everyone has this inborn capacity. Whether the latter can be realized depends on adequate nurturing and the conditions that are given by one's environment (Chong 2009).

Xunzi's (Chinese: *Xunzi* 荀子, 298–238 BC, Chan 1969) philosophy, on the other hand, is, in some sense, opposed to Mencius. He believes human nature is neither specifically good nor bad but simply our desires and feelings with which we as human beings are born with, and that initially lack an inborn 'compass' for what is right (Chong 2009; Hutton 2005). This lack eventually produces a kind of "basic selfishness" (Lai 2006:22; Allan 1997). He challenges the idea of a 'native endowment' for being good and views goodness as a "result of human artifice", *wei* 偽 (Chong 2009:196), or "deliberate effort"[8] (Hutton 2005), and in that sense, a result of "education and socialization" (Sim 200:140). Thus, external restraint in the sense of self-cultivation and refinement is necessary to prevent us from falling into wrongdoing (Hutton 2005). Furthermore, Xunzi distinguishes here between capacity and ability. For him having the capacity in the sense of a 'native endowment' does not necessarily lead to ability; there is no precondition necessary for learning ritual and having moral ability (Chong 2009)[9]. *Li* and moral principles are seen as a 'constitutive structure' to be worked on rather than being inborn, this involves significant effort on behalf of the human being to realize those (ibid.). Accordingly, learning, *xue*, in the *Xunzi* is as essential as in the *Lunyu* in the context of self-cultivation (Schwartz 1986). Developing a good nature requires constant practice and entails an intensive learning process.

---

[7] According to Liu (2013:57), *cai* could be also read as "potentiality" (cf. Schwartz 1985; Allan 1997), thereby coming closer to Aristotelian concepts. Originally, according to the earliest Chinese dictionary Shuo Wen, *cai* means "germinating grasses" (Liu 2013:57) or "seedling" (Allan 1997:111).

[8] By pointing to "deliberate effort" Xunzi's philosophy presented a clear counter-position to the school of thought as expressed in the *Laozi* for example, which is about 'non-action' in the sense of non-deliberate action (Hutton 2005).

[9] See here Xunzi's potter analogy; "Thus, when the potter shapes the clay to create the vessel, this is the acquired nature of the potter and not the product of anything inherent in his nature." (Chong 2009:198)

3. Ethical Answers from Confucianism to the Pandemic Crisis

What we can see from the above-presented ethical concepts in Confucianism is the strong emphasis on self-cultivation. Self-cultivation and learning are the ultimate starting point for actualizing one's (innate) capacities and becoming human (Zhang 2016). Thus, the concept of the human being in Confucianism is rather a "moral and social" one, going beyond the biological (Bai 2019:35). Only in our social relations we become truly human(e).

Linked to this perception of the human being, as being defined through social and moral aspects is the concept of human dignity. Although the term dignity is not present anywhere in Classical Confucian texts, there is a notion of dignity *qua* the endowment of inner virtues (the Mencian sprouts) one is born with that are unique to human beings, appreciation for this endowment, and the capacity to fully realize those virtues (Zhang 2016; Bloom 1998). In Confucian societies, fully realizing one's human potential and becoming *ren* by learning civilized (role-based) behavior especially through *li* and *yi* is equal to having dignity (Koehn and Leung 2004).

That every human being is endowed with these capacities – having a "common humanity" – entails some notion of equality and thus the need for mutual respect (Bloom 1998:94). Yet, to what extent a human being is able to develop her capacities can make a difference eventually (ibid.). Ni (2014:186) is more explicit: Dignity is not the result of something we possess commonly but "because we have a sense of what we can and should become". According to Zhang (2016:29) an "action is dignity-enhancing if it cultivates, practices or exhibits one's virtues; it is dignity-reducing (thus degrading) if it fails to exercise virtues or prevents anyone from cultivating or exercising virtues". Thus, the Confucian concept of the human being and human dignity is oriented towards progress of conscious self-refinement rather than being a given through mere biological features. Human dignity is an achievement (of self-cultivation) rather than a right or an entitlement (Ni 2014; Koehn and Leung 2004; Bloom 1998). As Ni (2014:182) points out: "There is no ground for anyone to claim unconditional entitlement for respectful treatment regardless of what oneself does". However, disregarding the need for mutual respect diminishes one's *yi* (appropriateness) and thus one's cultivation level towards humanity and dignity (Zhang 2016; Ni 2014:184): "The humiliation inflicted on us by others shows their lack of humanity, not our lack of dignity".

In the context of the pandemic, a concept of human dignity based on achievement rather than on entitlement reminds us of being more modest, and lenient with and respectful towards others. More solidarity could be promoted once we stop being occupied with mainly thinking of ourselves by claiming rights we feel entitled to and take for granted, and instead invest our productivity in becoming better human beings, which can only happen by properly and carefully conducting our social relations. The pandemic illustrated already the relentless effort medical personnel put in saving lives, risking to getting infected themselves; emerging communities of engaged individuals helping other people with higher infection risk with doing errands; and by the general population now carefully sticking to novel safety rules. This solidarity and mutual care would not have happened if individuals were merely interested in having their own rights and entitlements fulfilled, like for example their individual access to medical services or their individual freedom of movement. Thus, especially in challenging times, we need to be able to look beyond the individual's rights and entitlements, understanding the bigger picture of a peaceful, cooperative society, which is ultimately grounded in solidarity. Solidarity is rooted in mutual respect. Whether this notion of respect is derived from the Enlightenment idea of all human beings sharing the same capacity for reason (Kant) or the ancient Chinese idea of all human beings sharing the same capacity for becoming human(e), a good human being, may not be decisive here. Yet, the difference is that with the latter comes a more progress-oriented understanding of our own life, the need for (constant) learning in life, and perhaps the aspiration to truly becoming a 'good' human being.

4. Looking beyond Western Ethics: The Need to Combine both East and West in the Age of Globalization and Global Crisis

The pandemic is global, and thus we need to better understand the meaning of ethics in different cultures and the different approaches to ethics across the globe. Living in a globalized world, we should aspire to learn from each other, enriching our understanding of our life and the world as such by looking beyond the values we have been socialized with. There is no single 'best' ethics to solve all problems. Combining diverse ethical concepts from across the globe helps us to better solve pressing issues due to a variety of solutions.

Neither collectivism nor individualism is exclusively preferable, and so is dignity neither as an achievement nor as an entitlement exclusively desirable. Only a combination and balancing of concepts and approaches enables us to overcome the natural limitations inherent in one single ethics. For example, we could balance collectivism and individualism by emphasizing solidarity and reciprocity on the one hand, and by emphasizing empowerment of the individual to release her from collective pressure on the other hand. We could balance the different perspectives on human dignity by coming to understand the need for constant learning and self-refinement as a purpose in life, for ourselves and for our social community on the one hand, and the need to protect human beings against infringements on the other hand.

References

Allan 1997. Allan, Sarah. Way of Water and Sprouts of Virtue. New York: State University of New York (SUNY) Press 1997

Bai, 2019. Bai, Tongdong. Against Political Equality: The Confucian Case. New Jersey: Princeton University Press 2019

Bloom 1998. Bloom, Irene. In W.T. De Bary, and W. Tu (Eds) Confucianism and Human Rights. New York: Columbia University Press 1998 94–116

Chan 1969. Chan, Wing-Tsit. A Source Book in Chinese Philosophy. New Jersey: Princeton University Press 1969

Chan 1967. Chan, Wing-Tsit. Chinese theory and practice, with special reference to humanism. In C. A. Moore (Ed) The Chinese mind: essentials of Chinese philosophy and culture. Honolulu: University of Hawaii Press 1967 11–30

Chong 2009. Chong, Kim-Chong. Classical Confucianism (2): Meng Zi and Xun Zi. In B. Mou (Ed) Routledge History of World Philosophies: History of Chinese Philosophy. New York: Routledge 2009 189–208

Fung 1958. Fung, Yu-Lan. A short history of Chinese philosophy. New York: MacMillan 1958

Hennig 2016. Hennig, Alicia. Three Different Approaches to Virtue in Business — Aristotle, Confucius, and Lao Zi. Frontiers of Philosophy in China, 11 (2016) 4: 556–586

Hutton 2005. Hutton, Eric L. Xunzi: Introduction and Translation. In B. W. Van Norden, and P. J. Ivanhoe (Eds) Readings in Classical Chinese Philosophy). Indianapolis: Hackett Publishing Company 2005 2nd edition 255–310

Ivanhoe 2009. Ivanhoe, Philip J. Introduction. In I. Bloom (Transl), and P. J. Ivanhoe (Ed) Mencius. New York: Columbia University Press 2009 ix–xxii

Koehn and Leung 2004. Koehn, Daryl and Leung, Alicia S. M. Western and Asian Business Ethics: Possibilities and Problems. In K. Leung, and S. White (Eds) Handbook of Asian Management. New York: Kluwer Academic Publishers 2004 265–292

Lai 2006. Lai, Karyn. Learning from Chinese Philosophies: Ethics of Interdependent and Contextualised Self. Burlington: Ashgate Publishing Company 2006

Lin 1974. Lin, Yü-Sheng. The Evolution of the Pre-Confucian Meaning of Jen 仁 and the Confucian Concept of Moral Autonomy. Monumenta Serica 31 (1974): 172–204.

Liu 2013. Liu, Xiusheng. Mencius, Hume and the Foundations of Ethics. New York: Routledge 2013

Moore 1967. Moore, Charles A. Introduction: the humanistic Chinese mind. In C. A. Moore (Ed) The Chinese mind: essentials of Chinese philosophy and culture. Honolulu: University of Hawaii 1967 1–10

Ni 2014. Ni, Peimin. Seek and You Will Find It; Let Go and You Will Lose It: Exploring a Confucian Approach to Human Dignity. Dao 13 (2014):173–198.

Niedenführ and Hennig 2020. Niedenführ, Matthias and Hennig, Alicia. Confucianism and Ethics in Management. In C. Neesham, and S. Segal (Eds) Handbook of Philosophy of Management. Netherlands: Springer

Robinson 2016. Robinson, Douglas. The Deep Ecology of Rhetoric in Mencius and Aristotle. Albany: State University of New York Press (SUNY) 2016

Schwartz 1985. Schwarz, Benjamin. The World of Thought in Ancient China. Cambridge, MA, US: The Belknap Press of Harvard University Press 1985

Shun, K.-L. 2002. Ren 仁 and Li 禮 in the Analects. In B. W. Van Norden (Ed) Confucius and the Analects: New Essays. New York: Oxford University Press 2002 53–72

Sim 2007. Sim, May. Remastering Morals with Aristotle and Confucius. Cambridge, UK: Cambridge University Press 2007

Slingerland 2003. Slingerland, Edward. Confucius Analects: With Selection from Traditional Commentaries. Indianapolis: Hackett Publishing Company 2003

Slingerland 2009. Slingerland, Edward. Classical Confucianism (1): Confucius and the Lun-Yü. In B. Mou (Ed.) Routledge History of World Philosophies: History of Chinese Philosophy. New York, US: Routledge 2009 107–136

The Economist 2007. Confucius Makes a Comeback. The Economist, 17 May 2007. [URL:https://www.economist.com/letters-to-the-editor-the-inbox/2007/05/28/confucius-makes-a-comeback-may-19th, visited January 31, 2019]

Tu 1985. Tu, Weiming. Confucian Thought: Selfhood as Creative Transformation. New York, US: State University of New York (SUNY) Press 1985

Van Norden 2005. Van Norden, Brian W. Mengzi (Mencius): Introduction and Translation. In B. W. Van Norden, and P. J. Ivanhoe (Eds) Readings in Classical Chinese Philosophy. Indianapolis: Hackett Publishing Company 2nd edition 2005 115–160

Wren 1984. Wren, Christopher S. A Return to the Thoughts of Confucius. The New York Times, 14 October 1984. [URL: https://www.nytimes.com/1984/10/14/weekinreview/a-return-to-the-thoughts-of-confucius.html, visited January 31, 2019]

Yan 2001. Yan, Yunxiang. Practicing kinship. In S. Franklin, and S. McKinnon (Eds) Relative values: reconfiguring kinship studies. Raleigh: Duke University Press 2001 224–245

Yu 2006. Yu, Jiyuan. Yi: Practical Wisdom in Confucius Analects. Journal of Chinese Philosophy 33 (2006) 3: 335–348.

Yu 2007. Yu, Jiyuan. The Ethics of Confucius and Aristotle. New York: Routledge 2007

Zhang 2016. Zhang, Qianfan. Human Dignity in Classical Chinese Philosophy. New York: Springer Nature 2016

Alicia Hennig is holding a full research position as Associate Professor of Business Ethics at the department of philosophy at Southeast University in Nanjing, China. She obtained her PhD in philosophy and applied ethics (business ethics) from Technical University Darmstadt, Germany with co-supervision from Thomas Pogge (Yale, CT, US). During her PhD she worked at a leading private business school in Germany, Frankfurt School of Finance and Management, and published first working papers on China and business ethics.

Her current research focuses on Chinese philosophy and its application in organizations in the context of values, ethics and innovation. In addition to her research she also has practical working experience gained at Chinese as well as foreign companies in China.

The Foundation and Functioning of the World Emergency COVID19 Pandemic Ethics Committee

Darryl Macer, Eubios Ethics Institute, New Zealand, Japan and Thailand

Abstract

The rationale for the establishment of the World Emergency COVID19 Pandemic Ethics (WE-COPE) Committee is the global need for ethical reflection and practice in order to enact and review policies and practices that will save lives. The paper will examine the processes of this multidisciplinary group of 50 persons of global background who are independent of government, living in different countries under different conditions during the same COVID-19 crisis. Could this model actually be an independent forum to develop good practices, and how much were the produced statements on mask use, triage, and the other dozen topics, actually useful, and for whom?

Key words

Bioethics, COVID-19, Ethics Committee, Triage, Mask, War, Eubios

1. World Emergency COVID19 Pandemic Ethics Committee

These are difficult times. All around the world, tens of thousands of people, young or old, rich or poor, from all walks of life have died in grim situations of the COVID-19 pandemic, especially in places suffering from insufficient infrastructure, human resources, protective equipment, and/or lack of clear triage decision-making protocols. There have been instances of dumping of bodies in rental trucks next to elderly homes, of denial of access of critically ill persons to basic medical care from hospitals or giving up on treating the elderly (just because of their age).

In this paper I will illustrate the application of the theory of bioethics to practice through the construction and functioning of an international ethics committee. I will refer to the identification of topics of significance and the development of consensus statements on triage, use of masks and use of the war metaphor in COVID-19 as illustrations of the effectiveness of this forum to deliberate on transnational and global bioethics issues.

The World Emergency COVID19 Pandemic Ethics Committee (WeCope) [https://www.eubios.info/world_emergency_covid19_pandemic_ethics_committee] is a multidisciplinary group of over forty persons from a variety of professional backgrounds of cross-cultural and global background who are independent of government, living in different countries under different conditions during the same COVID-19 crisis. We are tasked with the following:

1) To act as an independent forum to gather accounts of the experiences and perspectives, especially concerning good practices, and alleged human rights abuses.

2) To consider the interface between the theory and practice of ethics around the world and the need for ethical initiatives in research, policy, and information sharing in the world emergency responses and aftermath of the COVID-19 pandemic.

3) To compile and produce reports and policy statements that may guide individuals, civil society organizations (both non-profit and for-profit), governments, and international entities in their responses to the global health emergencies linked to COVID-19, which have utility both in the current pandemic and further ones.

4) To be of service to those who seek our assistance, and to the most vulnerable among us.

5) To act quickly and issue reports and statements quickly.

At the first meeting of the WeCope Committee, we agreed on a Modality of Work and Outputs of the Committee. We tried both Zoom and Skype as platforms and decided after one

Zoom meeting to continue to use group Skype as an easier forum. It was important that it is accessible to significantly more people around the world because of national restrictions. At first, we have committee discussion on different issues and selection of the most important topics. The current list of topics is below, and occasionally new topics are added. Next we assign each topic to a small group of volunteers that should write the kind of document considered needed. The members of the subcommittee can add additional persons and experts to each subcommittee in order to expand the number of minds at work on each topic.

Documents include written statements and discussion documents and academic papers on specific issues, which may make recommendations on specific policy options. The papers are also descriptive documents comparing the situation, policies and ethical approaches in different countries, in response to specific questions. Then we see submission of the written document developed by the sub-group to the committee for further discussion and further inputs. Where appropriate a draft is also discussed in a Virtual Conference among an even broader group of peers and the public. After several rounds of editing and brain-storming the statement or paper is released. In the appendix to this paper are three Statements as examples.

There is added Value of the WeCope Committee compared to other Forums due to its independence, being multidisciplinary, cross-cultural and having a more global background. There are members from a wide variety of professional backgrounds living in different countries under different conditions during the same COVID-19 crisis. As a result, we can act and issue reports and statements quickly.

The members sign all statements (unless they abstain), and include: Dr. Thalia Arawi (Lebanon), Dr. Mouna Ben Azaiz (Tunisia) , Dr. Lian Bighorse (San Carlos Apache Nation, USA), Dr. Andrew Bosworth (Canada), Dr. Rhyddhi Chakraborty (India, UK), Mr. Anthony Mark Cutter (U.K.), Dr. Mireille D'Astous (Canada), Dr. Ayoub Abu Dayyeh (Jordan), Dr. Nilza Maria Diniz (Brazil), Dr. Hasan Erbay (Turkey), Prof. Nader Ghotbi (Japan), Prof. Abhik Gupta (India), Prof. Soraj Hongladarom (Thailand), Prof. Miwako Hosoda (Japan) , Prof. Dena Hsin-Chen Hsin (Taiwan), Dr. Anower Hussain (Bangladesh), Prof. Bang-Ook Jun (Republic of Korea), Prof. Hassan Kaya (South Africa), Dr. Sumaira Khowaja-Punjwani (Pakistan), Prof. Julian Kinderlerer (South Africa), Dr. Lana Al-Shareeda Le Blanc (Iraq), Prof. Marlon Lofredo (the Philippines), **Dr. Manuel Lozano Rodríguez (Spain)** , Prof. Darryl Macer (New Zealand), Prof. Raffaele Mantegazza (Italy), **Dr. Aziza Menouni (Morocco)** , Dr. Endreya Marie McCabe (Delaware Nation, USA), Prof. Erick Valdés Meza (Chile, USA), Dr. Ravichandran Moorthy (Malaysia), Prof. Firuza Nasyrova (Tajikistan), Dr. Suma Parahakaran (Malaysia) , Prof. Maria do Céu Patrão Neves (Portugal) , Prof. Deborah Kala Perkins (USA) , Prof. Osama Rajkhan (Saudi Arabia), Ms. Carmela Roybal (Tewa Nation, USA), Prof. Mariodoss Selvanayagam (India), Prof. Mihaela Serbulea (Romania) , Dr. Jasdev Rai Singh (England) , Dr. Raquel R. Smith (USA), Prof. Takao Takahashi (Japan), Dr. Ananya Tritipthumrongchok (Thailand), Dr. Kayo Uejima (Japan), Dr. Lakshmi Vyas (UK) , Prof. Yanguang Wang (China), **Prof. John Weckert (Australia),** Dr. Anke Weisheit (Uganda). There are further subcommittee members who may also sign particular statements that they contributed to.

2. Major themes identified for bioethical deliberation

More than a dozen topics were identified as topics for important deliberation related to the COVID-19 pandemic. I will later go into further detail on two of these topics, mask use and triage, and in the appendix include three statements. These will serve as illustrations. The list of subcommittees is:

3. Subcommittees that have completed their work:

1) Public Use of Masks and/ Face Covers as an Ethical Responsibility, and Imposition of Restrictions for People not Wearing Masks

2) Ethical guidelines for COVID-19 triage management

3) Statement against using the War Metaphor Other subcommittees with ongoing work:

4) State and governance in COVID-19

5) Autonomy and Responsibility within a public health emergency

6) Disaster Communication Ethics

7) Ethical Issues of COVID-19 for Indigenous Communities

8) Ethical Issues of COVID-19 for Persons living with Disabilities

9) COVID-19 and Refugees

10) Role of Faith Systems and Religions in COVID-19

11) Impact of COVID-19 Measures on Crime, Corruption, & Inequity of the Impacts of Control Measures

12) Lessons Learned in a Pandemic

13) Ethical Values and Principles for a New World Order (post COVID-19 crisis)

14) Environmental Implications of COVID-19

15) COVID-19 and Gender

16) COVID-19 and Education

There are regular virtual conferences including the series of **International Public Health and Bioethics Ambassador Conferences** organized by Eubios Ethics Institute every few weeks were dozens of persons have presented papers relating their experiences to bioethical theory and policy linked to COVID-19. Most of these papers have been published in *Eubios Journal of Asian and International Bioethics (EJAIB*; https://eubios.info/ejaib_journal). These public cross-cultural forums have been critical to develop reflection on bioethics more. Let us examine several topics in more detail to illustrate the linkage of theoretical principles of bioethics to practice.

4. Wearing Masks and the Precautionary Principle

The precautionary principle is widely recognized in international law, yet it was not used during the COVID-19 crisis by most governments, presidents, chief medical officers, national medical associations and even the World Health Organization (WHO). They have failed to apply this principle to a very simple public health measure that everyone can do to protect themselves and their community, wearing face covers and masks. At last by April 2020 there was a change of heart in these so-called wise people to change their previous paternalistic recommendations not to wear masks or face coverings, to now please wear face coverings or even face a penalty if you do not wear face coverings in some countries. I wish to address the question of moral responsibility for this erroneous advice that was provided by many medical professionals and medical associations. I would go so far as to suggest that these persons have blood on their hands and should be disturbed in their sleep at night. Tens of thousands of lives have been lost because of their recommendations not to wear masks, and this is increasing around the world as certain public figures still do not promote the use of face coverings and/or masks.

Actually many people thought that they should wear masks, and most in East Asia just went ahead to wear masks, but in Western countries and some others, people were specifically advised not to wear masks. This was counter to scientific evidence despite the false claims to advise people not to wear masks. For example, Jefferson et al. (2011) in a *Cochrane Review* of dozens of studies already had shown a decade ago that ordinary masks were effective, and recommended to wear masks. Wu et al. (2014) had already presented evidence from the SARS epidemic in Beijing that use of face masks by the public reduced risk of infection significantly for those who used them. It is no surprise that the community transmission of SARS-CoV-2 would also be reduced by use of masks and face covers, since it worked in the SARS-CoV-1 epidemic.

Fortunately, we can see some dramatic change of heart in the USA which has the highest number of infections and deaths from COVID-19. For example, on 29 February, the U.S. surgeon general Dr. Jerome Adams tweeted in capitals "STOP BUYING MASKS" and said that masks do not offer any benefit to the average citizen. On 3 April 2020 the U.S. Centers for Disease Control and Prevention recommended that Americans wear "cloth face coverings fashioned from household items or made at home from common materials ... as an additional, voluntary public health measure."

There have been criticisms of WHO by many persons about many things, but for me I cannot understand how they could ignore scientific evidence and be so reluctant to have people wear a face cover. In the WHO statement, "There is limited evidence that wearing a medical mask by healthy individuals in the households or among contacts of a sick patient, or among attendees of mass gatherings may be beneficial as a preventive measure. However, there is currently no evidence that wearing a mask (whether medical or other types) by healthy persons in the wider community setting, including universal community masking, can prevent them from infection with respiratory viruses, including COVID-19 (WHO 2020a)." They start to admit some use of masks, however, *"We can certainly see circumstances on which the use of masks, both home-made and cloth masks, at the community level may help with an overall comprehensive response to this disease."*

In 2019 WHO (2019) issued advice to wear masks in times of an epidemic and pandemic in WHO guidance on "Non- pharmaceutical public health measures for mitigating the risk and impact of epidemic and pandemic influenza". That statement recommends face mask use in the community for asymptomatic individuals in severe epidemics or pandemics in order to reduce transmission in the community; this is based on mechanistic plausibility for the potential effectiveness of this measure.

A study in Singapore in March 2020 had already demonstrated how asymptomatic persons were spreading the SARS-CoV-2 virus (Wei et al. 2020), which led to a change in the Singapore government's recommendations. However, the Singapore government had already ordered the Armed Forces to deliver 5.2 million masks to 1.3 million households across the city, on 1 February 2020, when Singapore had recorded just 13 cases of the coronavirus. There have been some medical voices against the voices of authorities not to wear masks. Burch (2020) wrote, *"Despite hearing that face masks "don't work," you probably haven't seen any strong evidence to support that claim. That's because it doesn't exist.",* and also provided some easy to use guidelines on how to make more effective face coverings. As Wei et al. (2020) wrote, *"The possibility of presymptomatic transmission of SARS-CoV-2 increases the challenges of COVID-19 containment measures, which are predicated on early detection and isolation of symptomatic persons."*

Even three weeks after Singapore, the American Medical Association President said, "there is "little benefit to wearing a mask", and "the CDC does not recommend that people wear face masks to protect themselves from respiratory viruses." This includes COVID-19" (Berg 2020a; 21 Feb). The American Medical Association (2020) "Statement on CDC's recommendation for public on cloth masks" on 3 April, 2020 accepted the public use of masks, and also it was reported that some healthcare institutions had been refusing to allow physicians from wearing their own mask when the physicians had made a medical judgment that their own mask was safer than the ones the institution had provided to them (Berg 2020b). There were reports that some institutions only had enough masks to provide one mask a day to their professionals. In some countries, there were reportedly even less masks.

There are still other authorities that remain against general mask use, such as European Centre for Disease Prevention and Control (2020) who wrote in their "Using face masks in the community" statement, "There is no evidence that non-medical face masks or other face covers are an effective means of respiratory protection for the wearer of the mask" At the same time they state, "For communication purposes, it is important to emphasize that the people who use face masks in the community want to protect their fellow citizens in case they are infected. They do not want to unknowingly spread the virus, and wearing a mask should not be misconstrued that they want to protect themselves from others. Wearing a mask is not an act of selfishness and should be promoted as an act of solidarity." Perhaps this is a way for medical authorities to save their public face while not further causing the deaths of citizens.

5. Individual responsibility and group solidarity

It has been quite a contrast to look at the policies announced in different countries over whether people should wear masks to protect themselves, and/or others from infection during the time of COVID-19. This is a very simple example to illustrate the evolution of individual responsibility and group solidarity, although it is related to rather diverse cultural traditions around the world. Personally, I found it very interesting because I lived in Japan for several decades and am very used to seeing people wear masks especially during the pollen season in the spring. It was also common sense that everyone would wear a mask if you had any infection to avoid spreading the disease to other people. Almost every household has masks as a regular item in their cupboards. Throughout 2020 East Asians have continued to use masks to attempt to prevent COVID-19 infection. In China, Hong Kong, Taiwan, South Korea and Japan mask-wearing has become the norm, with some stores refusing entry to those without face covers. Hong Kong authorities gave advice to wear masks in public on 24 January, and in China on 31 January. Taiwan had even stockpiled enough masks that they did not have a shortage.

When we compare the situation in different countries we can see a full range of policy statements and actual practice between countries (and/or individual institutions and commercial premises) which make it compulsory to wear a mask before you enter into a supermarket, or enter to a medical clinic, pharmacy or hospital, and countries who publicly state that you have no advantage to wear a mask so you shouldn't be wearing masks. Some of the countries with mandatory face mask use include Austria, Bosnia-Herzegovina, Czech Republic, Indonesia, Israel, Kenya, Morocco, Panama, Slovakia, Ukraine, Vietnam; and the island of Luzon, the Philippines, and the city of Jena in Germany. By June 2020 cities such as Los Angeles and New York City had made it compulsory. Some countries recommend using masks, but unless there are sufficient masks available a fabric face cloth can be used as an alternative. For some examples see Andelane (2020), Feng et al. (2020), Huo (2020), Ting (2020). I also found it interesting to be a mask wearer during mid-March 2020 in Geneva, London and Istanbul, noting that in all these places I was almost the only person wearing a mask. On my last day in Geneva on the 12 March I did see several other people wearing masks, and on a flight from Istanbul to Los Angeles on the 14 March surprisingly I was among 20% of the people wearing a mask on the flight – being one of 4% on the flight in the reverse direction 2 weeks earlier.

One of the rationales that the U.S. Centers for Disease Control provided for their previous statements to ask the public not to wear a mask, or statements not recommending to wear a mask earlier, was that there was a shortage of surgical masks and the mask should be provided to first responders, including medical staff because there was a shortage of masks in the country. It is interesting if that is the same rationale that is given in other countries, nevertheless it raises a number of individual and collective issues of expectations and responsibilities for public health. Since we know that in many viral infections of the respiratory tract there are many asymptomatic persons who can spread the virus, and that among young adults perhaps more than half the persons are asymptomatic, it is simple public health prevention to let people wear masks.

In article 4 of the Universal Declaration on Bioethics and Human Rights it states that human beings have both autonomy and responsibility and that these should be balanced. So when the government tells citizens who wanted to wear a mask that they should not wear a mask, it is providing a directive like a paternalistic big brother to tell citizens do not wear masks because we do not have enough masks and you should give your masks to the medical staff who really need it. They actually made calls that citizens should give any N-95 masks they have as a donation to medical staff. The same government was actually negligent not to have a national stockpile after decades of discussions of pandemic preparedness.

For those of us who felt that it was a matter of responsibility to wear a mask so as not to have any risk of infecting others, it's a very strange message from public health officials. The fact that when you go to a hospital even under normal circumstances medical staff are wearing masks suggest that mask have an important function in preventing infection. It would therefore seem to be unethical for the double standards to allow medical staff not to be infected by wearing masks, while also telling the public you can go to the supermarket and your essential work without a mask. They said the mask is not going to help you.

In fact, providing this misinformation is unethical for public health authorities to have recommended not to wear masks. It is also a complete contradiction that after two months of saying don't worry now they suddenly say, "Yes you need to wear a face covering when you go in public." This is such basic knowledge that actually I saw many people in the USA wearing masks and thus "contravening the advice of the CDC" throughout March 2020, especially immigrants in the USA from divergent spaces such as East Asia, Persia and Latin America.

There are also some other strange anomalies that I have observed, for example a mother of a 7 year old child inside a pharmacy who was picking up a drug prescription was told by the store that they would report her to the police if she did not bring the 7 year old in from his car seat to the pharmacy store. Apparently, he could not sit protected in the car and play video games on the telephone while his mother was waiting for the prescription to be picked up, and he should come into the pharmacy to be exposed to other customers who might be sick. I think that the mother made the ethical choice, although there is a law that children should not be left in a car, it was only 14C temperature and it was just for ten minutes with his consent. On the positive side however, I note that it seems that the police in California have been quite rational about the social distancing, when compared to some other Western style democracies that fine or imprison apparently healthy individuals who went out of their house. That is a topic for another paper, and of course physical distancing has had positive impacts in the pandemic.

6. An Erosion of Trust

When we have a public health emergency, trust is critical (Lofredo, 2020), citizens start to doubt public health officials who have earlier said they should not wear a mask or face covering. The same officials also tried to blame citizens who wanted to go to the beach or on a nature walk, and some parts of California closed beaches while saying there was no advantage to wear a mask.

Further epidemiological analysis will let us examine how many deaths were caused by the erroneous advice not to wear masks which has been admitted to now be inappropriate guidance from the health authorities. How much did this contribute to the spread of disease? Probably not washing hands was more of a factor, or failure to keep physical distance from each other. Ignorance may also have been a cause of a rapid rise in COVID-19. Given the need for economies to restart, and after a realization of the broader impacts of the recession caused by stay at home orders, the new normal will be to wear masks. This is not rocket science, but a lesson of SARS that many countries failed to learn. Let us see when governments will actually change their advice, and admit their mistake of telling persons not to wear masks. At least some governments, and some medical professionals, have now admitted their mistake and changed their policies.

In the WeCope Statement on Masks (Appendix) we can see recommendations over the use of masks as an issue of accountability for public health officials and medical professionals who told their patients and people don't wear masks because it doesn't help you. This is certainly an issue of individual responsibility and group solidarity, but I think everyone should wear a cover over their mouth and nose from the beginning. In the age of informed choice I did not expect erroneous paternalism to have arisen again in 2020.

7. Ethical foundations of triage

Another important medical issue that has emerged during the COVID-19 pandemic is triage. Literally hundreds of policies have been declared and shared. Triage is the sorting and allocation of treatment to patients, especially battle and disaster victims, according to a system of priorities designed to maximize the number of survivors. It involves articulation of a policy by medical administrators, and/or an assignment by medical professionals of degrees of urgency to persons with injuries or illnesses to decide the order of treatment when there is a large number of patients or casualties (Ghotbi et al., 2020). Generally, the persons who are thought to be saved through immediate medical attention will be treated first, others who can wait will be given a lower priority, and those who are unlikely to be saved will not be treated if lives can be saved in the first group. One of the most important reasons for the difficulty with emergency medical ethics is that the time required for emergency healthcare professionals to make decisions in case of any ethical conflict is limited (Erbay 2014). The provision of treatment depends on available resources. As an ethical minimum, patients who are in a medically futile situation must not be ignored, and can be provided with palliative care to ensure they are pain free. However, in extreme and/or resource poor situations there may be a shortage of all medicines including pain relieving medication (Ghotbi et al. 2020).

There have been reports of medical doctors excluding patients above a certain age (e.g.

above 80 years of age) from receiving life-saving treatments in overwhelmed Intensive Care Units (ICU) (Ghotbi et al. 2020). Rosenbaum (2020) describes the triage of patients during the COVID-19 pandemic in Italy, and refers to the use of old age as a factor to deny ventilator usage for two reasons: "to dedicate its limited resources to those who both stand to benefit most and have the highest chance of surviving". The example used is saving a 65-year-old patient instead of an 85-year-old patient because the saved patient would live longer and also have a bigger chance of being saved. The utilitarian approach to triage in this case implies saving considerably younger patients who have an apparent advantage in chance of survival (Ghotbi et al. 2020). The same paper suggests three principles for triage: separating clinicians providing care from those making triage decisions through a "triage officer" backed by an expert team of nurses and respiratory therapists, who communicate the decision to the clinicians, the patient and the family; regular review of decisions by a centralized monitoring committee to ensure that there are no inappropriate inequities; and regular review of the triage algorithm to update it based on new information (Rosenbaum 2020).

In the USA, the triage system for COVID-19 patients relies on two primary principles of saving the most lives and saving the most life years (Gutel 2020). Triage in USA follows secondary principles as well, such as prioritizing the treatment of healthcare workers engaged in the disaster response and consideration of the "life cycle status," which again favors the survival of younger patients (Gutel 2020). Berlinger et al. (2020) from the Hasting Center have referred to the ethical challenges of COVID-19 in the face of duties to care, to promote moral equity, to plan for uncertainty, to support workers and protect vulnerable groups, and to provide policy guidelines; they have also provided ethical guidelines for institutional ethics services responding to COVID-19. In the WeCope Committee paper we aimed to provide simple, practical, and defensible ethical guidelines for triage management of COVID-19 patients based on the principles of distributive justice, fairness, non-discrimination, and beneficence (Nader et al. 2020). As much as possible, guidelines and procedures should be established on the ground of a fair process approach and procedural justice (Kinlaw 2007). The WeCope Declaration on Triage is in the Appendix.

The duty to care has led many nations to call their healthcare workers heroes because they are risking their lives caring for COVID-19 patients amidst a lack of sufficient personal protective equipment (PPE) and other safeguards (Hsin and Macer, 2004). The refusal to treat could have a drastic effect on triage. The heroism of healthcare workers is the main source of support for COVID-19 patients, especially when protective personal equipment (PPE) is scarce and full protection is not available. To guide healthcare workers in their duties to care and treatment in a triage situation, the World Health Organization (WHO) released the Emergency Triage Assessment and Treatment guidelines that divides patients into three main categories: *emergency cases* who require immediate emergency treatment, *priority cases* who must be given priority in the queue for rapid assessment and treatment, and *non-urgent cases* who can wait their turn in the queue for assessment and treatment (WHO 2005).

Patrão Neves (2020) considers that the selection of patients based on personal characteristics (age, gender, profession, ethnicity, nationality, number of dependents, and so on) violates two fundamental ethical principles: the principle of human dignity which values every human being equally, and the principle of social justice which requires equal opportunities for all. Therefore, it is important to make a distinction between rationing and rationalization. Rationing may be ethically acceptable when the criteria of selection are transparent and refer to non-vital resources. Rationalizing refers to the most reasonable ('rational') use of limited resources solely under the criterion of making the most of it; the goal is optimization of available resources, making them as efficient as possible. Therefore, in life and death decisions, such as providing respiratory support for COVID-19 patients, rationalization may be the only ethical approach because it does not value some persons in detriment of others, but chooses the optimization of scarce resources (Ghotbi et al. 2020).

Conclusions

This paper outlines how the establishment of the World Emergency COVID-19 Pandemic Ethics (WeCope) Committee offers a useful opportunity for independent ethical reflection on questions of bioethics that face all communities during the COVID-19 pandemic. It also finds that a number of medical professionals, medical authorities, governments and the World Health Organization, have not performed as ethically as we would have expected during the COVID-19 epidemic and pandemic by advising members of the public not to wear masks to protect their own health and the health of those around them (Macer 2020). Although by April 2020 most authorities have changed their advice to recommend or even compel citizens to wear face coverings and masks when in public, we need to examine the question of failed moral responsibility and the accountability for this erroneous advice. There are also important ethical issues that are raised when we start to discriminate people on the basis of age, or other factors in triage, rather than relying simply on medical criteria to save life (Ghotbi et al. 2020).

Acknowledgements

I appreciate all members of the World Emergency COVID-19 Pandemic Ethics (WeCope) Committee, and other scholars for their shared wisdom and determination to improve our responses to COVID-19.

References

American Medical Association 2020. Statement on CDC's recommendation for public on cloth masks. (3 April, 2020). [URL: https://www.ama-assn.org/press-center/ama-statements/statement-cdc-s-recommendation-public-cloth-masks]

Andelane 2020. Andelane, Lana. Coronavirus: Countries where face masks are mandatory in COVID-19 fight, *Newshub* (7 April 2020). [URL: https://www.newshub.co.nz/home/world/2020/04/coronavirus-countries-where-face-masks-are-mandatory-in-covid-19-fight.html]

Berg 2020a. Berg, Sara. COVID-19: 6 key points physicians should share with patients. American Medical Association website (21 Feb 2020). Accessed on 6 April 2020 [URL: https://www.ama-assn.org/delivering-care/public-health/covid-19-6-key-points-physicians-should-share-patients]

Berg 2020b. Berg, Sara. COVID-19 safety: Don't bar physicians from wearing their own PPE. American Medical Association website. (2 April 2020). Accessed on 6 April 2020 [URL: https://www.ama-assn.org/delivering-care/public-health/covid-19-safety-don-t-bar-physicians-wearing-their-own-ppe]

Berlinger 2020. Berlinger, N., Wynia, M., Powell, T., Micah Hester et al. Ethical framework for health care institutions responding to novel coronavirus SARS-CoV-2 (COVID-19). Guidelines for institutional ethics services responding to COVID-19 *Managing uncertainty, safeguarding communities, guiding practice.* The Hastings Center (16 March 2020)

[URL: thehastingscenter.org/ ethicalframeworkcovid19]

Burch 2020. Burch, Adrien. "What's the Evidence on Face Masks? What You Heard Was Probably Wrong". Accessed on 6 April 2020 [URL: https://medium.com/better-humans/whats-the-evidence-on-face-masks-5f3c27a18cc]

Erbay 2014. Erbay, H. Some ethical issues in prehospital emergency medicine. *Turk J Emerg Med*, *14*(4), 193–198. [URL: https://doi.org/10.5505/1304.7361.2014.32656]

Feng 2020. Feng, Shuo et al. Rational use of face masks in the COVID-19 pandemic, *Lancet Respiratory Medicine*, Accessed on 6 April 2020.

Ghotbi 2020. Ghotbi, Nader., Lofredo, Marlon Patrick P., Patrão Neves, Maria do Céu., D'Astous, Mireille., Chakraborty, Rhyddhi., Bilir, Esra., Arawi, Thalia., Weisheit, Anke., Erbay, Hasan., Rai, Jasdev Singh., Cutter, Anthony Mark., Ben Aziz, Mouna ., Macer, Darryl R.J. 2020. Ethical guidelines for COVID-19 triage management. *Eubios Journal of Asian and International Bioethics*. 30(6) (June 2020): 201-207.

Gutel 2020. Gutel, Fred. Who Should Doctors Save? Inside the debate about how to ration coronavirus care. *Newsweek*. (3 April 2020). [URL: https://www.newsweek.com/2020/04/24/who-should-doctors-save-inside-debate-about-how-ration-coronavirus-care-1495892.html]

Hsin 2004. Hsin, H-S. D., Macer, D.R.J. Heroes of SARS: Professional Roles and Ethics of Health Care Workers. Journal of Infection 49: 210-5. [URL: https://www.eubios.info/Papers/sarsji.pdf]

Huo 2020. Huo, Jingman. Why There are so Many Different Guidelines for Face Masks for the Public, National Public Radio (April 10, 2020). [URL: https://www.npr.org/sections/goatsandsoda/2020/04/10/829890635/why-there-so-many-different-guidelines-for-face-masks-for-the-public]

Jefferson 2011. Jefferson T, Del Mar CB, Dooley L, Ferroni E, Al-Ansary LA, Bawazeer GA, van Driel ML, Nair NS, Jones MA, Thorning S, Conly JM. Physical interventions to interrupt or reduce the spread of respiratory viruses. *Cochrane Database of Systematic Reviews* 2011, Issue 7. Art. No.: CD006207. DOI: 10.1002/14651858.CD006207.pub4.

Kinlaw 2007. Kinlaw, Kathy, Levine, Robert. Ethical guidelines in pandemic influenza- recommendations of the ethics subcommittee of the advisory committee to the director. Centers for Disease Control and Prevention. (15 Feb, 2007). [URL: https://www.cdc.gov/od/science/integrity/phethics/docs/panflu_ethic_guidelines.pdf

Lofredo 2020. Lofredo, Marlon Patrick P. Social Cohesion, Trust, and Government Action Against Pandemics. *Eubios Journal of Asian and International Bioethics*. 30(3) (April 2020): 182-6.

Macer 2020. Macer, Darryl R.J. Wearing Masks in COVID-19 Pandemic, the Precautionary Principle, and the Relationships between Individual Responsibility and Group Solidarity. *Eubios Journal of Asian and International Bioethics*. 30(4) (May 2020): 201-207.

Patrão 2020. Patrão Neves, Maria. The ethical implications of 'rationing' vs. 'rationalization'. *Eubios Journal of Asian and International Bioethics* 30(4):131-133.

Rosenbaum 2020. Rosenbaum L. Facing covid-19 in Italy - ethics, logistics, and therapeutics on the epidemic's front line. New England Journal of Medicine. (18 March 2020) doi: 10.1056/ NEJMp2005492

Ting 2020. Ting, Victor. "To mask or not to mask: WHO makes U-turn while US, Singapore abandon pandemic advice and tell citizens to start wearing masks". South China Morning Post. (4 April 2020) [URL: https://www.scmp.com/news/hong-kong/health-environment/article/3078437/mask-or-not-mask-who-makes-u-turn-while-us]

Wei 2020. Wei W.E., Li, Z., Chiew, C.J., Yong, S.E., Toh, M.P., Lee, V.J. Presymptomatic Transmission of SARS-CoV-2 — Singapore, January 23–March 16, 2020. MMWR Morb Mortal Wkly Rep 2020;69:411–415. DOI: [URL: http://dx.doi.org/10.15585/mmwr.mm6914e1external icon]

Wu 2004. Wu, Jiang et al. Risk Factors for SARS among Persons without Known Contact with SARS Patients, Beijing, China. Emerg Infect Dis. (Feb. 2004); 10(2): 210–216. [URL: https://wwwnc.cdc.gov/eid/article/10/2/03-0730_article]

World Emergency COVID19 Pandemic Ethics (WeCope) Committee (23 April 2020), Wearing masks and face covers as social responsibility during the COVID-19 pandemic, *Eubios Journal of Asian and International Bioethics (EJAIB)* 30(5) (June 2020): 197-198. https://www.eubios.info

World Emergency COVID19 Pandemic Ethics (WeCope) Committee (31 May 2020), Statement on ethical triage guidelines for COVID-19, *Eubios Journal of Asian and International Bioethics (EJAIB)* 30(5) (June 2020): 198-201. https://www.eubios.info

World Health Organisation (WHO) 2005. Emergency triage assessment and treatment (ETAT). Manual for participants.

World Health Organisation (WHO) 2019. Non-pharmaceutical public health measures for mitigating the risk and impact of epidemic and pandemic influenza: WHO. Available from: https://apps.who.int/iris/bitstream/handle/10665/329438/9789241516839-eng.pdf

World Health Organization (WHO) 2020. Advice on the use of masks in the context of COVID-19. Interim guidance. (6 April 2020) [URL:https://apps.who.int/iris/bitstream/handle/10665/331693/WHO-2019-nCov-IPC_Masks-2020.3-eng.pdf?sequence=1&isAllowed=y]

Appendix 1: Wearing masks and face covers as social responsibility during the COVID-19 pandemic

• *Statement of the World Emergency COVID19 Pandemic Ethics (WeCope) Committee (23 April 2020)*

As experts in many fields, coming from many cultures and nations across the world, we declare that the scientific evidence is clear that there is an expected advantage to both individuals and those around them to wear proper face covers including masks in public during the COVID-19 pandemic.

In the early stages of the COVID-19 epidemic and pandemic, a number of medical professionals, medical authorities, governments and the World Health Organization (WHO) had denied there were advantages for wearing masks, opposed wearing them, and/or warned persons who wanted to wear masks that there was a risk of using them due to what they saw as general inappropriate use and/or providing a false feeling of safety. Unfortunately, in only a few countries mask use was encouraged by the governments, despite long standing evidence of their effectiveness (Jefferson et al., 2001; Wu et al., 2004).

There appear to have been two common reasons for opposing mask use. One is a genuine ignorance of their effectiveness, and another is fear in many countries that there were insufficient masks for medical staff. Whatever the reasons, the communication was often flawed, contradictory, unscientific, and/or deceptive, likely causing harm through increased numbers who were infected. This also has resulted in loss of public trust in health leadership and management in some places, at a time when trust is critical.

Although by April 2020 most authorities have changed their advice to actively recommend or even compel citizens to wear face coverings and masks when in public, the questions over failed public moral responsibility and the accountability for this erroneous advice should be looked at as a lesson of the COVID-19 pandemic. While some authorities order all persons to wear masks in public because of the social advantages, in case where there are limited supplies, or affordability, other face coverings may still protect against transmission. Also, we do not agree with fines or penalties against persons who do not wear masks in public spaces, but encourage honest communication and education.

The Precautionary Principle is widely recognized in international law, yet it was generally not applied well during the COVID-19 crisis. Many people thought that they should wear masks and we applaud their informed choice, as well as the advices of some governments to wear masks, and efforts to distribute masks to the public. Article 4 of the Universal Declaration on Bioethics and Human Rights states that human beings have both autonomy and responsibility and that these should be balanced. We also still urge all in positions of authority, at least not to discourage mask use by concerned persons, for any political, cultural, racial, economic or other reasons.

It has been quite a contrast in the policies announced in different countries over whether people should wear masks to protect themselves and others from infection during the time of COVID-19 (Macer, 2020). This is a very simple example to illustrate the evolution of individual responsibility and group solidarity, although it is related to rather diverse cultural traditions around the world. We urge governments to be transparent in their assessment of the epidemiological analysis and statistics, and truthful in their public communication to uncover the scale of damage caused by any erroneous advice to citizens who wanted to wear masks, but did not wear masks because of inappropriate guidance from the health authorities.

In a world where authorities ought to be representatives of the people they serve, and a reference for the informed choices that people make, truth, transparency and inclusion in partnership with civil society are essential, and the respect for social responsibility is an ethical imperative.

Members, World Emergency COVID19 Pandemic Ethics (WeCope) Committee:

https://www.eubios.info/world_emergency_covid19_pandemic_ethics_committee

Appendix 2: Statement on ethical triage guidelines for COVID-19

• *Statement of the World Emergency COVID19 Pandemic Ethics (WeCope) Committee (31 May 2020)*

Rationale

This is our statement, as experts from many fields, cultures and nations across the world, having realized that tens of thousands of people have died in grim situations of the COVID-19 pandemic not only from the lethal susceptibility that some people have to this novel virus, but also because of insufficient infrastructure, human resources, protective equipment, and/or a lack of clear triage decision making protocols. The severe shortage of resources in response to the overwhelming number of patients needing life-saving treatment has reduced the ability of most healthcare systems to organize a reasonable and ethical method for triage. There have been instances of denial of access of critically ill persons to basic medical care from hospitals, excluding patients above a certain age from receiving life-saving treatments in overwhelmed Intensive Care Units (ICU), and instances where the poor and underprivileged were not given equal and fair access to quality healthcare.

In this context as an independent, multidisciplinary and cross-cultural committee, we urge all to reflect again on the moral foundations of the widely accepted principle of triage, and the reality of healthcare systems unable to cope with the pandemic. We here provide simple, practical, and defensible ethical guidelines for triage management of COVID-19 patients based on the principles of love of life, respect for human dignity, distributive justice, fairness, non-discrimination, shared decision making, and beneficence. The ethical challenges of COVID-19 include observance of the duties to care, promotion of moral equity, planning for uncertainty, support for healthcare workers, protection of vulnerable groups, and provision of practical and ethical policy guidelines. Under no circumstances should the existence of the triage protocol justify negligent public health strategies.

Recommendation 1: *People need to know the ethical basis and moral justification when they, or their loved ones, are denied treatment or access to scarce resources such as ventilators or denied admission to a hospital.*

Ethical foundations of triage

Triage is the sorting and allocation of treatment to patients, according to a system of priorities designed to maximize the number of survivors. It involves articulation of a policy by medical administrators, and/or an assignment by medical professionals of degrees of urgency to patients to decide the order of treatment when there is a large number of them. There are different ethical theories to guide the process of triage in hospitals overwhelmed by COVID-19 patients in need of life-saving treatment. Egalitarianism seeks to treat patients equally; utilitarianism aims to maximize the greatest benefit to the greatest number, measured by the remaining life years that a decision may save; and prioritarianism argues for treating the sickest first, which is the usual practice at emergency rooms in the majority of healthcare settings.

Particularities of triage for COVID-19

Generally, patients who may be saved through immediate medical attention are treated first; others who can wait are given a lower priority, and those who are unlikely to be saved may not receive treatment with scarce resources that are needed to save lives in the first group. The provision of treatment, therefore, depends on available resources. The difficulty with emergency medical ethics is that the time required for emergency healthcare professionals to make decisions in case of any ethical conflict is limited. Patients may thus be divided into the three categories of *emergency cases* who require immediate treatment, *priority cases* with priority in the queue for rapid assessment and treatment, and *non-urgent cases* who can wait their turn in the queue for assessment and treatment. In COVID-19, the separation of *emergency cases* from others is based on the presence of serious respiratory distress, severe dehydration or shock, mental status changes, and chest pain. In light of reports of people who were not admitted to hospital, rapidly deteriorating when left unsupervised at home, ignoring the care of COVID-19 patients should be carefully examined in the context of the duty of care.

Ethical objections to selection of patients

Selection of patients based on personal characteristics (age, gender, profession, ethnicity, nationality, number of dependents, disability, and so on) violates two fundamental ethical principles: the principle of human dignity which values every human being equally, and the principle of social justice which requires equal opportunities for all. None of the risk factors for predicting a grave outcome in COVID-19 has been proved as definitive in terms of prognosis and thus treatment should not be denied based on an underlying condition. Using old age as an excuse to deny treatment is discriminatory, unethical, and in contradiction with basic social and cultural values. The use of a 'simple cut-off' policy on age constitutes direct discrimination because comorbidities may put a younger person at a disadvantage compared with an older but healthier patient. There should neither be any race, gender or culture-based discrimination so that everyone is treated fairly, as all human beings have inherent dignity.

Recommendation 2: Triage committees should be formed in hospitals in preparation for times of crisis, to help assist healthcare professionals decide which patients would get scarce resources based on clinical data.

Triage committees in the context of ethics committees

The healthcare system should establish independent, multi-disciplinary ethics committees, if they do not already exist. Bioethics and triage committees should wherever possible make the difficult decisions, not the bedside health professionals who will keep doing their best for each and every patient. The triage committee should be a small but always available group of 3 highly respected professionals, with two healthcare professionals, for example a physician and a nurse, plus an ethicist. The availability of an ethics committee 24/7 helps in making unbiased decisions and reduces the burden of choice on the healthcare team, who at the time of triage are tasked with saving as many lives as possible.

It has been accepted for years in triage that the most important criterion is survivability, so that only patients who are unlikely to live, even with medical intervention, would be kept off scarce resources such as ventilators, and the highest priority would be for patients who are likely to recover with ventilator support. Ideally, the committee should examine each patient anonymously, and factors like race, ethnicity, and status should not influence their decision. If the committee gives a priority for children who are in the early phases of a normal lifespan compared to an older person in otherwise identical circumstances, it should be a public policy decision of the wider community, noting that it is a form of ageism. as discussed above. Fairness as well as transparency over triage rules are important so that the public can trust the healthcare system in respect with rationing decisions.

Independence of review and resources

We recommend separating the clinicians providing care from those making triage decisions through a "triage officer" who communicates the decision to the clinicians, patients and their family, regular review of decisions by a centralized monitoring committee to ensure that there are no inappropriate inequities, and regular review of the triage algorithm to update it based on new information. Sufficient resources should be provided to enable such a system including shared decision making, especially now with the hindsight that we have after months living with COVID-19.

Recommendation 3: The protection of the vulnerable is a core ethical principle.

There should be an upfront commitment to core values at the start of any triage statement. Under certain circumstances, triage is needed to optimize the benefit of the healthcare system to the citizens, when the number of severely sick patients needing intensive care is more than the capacity of the healthcare system to try and save them all. Some frail patients may not be good candidates for aggressive live-saving treatments, especially when the chance of success is dim. We recommend trying to have an informed discussion with frail patients and relatives of the patient before making difficult decisions.

Palliative care

Triage should prioritize patients who are most likely to benefit from intensive care, in order to maximize the number of lives that can be saved. Triage policies must consider palliative care for patients whose triage decision does not include life-sustaining care, as well as those who are likely to die from COVID-19. Patients who are in a medically futile situation must not be ignored, and can be provided with palliative care to ensure they are pain free. The available usual basic care considered as non-extraordinary measures, such as food or fluids should not be withheld, either. When patients are severely affected by pre-existing conditions, end-of-life care ethics do not necessarily consider that treatment should be initiated, when it may result in additional suffering, burden or distress for patients. If treatments are expected to aggravate patient suffering, level of care decisions may allow the choice of palliative care without aggressive treatment. Openness and transparency of communication facilitate the difficult discussions about end-of-life decisions. Efforts need to be made to allow family members to be present at the time around the end of life, as regrettably many persons have passed away separated from family members.

Recommendation 4: Age, gender, race, ethnicity, existing disabilities, morbidities and/or chronic background conditions should not be used to exclude and/or deny the needed treatment or care to COVID-19 patients.

Only certain situations may be ethically considered as a priority in triage. Such a consideration should be based on clinical and objective factors, and comply with the protocol approved by a hospital, regional, or national ethics committee[1], in consultation with the broader

---

[1]   In some countries there may be national laws that restrict the choices suggested in these recommendations; however, these are addressed to persons at all levels including policy makers, administrators, practitioners, patients and family members. We do not suggest persons break their national laws, but reflect and consider legal and administrative reforms.

community, as follows:[2]

a] A competent patient may make an autonomous decision on level of care, such as choosing palliative care over intubation/ventilator use when the chance of success is very low. Patients can also provide an advance directive, or a 'durable' power of attorney as their surrogate, in case they succumb into a more serious situation in later stages.

b) After a patient has been provided with mechanical ventilation, the ventilator may not be withdrawn unless the treatment is determined to be futile and it is needed to try and save another patient who may benefit from it.

c) Do-not-resuscitate-orders are an ethically acceptable practice for patients when medical doctors have good reason to judge resuscitation would be futile.

d) When a number of patients are being considered for allocation of a rationed resource such as ventilators, priority is with those who are more likely to benefit from it. Estimation of likely healthy life-years saved may be included in determination of the potential benefit. This is the only situation where age may be considered, not to deny treatment, but to decide saving whom may significantly increase the life-years saved. The difference in the predicted healthy life years saved should be significant to justify such a consideration.

e) Healthcare workers engaged in the care of COVID-19 patients who get sick and need a rationed resource such as ventilators, can be given priority over non-healthcare workers, because saving them will be to the benefit of many other patients.

f) Prioritization in the form of affirmative action may be considered by the committee as discussed above under *"Ethical Objections to Selection of Patients"*.

g) Prioritization in the form of affirmative action may be considered for other emergency responders who become sick while performing their duties to save the lives of others.

Members, World Emergency COVID19 Pandemic Ethics (WeCope) Committee:

https://www.eubios.info/world_emergency_covid19_pandemic_ethics_committee

---

[2] Deviations from the protocol should be accepted only when approved by an ethics committee, but we note that in some places across the globe, there may be critical human resource constraints. We also note that including a representative of patients' rights groups in triage committees may be an advantage.

Appendix 3: A Call to Cease the Use of War Metaphors in the COVID-19 pandemic
• *World Emergency COVID19 Pandemic Ethics (WeCope) Committee (14 June 2020)*

Preamble
As an independent, multidisciplinary and crosscultural committee, comprised of experts from cultures and nations across the world, we urge all to reconsider their language, stating:

Recommendation 1: In communications relating to COVID-19 and coronavirus, any reference or metaphor belonging to the semantic context of war must be avoided.

War is sweet for the inexperienced, said Erasmus of Rotterdam. Using the metaphor of war to describe a pandemic means underestimating war, taking it as a challenge or a fight, almost normal, and quite natural. What we are facing is not an enemy who has a clear will to destroy us; it is a virus, a natural organism with no personal will, and if anything has enhanced its destructive action, it is years of unfortunate ecological management by the humans. There is no invasion from another planet to this world. Everywhere, and especially those with less resources, are paying the price of a globalization without a soul, without respect for natural resources and unfortunate ecological mismanagement by human beings.

The use of the war metaphor is extremely dangerous because it risks transforming preventive public health procedures into instruments of social control. The emergency of war requires total mobilization against the human enemy, and not taking responsibility for the damage that can be caused to other people, as in the case of the pandemic. There is no one to kill in a pandemic, but there are many to defend against the possibility of an infection. It is not a question of acting aggressively against another person or even defending yourself from another person, but of defending others from ourselves.

In warfare, gas masks are used to defend us from a weapon used by other people, but masks in a pandemic are mainly used to protect others from our potential breathing out of infectious droplets. The situation is exactly the opposite of war: the use of face masks is an act of love towards others, not an act of defense against an enemy. We are asked to keep our distance not from our enemies but from our friends aiming to isolate the virus. We are not building physical trenches but social barriers that allow the well-being of others and limit the damage that we could do.

Recommendation 2: Particularly with regard to communications aimed at children and adolescents, it is necessary to differentiate the situation caused by the virus from that of war, with detailed examples.

The use of the war metaphor is especially dangerous in education. Telling the kids that we are at war means presenting war as a natural response to an emergency, with an aggression that is not appropriate. Children have the right to grow in a safe and healthy planet where there are sensible ways of uplifting one another's morale for managing a pandemic that do not terrorize their lives. The language of the government and leaders must give inspiration to the youth and the next generation without using the pandemic to instill fear in people. Words affect people psychologically and emotively and have psychological consequences. The virus has not attacked us out of an evil deed; it is taking advantage of the mistakes in human approach to the nature with rapid globalization on a fragile base. But war is nothing natural; it is the worst of the choices that human beings can make and must never be used as a metaphor to define what is instead a strategy of resistance against a virus that must find us united as brothers and sisters, without ever using the word enemy.

Recommendation 3: It is necessary to avoid any form of stigmatization towards those who do not respect the health rules, inviting them to change their behavior but without pointing to them as enemies.

Any form of stigma distracts public opinion from the real goal of fighting the novel coronavirus but not groups of humans whatever their behavior. Furthermore, stigmatization produces an effect of infantilization: one is led to believe that the population as a whole is unable to comply with the rules and that there are particular groups that do not have this ability. This can lead to discriminatory behavior, including ableism, ageism, classism up to actual racism. Stigmatization can cause a shift in the way one thinks and there are behavioral consequences.

Recommendation 4: Safety and preventive measures must always be presented as emergency measures against the virus and their duration must be limited to the period of time necessary for the safety of the community.

Michel Foucault's analysis of the political management of plague and leprosy are pertinent. These diseases, spread throughout Europe, were used for social control purposes; it was the territory, in its physical subdivision and the regulation of spaces, that constituted an instrument of control and became more and more pervasive. When in the 17th century a sphere of intimacy took form, almost immediately the political tactics for violating it were created. In the current situation, it is necessary to be cautious in the analysis; credibility should not be given to the conspiracy readings. It is necessary to understand that every standard and every control device, put in place exclusively for health reasons, may lend themselves to be used for other reasons, unless citizens become democratically aware of the situation and pay close attention to what may happen in the future. For instance, the automatic download and installation of tracking software for contact-tracing without an active opt-in option should be critically evaluated.

Using a safety device such as a face mask, or maintaining a safe physical distance, when implemented through understanding and awareness, is different from being subject to an imposed standard. Wearing a face mask so as not to harm someone else is a profoundly moral act; it is not a question or paranoia of others as possible danger, but on the contrary, of attenting to our own behavior in respect to the wellbeing of others. This should constitute the transition from passively accepted norms to internalized norms with the fulcrum on the relationship between the self and the other, during the pandemic.

Recommendation 5: Research should be conducted to find the most suitable language to define the attitude of human beings towards the pandemic. One possible choice could be the term resistance.

In an emergency, each person should put in place personal and collective resistance strategies, so it is a matter of resisting the virus from a medical point of view but also of behaving in such a way as not to harm other persons.

Very often when we speak of individual responsibility we consider ourselves as isolated individuals, a kind of abstraction, owner of rights and duties. The link between responsibility and autonomy is sometimes so close that the fulfillment of one's duties seems to be indifferent from the relationship with others, as in "I do my duty to be able to enjoy my rights", the focus is on 'me' and 'my' duties and rights.

The coronavirus emergency has reversed the situation; I wear a face mask so as not to harm other people, and I keep social distances first of all because I could hurt others. The ethics of the self, to be defended at all costs, as if it were a city besieged by the enemy, has been turned upside down in the ethics of the other. We ask children to stay at home not because they are particularly at risk, but especially to protect their grandparents; all this could be a reversal of the relationship between individual and community. It is not the community that imposes rules on the individual, who perceives them as limitations, but it is the individuals who limit themselves because this is the only way to belong to a community. I don't come first, and strictly speaking, nor does the other, but the relationship between the self and the other is the foundation of everything.

It is the relational aspect of COVID-19 and its preventive measures, which must be at the center of ethical reflection. The community is not made up of wandering atoms, of people who fear the other, but of relationships that redefine the subjects within them, in their micro- and macro- relationships which then build the social totality, in which the recognition of the other is the premise for self-recognition of the ego.

Inter-connective metaphors should bring cohesiveness and encouragement during a pandemic. One should not experience loss of control or feel disempowered, nor should they feel that there is a possibility of non-compliancy from their perspective. The pandemic can be a turning point for many citizens to develop new ways of thinking, to encourage cooperation to contribute positively to everyone's well-being instead of reinforcing the possibility of others being victimized while dealing with preventive measures. Social measures should foster a sense of encouragement and a greater sense of responsibility. The operational models and dynamics from a social consciousness perspective should be fostering and nurturing especially for preventive measures for health and well-being.

Signed by all Members, World Emergency COVID19 Pandemic Ethics (WeCope) Committee

https://www.eubios.info/world_emergency_covid19_pandemic_ethics_committee

References

Lawn, S., Delany, T., Pulvirenti, M., Smith, A., & McMillan, J. (2016). Examining the use of metaphors to understand the experience of community treatment orders for patients and mental health workers. *BMC psychiatry*, *16*, 82. https://doi.org/10.1186/s12888-016-0791-z

Darryl Macer, Ph.D., Hon.D., is Director, Eubios Ethics Institute, New Zealand, Japan and Thailand, Email: darryl@eubios.info.

The Hidden Cost of Social Isolation

Irene M. Miller, Independent Scholar, USA

Abstract

Isolation and social distancing are unnatural states and come at considerable cost. All viruses will follow their natural courses. We must weigh the proportionality of the cost of the preventive measures to the cost of the disease. Dare we question possible misconceptions? My medical experiences in the USA, China and Africa give rise to my concern over unrealistic expectations regarding blanket testing or even waiting for a vaccine before easing social distancing. Triage is an age old ethical concern, not new to the present situation. Do we allow fear to make our lives less humanistic? Only courage will allow change and preserve our human dignity.

Key words

isolation, fear, courage, mutations.

> *The wise man's teachings are unlike conventional ones*
> *And invalidate common misconceptions.*
> *He spontaneously supports nature*
> *And cannot act otherwise. Lao Zi*[1]

In life we are taught to follow what is commonly accepted and it would seem appropriate that presently we all live in a national confinement. For twelve weeks now no one has come to my house, I cannot go to anyone else's house, and in total isolation I eat my every meal. Does the fear of a virus justify such a blanket alteration of the normal rhythm of life? This prolonged unnatural state, with no end in sight, is not without effects.

A virus will go where it wants and will run its course. The massive lock downs likely prolong its course. Counting the cost of this edict, the millions of lives affected by new poverty secondary to job losses (40 million alone in USA), the uncountable people, who fearful of using the medical facilities succumbed to the devastating effects of untreated illnesses, as well as the many, many elderly who are cut off from the loving, healing touch of family and community, as well as the increased rate of depression and suicide, the increased child and domestic abuse, the economic collapse, and so much more. All of this because of the fear of spread of a virus, of which the vast majority recovers, 35 % are asymptomatic and not even aware that they had been infected? The latest reported death rate from the CDC is 0.4 %, mostly in the elderly.

In California there has been a 50 % reduction of heart attack admissions, many hospitals are half empty, nurses are being furloughed. Might there be a misconception in our handling this? Is the imposition of distancing on every citizen, regardless of whether they live in rural or in densely populated metropolitan areas, necessary? There are countries that have not imposed alockdown and they are surviving without catastrophe. Many citizens worldwide voice concern over the infringement of personal freedom. Is isolation still a valid concept?

Is the claim, that we suffer so that the minority might live, still valid, when this minority we are trying to protect, the elderly and weak, and the children, on whom our future depends, suffer disproportionately?

---

[1] Hou Cai 2017, The Guodian Bamboo Slips, ed. Miller IM, Sass HM, Zürich, Lit, p. 37.

I entered the medical profession as an adult, a cellist and having raised a family. It was with the clear understanding that I will help all who are ill, and that included entering in dangerous and uncontrolled situations. Always conscience was my guide and became second nature, triage is part of medical practice. Did I suffer needle sticks during surgery in the early stages of AIDS, when no treatments were available? Yes, I did. Did I bring the trays of food to the AIDS patient, when no nurse would enter that room? Yes, already then the fear of the unknown had been great. Did I go up an elevator to the upper floors of a burning highrise on Wall Street to administer medical aid, when everyone was fleeing down the staircases? I only feared for my young nurse, who accompanied me. When I practiced in rural China near the Himalayans, without running water to wash hands or clean surfaces, I saw and treated all who came and were sick. In my work on Indian Reservations I faced no unusual dangers and was very impressed with the sense of trust and closeness within their families. Even their very small children were trusting of me, when examining them, while almost every other baby will cry, these children did not exhibit fear and mistrust.

Working and living in Uganda I oriented the new WHO doctors to the health hazards of the region, including snake bites. They had arrived to study a new Ebola outbreak. In Kampala's Makareri University Hospital, at an international meeting on Ebola, I learned that the virus quickly mutates, losing virulence in transmission from man to man, so that local outbreaks eventually die down. This was in the 1990s and research since believes that mutations are somewhat slower, complex computer models still trying to determine a more precise estimate. But it is now known that asymptomatic Ebola patients exist. The mutation rate of other viruses is also difficult to catch up with. There were years, in which the flu vaccine may have been less than 30% effective, because of the rapid mutations.

Long experience has taught me that tests can have many false positives and negatives, and have to be coupled with clinical findings. Why are we clamoring to test all people? Are we waiting to end lock downs until an effective vaccine can be found? Can it be found? Already while in Uganda every effort was made to find and test a vaccine for HIV and for Malaria. To this day every two minutes a child dies from Malaria, more than 200 million new cases annually (WHO), yet no effective vaccine has been found. And we fret ourselves over the present infection rate of a passing virus of about 4 million, of which a third does not even know they had it and with a death rate of 0.4 %?[2]

Why my concern with the effects of altering the natural rhythm of life? Living in a prolonged state of isolation and social distancing brings harm, psychological and physical.

What makes us human?   Without human touch and loving nurture a newly born life will die. This human connection, closeness, and our interactions with each other, will let us thrive and grow here on earth till the end of our days. Multiple physiologic actions occur, when we look into some one's eyes and face, when we feel the touch of a human hand or hear the real sound of a familiar voice. Our own electromagnetic fields benefit from the intersection with that of others.   Community and civility are built on these pillars. Our human spirit is thought and speech, inquiry, the question. Different perspectives keep our thinking fluid. We want to understand and need social intercourse. As children we learn through play. How can we now allow them to be locked into their own apartment for months at a time? There has been a great increase in childhood depression. Without interaction with their peers, how can they find out what the real world is like? How can they become socialized and physically strong? We also know that screen time can be harmful, if not balanced with real life experiences. Now, all is to become

---

[2]   CDC new models for publication 5/22/2020.

screen time, even their schooling. As virtual life becomes the norm in supplanting real life, this poses risks for all. What is a virtual school lesson compared to the classroom full of children with a teacher responding to their needs and questions? Where can our children and we now gather real life experience? What is a "live" concert on your computer screen compared to a real live performance? Yes, we are emotional beings, live music touches that part in us, moves us and allows dreams to take on some form, nourishes our soul and keeps us human.

Do we dare to allow fear to deprive us of all this? When we cower in fear we begin to live a less humanistic life. Even our immune systems are affected by prolonged fear. Where is our courage? There is no place on earth where our safety is guaranteed or certain. Where can you be safe from the sudden devastating effects of a cerebral hemorrhage or stroke, heart attack, cancer or car crash? Only with courage and the encouragement of others can we face each new day and live with these constant vulnerabilities in life, as well as accept the certainty of the relentless incremental decline of physical health and strength with aging. Now, for fear of a virus we are losing our courage and withdraw into our chambers by ourselves. It is a withdrawal from life. Cervantes once said: 'He, who loses wealth loses much. He, who loses a friend loses more; but he who loses his courage loses all'.[3]

This year, May 8th 2020, many nations celebrated the 75th year of the end of WW2, now called Liberation Day. When I saw again the photos on the news of the total destruction, which I do remember well from my childhood, the rubble all around from the bombings, the millions killed, the millions homeless, neither food nor water or heat, I worry less about the great economic losses and breakdowns of the present. What gave all the women in Germany the strength to pick up the rubble and sort the bricks? Their men had either been killed or were in prison camps. They and their children were hungry. It was plain old courage. Where did it come from? Courage is the quality of mind and spirit, which enables us to face danger and difficulties without fear. The word is derived from cuer, the heart, cor-age. In these broken women this courage came from within and from living a day at a time. We did not worry about next month or next year. Can we permit fear to cripple our way of life?

Our days are always numbered. Each birth signals a death down the road. That is the truth. We reject the natural cycle of birth and death and worship living long past our time. We think it fine, when people, herded in care facilities turn 100, totally dependent on others for care, while often unaware of where they are any more. Do we live so affluently, that we forget we cannot live forever? What have life expectancy and longevity to do with quality of life?

Is there hope for future learning? May we learn? Are we willing to address the many vulnerabilities in our health systems, food chains, and more, that corona virus has exposed? Are we blinded by the computer's capability to spew out mountains of data and projections, numbers too hard to grasp with our common understanding? The computer's predictions and multiplications of viral spread and second waves have become conventional thought. Is now the time to abandon common sense and experience? Have our ethical convictions still an audible voice within us?

We seem to be getting more rest with no place to go. We seem to be eating more locally produced, healthier food. Might we see less obesity? Air pollution is drastically reduced with less travel. May we see less respiratory disease? Better climate control? Can we return to a more tempered life style? Can we become more family focused, more meals cooked at home and eaten together by the whole family? Are we willing to change to return to a more humanistic life? Will we be kinder to the needy, less greedy? Can we be content with less? Even though

---

[3] Cervantes, Spanish novelist 1546-1616.

the land may be in disarray, are we willing to cultivate more decency and kindness in ourselves and our children?

'Living in simplicity would restore nature's rhythm and they would become content. Contentment brings with it its own peace and stability'[4]. And may we never again take for granted the round of friends at our dinner table with its lively conversations and companionship.

Irene M. Miller, celloimm@aol.com, born in Berlin, a cellist, has practiced medicine in USA, China and Africa. Now retired, she lives in New Hampshire.

---

[4] Hou Cai 2017:39.

Ethics in times of Corona: Should close relatives of persons with COVID-19 be allowed to visit their loved ones in the hospital?

David Martin, University of Witten/Herdecke, Germany

Abstract

Starting from a personal situation of the author, whose 54 year-old friend is on the intensive ward with severe COVID-19, with a wife and two teenage children at home with mild COVID-19, hospital visitor policies are discussed. The discussion starts from personal standpoints and then reaches out to include international literature on the matter. Virtual communication and human resourcefulness make many things more acceptable and new aspects possible. However, solutions should be as individually and locally tailored as personal responsibility and circumstances allow.

Key words

Visitor policies, individual solutions

Introduction

Given that most of us are flooded with numbers and their interpretations, this chapter will depart from a single, very personal situation. Ethics in medicine is, in fact often a question of sitting together and giving a particular situation in the hospital or in the practice some deep thinking from various perspectives.

1. Situation

As I am writing this, a friend of ours, 54 years old, slightly obese, with asthma and living in a polluted city, but with no other risk factors, is in a university hospital with oxygen and non-invasive respiration support. Diagnosis: acute COVID-19 with bilateral pneumonia. I hope he will not need artificial respiration.

His wife and two teenage children are not allowed to visit him. Is this ethical? My immediate reaction was: no.

2. Personal thoughts

Ethics is not about immediate reactions, however; it is about a thorough consideration of the matter from all sides. Conventionally, ethics is about considering our basic values, deriving norms and regulations from values and conditions, and finally adapting and applying them to a specific situation or particular domain of action. Less conventionally, ethics is about empowering and trusting each community and each individual to find good solutions for their specific situations.

My immediate reaction was: "no, prohibiting a person to visit their loved one in hospital is not ethical, especially if this loved one is on the verge of death." This immediate reaction is based on my perspective from Germany. Our hospitals are rather empty at the moment. While the staff is busy, I am sure they could, at particular times, make arrangements for relatives to properly drape themselves so as to reduce contagion risk to a minimum. Perhaps the staff may even gain time by being able to delegate some tasks to the relatives. But whether the relatives can be of practical help or not is perhaps irrelevant considering the pure human importance of being present for a loved one who is suffering or dying. A further consideration is that the presence of a loved one can help a patient be more relaxed, have less stress and thereby need less painkillers, less oxygen and have a better course of disease. Stress affects the microbiome (Pena Cortes u. a. 2018) and may negatively affect the course of infections such as HIV (Antoni 2003)(Evans u. a. 1997), wound infection (Rojas u. a. 2002) and wound healing (Christian u. a. 2006). A search for studies on COVID-19 and stress retrieved no studies on the matter to date.

The above-mentioned friend is in Chile, however. There, the hospitals are overcrowded, his wife and two children have fever and mild symptoms of COVID-19. Would it be ethical to allow them to enter the hospital? Perhaps not: The staff may already be at its limit. The wife or children may be super spreaders and could potentially infect the whole, crowded ward of a hospital in Santiago de Chile. Further, the hospital may already have a shortage of isolation equipment such as sterile clothing, masks and goggles. Finally, given the possibility of virtual audio-visual communication, new ways of partially bridging the communication gap may be possible, lessening the burden of not being with each other. Thus I have come to the conclusion that yes, it may be ethical for a person not to be able to visit a severely ill relative with COVID-19 in some hospitals in some circumstances.

My wife, who developed and leads the Corona Clinic in Tübingen, Germany, does not share my new opinion: On a normal ward she would let all three members of the close family visit him, and on the intensive ward she would still let his wife and both teenaged children visit their husband/father, one after the other. She says the family could acquire protective sterile clothing, a mask, goggles, and gloves. She says goggles would be important even though the woman and both children already have COVID-19 as goggles prevent them from putting their fingers in their eye area and then spreading infectious tear fluids. My wife has been seeing patients with Sars-CoV-2 infections all day long for several weeks. She wore sterile clothing, goggles and a mask and neither she nor anyone on her team has contracted COVID-19 or developed antibodies against Sars-CoV-2 to date. So using the same degree of protection, she cannot see why the relatives should not be allowed to visit their father: Why should the diagnostic procedures and triaging in her Corona Clinic be more important than the care of and attention to a loved one in the hospital? If every supermarket has someone standing at the entrance to make sure people are abiding to hygiene regulations, why not the same in hospital entrances? Since most countries do not wish to provide the clothing, goggles and mask free of charge, a store at the entrance could sell them at an acceptable price.

A further argument for allowing visitors who themselves were Sars-CoV-2/COVID-19 positive is that in the second week after outbreak of the symptoms, the risk of infecting others drops to nearly zero, hence many relatives will then no longer be a danger to themselves or others (He u. a. 2020, 19; To u. a. 2020). Our personal experience is that this is often not taken into consideration, leading at times to absurd contact prohibitions.

3. How things are dealt with internationally

Hospital visiting policies are not dealt with uniformly, which, from an ethical point of view is appropriate since hospitals have different conditions and are in different contexts. The nurses should be given a strong say in the matter (\Ag\aard und Lomborg 2011). In Germany, visits to old people's homes and nursing homes, hospitals and facilities for the disabled were prohibited in March, April and Mai 2020. Exceptions were only made for very special cases, such as in the palliative care area, when parents visit their children at the children's hospital ward or in the pleasing case of births. These regulations are now slowly being loosened.

From mid-March onwards, the German BIVA care protection association, which represents the interests of people in need of care nationwide, received a dramatically increasing number of calls for help. Relatives of the seriously ill and dying reported that they too were turned away at the front doors of nursing homes. The visiting bans were interpreted very restrictively because of the great uncertainty and fear of infected residents or staff. In an online survey by the BIVA, 90 percent of those questioned stated that they no longer had the opportunity to see their relatives (Ott o. J.).

A survey of the websites of all 472 National Health Insurance contracted hospitals in Taiwan revealed that in April 2019, 276 hospitals had posted new visiting policies on their websites. Visits to ordinary wards were forbidden in 83 of those hospitals. Among the 193 hospitals that had new visiting policies and still allowed visits to ordinary wards, 73.1% restricted visitors to two at a time and 54.9% restricted visits to two visiting slots per day. Furthermore, history taking regarding travel, occupation, contacts, and cluster information was mentioned by 82.4% of these 193 hospitals, body temperature monitoring by 78.2%, hand hygiene by 63.2%, and identity checks by 51.8% (Liu u. a. 2020).

Studies from other countries are lacking.

Many creative, mainly virtual, solutions are being thought about and put into practice to enable meaningful communication between family caregivers and residents of short and long-term care facilities (Hado und Friss Feinberg 2020). In Italy "WhatsApp" enabled family members to participate in clinical rounds. In a small survey, family members had a good impression, indicating that the virtual presence could replace real presence well or very well at times. However, the real presence at bedside was considered irreplaceable. They perceived that their loved one, when admitted to hospice, had to say good-bye in presence before dying (Mercadante u. a. 2020).

4. Final considerations

This chapter departed from a personal situation and returns to it. In the case of the 54-year-old friend the family easily accepted the fact that they were not able to visit him. The staff enabled chats, calls and video-calls several times per day and even took pictures for the relatives. Being able to see and hear the very weak but optimistic voice of their husband/father has made the situation tolerable – up to now: he is still on the intensive ward.

As often in ethics, the answer does not have to be a strict "yes" or "no" ruling for all situations. Depending on circumstances, hospital districts, hospitals and even single wards and parts of wards in a hospital should be allowed to make their own choices on visiting policies – and adapt them to the circumstances. Ultimately, ethical thinking is a thinking that adapts highest personal and human values with agility to specific circumstances. Hence, we are all called, at all times, to be our own ethics committees and to participate in social ethic processes.

My personal experience in writing this chapter is the realization that I was perhaps too quick in changing my mind. My gut feeling had always been "no, it is not right for loved ones to not be able to see their relatives in hospital". However, as soon as I began writing about it, the concepts "crowded hospital", "lack of masks etc." and "infectious relatives", quickly swung me to accepting a strict no-visitor regulation in the Chilean hospital, even though I had little insight into the concrete situation. A look at how politicians are dealing with COVID-19 worldwide gives me the feeling that I may not be the only one to have such reflexes: Many of us making decisions "from the top" tend to chronically underestimate human resourcefulness, be it immunological, social or spiritual. The more we acknowledge *and develop* these resources in ourselves and others, the less regulations we will need to impose externally on ourselves and others.

It was only after further delving into the matter with others that I realized that, as far as staffing and equipment allow, we should have the courage, as individuals and as a global society, to maintain the value of personally being with a loved one in the hospital. Especially a person who is on the verge of death should, under all circumstances and with utmost effort, be enabled to be in the presence of their loved ones. With some love and ingenuity, we will realize as medical staff and hospital managers that this is, in fact, almost always feasible. It is important to realize here that the visiting rules announced by hospital directors and governments usually entail the possibility of making exceptions. We should be aware of our freedom of action, cultivate it, and maintain it by making sensible and responsible use of it.

References

\AAg\aard, Anne Sophie, und Kirsten Lomborg. 2011. „Flexible family visitation in the intensive care unit: nurses' decision-making". *Journal of clinical nursing* 20(7–8): 1106–1114.

Antoni, Michael H. 2003. "Stress management effects on psychological, endocrinological, and immune functioning in men with HIV infection: empirical support for a psychoneuroimmunological model". *Stress* 6(3): 173–188.

Christian, Lisa M. u. a. 2006. "Stress and wound healing". *Neuroimmunomodulation* 13(5–6): 337–346.

Evans, Dwight L. u. a. 1997. "Severe life stress as a predictor of early disease progression in HIV infection". *American Journal of Psychiatry* 154(5): 630–634.

Hado, Edem, und Lynn Friss Feinberg. 2020. "Amid the COVID-19 Pandemic, Meaningful Communication between Family Caregivers and Residents of Long-Term Care Facilities is Imperative". *Journal of Aging & Social Policy*: 1–6.

He, Xi u. a. 2020. "Temporal dynamics in viral shedding and transmissibility of COVID-19". *Nature medicine* 26(5): 672–675.

Liu, Ya-An u. a. 2020. "Hospital visiting policies in the time of coronavirus disease 2019: A nationwide website survey in Taiwan". *Journal of the Chinese Medical Association*. https://www.ncbi.nlm.nih.gov/pmc/articles/PMC7199773/ (30. Mai 2020).

Mercadante, Sebastiano u. a. 2020. "Palliative care in the time of COVID-19". *Journal of Pain and Symptom Management*.

Ott, Helena. „Besuchsverbot in Pflegeheim: Menschen verzweifeln". *Süddeutsche.de.* https://www.sueddeutsche.de/politik/coronavirus-pflegeheime-besuchsverbot-sterben-1.4871274 (30. Mai 2020).

Pena Cortes, Luis Carlos u. a. 2018. "Development of the Tonsil Microbiome in Pigs and Effects of Stress on the Microbiome". *Frontiers in Veterinary Science* 5. https://www.ncbi.nlm.nih.gov/pmc/articles/PMC6156429/ (1. Februar 2020).

Rojas, Isolde-Gina, David A. Padgett, John F. Sheridan, und Phillip T. Marucha. 2002. "Stress-induced susceptibility to bacterial infection during cutaneous wound healing". *Brain, behavior, and immunity* 16(1): 74–84.

To, Kelvin Kai-Wang u. a. 2020. "Temporal profiles of viral load in posterior oropharyngeal saliva samples and serum antibody responses during infection by SARS-CoV-2: an observational cohort study". *The Lancet Infectious Diseases*.

David Martin, born 1973 in Vermont, USA, grew up in the USA, France and England. He is a pediatrician, pediatric endocrinologist, oncologist, diabetologist and hematologist. He holds the Gerhard Kienle Chair of Medical Theory, Integrative and Anthroposophic Medicine at the University of Witten/Herdecke and leads the pediatric endocrinology, diabetology and integrative pediatric oncology services in the Filderklinik, an anthroposophic hospital in Germany. He has received several prizes for his research in the field of growth, skeletal development and endocrinology and is Counselling Professor of the German National Academic Foundation. He is the founder and director of www.feverapp.org, www.warmuptofever.org, and the Clinical Foundation Course of the Eugen-Kolisko Academy www.kolisko-academy.org, faculty of www.anthroposophic-drs-training.org, scientific director of http://icihm.damid.de/en_and is co-founder and co-director of www.lebens-Weise.org and www.medienfasten.org. Contact: Chair of Medical Theory, Integrative and Anthroposophic Medicine, Department of Health, University of Witten/Herdecke. David.Martin@uni-wh.de.

The Corona Virus pandemic and the Al-majiri system in Nigeria: protecting the extra vulnerable

Peter F. Omonzejele, University of Benin, Nigeria

Abstract

In many parts of the world the poor and uneducated are more vulnerable in a health crisis, just as in this COVID-19 pandemic. The Al-Majiris in Benin and other States of Western Africa are extra vulnerable to harm and exploitation due lack of education and citizen rights, governmental self-interests and corruption and infrastructure deficits.

Key words

Al-majiris, extra vulnerability, pandemic, political interests, poverty, vulnerability, West-Africa.

Introduction

The Corona virus pandemic was discovered in the China in the last quarter of 2019. From there, it gradually spread to other parts of the world, including Nigeria. Efforts to contain the spread of the virus exposed infrastructural deficits in many countries, especially those in West Africa. For instance, many West African countries had very few ventilators, some did not even have well-equipped isolation centers in place, inadequate healthcare workers, non-availability to shortage of personal protective equipment, etc. *Ab initio*, it was clear to governments in the West African region that the only reasonable option available to them was prevention rather than management of the disease. Hence, they took the decision to close international borders (air and land) to foreigners since almost all reported cases of COVID-19 in the region were imported. In addition, and in line with the World Health Organization (WHO) guidelines, they used print and electronic media to direct their citizens on regular hand washing with soap and water, the use of hand sanitizers, mandatory use of face masks, social and physical distancing, restriction of movements (lockdowns) and ban on inter-state travels. Adherence to those guidelines in West African countries grappling with infrastructural deficits, prevalent poverty and corrupt practices by enforcement agents made compliance difficult.

Practical challenges

In Western countries, availability of water is taken as a given and for granted. This is not the case in many countries of the world. For example, in West African countries, clean water is a scarce commodity. This means that hand washing with water and soap could be a challenge in settings where water is a scarce resource. The implication is that despite the general agreement that proper hand washing kills bacteria and viruses, unfortunately, 'water is a rarity- especially in the rural areas - and most West Africans, be they in the rural or urban areas, have never seen an air dryer used for the purpose of drying one's hands after washing' (Omonzejele 2014,418). It then means that even if citizens in that region wish to drink or adhere to the guideline on hand washing, they simply cannot do so if there is no water. This is one of the practical challenges to combating COVID-19 in the region. Needless to say, in a region where there is endemic poverty, very few people can afford the regular purchase and consistent use of alcohol-based hand sanitizers.

One of the globally recognized ways of curtailing COVID-19 is to lock down whole cities, provinces and sometimes even countries. For instance, China locked down the city of Wuhan for an extended period of time. This certainly slowed down the spread of the virus to other parts of China. Countries such as, France, Spain, Italy, the United States of America, the United

Kingdom were locked down at some point as a way of curtailing the raging spread of the virus. One common denominator with all those countries is that they made palliatives available to their citizens and residents. In addition, they made stimulus packages available to small and medium scales entrepreneurs. Unfortunately, in many West African countries, palliatives were not available, and were available; it was so little for such palliatives to have any effect on the economic consequences of a lock down. In some cases, it was out rightly politicized. The consequence was that it then became difficult to enforce lock downs as people had to make the bitter choice between dying from the pandemic or from hunger. Most people chose to die from the pandemic. Hence, government directives on lock downs were flagrantly disobeyed. The logic is simple: a starving person without support and safety net cannot be expected to remain at home. Particularly hit were those who are daily wage earners, such as; artisans, traders, small business owners, etc. This was and still is a practical challenge in combating the COVID-19 pandemic in West Africa, including Nigeria.

At the level of managing the COVID-19 in health facilities in West Africa, the pandemic further exposed the weak health infrastructure in that region. According to Roca et 2020, e631: 'Many West African countries have poorly resourced health systems, rendering them unable to quickly scale up an epidemic response. Most countries in the region have fewer than five hospital beds per 10 000 of the population and fewer than two medical doctors per 10 000 of the population (based on WHO global health observatory data), and half of all west African countries have per capita health expenditures lower than US$50 (based on WHO global health expenditure data. In contrast, Italy and Spain have 34 and 35 hospital beds, respectively, per 10 000 of the population, 41 medical doctors per 10 000 of the population, and US$2840 and US$2506 per capita expenditure. Despite having young populations (old age is a major risk factor for severe forms of COVID-19 and mortality), some west African countries have rates of other risk factors similar to European countries.' This shows the dire and challenging health circumstances in the West African region.

At the level of care for those who have contracted the COVID-19 disease, *ab initio*, everyone knew it was going to constitute a challenge. Within the first month of managing patients for the condition, there were shortages of test kits, ventilators, personal protect equipment, etc. At some point, the old saying that necessity is the mother of invention came to bear. For instance, in Senegal with only 50 ventilators nation-wide, scientists, in collaboration with Mologic, a British biotech company 'developed a COVID-19 test kit that cost $1 and a ventilator which cost $60. The kit can deliver results in 10 minutes and can be used at home like a pregnancy kit' (Oguntola 2020). This is against imported ventilators that cost $16,000 for one. Nigerian engineers and scientists in tertiary institutions have also been reported to have manufactured low-cost ventilators as well. In the meantime, the Chinese government, the European Union, business organizations and wealthy individuals provided assistance in the form of medical equipment, technical assistance and much needed financial support, among other things, to build standard isolation centers. However, despite material and financial supports received to combat the pandemic, a category of people that has been mistreated and must be considered extra vulnerable victims of the pandemic- are the al-majiris.

The al-majiris: protecting the extra-vulnerable in the COVID-19 pandemic

Al-majiris are found in several countries in Western Africa. In Nigeria, they are predominantly located in the northern part of that country. The term al-majiri is used to refer to 'school age children who leave the comfort and parental care to seek knowledge in nearby towns and cities (Usman 1981, 24). In general, the system was held in high esteem in that region, at least,

before the pre-colonial era. However, when the British arrived, they introduced Western education and de-emphasized the al-majiri system obtainable in northern Nigeria. For the British to
achieve the desired objective, it starved the al-majiri system of state funding (Shittu and Olaofe
2015, 38). After which those who ran the system did so at their own expense without state support, and the system no longer carried with the awe it used in the past. Instead: 'The word, al-
Majiri, which used to command respect, sympathy and solidarity, nowadays generates obnox-
ious feeling in the public domain. What quickly comes to the mind of many people whenever
the word is uttered is the image of malnourished and destitute school age-street children, who
constitute public nuisance and security threat to the society'. (Alechenu 2012*).

From that point, the al-majiris were more or less vulnerable persons who were randomly
utilized by influential persons and politicians for their own purposes and benefits.. When they
are considered of no benefit or use to them (politicians and other influential persons), they were
disposed of. This is the reason why states in Nigeria that had previously used them for their
electoral value, all of a sudden no longer wish to have them in their states due to the COVID-19
pandemic ravaging the globe. For instance, Governors of Kano and Kaduna states of Nigeria
have sent the al-majiris away from their regular states of resident because of the COVID-19 to
other states (Mohammed and Maishanu, 2020). In like manner, States in Southern Nigeria continue to send away trucks loaded with al-majiris back to their previous states of resident in
northern Nigeria. These mistreatments caused further abuses to the al-majiris and exposed their
vulnerability.

What does it mean to be vulnerable? To be vulnerable is to be unable to protect one's interests from harm and exploitation. According to the Council for International Organization of
Medical Sciences (CIOMS 2002), vulnerable people are '...those who are relatively or absolutely incapable of protecting their own interests because they may have insufficient power, intelligence, education, resources, strength, or other needed attributes to protect their own interests. The al-majiris in Nigeria perfectly fit into this definition. However, Omonzejele (2014,
263-264), had made a distinction between intrinsic and contextual forms of vulnerability. Contextual forms of vulnerability refer to situations in which the inability to protect one's own interests emanates from social, cultural, political, or economic circumstances. In this case, the
cause of vulnerability is extraneous. For instance, the lack of access to essential medicines in a
rural village in Kano or Sokoto is a social, economic or political circumstance specific to those
in that rural area, and not to all citizens of Kano or Sokoto states. It is within this context; one
must understand the extra-vulnerability burden placed on the al-majiris of northern Nigeria. And
since 'the al-majiri fall among the category of extremely poor children in Nigeria' (Isiaka 2015,
10), then they must be considered as contextually vulnerable. However, the COVID-19 pandemic general the vulnerability of the region, but the al-majiris with special identifiable vulnerability went beyond those of the general population, it is for that reason that the al-majiris
should be considered as extra-vulnerable. In fact, Kottow (2003, 461) has argued that this form
of destitute vulnerability should be referred to as susceptibility. This is because it appears the
concept of vulnerability is incapable of capturing extreme forms of vulnerability beyond the
general vulnerabilities of others in the same community, country or region. It is for this reason
that the concept of susceptibility might be employed to capture the destitution of the al-majiris
in the face of the COVID-19 pandemic. What then is the difference between the concepts of
vulnerability and susceptibility?

The distinction between the concepts of vulnerability and susceptibility does not work in
many languages. It is even a possibility that such a distinction only works in English. Nevertheless, an exposé of the concept of susceptibility is important for two reasons. First, it helps to

establish that the concept of vulnerability has short-comings in preventing potentially harmful group of people, such as the al-majiris, and which cannot be morally justified. But second, it also establishes that despite its short-comings it is doubtful that the concept of susceptibility is a viable alternative, hence, I introduced the term the extra-vulnerable.

The idea of susceptibility is relatively new in bioethics. However, the term has been in use in main stream medical practice for a long time. Kottow introduced the concept of susceptibility into bioethics because he believes that all human beings are vulnerable, but not all human beings are susceptible. According to Kottow (ibid), the concept of vulnerability is a universal phenomenon identifiable in all humans. This makes the concept somewhat difficult and nebulous at the point of application in terms of those who need special protection due to potential added exposure to harm.

It is for that reason that Kottow sought for a more appropriate term or concept in place of (or to be used alongside) the rather better-known concept of vulnerability. This is because there is no doubt beyond universal vulnerability that there are people who are more exposed to harm and injury in specific ways than others (MacIntyre, 1999: 462). For instance, O'Neill (1996: 462) states that all humans are "persistently vulnerable in ways typical of the whole species", and that consequently they all require protection of some sort. In the same vein that due to infrastructural deficit in the West African region, all citizens in that region are vulnerable to the virus in a way citizen in wealthy nations are not. Further still, there are categories or group of people, such as the al-majiris that are even more vulnerable to the virus even within and amongst the already general vulnerability in that setting. This means that, there is a further need to protect those who are 'deeply, variably and selectively vulnerable in specific circumstances, a state of destitution that needs to be addressed with sensitivity to and rejection of harm these individuals are prone to'. Kottow refers to this distinct form of vulnerability indicated by MacIntyre and O'Neill as a state of susceptibility, which he argues is different from the state of general vulnerability. Kottow (2003: 463) makes the distinction between both conditions as: 'Vulnerability can be reduced by equal protection to all members of society under a principle of justice. Susceptibility is a determined state of destitution and therefore can only be reduced or neutralized by measures that are (a) specifically designed against the destitution in question, and (b) actively applied. The susceptible, like the sick, requires targeted treatment to palliate their misery'. - Kottow (ibid.) explains further that the state of susceptibility exposes the affected to additional harm, a condition which can only be ameliorated by addressing the specific nature of the condition and that: 'In a nutshell, the vulnerable are intact but at risk, in the same way a fine piece of porcelain is unblemished but highly vulnerable to being damaged. The susceptible are already injured, they already suffer from some deficiency that handicaps them, renders them defenseless and predisposed to further injury; their wounds lower the threshold to additional suffering'.

Kottow also (ibid. 463) indicates further that, it would be 'a misdiagnosis of consequence' to treat the susceptible as vulnerable. According to him, this is because governments generally provide protective rights based on the notion of general human vulnerability. But those general protective rights do not protect the susceptible. General protective rights could only be of use to the susceptible if such protections were 'personalised' and specific. What Kottow intends to state here is not quite clear, as protective rights are generally not given to humans on the basis of general vulnerability; if they were why would there be special protections for the elderly suffering from Alzheimer? The latter are given government protections too. What could be deduced from Kottow argument as it pertains to the al-majiris is that they need personalized protection from COVID-19 because of their specific destitution. Based on this line of argument, a moral wrong was done to the al-majiris when they were not granted care based on the susceptibility to the COVID-19. Lack of care for them dashed their expectations, as they had legitimate expectations which were dashed with serious consequences. This is because the al-majiris are people who have already suffered harm. According to Kottow, one simply does not harm the already seriously harmed if one can avoid it. And to do so requires the distinction between vulnerability and susceptibility. For Kottow (ibid. 462) a clearer way of understanding harm caused to people in dependency circumstance is to identify and recognize the distinction between the concepts of vulnerability and susceptibility. Regardless, of the applicable concepts to the circumstances of the al-majiris, what is important to note is that a situation where al-majiris were treated as cartels to be moved around and tossed about by states in Nigeria is morally acceptable and condemnable. Given their state of destitution, it will suffice for us to categorize them as the extra vulnerable needing further protection, beyond that of others, from the COVIDE-19 disease.

Conclusion

The al-majiris' hardship derives from a lack of care and funding from region governments. This is responsible for their contextual vulnerability associated with the al-majiris as occasioned by their destitution. West African governments in general and the Nigerian government in particular must make conscious decision to revitalize the al-majiri educational system by making funds available to local government authorities for it.

The al-majiris, like other citizens of Nigeria, have the right to reside in any state of their choice in the Nigerian federation, and there is no reason why the al-majiris should be denied of this right. It is a constitutional violation when state governors forcefully move them away from their states because (according to such governors) they are perceived to be potential carriers of the COVID-19 disease. This is even more morally burdensome when we know that these same state governors utilize the al-majiris for their electoral worth. Each one of the al-majiris ought to be treated as an end, and not utilized by politicians as means to achieving their selfish political interests.

References

Alechenu, J. April 29, 2012. "The odds against the Almajiri Education," *The Sunday Punch*, 59.

Isiaka, T.O. 2015. A pilot study of the challenges of infusing al-majiri educational system into the universal basic educational programme in Sokoto State, Nigeria. *Journal of Education and Practice* 6 (16): 10.

Kottow, M. 2003. The Vulnerable and the Susceptible. *Bioethics.* 17: 5-6.

MacIntyre, A. 1999. Dependent Rational Animals. In. M. Kottow. 2003. The Vulnerable and the Susceptible. *Bioethics.*17.5-6.

Mohammed, I and Maishanu, A. May 10, 2020. Kano, Kaduna provide COVID-19 status of hundreds of returned almajiris. *Premium Times* https://premiumtimesng.com.(accessed 15th July 2020)

Oguntola, T. 2020. Senegal scientists develop $1 COVID-19 testing kit, $60 ventilator. *Nigeria Leadership Newspaper.* http://leadership.ng (accessed 2nd May 2020).

Omonzejele, P.F. 2014. Ethical challenges posed by the Ebola virus epidemic in West Africa. *Journal of Bioethical Inquiry* 11 (4): 418.

Omonzejele, P.F. 2014. Understanding the concept of vulnerability from a Western Africa perspective. In: Teays, W. Gordon, J-S and Renteln, AD. *Global Bioethics and Human Rights-Contemporary Issues*. New York. Romwan & Littlefield.

O'Neill, O. 1996. Towards Justice and Virtue. In: M. Kottow. The Vulnerable and the Susceptible. *Bioethics*. 17.5-6.

Roca, A. M. Martinez-Alvarez, A. Jarde, E. Usuf, H. Brotherton, M. Bittaye A. Samateh, M. Anthonio, J. Vives-Tomas, and U. D'Alessandro. 2020. COVID-19 pandemic in West Africa. *The Lancet Global Health* 8 (5): e631.Shittu, A and Olaofe, M. 2015. Situations of the al-majiri system of education in contemporary Nigeria: matters arising. *IlorinJournal of Religious Studies* 5 (2): 38

Usman, YB. 1981. *Transformation of Katsina 1400-1885*, (Zaria: Ahmadu Bello University Press Ltd), 24.

Peter Omonzejele, PhD, is a philosopher and bioethicist. He trained in bioethics at the University of Witwatersrand, Johannesburg, South Africa and at the University of Central Lancashire, Preston, England. He is Professor of Cross-Cultural Bioethics in the Department of Philosophy, University of Benin, Benin-City, Nigeria. – pfomonzejele@yahoo.com.

Science and Ethics in Times of Crisis

Željko Kaluđerović, University of Novi Sad, Serbia

Abstract

The author is of the opinion that in the era of rapid strengthening of social and technological effects of science, it is necessary to ethically codify the issue of social responsibility of scientists which, in order to be adequately internalized, must be an integral part of their upbringing and education from the earliest days. Corresponding interdisciplinary, multidisciplinary, transdisciplinary and pluriperspective approach, as well as the awareness of the essential compatibility of scientific freedom and responsibility, finally, should result in a different and more sophisticated attitude of scientists themselves towards the possibilities of their own discipline and significance of its effects.

Key words

science, ethics, crisis, principles, values, freedom, responsibility

> *Studies flourish, minds are awakening, it is a joy merely to be alive!*[1]

Said the famous humanist and a friend of Desiderius Erasmus Roterodamus, Ulrich von Hutten, already in the 16th century to depict the intellectual excitement of people of the New Age. Almost a century after Hutten, a great English philosopher Francis Bacon moderately, but in line with the optimism of the epoch, notes that the happiness of his time is that little vessels, like the celestial bodies, should sail round the whole globe, and that these times may just use *plus ultra* where the ancients used *non plus ultra*. Bacon claims that the true purpose of any science is the practical use. In *The New Organon*, he states that the true and legitimate goal of sciences is nothing else but to endow human life with new discoveries and resources. In other books, Bacon will vary the same idea, and as the goal of science he states "to serve human welfare", "to succeed in helping to eliminate the difficulties of human life", or "continually enriching humanity with new deeds and forces".

The practical benefit that he stands for is the dominion of man, i.e. mankind over nature. Unlike some of his contemporaries who wanted to regulate the relations with nature by means of mysticism, magic, or astrology, Bacon was at a position that the dominion over nature can only be achieved by the scientific knowledge of nature's causality:

> Human knowledge and human power meet at a point; for where the cause isn't known the effect can't be produced[2]

The dominion over nature, i.e. practical benefit, he considered to be the basic and ultimate, and not the immediate and current goal of science. Intending to dissociate himself from the interpretation of his philosophy in the sense of harsh practicality and pragmatism, Bacon has even argued that "the acts should be made more like pledges of truth than as contributing to the comforts of life", and that contemplating things as they are, without superstition or imposture, error or confusion, is in itself worthier than all the practical upshots of discoveries.

The German physicist and philosopher Werner Heisenberg in *Physics and Beyond*, more than three and a half centuries after Bacon wrote:

> Science is made by men, a self-evident fact that is far too often forgotten. If it is recalled here, it is in the hope of reducing the gap between the two cultures, between art and sci-

---

[1] Ward, Joseph H 2018. *The Hand of Providence*. Frankfurt am Main: Outlook Verlag GmbH. 67.

[2] Bacon, Francis. *The New Organon: or True Directions Concerning the Interpretation of Nature*. [http://www.earlymoderntexts.com/assets/pdfs/bacon1620.pdf, visited June 2, 2020] 4.

ence. ... Science rests on experiments; its results are attained through talks among those who work in it and who consult one another about their interpretation of these experiments. Such talks form the main content of this book. Through them the author hopes to demonstrate that science is rooted in conversations. ... Human, philosophical or political problems will crop up time and again, and the author hopes to show that science is quite inseparable from these more general questions.[3]

Most often we lose sight of this self-explanatory fact, although it represents a crucial point in the approach to the phenomenon of science and scientific creation, and generally in the scientific attitude of man to the world. Warning and insisting on an almost trivial matter probably would not make any sense at all, had it not been generally forgotten, although it is fundamental in the entire scientific development and its overall role and meaning. Tracing Martin Heidegger, it could be said that the oblivion of the essential is a precondition and the assumption of any opinion,[4] and probably in that sense, Heisenberg warns of the necessary oblivion of the most understandable fact that science is made by humans. This oblivion is the assumption of the entire scientific and technical[5] progress, that is, of all models of scientific approach to life, i.e. reality. Without it, probably there would be no intense progress as recorded in the last few centuries in European history. Science, therefore, is an ambivalent and ambiguous phenomenon, which is its characteristic that is both inherent in the European culture and civilization, and at the same time allows it to expand and rise to a planetary and universal level.

Ambivalence is noticeable in almost every scientific act and every scientific result.[6] It could be said when genetics, atomic physics, or some other contemporary discipline is concerned that, to a significant extent, mankind as a community of a single kind of beings depends on them, or furthermore, that the fate of the planet itself, or its survival actually depend on its results. The achievements of these disciplines facilitates development in both directions almost to the same extent: namely, the results of scientific achievements, although they primarily tend towards progress and achievement of the highest human values, at the same time, they may generate adverse, even catastrophic consequences.

Herbert Marcuse, at one stage, even thought that the scientific and technical process almost completely got out of the human control, and that the dilemma whether the planet would survive or fail will be decided by pure coincidence.[7] Closer to the truth, according to the author, is the fact that despite all ambivalence, scientific achievements are still under the control of men, and that in different modes this control can be more efficient and more differentiated in the future.

---

[3] Heisenberg, Werner 1971. *Physics and Beyond*. New York, Evanston, and London: Harper & Row, Publishers. XVII.

[4] Heidegger, Martin 1969. *Identity and Difference*. New York, Evanston, and London: Harper & Row, Publishers. 42-74.

[5] Today, the phrase scientific and technical is often used, although it should not be forgotten that only the modern epoch has enabled and established this commonality of "science" and "technique". In earlier times, this almost implicit blend of science and technique was not self-evident. Although, for example, the invention and use of a steam engine caused the first industrial revolution, it was not the result of scientific discovery, but rather a technical invention created with a very clear practical application in crafts, agriculture and mining. It can be assumed that science will return to its source in the future, i.e. to the, search for the truth, while the technique will focus on the correction of the world in terms of creating adequate assumptions and conditions for the improvement of human life.

[6] Albert Einstein used to say that science is a powerful instrument. Whether this instrument is used in the glory of mankind or for its ruin depends on mankind, and not on the instrument. See: Infeld, Leopold 1983. *Albert Ajnštajn*. Beograd: Nolit.

[7] Marcuse, Herbert 2002. *One-Dimensional Man*. London: Taylor Francis Ltd

That is why the issue of responsibility[8] of the scientist is of crucial importance, it is a fundamental issue of their actions, and not an auspicious issue that can but needn't be linked to what is happening in the field of science. In other words, this issue must be the starting point of any scientific act, with full awareness of possible abuses and negative consequences that could follow from almost any result. The lack of full awareness of responsibility can be illustrated by disproportionately high investment in scientific programs and projects that have practical application, and significantly less funds in the so-called pure science, i.e. fundamental research, or in social and humanistic sciences which do not generate immediate benefits but allow the development of science as such.

On the wave of complacency with the technical and technological progress which the XX and the XXI centuries have brought, as if it has been forgotten that science and philosophy began with wonder or admiration.[9] At first, wonder was related to the unusual phenomena that stood before people's eyes, and then transferred to larger things, such as celestial bodies, and reached the wonder about the creation of the whole universe. Wonder, of course, also contains in itself a dimension of ignorance, which, again, is most often related to the ignorance of the cause. People have always been amazed when they see a consequence and cannot find the cause of its occurrence. The awareness of this ignorance often occurs when a person concludes that something is happening in a way that is opposite to the usual one. An example that Aristotle presents are the marionettes which no one expects to move or dance according to an appropriate tune (*Met.*983a12-15). Then it becomes clear that there is some hidden cause. Man's natural aspiration for knowledge, assisted by some sort of fear of ignorance, as well as by the necessary amount of boldness, urges people to look for the causes of these phenomena.

Similar processes occur when solving geometric, astronomical or microbiological problems, for instance. Undoubtedly, the dramatic changes in the world over recent decades have been the result of scientific developments, but it should be borne in mind that this is not the primary goal of science. The significant motive for people to start dealing with science was, and it undoubtedly should also be today, the search for the truth. In Stagirites' words - knowledge for the purpose of knowledge. In this connection of motives that are related to the truth and search for it, as well as its practical pretensions, the essential dual value of science and scientific development can be detected. The modern world is undoubtedly marked by the prevalence of the latter, practical aspect of science, or the efficiency of applying its results in everyday life of people, so the attention of science and scientists is most often focused on achieving as good a result as quickly as possible.

Another German physicist and philosopher, Carl Friedrich von Weizsäcker, is right in saying that as long as concern and consideration are not equally applied both to the results and negative consequences of a scientific experiment, the human race will not be mature enough to

---

[8] For more details on the concept of responsibility consult: Čović, Ante 2009. Biotička zajednica kao temelj odgovornosti za ne-ljudska živa bića. In: Čović, Ante, Gosić, Nada, Tomašević, Luka. eds. *Od nove medicinska etike do integrativne bioetike.* Zagreb: PERGAMENA / Hrvatsko bioetičko društvo. 33-46; Lerga Rinčić, Iva 2007. *Bioetika i odgovornost u genetici.* Zagreb: PERGAMENA

[9] See in particular: *Metaphysics* 982b11-21. About wonder as something that initiates philosophizing, Stagirites writes in the manuscript *On the Heavens* 294a11-28, as well as in other places (Consult: Bonitz, Hermann 1975. *Index aristotelicus* (Vol. 5). Berlin: Walter de Gruyter & Co. 323a45-59). Plato also writes about the same topic, e.g., at *Theaetetus* 155d and *Philebus* 14c-e. At Plato, the wonder is, primarily, oriented to ideas (*Parmenides* 129c), while for Aristotle this is the case with the sensuous world (as can be seen from his note at *Parts of Animals* 645a5-17, where at the end of the passage (*PA*645a16-17) he states: *Every realm of nature is marvellous* (ἐν πᾶσι γὰρ τοῖς φυσικοῖς ἔνεστί τι θαυμαστόν). Aristotle 1991. *Parts of Animals.* In: Barnes, Jonathan. ed. *The Complete Works of Aristotle I.* Princeton: Princeton University Press. 1004

live in a technical civilization.[10] The utilitarian moment, of course, has not been an eternal feature of science and scientific development. It has acquired that aspect through certain historical circumstances and conditions which characterize the spirit of time, especially in the last hundred years. The search for truth, wonder and curiosity,[11] as indicated, represent a permanent feature of scientific activity, something without which science simply cannot exist. The practical side, on the other hand, is on the margins of science, while the questions about the essence of man and the human world are its permanent preoccupation. These specific human questions play a major role in any scientific process, research, and experiment. Their presence certainly influences the results of contemporary sciences.[12]

In that sense, Edmund Husserl wrote the following in The Crisis of European Sciences and Transcendental Phenomenology:

> The specifically human questions were not always banned from the realm of science; their intrinsic relationship to all the sciences – even to those of which man is not the subject matter, such as the natural sciences – was not left unconsidered. As long as this had not yet happened, science could claim significance – indeed, as we know, the major role – in the completely new shaping of European humanity which began with the Renaissance. Why science lost this leadership, why there occurred an essential change, a positivistic restriction of the idea of science – to understand this, according to its deeper motives, is of great importance for the purpose of these lectures.[13]

It could be said that the original idea of science in its form of wonder and curiosity is more beneficial for man than all practical discoveries that undoubtedly radically change the world and establish often an unexpected reality for man himself. The trouble is that the newly established reality can never satisfy the human nature, that the scientific and technical universe has expelled precisely that which this nature is searching for and what it feels like its original domestication. On the other hand, all technical and technological achievements with practical application are the result of purely theoretical, purely scientific research, and not of some sort of rational plan of the scientists themselves. The basis is the effort to discover the marvelous order in nature,

---

[10] Weizsäcker, Carl Friedrich von 1986. *Die Verantwortung der Wissenschaft im Atomzeitalter*. Göttingen: Vandenhoeck & Ruprecht

[11] See also concluding considerations of Immanuel Kant's *Critique of Practical Reason*: *Two things fill the mind with ever new and increasing admiration and awe, the oftener and the more steadily we reflect on them: the starry heavens above and the moral law within. ... The former view of a countless multitude of worlds annihilates as it were my importance as an animal creature, which after it has been for a short time provided with vital power, one knows not how, must again give back the matter of which it was formed to the planet it inhabits (a mere speck in the universe). The second, on the contrary, infinitely elevates my worth as an intelligence by my personality, in which the moral law reveals to me a life independent of animality and even of the whole sensible world, at least so far as may be inferred from the destination assigned to my existence by this law, a destination not restricted to conditions and limits of this life, but reaching into the infinite.* Kant, Immanuel. *Critique of Practical Reason*. [https://www.gutenberg.org/files/5683/5683-h/5683-h.htm, visited June 2, 2020].

[12] Including mentioned genetics. Starting from the first researches by Gregor Mendel in 1865, through the explanation of DNA molecule structure by James Watson and Francis Crick in 1953, cloning of sheep Dolly in 1997, until the project of sequencing of the human genome that was launched at the end of 1990 and the drawing up of the human genome map in 2003. Consult: Delić, Ninoslav, Stanimirović, Zoran 2004. *Principi genetike*. Beograd: Elit Medica. See: Kaluđerović, Željko 2018a. Bioethics and Hereditary Genetic Modifications. *Conatus - Journal of Philosophy* 3(1): 31-44; Kaluđerović, Željko 2010. Bioethical analysis of the United Nations Declaration on Human Cloning. *JAHR* 1(1): 39-50

[13] Husserl, Edmund 1970. *The Crisis of European Sciences and Transcendental Phenomenology*. Evanston: Northwestern University Press. 7

and practical pretensions would only disable these great scientific ambitions.[14]

The modern civil era is based on the logocentric and homocentric image of the world, whose meaning, on Aristotle's trail, is derived from high trust in human understanding and reason abilities. The Stagirites, moreover, emphasizes that *logos* abilities can only be attributed to people.[15] By affirming that only man has a gift of speech among all living creatures (λόγον δὲ μόνον ἄνθρωπος ἔχει τῶν ζῴων, *Pol*.1253a9-10), he emphasizes the difference between humans and other living beings also in the segment of the organized community for life.

By defining man as the only living being who has a speech,[16] the Aristotle at the beginning of *Politics*, in fact, exhibited one of his three known original definitions of man. The second definition of man is that he is the only living being able to differentiate between good and evil (ἀγαθοῦ καὶ κακοῦ), i.e. just and unjust (δικαίου καὶ ἀδίκου) (*Pol*.1253a15-18). The third, and certainly best known, Stagirites' definition of man is that he is by nature a social animal or a political animal (ἄνθρωπος φύσει πολιτικὸν ζῷον, *Pol*.1253a2-3). Man is "by nature", i.e. by his original structure, which distinguishes him from other natural species, a being that can realize its own humanity only in a community with other people. This communality of people is not identical with the communality of ants, bees or some other animals that also live in organized forms of living. According to Aristotle, people base their own communality on *logos* in the community as a community, by regulating it by agreed and accepted rules, customs, and laws.

The anthropocentricity[17] of this and such *Weltanschauung* is an important reason why our dominant technical civilization did not develop in harmony with nature, but much more often in opposition to it. No human act in the past was able to substantially affect the spontaneity of the existence of our planet. As much as man was changing the natural environment in which he lived, this did not leave a greater trace on Earth itself. The rapid development of technique in this as well as in the last century put man in a completely new moral situation. The new situation is reflected in the fact that modern man must assume responsibility for the effects that are not the result of the actions of any individual, but represent the collective act, an act, in Husser-

---

[14] British physicist Ernest Rutherford, who defined the nuclear nature of atoms in 1932, said that physicists were not seeking for new energy sources or new and usable elements. The real reason for what they did lies in the impulse and fascination of research and the discovering of the deepest secrets of nature.

[15] The dignity of an individual is viewed from the perspective of the reasonability of one's nature, and such nature is attributed only to man. Only man is liberated from the empire of the goals, while the so-called non-human living entities related to connections and relations that exist in nature. Only man is aware of himself and is able to distance himself from himself for the benefit of higher goals, to relativize his own interests, up to self-surrendering (Consult: Derrida, Jacques 2002. The Animal That Therefore I Am (More to Follow). *Critical Inquiry* 28(2): 369-418). It gives him, as a moral being, the absolute status that establishes his indescribable dignity, which gives him the right not to be "enslaved" by anybody and being a moral being, no to be deprived of his own goals. Human dignity is often associated with Kant's second formulation of the categorical imperative: *Act so that you use humanity, as much in your own person as in the person of every other, always at the same time as end and never merely as means.* Kant, Immanuel 2002. *Groundwork for the Metaphysics of Morals*. New Haven and London: Yale University Press. 46-47. See: Eterović, Igor 2017. *Kant i bioetika*. Zagreb: PERGAMENA, Cent. za int. bioet. Fil. fak. Sveučilišta u Zagrebu. 104-110

[16] Denial of *logos* abilities of animals is not an incidental thing in various Aristotle's writings, but a fact of crucial importance in his observations. It was conducted in the Stagirites' *corpus* in two ways. Directly, by denying animals the ability to have any of these abilities, and indirectly by emphasizing that logical abilities can be attributed exclusively to humans. Consult: Калуђеровић, Жељко, Миљевић, Ана 2019. Стагиранин, Ерешанин и нељудска жива бића. *ARHE* XVI(31): 105-131

[17] About the roots of anthropocentrism see author's article: Kaluđerović, Željko. Hellenic Anticipations of Homocentrism. *Forthcoming*. Consult as well: Krznar, Tomislav 2016. *U blizini straha*. Karlovac: Veleučilište u Karlovcu. 63-76

lian terms, "of anonymous functioning subjectivity".[18]

The effects of modern technique suggest a completely new situation for traditional social and humanistic sciences, since the postulate of an anthropocentric image of the world is essentially derogated in the sense that people as species are unquestionable in their existence on the Earth. Ensuring the survival of the human species in the foreseeable future is a task to whose achievement new knowledge in some of them should contribute, especially in ethics[19] or bioethics.[20] In order for this fact to be confirmed, they need to re-examine the power of technique, whose deeds thus acquire a philosophical sign, given the importance they have in the lives of the human species.

In the meantime, nature has begun to vigorously "protest" against excessive human activity by changing the climate on Earth ("global warming"), but also by increasing the number of diseases and plagues in humans and animals.[21] Burning stakes during the crisis[22] of so-called "Mad Cow", "Bird Flu", "Swine Flu" diseases, "African swine fever", or the latest "Coronavirus (COVID-19)",[23] to name some, are just a warning to people and a hint of much more serious problems they may face. As an imperative, a new order in life is introduced, where one will become aware that the Earth can no longer tolerate man's often ruthless acts, but requires the cooperation of man with the world surrounding him.

---

[18] Husserl, Edmund 1970. *The Crisis of European Sciences and Transcendental Phenomenology*. Evanston: Northwestern University Press. 111-114

[19] About ethics as a philosophical discipline on morality see: Kaluđerović, Željko 2016. Pretpostavke nastanka morala. *Bošnjačka pismohrana* (Zbornik radova Simpozija "Gdje je nestao - moral") 15(42-43): 135-147

[20] The "father" of European bioethics Fritz Jahr coined the original term Bioethics and formulated a Bioethics Imperative: *'Respect every living being on principle as an end in itself and treat it, if possible, as such!'*. Jahr, Fritz 2012. Reviewing the ethical relations of humans towards animals and plants. In: Muzur, Amir, Sass, Hans-Martin. eds. *Fritz Jahr and the Foundations of Global Bioethics. The Future of Integrative Bioethics*. Berlin – Münster – Wien – Zürich – London: Lit Verlag. 4. Consult also: Zagorac, Ivana 2018. *Bioetički senzibilitet*. Zagreb: PERGAMENA, Znan. cent. izvr. za int. bioetiku. 155-167

[21] Some of the leading authors, whose views are representative of contemporary discussions about the new regulation of the relationship between humans and animals are undoubtedly Peter Singer (Singer, Peter 2011. *Practical Ethics*. New York: Cambridge University Press; Singer, Peter 2001. *Writings on an Ethical Life*. New York: HarperCollins Publishers Inc), Tom Regan (Regan, Tom 2004. *The Case for Animal Rights*. Berkeley: University of California Press; Regan, Tom 1982. *All That Dwell Therein*. Berkeley: University of California Press) and Klaus Michael Meyer-Abich (Meyer-Abich, Klaus M 1997. *Praktische Naturphilosophie*. München: C. H. Beck; Meyer-Abich, Klaus M 1984. *Wege zum Frieden mit der Natur*. München und Wien: Hanser). They, to put it briefly, believe that animals are beings capable of suffering, which have their own interests and needs that are partly similar to the basic needs of men; if there is such a similarity, then, the principle of equality requires that the interests of animals are respected equally as the similar interests of humans; animals finally have their own value, which for some derives from their consciousness, while for others additional importance lies in the kinship of humans and animals. For more details see: Kaluđerović, Željko. The Reception of Non-Human Living Beings in Philosophical and Practical Approaches. *Epistēmēs Metron Logos. Forthcoming.*

[22] The word "crisis" originates from the Greek feminine noun κρίσις and has at least four groups of meanings: "separating", "distinguishing", "decision", "judgement", "choice", "election"; "judgement of a court", "trial", "suit", "condemnation", "dispute"; "event", "issue", "turning point of a disease"; "middle of a spinal column". Consult: Liddell, Henry G., Scott, Robert, Jones, Henry S 1996. *A Greek-English Lexicon*. Oxford: Oxford University Press. 997.

[23] Professors Hans-Martin Sass and Martin Woesler rightly write and ask in their call for papers the following: *Having overcome world wars and the cold war, this exceptional time now throws us back on questions we did not imagine to be asked again – and it opens a cosmos of ethical questions: What is human dignity? What makes a human human? The forced quarantaine has offered time to reflect. Can we learn from the pandemic? How can we face this challenge, if it will return, e.g. with a 2ⁿᵈ wave? And if the virus can be defeated: Should we change our way of life and how can a more humanistic life look?*

The usual behavior of a typical scientist, especially in natural and technical sciences, until relatively recently was characterized by simplified utilitarian reasoning and scientific reductionism, thinking and decision making on science in its narrowest part, excluding or faintly mentioning the cooperation between different areas and the compatibility of their methods. Fortunately, there are more and more scientists who change the original attitude and it can also be said due to the holistic approach of certain social and humanistic sciences, and they begin to look at problems more comprehensively, taking into account knowledge from multiple disciplines when making conclusions on the use or non-use of certain methodology and technique. The smallest common denominator of all people should, or in fact, would have to be the attitude of Hans Jonas in his paper *The Imperative of Responsibility*:[24]

We should not compromise the conditions for an indefinite continuation of humanity on earth.[25]

It is not to be expected, however, that scientists will abandon their projects because of the potential dangers of future inventions, nor are things so black that Peter Sloterdijk should be followed in the conclusion that anything that anyone does today in the space that is under the influence of technical advancement, has been put into the function of general military strategies, including, according to him, the technological progress itself.[26]

The process of spreading scientific and technical achievements is an anthropological phenomenon that is difficult to stop, because it is considered to be the ontological determinant of the modern man. The society truly has a complex task to balance between the scientific freedom of research[27] and the responsibility of preserving social norms and social values.

Scientific freedom ... is an acquired right, generally approved by society as necessary for the advancement of knowledge from which society may benefit. ... Scientific freedom and responsibility are basically inseparable.[28]

The existing largely heteronomous prohibitions, although necessary, are not sufficient if the scientists themselves do not develop the awareness that they should follow the general humanistic moral principles and principles of scientific criticality. In complex times of strengthening social and technical and technological effects of science, it is necessary to ethically codify the issue of social responsibility of scientists, which because of its adequate internalization must be an integral part of their *paideia* from the earliest days. It is very important that scientists and philosophers in their conclusions and insights which, especially in humanities, often have the character of value beliefs, do not go below the achieved civilization standards of ethical and moral culture, and that they consider various topics with due care and awareness of the dilem-

---

[24] See as well: Jurić, Hrvoje 2010. *Etika odgovornosti Hansa Jonasa*. Zagreb: PERGAMENA. 153- 165

[25] Jonas, Hans 1990. *Princip odgovornosti*. Sarajevo: Veselin Masleša. 28

[26] Sloterdijk, Peter 2001. *Critique of Cynical Reason*. Minneapolis London: University of Minnesota Press

[27] Article 12b Universal Declaration on the Human Genome and Human Rights reads: *Freedom of research, which is necessary for the progress of knowledge, is part of freedom of thought. The applications of research, including applications in biology, genetics and medicine, concerning the human genome, shall seek to offer relief from suffering and improve the health of individuals and humankind as a whole.* Universal Declaration on the Human Genome and Human Rights. [http://unesdoc.unesco.org/images/0012/001229/122990eo.pdf, visited June 2, 2020]

[28] AAAS Committee on Scientific Freedom and Responsibility *Scientific Freedom and Responsibility* 1975. Washington, DC: American Association for the Advancement of Science. [https://www.aaas.org/sites/default/files/SRHRL/PDF/1975-ScientificFreedomResponsibility.pdf, visited June 2, 2020] 5

mas that can be encountered in their professional work.[29] An appropriate interdisciplinary, multidisciplinary, transdisciplinary and pluriperspective approach, as well as the awareness of the essential compatibility of scientific freedom and responsibility, should ultimately result in a more delicate and responsible attitude of the scientists themselves towards the possibilities of their own scientific discipline and the significance of its effects.

References

AAAS Committee on Scientific Freedom and Responsibility *Scientific Freedom and Responsibility* 1975. Washington, DC: American Association for the Advancement of Science. [https://www.aaas.org/sites/default/files/SRHRL/PDF/1975-ScientificFreedomResponsibility.pdf, visited June 2, 2020] 5

Aristotle 1991. *Metaphysics*. In: Barnes, Jonathan. ed. *The Complete Works of Aristotle II*. Princeton: Princeton University Press.

Aristotle 1991. *On the Heavens*. In: Barnes, Jonathan. ed. *The Complete Works of Aristotle I*. Princeton: Princeton University Press.

Aristotle 1991. *Parts of Animals*. In: Barnes, Jonathan. ed. *The Complete Works of Aristotle I*. Princeton: Princeton University Press. 1004

Aristotle 1991. *Politics*. In: Barnes, Jonathan. ed. *The Complete Works of Aristotle II*. Princeton: Princeton University Press.

Bacon n.d. Bacon, Francis. *The New Organon: or True Directions Concerning the Interpretation of Nature*. [http://www.earlymoderntexts.com/assets/pdfs/bacon1620.pdf, visited June 2, 2020] 4

Bonitz 1975. Bonitz, Hermann. *Index aristotelicus* (Vol. 5). Berlin: Walter de Gruyter & Co. 323a45-59

Čović 2009. Čović, Ante. Biotička zajednica kao temelj odgovornosti za ne-ljudska živa bića. In: Čović, Ante, Gosić, Nada, Tomašević, Luka. eds. *Od nove medicinska etike do integrativne bioetike*. Zagreb: PERGAMENA / Hrvatsko bioetičko društvo. 33-46

Derrida 2002. Derrida, Jacques. The Animal That Therefore I Am (More to Follow). *Critical Inquiry* 28(2): 369-418

Đelić 2004. Đelić, Ninoslav, Stanimirović, Zoran. *Principi genetike*. Beograd: Elit Medica

Eterović 2017. Eterović, Igor. *Kant i bioetika*. Zagreb: PERGAMENA, Cent. za int. bioet. Fil. fak. Sveučilišta u Zagrebu. 104-110

Heidegger 1969. Heidegger, Martin. *Identity and Difference*. New York, Evanston, and London: Harper & Row, Publishers. 42-74

Heisenberg 1971. Heisenberg, Werner. *Physics and Beyond*. New York, Evanston, and London: Harper & Row, Publishers. XVII

Husserl 1970. Husserl, Edmund. *The Crisis of European Sciences and Transcendental Phenomenology*. Evanston: Northwestern University Press. 7, 111-114

Infeld 1983. Infeld, Leopold. *Albert Ajnštajn*. Beograd: Nolit

---

[29] Consult also: Kaluđerović, Željko 2018b. Held's Conceptualization of Globalization Process. In: Arabatzis, Georgios, Protopapadakis, Evangelos D. eds. *Thinking in Action*. Athens, Hellas: The NKUA Applied Philosophy Research Laboratory. 53-67

Jahr 2012. Jahr, Fritz. Reviewing the ethical relations of humans towards animals and plants. In: Muzur, Amir, Sass, Hans-Martin. eds. *Fritz Jahr and the Foundations of Global Bioethics. The Future of Integrative Bioethics*. Berlin – Münster – Wien – Zürich – London: Lit Verlag. 1-4

Jonas 1990. Jonas, Hans. *Princip odgovornosti*. Sarajevo: Veselin Masleša. 28

Jurić 2010. Jurić, Hrvoje. *Etika odgovornosti Hansa Jonasa*. Zagreb: PERGAMENA. 153- 165

Kaluđerović 2010. Kaluđerović, Željko. Bioethical analysis of the United Nations Declaration on Human Cloning. *JAHR* 1(1): 39-50

Kaluđerović 2018a. Kaluđerović, Željko. Bioethics and Hereditary Genetic Modifications. *Conatus - Journal of Philosophy* 3(1): 31-44

Kaluđerović 2018b. Kaluđerović, Željko. Held's Conceptualization of Globalization Process. In: Arabatzis, Georgios, Protopapadakis, Evangelos D. eds. *Thinking in Action*. Athens, Hellas: The NKUA Applied Philosophy Research Laboratory. 53-67

Kaluđerović 2016. Kaluđerović, Željko. Pretpostavke nastanka morala. *Bošnjačka pismohrana* (Zbornik radova Simpozija "Gdje je nestao - moral") 15(42-43): 135-147

Калуђеровић 2019. Калуђеровић, Жељко, Миљевић, Ана 2019. Стагиранин, Ерешанин и не-људска жива бића. *ARHE* XVI(31): 105-131

Kant 2020. Kant, Immanuel. *Critique of Practical Reason*. [https://www.gutenberg.org/files/5683/5683-h/5683-h.htm, visited June 2, 2020]

Kant 2002. Kant, Immanuel. *Groundwork for the Metaphysics of Morals*. New Haven and London: Yale University Press. 46-47

Krznar 2016. Krznar, Tomislav. *U blizini straha*. Karlovac: Veleučilište u Karlovcu. 63-76

Lerga Rinčić 2007. Lerga Rinčić, Iva. *Bioetika i odgovornost u genetici*. Zagreb: PERGAMENA

Liddell 1996. Liddell, Henry G., Scott, Robert, Jones, Henry S. *A Greek-English Lexicon*. Oxford: Oxford University Press. 997

Marcuse 2002. Marcuse, Herbert. *One-Dimensional Man*. London: Taylor Francis Ltd

Meyer-Abich 1997. Meyer-Abich, Klaus M. *Praktische Naturphilosophie*. München: C. H. Beck

Meyer-Abich 1984. Meyer-Abich, Klaus M. *Wege zum Frieden mit der Natur*. München und Wien: Hanser

Plato 1989a. *Parmenides*. In: Hamilton, Edith, Cairns, Huntington. eds. *The Collected Dialogues of Plato*. Princeton: Princeton University Press

Plato 1989b. *Philebus*. In: Hamilton, Edith, Cairns, Huntington. eds. *The Collected Dialogues of Plato*. Princeton: Princeton University Press

Plato 1989c. *Theaetetus*. In: Hamilton, Edith, Cairns, Huntington. eds. *The Collected Dialogues of Plato*. Princeton: Princeton University Press

Regan 1982. Regan, Tom. *All That Dwell Therein*. Berkeley: University of California Press

Regan 2004. Regan, Tom. *The Case for Animal Rights*. Berkeley: University of California Press

Singer 2011. Singer, Peter. *Practical Ethics*. New York: Cambridge University Press

Singer 2001. Singer, Peter. *Writings on an Ethical Life*. New York: HarperCollins Publishers

Inc

Sloterdijk 2001. Sloterdijk, Peter. *Critique of Cynical Reason*. Minneapolis London: University of Minnesota Press

Universal   Declaration   on   the   Human   Genome   and   Human   Rights. [http://unesdoc.unesco.org/images/0012/001229/122990eo.pdf, visited June 2, 2020]

Ward 2018. Ward, Joseph H. *The Hand of Providence*. Frankfurt am Main: Outlook Verlag GmbH. 67

Weizsäcker 1986. Weizsäcker, Carl Friedrich von. *Die Verantwortung der Wissenschaft im Atomzeitalter*. Göttingen: Vandenhoeck & Ruprecht

Zagorac 2018. Zagorac, Ivana. *Bioetički senzibilitet*. Zagreb: PERGAMENA, Znan. cent. izvr. za int. bioetiku. 155-167

Željko Kaluđerović (1964, Vrbas, Serbia) is employed as Full Professor at the Department of Philosophy at the Faculty of Philosophy of the University in Novi Sad, Serbia (subjects: Hellenic Philosophy, Hellenistic-Roman Philosophy, Ethics, Bioethics, Journalistic Ethics and Philosophy of Morality), and at the Department of Philosophy and Sociology at the Faculty of Philosophy of the University in Tuzla, Bosnia and Herzegovina (subjects: Ancient Greek Philosophy and Political Philosophy).

Books: Aristotle and Presocratics (2004), Hellenic Concept of Justice (2010), Presocratic Understanding of Justice (2013), Philosophical Triptych (2014), Dike and Dikaiosyne (2015), Early Greek Philosophy (2017) and Stagirites (2018).

He has published more than 120 papers and reviews in different science and philosophy journals in Bosnia and Herzegovina, Croatia, Germany, Greece, Hungary, Montenegro, North Macedonia, Romania, Serbia, Turkey and USA. Kaluđerović took part in around 55 international symposiums and in one international congress (9th World Congress of Bioethics).

He is an editor in chief of the Journal of Philosophy *Arhe* (Novi Sad), coordinator of the Center for Bioethics at the Department of Philosophy, Faculty of Philosophy, University in Novi Sad and a member of several editorial boards of journals and proceedings, organizational, scientific and program committees of various international conferences and symposiums. E-mail contact: zeljko.kaludjerovic@ff.uns.ac.rs.

Pandemic as a Symptom

Hrvoje Jurić, University of Zagreb, Croatia

Abstract

Besides medical and public health questions, pandemic of coronavirus 2020 raised some serious philosophical, (bio)ethical, social, economic, political and legal questions which are not essentially new, but they appear in a new light, such as those on the concepts of life and health, as well as on the issues of freedom, autonomy and responsibility. Therefore, in this paper I discuss "pandemic as a symptom" of deeper problems that contemporary civilization, culture and society are faced with. For the purpose of discussing the thesis, I recall some older and recent works which could be useful in this regard.

Key words

philosophy, pandemic, health, state of exception, freedom, responsibility

1. Early Theoretical Discussions on the Coronavirus Pandemic

Already in the first several months of epidemic/pandemic of coronavirus (SARS-CoV-2 virus which causes COVID-19 disease), i.e. in the first months of the year 2020, it became clear that pandemic raises not only medical and public health questions, but also some serious philosophical, (bio)ethical, social, economic, political and legal questions. These questions are not essentially new, but the old questions appear in a new light.

Early theoretical discussions on coronavirus pandemic included distinguished philosophers who mostly expressed their thoughts on the current situation on the basis of their own theses presented in earlier works for which they became respected and well-known. However, some of them might have been better off listening to Georg Wilhelm Friedrich Hegel – who in his *Grundlinien der Philosophie des Rechts* (1820) said that philosophy as "the owl of Minerva takes its flight only when the shades of night are gathering" (Hegel 2001:20) – i.e. that they did not fly into the media prematurely, because for the sake of their own theses and conclusions they overlooked some facts and underestimated the scale of the crisis. But this does not mean that their texts have become irrelevant, because it was useful, for example, that the first of them I mention, the Italian philosopher Giorgio Agamben, reminded us of his theses on the "state of emergency" as a state that became regular and "lasting practice of government" which implies "the provisional abolition of the distinction among legislative, executive, and judicial powers" (Agamben 2005:7) and means that the boundary between law enforcement and law breaking becomes fluid.

In his short article "The State of Exception Provoked by an Unmotivated Emergency" (Agamben 2020), published on 26 February 2020 in the Italian daily newspaper *il manifesto*, Agamben warns of the danger that the rapid restriction of human freedom, which began with the pretext of terrorism and extended due to coronavirus, will continue to spread, because in a state of collective fear and panic citizens unconditionally accept the state's restriction of freedom in the desire for security, and this desire was created by the state, which is now intervening to satisfy it. Agamben's article provoked numerous reactions, documented on the website of the *European Journal of Psychoanalysis* (https://www.journal-psychoanalysis.eu/coronavirus-and-philosophers/), where they have been transmitted (and translated into English) mostly from the Italian online journal *Antinomie*. The debate first involved the French philosopher Jean-Luc Nancy, the Italian philosophers Roberto Esposito and Sergio Benvenuto, and the Indian philosophers Divya Dwivedi and Shaj Mohan. In the second wave, the Italian philosophers Rocco Ronchi and Massimo De Carolis joined this discussion, and the second time Benvenuto, Mohan and Nancy also commented. Nancy also published an article in the French daily newspaper

Libération on 24 March 2020, entitled "Communovirus", which is a term borrowed from an unnamed Indian friend, which describes a "virus coming from communism" (from China) and which "communizes" us, as opposed to the "corona" ("crown") "which evokes old monarchical or imperial histories" (Nancy 2020). Agamben himself, who boiled over this controversy, published four more articles during March and April 2020. His writing activity was certainly prompted by numerous criticisms, and perhaps the need for self-criticism, because – although he did not give up his original theses and conclusions – at the beginning of his first text, in describing the Italian epidemic situation, "frenetic, irrational and entirely unfounded emergency measures adopted against an alleged epidemic of coronavirus" (Agamben 2020), which a few months later in Italy probably no one would have signed, and perhaps he himself would not, although he did not completely disputed the suspicion about the scope and intensity of these measures.

All of the above articles expressed the view that, in addition to the health aspects of the situation in the short term, it is necessary to think about the political and economic aspects in the long term, as warned also by the French philosopher Alain Badiou (Badiou 2020) and especially the prolific Slovenian philosopher Slavoj Žižek who published, in less than two months, around ten texts on the issues of pandemic and, already in April 2020, a book entitled *Pandemic! COVID-19 Shakes the World* (Žižek 2020).

A kind of summary of the main topics of discussion (which are viewed differently by different authors) can be found in the article "The World After Coronavirus" by Israeli historian and intellectual bestseller Yuval Noah Harari, which was published in *The Financial Times* on 20 March 2020: "In this time of crisis, we face two particularly important choices. The first is between totalitarian surveillance and citizen empowerment. The second is between nationalist isolation and global solidarity." (Harari 2020)

Besides all the above, there is another important issue which, unfortunately, was not in the forefront of the world discussions on pandemic, and which the Australian-American philosopher Peter Singer and Italian philosopher Paola Cavalieri drew attention to with their article, published on 2 March 2020, on the Internet platform *Project Syndicate*. Singer and Cavalieri, both (and especially Singer) pioneers in the fight for the rights and liberation of non-human animals, rightly say that very few people mention, let alone consider, the causes of the pandemic, and state: "Both the 2003 SARS (severe acute respiratory syndrome) epidemic and the current one can be traced to China's 'wet markets' – open-air markets where animals are bought live and then slaughtered on the spot for the customers. Until late December 2019, everyone affected by the virus had some link to Wuhan's Huanan Market." (Singer, Cavalieri 2020)

Analysing the problem in both a narrower and a broader context, these authors – aware of the economic and cultural consequences of their conclusion – say: "Markets at which live animals are sold and slaughtered should be banned not only in China, but all over the world." (Singer, Cavalieri 2020)

This demand is certainly much milder than the demands that these authors normally point out and that are aimed at the complete abolition of all forms of exploitation, torture and killing of non-human animals and at a general change in the human attitude towards them. But it is also certain that with their text Singer and Cavalieri shed light on a topic that, no matter how much media pressure directs us in other directions, we should think about when considering this and other epidemics/pandemics. This topic can be summarized, although not completely precisely, as – ecological causes of the emergence and development of epidemics and pandemics, which should be considered in a broader bioethical perspective. Similar attitudes expressed authors of the books that should be considered again in the light of the current pandemic: Sonia Shah, an Indian-American scientific journalist and author of the book *Pandemic: Tracking Contagions, from Cholera to Ebola and Beyond* (Shah 2016), and Rob Wallace, an American biologist and author of the book *Big Farms Make Big Flu* (Wallace 2016). In interview published on 11 March 2020 on the website of German magazine *Marx 21*, Wallace said:

"The increased occurrence of viruses is closely linked to food production and the profitability of multinational corporations. Anyone who aims to understand why viruses are becoming more dangerous must investigate the industrial model of agriculture and, more specifically, livestock production. *Who is to blame?* I said industrial agriculture, but there's a larger scope to it. Capital is spearheading land grabs into the last of primary forest and smallholder-held farmland worldwide. These investments drive the deforestation and development leading to disease emergence. [...] As a result, many of those new pathogens previously held in check by long-evolved forest ecologies are being sprung free, threatening the whole world." (Wallace 2020)

If we add to this the information that has leaked to the media, which speaks of a causal link between air pollution in certain Chinese and Italian regions and the number of patients and deaths from coronavirus infection, which attacks primarily the respiratory system, environmental variables we will have to consider more than we have done so far.

2. Broader Framework for a Theoretical Discussion on the Coronavirus Pandemic

If we want to better understand the background of the discussion that was initiated by Giorgio Agamben, we need to look not only at the Agamben's and Nancy's works such as *Homo Sacer* (Agamben 1998) and *State of Exception* (Agamben 2005) or *The Inoperative Community* (Nancy 1991), *Being Singular Plural* (Nancy 2000a) and *The Intruder* (Nancy 2000b), but also at the classical work of biopolitical literature, *Discipline and Punish: The Birth of the Prison* by French philosopher Michel Foucault, published in 1975 (Foucault 1995), because the whole work, and especially the chapter "Panopticism" (Foucault 1995:195-228), is indispensable for exploring the way in which the restriction of freedoms and rights, control, "normalization", discipline and sanctioning work. Foucault's book describes in detail the mechanisms that have been completely exposed thanks to the recent situation.

On the other hand, if we want to better calibrate the discussion on bioethical aspects of recent pandemic, we should look at some books which today seem *more current than at the time* when they were published, such as *Disaster Bioethics: Normative Issues When Nothing Is Normal*, edited by Dónal P. O'Mathúna, Bert Gordijn and Mike Clarke (O'Mathúna, Gordijn, Clarke 2014), *Worst Case Bioethics: Death, Disaster, and Public Health* by George J. Annas (Annas 2010), and *Philosophy of Epidemiology* by Alex Broadbent (Broadbent 2013).

However, complexity of the current situation and need for both broader perspectives and deeper insights could direct us toward one of the most interesting thinkers and authors in the field of discussions on the issues related to health and society – Ivan Illich.

In his book *Medical Nemesis: The Expropriation of Health* from 1975 Illich put forward and sought to clarify and prove the thesis that professional medical practice had become a major threat to health and that the medical system had begun to pose a serious threat to health. How was it possible to put forward such a thesis in the face of the rapid progress and unprecedented successes of modern medicine, the eradication of some and the suppression of other diseases, and the prolongation of human life and the improvement of the quality of human life? The very title of this book suggests the answer: the "dark sides" of modern medicine should also be taken into account. Namely, *Nemesis* is an ancient Greek goddess who governs the destiny of man, distributing life and death, happiness and unhappiness, health and disease. She is the goddess of revenge who evaluates and charges human deeds according to merits. "Medical Nemesis" means, therefore, the revenge of modern medicine for the deviations that have occurred in the sphere of health and life with regard to the original tasks of medicine and healing, which Illich recalls. He wants to say that medicine is no longer, as it has been for most of human history, an aid in overcoming disease and acquiring or maintaining health, but has completely mastered human health and life. It is the "expropriation of health" from the subtitle of Illich's book. Medicine has imposed itself as an inevitable mediator between the individual and his health and life and has alienated the individual from his own health and life. If we ask ourselves what health and life are – the answer we must (and can) get only from medicine. Illich calls this the "medicalization" of health and life. Health and life no longer exist without medicine; personal experience of one's own existence (physicality, health, life) is exchanged for medical diagnosis. But apart from this "hegemonic" or even "tyrannical" aspect, Illich criticizes modern medicine at a lower level, in terms of its effectiveness, because it not only fails to fulfil its promises of curability of all diseases and "delaying death", but also produces new diseases, which is called "iatrogenesis". Illness production, or medicalization of some natural physical and mental states, according to Illich, encourages "medically sponsored behaviour and delusions" which "restrict the vital autonomy of people by undermining their competence in growing up, caring for each other, and aging, or when medical intervention cripples personal responses to pain, disability, impairment, anguish, and death" (Illich 1976: 271). Examples of Illich's theses from the 1970s today could be the "pandemics" of osteoporosis, hyperlipidemia and depression, and perhaps pandemics of influenza or coronavirus, because they are a direct or indirect consequence of the dehumanized and alienated industrial organizations of medicine, society and human life.

Fifteen years after *Medical Nemesis*, in 1990, Illich gave a lecture in Hanover that was later published under the title "Health as One's Own Responsibility – No, thank you!" (Illich 1992a). The "new" Illich recognizes and admits (both in that text and in some other texts from that period) that in *Medical Nemesis* he was too lenient towards modern medicine, i.e. insufficiently radical in its critique, and revises his conclusions. It is no longer so much a critique of the health care system, medicine as a science and practice, and other social systems and institutions, as a critique of the very concepts on which both modern medicine and modern society are based. That older Illich says: "I am convinced that health and responsibility belong to a lost past and that, since I am neither a romantic, a visionary, nor a drop-out, must renounce both of them […] I live in a manufactured reality ever further removed from creation. And I know today what that signifies, what horror threatens each of us. A few decades ago, I did not yet know it. At that time, it seemed possible that I could share responsibility for the re-making of this manufactured world. Today, I finally know what powerlessness is. Responsibility is now an illusion. In such a world, 'being healthy' is reduced to a combination of the enjoyment of techniques, protection of the environment, and adaptation to the consequences of techniques, all three of which are, inevitably, privileges." (Illich 1992a:3)

Illich does not deny the importance of health and responsibility as landmarks established autonomously and creatively by living individuals and convivial communities, but rejects "health" and "responsibility" as ideological slogans and phrases, as "values" prescribed by the ruling technological-economic-social-political system, i.e. rejects them as "axiomatic certainties" which, when investigated more deeply, are revealed "as deeply sickening, disorienting phenomena" (Illich 1992a:4). The explanation of his "no" (which seems to have been written for the spring of 2020) is the following: "I particularly don't say my 'No!' to a new ethics of responsibility for health because I see in modern sickness and dying occasions for finding oneself. The suggestion that we ought to accept the unavoidable epidemics of the post-industrial age as a higher kind of health is an impudence currently fashionable among pedagogues. But such instruction in suffering and dying is shameful. Care through bereavement counselling, education for dying, and the making of health plans aims directly at the destruction of the traditional art of suffering and dying, practices developed over hundreds of years. What sickens us today is something altogether new. What determines the epoch since Kristallnacht is the growing matter-of-fact acceptance of a bottomless evil which Hitler and Stalin did not reach, but which today is the theme for elevated discussions on the atom, the gene, poison, health and growth. These are evils and crimes that render us speechless. Unlike death, pestilence and devils, these evils are without meaning; they belong to a non-human order. They force us into impotence, helplessness, powerlessness, ahimsa. We can suffer such evil, we can be broken by it, but we cannot make sense of it, cannot direct it. Only he who finds his joy in friends can bear up under it. Our 'No!' is thus a universe apart from every 'Yes' to the secondary accompaniments of progress. [...] And finally, it would be either stupid or malevolent to label the no of which I speak as cynical indifference. Quite the contrary! In the forefront of our thoughts stand the many – innumerable people for whom four decades of development destroyed the cultural, technical and architectural space in which the inherited arts of suffering and dying were formerly nurtured." (Illich 1992a:3)

Instead of health and responsibility as orientation marks in the art of living and dying, today health is imposed on us "as function, process, mode of communication, [...] as an orienting behaviour that requires management" and responsibility "is reduced to a legitimizing formality" (Illich 1992a:4). In the spring of 2020, in the billions of strictly controlled pandemic solitary confinements soaked in paranoia, one should think about Illich's "diagnosis" of responsibility and health: "Being asked for responsibility is, when seen more clearly, a demand for the destruction of sense and self. [...] One cannot feel healthy; one can only enjoy her own functioning in the same way as one enjoys the use of her computer. To demand that our children feel well in the world that we leave them is an insult to their dignity. Then to impose on them responsibility for this insult is a base act. [...] Therefore, I find it reprehensible that the self-appointed health experts now emerge as caring monitors who, with their slogans, put the responsibility of suffering onto the sick themselves." (Illich 1992a:4)

What advice could we draw from Illich's thoughts in the midst of a coronavirus pandemic? To mock public health and political measures, designed to reduce the risk of contracting the virus, by discarding protective masks and gloves and hugging and kissing bystanders? No, because this is not an infantile "rebellion without a cause" at all, but a call to critically confront what is happening with health, life, human, humanity, and humanness, and a call not to look at the powerful authorities, who will "strictly but justly" say what actually is and how it should be, but to our own (individual and common) experience of being and need. Illich would perhaps tell us today that each for himself and all of us in our living human communities need to open the heavy curtain that shields human thought and action potentials, in order to rehabilitate those repressed, almost destroyed potentials.

What is SARS-CoV-2 and COVID-19 anyway? How and why did this coronavirus originate? How and why does it spread? What is the difference between infection and disease, epidemic and pandemic? Who defines it and for what purpose? How should we behave in relation to that? Illich, probably, would not deal too much with such questions, but he would certainly suggest that the answer to such questions should be reached by a detour, not by media-political shortcuts. Along the way – if we are patient enough and if we do not delude ourselves that a risk-free life is possible – we could discover what health and responsibility really mean. In any case, life, health, disease, dying and death should be guarded and preserved from total and totalitarian expropriation carried out by the specters of "medicine", "society", "state" and "technology", in order to evade medical, social, political and technological iatrogenesis.

Illich neither problematized only public health and medical facts, projections and recommendations, nor only the political measures that refer to it, nor even the visible or invisible political-ideological framework in which it takes place, but radically questioned the concepts and the values on which all of the above rests. For example, health and responsibility, concepts that we irresponsibly take for granted.

3. Consequences and Implications of the Coronavirus Pandemic

After several months of coronavirus crisis, at least three things are certain:

3.1. The coronavirus pandemic will be remembered as one of the key phenomena of the 21st century, together with a deepening ecological crisis and rapid climate change; the incessant and the world (according to its actors and effects) wars and the renaissance of terrorism; mass migrations of the population, primarily from Asia and Africa to Western Europe and from Central and South to North America; the digital revolution and the destructive and dehumanizing effects of automation; and the advance of neoliberal capitalism with repercussions on democracy. What all these phenomena have in common is that they are global and not new; new is only a way of their mass media presentation which inflates them to the breaking point, transforming societies into what Sloterdijk called "systems of care" and "stress communes" (Sloterdijk 2016). By emphasizing the aspect of mass media, we do not want to say that the mentioned "key phenomena of the 21st century" do not exist, but that they should be viewed contextually and critically. A pandemic is not just a matter of a disease caused by a certain virus, but it is also a *symptom* of deeper global social diseases such as the ones previously listed.

Given the high concentration of events, i.e. the mass production of events, and given the recent pandemic, we can indeed agree with Agamben's statement of "state of emergency" as a "legal form of what cannot have a legal form", including "juridical measures that cannot be understood in legal terms" (Agamben 2005:1). The state of emergency, according to Agamben, "tends increasingly to appear as the dominant paradigm of government in contemporary politics" and "unstoppable progression of what has been called a 'global civil war'" (Agamben 2005:2) is the perfect opportunity to realize such tendency.

3.2. The appearance of the coronavirus, and then the proclamation of the state of epidemic and pandemic, is equally a medical (virological, immunological, epidemiological, public health) and political (social, economic, legal, media) issue. This is actually obvious, but it should still be pointed out because these two interconnected dimensions are confused and merge into one. Namely, the whole issue of a pandemic is often reduced to the medical dimension, and the political dimension is "drowned" into it, i.e. the political dimension is presented as medical. First of all, expert opinions and recommendations should be distinguished from political decisions, regulations and sanctions. Moreover, the mere declaration of an epidemic or pandemic is already a political decision, made on the basis of medical facts; hence, the political form of a particular public health situation. Epidemiologists may believe that a total ban on the movement of citizens is the best solution to the problem of the spread of the virus, but the decision on what to do, with the responsibility it carries, is made by the political authorities. Political authorities obviously like to share their responsibility with the medical profession – these days even to the extent that it gives the impression that politics has left power to the medical profession and that a kind of "expertocracy" has been introduced – but it is more about the instrumentalization of the medical profession and experts by ruling political structures. Anyway, this kind of "political epidemiology" or "virological politics" is hastily introducing measures that are extremely restrictive and problematic not only from an ethical but also from a legal perspective, as even more conservative lawyers warn. On the other hand, in various countries, for various reasons, strict epidemiological measures are casually relativized, although the risk of infection has not passed, but the numbers of infected, sick and dead are higher than ever. In fact, a casual relativization of repressive measures relativizes repressive measures as a whole.

3.3. After this global "earthquake" caused by the pandemic, nothing will be the same and we will feel the consequences of what is happening today for a long time.

These are primarily health consequences, but not only those related to virus infection, disease and death, but also those related to emotional stability and mental health. Those who suffered from certain problems before the pandemic are especially endangered, but psychological crises will also affect many who previously fell into the category of "normal". As some psychologists and psychiatrists warn these days, long-term isolation, exposure to daily political, social and media pressure, and living in this lifestyle in general could result in a pandemic of mental disorders. The intimate anxieties and paranoia to which people are easily subjected are emphasized, and the nature of the pandemic is such that very little can be determined and predicted (with all the confidence of experts), so that it is accompanied by extreme uncertainty. And uncertainty in some ways could be worse than disaster, just as anxiety could be worse than fear.

The second group of easily predictable consequences of pandemic situation includes economic consequences. In this regard, the pandemic will mostly affect those who are vulnerable already in normal circumstances: the unemployed, lower paid workers, illegal workers, precarious workers, workers in private companies, etc., and their families, with all loans, debts, foreclosures and other problems. According to official data (and in reality it was probably even worse), in just twenty days of the pandemic crisis in Croatia, almost 15,000 people lost their jobs, while in the same period in the United States about 10 million people were fired. The trend will undoubtedly continue as long as measures that prevent the work of many companies are in place, with the consequences of what it seems now will not be able to be remedied, but, in combination with other consequences, will be a kind of social post-traumatic stress disorder, difficult to cure. Small private companies and crafts, family farms and workers' cooperatives will also be affected. But it is certain that capitalist system will not be endangered, which can be heard as a question these days, nor will the current situation lead to the "death of neoliberal capitalism", as some predict.

In the third group of consequences are the current and predictable political consequences, due to which the pandemic is both a health and a political threat. In this respect, the most visible are the repressive and increasingly repressive measures introduced by the world states in 2020, which concern not only freedom of movement and the right to assembly, but also the right to privacy and freedom of opinion and expression. Health and political authorities will say that it is obvious why certain repression is necessary and that there are good reasons for it – moreover, most citizens of the world are successfully convinced of it – but still a question should be asked that seems equally obvious: if, "with a good reason", fundamental human rights may be relativized and violated, what guarantees us that this will not be done in other situations, when other "good reasons" are found? And who is called or authorized to define which reason is sufficiently "good"? In other words: does this situation really give us good enough reasons to relativize and violate fundamental human rights? Also: when a call for freedom, autonomy, rights, responsibility and solidarity can be (and should be) silenced in order to achieve certain benefits? Given these issues, the current political and social measures, which differ globally only in nuances, could be assessed as excessive and we should ask ourselves, primarily, who measures and what is actually measured by these measures at all.

There is reasonable doubt that some measures introduced in the state of emergency will survive the "war against coronavirus" and remain in force, perhaps in a milder form, even when the immediate threat of the virus passes, or that the current pandemic militarization of society will accelerate the rapid erosion of democracy. Recent erosion of democracy worldwide is not only caused by "sin" (pressure from states and capital), but also by "omission" (lack of resistance from people, i.e. communities and individuals). Namely, the state of emergency, even if it is not declared, could disrupt the already fragile interpersonal relations by manipulatively generating caution, suspicion and paranoia, while restricting all and completely suspending some human rights, thus creating an extremely unusual situation for both individuals and communities. Historical experience confirms that once human rights and freedoms are abolished, they are never restored overnight, but they must be "invented" again after a social catastrophe, i.e. they must be fought for again. That is why we must be extremely suspicious of "pandemic measures", no matter how many minuses they manage to prevent with pluses in a medical-political "cost-benefit analysis".

Either way, we should listen carefully to those already quoted and recommended as good interlocutors to discuss the causes and consequences of this pandemic. In *State of Emergency*, Giorgio Agamben says: "This transformation of a provisional and exceptional measure into a technique of government threatens radically to alter – in fact, has already palpably altered – the structure and meaning of the traditional distinction between constitutional forms. Indeed, from this perspective, the state of exception appears as a threshold of indeterminacy between democracy and absolutism." (Agamben 2005:2-3)

Although Agamben believes that the state of emergency as a political paradigm has been in force for a long time, a situation such as the situation of today exposes this constellation and its danger is more visible than usual. In the aforementioned article, Yuval Noah Harari says: "Many short-term emergency measures will become a fixture of life. That is the nature of emergencies. They fast-forward historical processes. Decisions that in normal times could take years of deliberation are passed in a matter of hours. Immature and even dangerous technologies are pressed into service, because the risks of doing nothing are bigger. Entire countries serve as guinea-pigs in large-scale social experiments. What happens when everybody works from home and communicates only at a distance? What happens when entire schools and universities go online? In normal times, governments, businesses and educational boards would never agree to conduct such experiments. But these aren't normal times." (Harari 2020)

The dangers that Harari talks about – significant changes, primarily in the spheres of work and education – are also seen by Sergio Benvenuto: "After all, the effects of this epidemic will strengthen a tendency that would have in any case prevailed, and of which 'working remotely' or 'wfh', working from home and avoiding the office, is only one aspect. It will be less and less common for us to wake up in the morning and board public or private vehicles to reach the workplace; more and more we will work on our computers from our homes, which will also become our offices. And thanks to the Amazon and Netflix revolutions, we will no longer need to go out to do the shopping or to theatres to see movies, nor to buy books in bookshops: stores and bookshops (alas) will disappear and everything will be done from home. Life will become 'hearthed' or 'homeized' (we already need to start thinking up neologisms). Schools too will disappear: with the use of devices like Skype, students will be able to attend their teachers' lessons from home. This generalized seclusion caused by the epidemic (or rather, by attempts to prevent it) will become our habitual way of life." (Benvenuto 2020)

Benvenuto's dystopian projection does not apply and will not soon apply to all people. We know that many people, due to the nature of their jobs, do not have the opportunity to "work from home", no matter what catastrophe occurs. But in some spheres of the social life and some parts of the population at the global level, this Benvenuto's scenario is very certain and has already been partially realized. And if it turns out that education and many other social activities can really function "remotely", with the help of extremely controlled digital systems, this could in the near future be an argument for reducing public investment in these sectors. But even if this is not the case, the rapid technicization, digitization and virtualization of social life should be viewed with scepticism, not enthusiasm.

In the already quoted interview, Rob Wallace, in addition to criticizing the current pandemic-political measures, also presents a proposal "what to do" and on the basis of what this could be achieved: "Using an outbreak to beta-test the latest in autocratic control post-outbreak is disaster capitalism gone off the rails. In terms of public health, I would err on the side of trust and compassion, which are important epidemiological variables. Without either, jurisdictions lose their populations' support. A sense of solidarity and common respect is a critical part of eliciting the cooperation we need to survive such threats together. Self-quarantines with the proper support–check-ins by trained neighbourhood brigades, food supply trucks going door-to-door, work release and unemployment insurance–can elicit that kind of cooperation, that we are all in this together." (Wallace 2020)

On a global scale, such a call for solidarity is also a call for rehabilitation of the old regulative ideas of "liberté, egalité, fraternité". Peter Sloterdijk in his book *You Must Change Your Life* from 2009 says that "the understanding that shared life interests of the highest order can only be realized within a horizon of universal co-operative asceticisms – will have to assert itself anew sooner or later. It presses for a macrostructure of global immunizations: co-immunism." (Sloterdijk 2013:451-452).

4. Conclusion

While such an impression may have been created, this paper is not intended as a call for civil disobedience to prescribed public health measures to prevent the spread of infection by coronavirus. As always when it comes to civil disobedience, it is a matter of one's own attitude, decision, action, and responsibility. However, it is necessary to think critically about what is happening right now and what might happen to us after the end of this pandemic, which is another kind of disobedience, a "disobedience of higher level". What does such kind of disobedience mean, what does critical thinking mean, and what does respective responsibility mean – could be illustrated by the following quote taken from the book *In Defense of Anarchism* by the American philosopher Robert Paul Wolff, published in 1970: "Taking responsibility for one's actions means making the final decisions about what one should do. For the autonomous man, there is no such thing, strictly speaking, as a command. If someone in my environment is issuing what are intended as commands, and if he or others expect those commands to be obeyed, that fact will be taken account of in my deliberations. I may decide that I ought to do what that person is commanding me to do, and it may even be that his issuing the command is the factor in the situation which makes it desirable for me to do so. For example, if I am on a sinking ship and the captain is giving orders for manning the lifeboats, and if everyone else is obeying the captain because he is the captain, I may decide that under the circumstances I had better do what he says, since the confusion caused by disobeying him would be generally harmful. But insofar as I make such a decision, I am not obeying his command; that is, I am not acknowledging him as having authority over me. I would make the same decision, for exactly the same reasons, if one of the passengers had started to issue 'orders' and had, in the confusion, come to be obeyed." (Wolff 1998:15-16)

What does this mean for us as "pandemic people"? Maybe the following: one should, of course, guard against infection, for the sake of oneself and others, responsibly and in solidarity, but one should also guard against galloping manipulations and preserve mental health and emotional stability, in order to preserve freedom and autonomy. It is necessary to preserve the reason so that a question can be asked, so that an objection can be made, so that an answer can be reached which, if the answer is good, leads to new questions. It is especially important in the times of "infopandemic", which is much older than the coronavirus, but the current crisis makes it explicit and intensifies it.

That is why we need the "epistemological asceticism" that the mentioned Ivan Illich, in an interview published under the title "Against Health", recommended as a way to renounce "axiomatic certainties" (Illich 1992b). Regarding this, cultivated scepticism is a therapy against confusion and a vaccine against a pleasant but essentially destructive acceptance of certainty, in the sense in which Illich said: "Every era is like a firmament, with its conceptual fixed stars, under whose direction the ideas, but also the material experiences of the era come to existence. These basic concepts I call certainties, I should rather say assumptions which sound so obvious that no one examines them." (Illich 1992b:6).

Since the firmament of our era will not collapse even under the pressure of a pandemic, we have no choice but to continue to make an effort to radically question certainties. And even more than before, because the great crises of our epoch neither annul each other nor ever end, but pile on the top of each other and pervade each other with the passage of time to the point of indistinguishability. Even if the pandemic soon subsides, we will be sick for a long time thanks to it. In the sense in which we have called this pandemic a symptom of a much deeper-rooted disease of humanity, we may even be incurably ill. Nevertheless, depression and despair now seem like excessive luxury. Not everything is lost, unless we admit discouragedly that we are completely lost and that in that loss everyone is alone, hopelessly "socially distanced" and "self-isolated". Ivan Illich, when asked if, given the depressing scenarios he presents, he also sees any hope, he replied: "Yes. And it is not only strong, it is also often fulfilled. This scenario of which I have spoken, in which we are isolated if we seek and preserve meaning, is also an occasion for an intensity of friendship which would hardly be imaginable in a world of inherited ties, familiar culture, middle class values, wealth and security. This is my hope. Otherwise I have none." (Illich 1992b:7)

References

Agamben, Giorgio. Homo Sacer: Sovereign Power and Bare Life. Stanford: Meridian 1998.

Agamben, Giorgio. State of Exception. Chicago, London: The University of Chicago Press 2005.

Agamben, Giorgio. Lo stato d'eccezione provocato da un'emergenza immotivata. il manifesto, February 26, 2020. [URL: https://ilmanifesto.it/lo-stato-deccezione-provocato-da-unemergenza-immotivata/, visited June 1, 2020.]

Annas, George J. Worst Case Bioethics: Death, Disaster, and Public Health. New York: Oxford University Press 2010.

Badiou, Alain. On the Epidemic Situation. Verso, March 23, 2020. [URL: https://www.versobooks.com/blogs/4608-on-the-epidemic-situation, visited June 1, 2020.]

Benvenuto, Sergio. Welcome to Seclusion. European Journal of Psychoanalysis, March 2, 2020. [URL: https://www.journal-psychoanalysis.eu/coronavirus-and-philosophers/, visited June 1, 2020.]

Broadbent, Alex. Philosophy of Epidemiology. New York: Palgrave Macmillan 2013.

Foucault, Michel. Discipline and Punish: The Birth of the Prison. New York: Vintage Books 1995.

Harari, Yuval Noah. The World after Coronavirus. The Financial Times, March 20, 2020. [URL: https://www.ft.com/content/19d90308-6858-11ea-a3c9-1fe6fedcca75, visited June 1, 2020.]

Hegel, Georg Wilhelm Friedrich. Philosophy of Right. Kitchener: Batoche Books 2001.

Illich, Ivan. Medical Nemesis: The Expropriation of Health. New York: Pantheon Books 1976.

Illich, Ivan (a). Health as One's Own Responsibility – No, Thank You! The Ellul Studies Forum 5 (1992) 1:3-5.

Illich, Ivan (b). Against Health: An Interview with Ivan Illich. The Ellul Studies Forum 5 (1992) 1:6-7.

Nancy, Jean-Luc. The Inoperative Community. Minneapolis: University of Minnesota Press 1991.

Nancy, Jean-Luc (a). Being Singular Plural. Stanford: Stanford University Press 2000.

Nancy, Jean-Luc (b). L'Intrus. Paris: Galilée 2000.

Nancy, Jean Luc. Communovirus. Libération, March 24, 2020 [URL: https://www.liberation.fr/debats/2020/03/24/communovirus_1782922, visited June 1, 2020.]

O'Mathúna, Dónal P.; Gordijn, Bert; Clarke, Mike. Disaster Bioethics: Normative Issues When Nothing Is Normal. Dordrecht: Springer 2014.

Shah, Sonia. Pandemic: Tracking Contagions, from Cholera to Ebola and Beyond. New York: Farrar, Straus and Giroux 2016.

Singer, Peter; Cavalieri, Paola. The Two Dark Sides of COVID 19. Project Syndicate, March 2, 2020. [URL: https://www.project-syndicate.org/commentary/wet-markets-breeding-ground-for-new-coronavirus-by-peter-singer-and-paola-cavalieri-2020-03?barrier=accesspaylog, visited June 1, 2020.]

Sloterdijk, Peter. You Must Change Your Life: On Anthropotechnics. Oxford, Malden: Polity Press 2013.

Sloterdijk, Peter. Stress and Freedom. Oxford, Malden: Polity Press 2016.

Wallace, Rob. Big Farms Make Big Flu: Dispatches on Infectious Disease, Agribusiness, and the Nature of Science. New York: Monthly Review Press 2016.

Wallace, Rob. Coronavirus: Agribusiness Would Risk Millions of Deaths. Marx 21, March, 11, 2020. [URL: https://www.marx21.de/coronavirus-agribusiness-would-risk-millions-of-deaths/, visited June 1, 2020.]

Wolff, Robert Paul. In Defense of Anarchism. Berkeley, Los Angeles, London: University of California Press 1998.

Žižek, Slavoj. Pandemic! COVID-19 Shakes the World. New York, London: OR Books 2020.

Hrvoje Jurić, PhD, born in 1975 in Bihać, Bosnia and Herzegovina, studied Philosophy and Croatian Culture at the University of Zagreb (University Centre for Croatian Studies), earned his PhD degree 2007 in Philosophy at the University of Zagreb (Faculty of Humanities and Social Sciences), worked since 2000 in the Department of Philosophy of the Faculty of Humanities and Social Sciences, University of Zagreb, since 2019 as Full Professor of Ethics and Bioethics. Head of the Department of Philosophy (2016-2020) and Head of Department's Chair of Ethics (since 2015). Chief Secretary of the international conferences "Days of Frane Petrić" (2002-2006) and "Lošinj Days of Bioethics" (since 2002). Since 2014 Chief Secretary of the Centre of Excellence for Integrative Bioethics, which embraces seven Croatian bioethical institutions. President of the Croatian Bioethics Society (2016-2020). Since 2017 Head of the University Centre for Integrative Bioethics of the University of Zagreb. Since 1999 Deputy Editor of the philosophical journals "Filozofska istraživanja" and "Synthesis philosophica". - hjuric@yahoo.com.

Good Clinical Practice compliance in pandemic COVID-19: It is feasible?

Salvador Ribas, International Society for Clinical Bioethics, Spain

Abstract

In March 2020 special guidelines to monitor, control and guide protection against COVID-19 were issues by the European Medicine Agency (EMA) and the US Food and Drug Administration (FDA) for clinical trials management in Good Clinical Practice (GCP) to facilitate and improve global clinical research and protect patients and research persons. These 13 GCP principles will be analyzed in detail regarding protection of subjects involved, data, reporting and management.

Key words

COVID-19, Good Clinical Practice, compliance, preparedness, quality by design.

Introduction

As of March 11, 2020 coronavirus disease (COVID-19) was declared as pandemic by the World Health Organization (WHO), same scenario as filmed in Contagion (2011) by Steven Soderbergh. As result, the impact of COVID-19 on ongoing and new clinical trials was, and still is, enormous in the entire globe: increasing demands on nurses, physicians, and the healthcare services, restrictions of study visits to the hospital, difficulties in distributing the investigational medicinal product, difficulties for investigators to schedule visits and conduct safety evaluations, as summary, difficulties in guarantee trial participant safety and data reliability in the global clinical research.

Due to this scenario, urgent guidelines were published on March this year by the European Medicine Agency (EMA) and by the Food and Drug Administration (FDA) in order to minimize the impact of COVID-19 on clinical trials and implement extraordinary measures on the management of clinical trials[1], and similar guidelines were published by National Competent Authorities[2]. The persistent emergence of ethical conflicts in healthcare and clinical research in the current COVID-19 pandemic has forced all regulatory bodies to issue instruments that facilitate the decision making process in the field of clinical trials, as for example to convert physical study visits into phone or video calls, allow study visits to be conducted at alternative locations, extend the duration of the clinical trial, or to consider a temporary halt of the clinical trial[3].

How to protect patient safety and minimize and mitigate the impact of COVID-19 on clinical trials are the two urgent main tasks in order to continue the research on new drug development and guarantee new treatments for our societes. EMA and FDA guidelines are good initiatives, but we cannot forget main mantra for clinical trials: Guidelines for Good Clinical Practice (GCP).

---

[1] EMA. Guidance on the Management of Clinical Trials during the COVID 19 (Coronavirus) pandemic, version 1.0, March 20, 2020; version 2.0, March 27, 2020; and version 3.0, April 28, 2020. FDA Guidance on Conduct of Clinical Trials of Medical Products during COVID-19 Pandemic. Guidance for Industry, Investigators, and Institutional Review Boards, March 2020, and updated on March 27, April 2, April 16, May 11, May 14, June 3, and July 2, 2020.

[2] See for example: Medicines and Healthcare products Regulatory Agency. Managing clinical trials during Coronavirus (COVID-19). Available on: https://www.gov.uk/guidance/managing-clinical-trials-during-coronavirus-covid-19.

[3] EMA. Guidance on the Management of Clinical Trials during the COVID 19 (Coronavirus) pandemic, version 3.0, April 28, 2020.

1. GCP Principles During The COVID-19 Pandemic

GCP are defined as "an international ethical and scientific quality standard for designing, conducting, recording, and reporting trials that involve the participation of human subjects. Compliance with this standard provides public assurance that the rights, safety and well-being of trial subjects are protected, consistent with the principles that have their origin in the Declaration of Helsinki, and that the clinical trial data are credible"[4], and are referenced in international and local legislation[5], therefore legally enforceable.

E6(R1) GCP was published on 1996[6], and it was recently amended on 2016 being effective on June 2017 to encourage implementation of improved approaches to clinical trial design, data recording, and reporting.

GCP includes 13 principles with unique goals: subject protection and data reliability. The rights, safety and well-being of patients or healthy volunteers for medical research must be protected and data collected must be credible. In the current COVID-19 pandemic scenario it is clear that research staff, investigators, nurses, technicians, pharmacists are faced with a new challenge: comply with these principles during these unusual circumstances. It is feasible?

The first principle states that clinical trials should be conducted in accordance with the ethical principles that have their origin in the Declaration of Helsinki developed by the World Medical Association, and the second one add the following: "before a trial is initiated, foreseeable risks and inconveniences should be weighed against the anticipated benefit for the individual trial subject and society"[7]. We have here two key terms: individual trial subject/participant and society, is it feasible to benefit both? This not something new bioethics experts. The first bioethics centers were created in 1969 (Institute of Society, Ethics and the Life Sciences, Hastings Center) and 1971 (Joseph and Rose Kennedy Institute of Ethics for the Study of Human Reproduction and Bioethics) in the United States, and at this time the Belmont Report was published, proposing three fundamental ethical principles that aimed to protect patients and justify actions in clinical research: the principle of respect for people (autonomy), the principle of beneficence, and the principle of justice[8]. Therefore we can assume GCP principles 1 and 2 are covering the principle of respect for autonomy, and the principle of justice. The principle of beneficence can be found on the third GCP principle: "rights, safety, and well-being of the trial subjects are the most important considerations and should prevail over interests of science and society"[9].

During COVID-19 pandemic period, is it feasible to comply with those principles? We

---

[4] ICH Guideline E6(R2) Guideline for Good Clinical Practice, 2016. Introduction.

[5] Directive 2001/20/EC of the European Parliament and of the Council of 4 April 2001 on the approximation of the laws, regulations and administrative provisions of the Member States relating to the implementation of good clinical practice in the conduct of clinical trials on medicinal products for human use. Directive 2005/28/EC of 8 April 2005 laying down principles and detailed guidelines for good clinical practice as regards investigational medicinal products for human use, as well as the requirements for authorisation of the manufacturing or importation of such products. Regulation (EU) No 536/2014 on clinical trials on medicinal products for human use, and repealing Directive 2001/20/EC. EC Guideline C(2019) 7140 final on Good Clinical Practice specific to Advanced Therapy Medicinal Products.

[6] ICH Guideline E6(R1) Guideline for Good Clinical Practice, 1996.

[7] ICH Guideline E6(R2) Guideline for Good Clinical Practice, 2016, page 9.

[8] The National Commission for the Protection of Human Subjects of Biomedical and Behavioral Research. *The Belmont report: ethical principles and guidelines for the protection of human subjects of research.* Washington DC: Department of Health, Education, and Welfare, 1979.

[9] ICH Guideline E6(R2) Guideline for Good Clinical Practice, 2016, page 9.

should expect this, however difficulties in compliance are not trivial. The Committee for Human Medicinal Products (CHMP) recognizes that patient safety is the most important value and in order to guarantee beneficence and trial participant safety two key issues must be assessed: COVID-19 potentially affecting trial participants directly, and COVID-19 related measures affecting clinical trial conduct[10].

It is assumed that safety of trial participants is the highest priority in clinical trials, but in the current COVID-19pandemic, societies and their survival are also priority. In that sense, priority is given to clinical trials for the prevention and/or treatment of COVID-19 and COVID-19-related illnesses. Moreover, in the current COVID-19 pandemic scenario, infection of healthy volunteers must be considered as a real possibility.This is supported by the WHO publishing a guidance for scientists, ethics committees, and regulators in deliberations regarding human challenge studies.[11]

New open questions are derived from the fourth GCP principle: "the available nonclinical and clinical information on an investigational product should be adequate to support the proposed clinical trial"[12] Currently, do we have adequate data to support clinical trials to treat COVID-19? With this principle we have a new key element: data.

Relevant initiatives supported by the European Commission have been started in order to guarantee open access to all data[13-14] following the FAIR principles: data should be findable, accessible, interoperable, and re-usable (FAIR)[15]. In this time of COVID-19 pandemic, it is this feasible? Sponsors and researchers will guarantee open access to all data collected? This data will be accessible?

Lastly, in addition to the fourth GCP principle and FAIR principles, researchers must be compliant with EU principles on data protection: transparency, purpose limitation, data minimization, accuracy, storage limitation, integrity, confidentiality and accountability[16].

Data has become the most valuable resource as published in the journal The Economist: "The world's most valuable resource is no longer oil, but data"[17]. If so, then, which principle must be protected: beneficence/trial participants safety or justice/data collection in benefit all societies. It seems clear as stated by the EMA that trial participation must be the priority: "It is expected that the sponsor performs a risk assessment of each individual ongoing trial and the investigator of each individual trial participant and implement measures, which prioritize trial participant safety and data validity. In case these two conflicts, trial participant safety always prevails"[18]

As summary for now, we can assume GCP principles two and three are supporting protection of trial participants and societies, whereas GCP principle four guarantees clinical trials are

---

[10] Committee for Human Medicinal Products (CHMP). Points to consider on implications of Coronavirus disease (COVID-19) on methodological aspects of ongoing clinical trials draft, March 25, 2020.

[11] WHO. Key criteria for the ethical acceptability of COVID-19 human challenge studies, May 6, 2020.

[12] ICH Guideline E6(R2) Guideline for Good Clinical Practice, 2016, page 9.

[13] Available on: https://www.openaire.eu/

[14] Available on: https://bip.covid19.athenarc.gr/

[15] Available on: https://www.go-fair.org/

[16] European Data Protection Supervisor (EDPS). A Preliminary Opinion on data protection and scientific research, January 6, 2020.

[17] The Economist, May 6, 2017.

[18] EMA Guidance on the Management of Clinical Trials during the COVID 19 (Coronavirus) pandemic. Last updated on April 28, 2020, page 7.

supported by adequate data and evidence. However in order to make principle four effective, compliance with protocol and procedures is required, and that is why the following GCP principles five and six are required to guarantee trial participant safety and data reliability: "clinical trials should be scientifically sound, and described in a clear, detailed protocol"[19], GCP principle five, and "should be conducted in compliance with the protocol"[20], GCP principle 6. In other words compliance with protocol and study-specific procedures is the key element in order to guarantee patient safety and data credibility.

It is assumed with the current COVID-19 pandemic a larger number of protocol deviations than normal will occur, and deviations should be reported by investigators and sponsors. In addition, the EMA has declared that during inspections GCP inspectors will take a proportionate approach when such deviations are reviewed, recognizing that the best interest of the trial participants is maintained, and the trial participants are not put at undue risk[21]. Deviations should be assessed, but then how data will the remaining data be credible? The quality of data collected during the COVID-19 pandemic will be reliable and credible in order to guarantee adequate clinical trials and develop efficient drugs and vaccines. It is feasible?

Research staff is responsible to conduct study-specific procedures and collect data, and that's why GCP principle seven and eight are linked to the previous principles. As stated in the GCP principle, medical decisions made on behalf of subjects should always be the responsibility of a qualified physician, and each individual involved in conducting a trial should be qualified by education, training, and experience to perform his or her respective task(s)[22], however it is well known that the content and training on GCP requirements may differ in each country. In addition, the impact of COVID-19 has causes many retired doctors to return to work, and a large number of medical students are also involved in the COVID-19 response. In the COVID-19 pandemic, is it feasible for sites to always have a qualified researcher involved in all clinical trial-related decisions?

The next GCP principle is focused on the informed consent: a freely given informed consent should be obtained from every subject prior to clinical trial participation. In this regards, regulatory authorities agree informed consent procedures must be followed and the process must be properly documented, however due to the COVID-19 pandemic sites were forced to change the informed consent process. In that sense, regulatory agencies agree on that "If written consent by the trial participant is not possible (for example because of physical isolation due to COVID-19 infection), consent could be given orally by the trial participant in the presence of an impartial witness", and/or "in case of acute life-threatening situations, where it is not possible within the therapeutic window to obtain prior informed consent from the trial participant (or her/his legal representatives(s)), informed consent will need to be acquired later"[23]

If GCP principle 9 is clearly an instrument to protect trial participants, the next one is principle supporting data reliability. Accordingly, this principle, clinical trial information should be recorded, handled, and stored in a way that allows its accurate reporting, interpretation and verification, and this applies to all records irrespective of the type of media used. During the current

---

[19] ICH Guideline E6(R2) Guideline for Good Clinical Practice, 2016, page 9.

[20] ICH Guideline E6(R2) Guideline for Good Clinical Practice, 2016, page 9.

[21] EMA Guidance on the Management of Clinical Trials during the COVID 19 (Coronavirus) pandemic, version 3.0 April 28, 2020, page 17.

[22] ICH Guideline E6(R2) Guideline for Good Clinical Practice, 2016, page 9.

[23] EMA Guidance on the Management of Clinical Trials during the COVID 19 (Coronavirus) pandemic. Last updated on April 28, 2020, page 11.

COVID-19 pandemic, monitoring visits, audits, and inspections have been stopped, and have been conducted remotely, therefore data cannot be verified as usual. The impact of COVID-19 on GCP principle 10 still is unknown and the results will be only be understood once clinical research associates, auditors, and inspectors are able to resume site visits. It is well accepted that data collection cannot be stopped and should continue in order to not interrupt drug development, however, as the CHMP defend, potential risks for patients when undergoing study-specific procedures must take priority in decisions[24,] ;trial participant safety is the main value to be protected, prior data collection.

Source data should be attributable, legible, contemporaneous, original, and accurate (ALCOA principles), but also should be complete, consistent, enduring, and available when needed (ALCOA+)[25]. Regulators have provided alternative methods to be complaint with ALCOA principles like the use email correspondence as signature in such case wet-ink signatures are not possible[26], but to what extent the COVID-19 pandemic will impact source data is unknown. During the current COVID-19 pandemic, researchers should follow GCP, FAIR, and ALCOA+ principles;there is no alternative if societies want to continue to develop drugs with adequate data.

In addition, we cannot forget the data should kept confidential as per the next GCP principle (10)#, confidentiality of records must be protected, respecting patient privacy and in accordance with the applicable national regulatory requirement(s), and again the same question: is it feasible?

COVID-19 also has impacted the GCP principle focused on the study drug: the study drug should be handled, and stored in accordance with applicable Good Manufacturing Practice, and should be used in accordance with the approved protocol. Is this feasible when study drug cannot be dispensed at site?

Finally, we have the last GCP principle: "Systems with procedures that assure the quality of every aspect of the trial should be implemented." Aspects of the trial that are essential to ensure human subject protection and reliability of trial results should be the focus of such systems.

2. Mastering Common Bioethical Issues Among Moral Strangers

Daniel Buchanan argued that bioethics has three main functions: identifying and defining existing ethical conflicts; providing systems or methods to think about new emerging ethical conflicts in the field of medicine; and helping scientists and physicians to make decisions[27]. In the current COVID-19 pandemic, regulatory agencies have identified new emerging issues on the management of clinical trials, and new guidelines/methods have been published in order to continue research in developing new drugs and vaccines.

H. Tristram Engelhardt assumes that our contemporary society is constituted by relationships between moral strangers, between people who do not share the same morality, and proce-

---

[24] Committee for Human Medicinal Products (CHMP). Points to consider on implications of Coronavirus disease (COVID-19) on methodological aspects of ongoing clinical trials draft, March 25, 2020, page 2.

[25] EMA/INS/GCP/454280/2010. GCP Inspectors Working Group (GCP IWG). Reflection paper on expectations for electronic source data and data transcribed to electronic data collection tools in clinical trials.

[26] Medicines and Healthcare products Regulatory Agency. Managing clinical trials during Coronavirus (COVID-19). Available on: https://www.gov.uk/guidance/managing-clinical-trials-during-coronavirus-covid-19.

[27] Daniel Callahan. "Bioethics as a discipline." *Hastings Center Studies*, n°1 (1973): 68.

dural bioethics allows coexistence between moral strangers[28]. Research staff, and all stakeholders involved in clinical research are in fact moral strangers, and GCP principles, like bioethical principles, helps to create a common mantra in the benefit of trial participants and data reliability.

Conclusion

In bioethics, ideas of right and good decisions have often been subordinated to procedural standards[29], and the same occurs in the field of clinical research: decisions in research should be subordinated to the protocol and study-procedures, in order words, compliance must be guaranteed.

We are faced with a primary understanding of clinical research: the procedural approach focused on guidelines, good, and best practices. However, unlike GCP principles, clinical research associates, auditors, and inspectors from National Competent Authorities (compliance experts) are ensuring that the standards of GCP are applied and they may/must play a key role in maintaining a substantive approach that allow drug companies to protect trial participants and society's interest. Such compliance experts can overcome the gap that exist between guidelines, principles, procedures and their application to the clinical research in pandemic COVID19. Compliance experts should play a key role in providing context to the systems and clinical trial procedures, and guarantee quality in clinical research. A well-designed protocol should guarantee the rights amd safety of the paitent throughthe consistent procedures and practices.

The essential trait of the procedural approach is that it focuses on the formulation of procedures that help solve issues in clinical research while respecting GCP principles. A correct action depends on compliance to the procedure, thus the responsibility does not fall on the investigator, but on the protocol and its design, therefore quality by design is the key new element to be reinforced in the next coming ICH E6(R3) to protect trial participant safety and data reliability in the clinical research.

References

Belmont 1979. The National Commission for the Protection of Human Subjects of Biomedical and Behavioral Research. *The Belmont report: ethical principles and guidelines for the protection of human subjects of research.* Washington DC: Department of Health, Education, and Welfare, 1979.

Callahan 1973. Callahan, Daniel. "Bioethics as a discipline". *Hastings Center Studies*, n° 1 (1973): 66-73.

CHMP 2020. Committee for Human Medicinal Products (CHMP). Points to consider on implications of Coronavirus disease (COVID-19) on methodological aspects of ongoing clinical trials draft, March 25, 2020.

EC 2001. Directive 2001/20/EC of the European Parliament and of the Council of 4 April 2001 on the approximation of the laws, regulations and administrative provisions of the Member States relating to the implementation of good clinical practice in the conduct of clinical trials on medicinal products for human use.

---

[28] Tristram H. Engelhardt. *The foundations of bioethics.* New York: Oxford University Press, 1986.

[29] Mark Siegler. "The progression of medicine. From physician paternalism to patient autonomy to bureaucratic parsimony". *Archives of Internal Medicine* n°145 (1985): 714.

EC 2005. Directive 2005/28/EC of 8 April 2005 laying down principles and detailed guidelines for good clinical practice as regards investigational medicinal products for human use, as well as the requirements for authorisation of the manufacturing or importation of such products.

EC 2014. Regulation (EU) No 536/2014 on clinical trials on medicinal products for human use, and repealing Directive 2001/20/EC. Last update: into application during 2020

EC 2019. EC Guideline C(2019) 7140 final on Good Clinical Practice specific to Advanced Therapy Medicinal Products

EDPS 2020. European Data Protection Supervisor. A Preliminary Opinion on data protection and scientific research, January 6, 2020.

EMA 2010. EMA/INS/GCP/454280/2010. GCP Inspectors Working Group (GCP IWG). Reflection paper on expectations for electronic source data and data transcribed to electronic data collection tools in clinical trials.

EMA 2020. EMA Guidance on the Management of Clinical Trials during the COVID 19 (Coronavirus) pandemic. Last updated on April 28, 2020.

Engelhardt 1986. Engelhardt, H. Tristram. *The foundations of bioethics*. New York: Oxford University Press, 1986.

FDA 2020. FDA Guidance on Conduct of Clinical Trials of Medical Products during COVID-19 Pandemic. Guidance for Industry, Investigators, and Institutional Review Boards, March 2020.

ICH 2016. ICH Guideline E6(R2) Guideline for Good Clinical Practice, 2016.

Siegler 1985. Siegler, Mark. "The progression of medicine. From physician paternalism to patient autonomy to bureaucratic parsimony". *Archives of Internal Medicine*, n°145 (1985): 714.

UK 2020. Medicines and Healthcare products Regulatory Agency. Managing clinical trials during Coronavirus (COVID-19). Available on: https://www.gov.uk/guidance/managing-clinical-trials-during-coronavirus-covid-19.

WHO 2020. WHO. Key criteria for the ethical acceptability of COVID-19 human challenge studies, May 6, 2020.

Salvador Ribas holds a PhD in Philosophy from the University of Barcelona; he is Manager for Quality Assurance in clinical trials, a Board Member of the Spanish Quality Assurance Society (SEGCIB), and also Vice-President of the International Society for Clinical Bioethics (ISCB); salvador.ribas@gmail.com.

Autonomy and Trust:
Conclusions from the Greek Model of
Management of the COVID-19 Pandemic

Eleni Kalokairinou, Aristotle University of Thessaloniki, Greece

Abstract

The aim of this paper is to bring out the particular way in which Greece has managed the COVID-19 Pandemic and to underline that, while certain countries seemed to either violate human measures (e.g. China), or to respect human freedom and autonomy at the expense of public health and life (e.g. Sweden), the Greek Model succeeded in striking the golden medium between respecting human autonomy and rights on the one hand and protecting public health on the other. The way the Greek Model achieved this was by employing a "richer" notion of autonomy, which obeys universal laws, and as such leads to mutual trust. It is precisely this mutual trust that people showed to themselves and to one another that has proved the particular model of managing the pandemic successful.

Along its long history, human society has quite often been devastated by plagues, epidemics and pandemics. Thucydides, the ancient Greek historian, mentions and describes in his *History of the Peloponnesian War* the plague that befell Athens during the second year of the Peloponnesian War in 430 B.C.[1] Among the people who died, according to some calculations between 75.000-100.000 people, have been included Pericles, the famous inspirer of the ancient Greek democracy and his two sons.

Many epidemics and/or pandemics have occurred in human society since then. In modern times plagues were widespread in Europe. Among them we can mention the epidemic of London in 1532, with another outburst in 1535. The Tyrolese town of Stertzing was also affected by the plague of 1534. The authorities of the town issued the *Ordinance* throughout the duration of the deadly plague by virtue of which they attempted to implement measures of social distancing among people. Paracelsus, a Swiss physician, 1493-1541, composed a tract, *On the Plague in Stertzing* in which he condemned the methods and advice of his contemporary physicians and made his own suggestions.

In the contemporary era quite a few pandemics have struck human society, the most devastating of them being the Spanish Influenza in 1918-1919 that killed between 20-50 million of people all over the world.[2] Still, many other epidemic/pandemic diseases have struck societies like, to mention a few, cholera, Ebola virus disease, Influenza pandemic or seasonal, Mers-CoV, Novel Coronavirus (2019-nCoV), Plague and Sars.[3]

Coronavirus disease 2019 (COVID-19) is a virus that affects the respiratory system of man and, if not taken care of, may prove fatal. Last December the World Health Organization was informed about a number of cases with severe respiratory problems in the town Wuhan, capital of Hubel, China. The virus was spread very quickly, the number of cases were dangerously increased, the Chinese started having great numbers of casualties. In Europe, Italy was among the first countries that was infected by the disease. The first cases were detected to have imported the disease in Lombardy, in the north of the country, after a commercial trip to China. In a very short period of time, there was an outburst of the coronavirus disease in the north district of Italy.

Gradually, all other European countries started having their first covid-19 cases and casual-

---

[1] Thucydides, *History of the Peloponnesian War*, Book 2, 52.

[2] https://www.euro.who.int/en/health-topics/communicable-diseases/influenza/pandemic-influenza/past-pandemics.

[3] https://www.who.int/emergencies/diseases/en/.

ties. In Greece the first covid-19 cases were imported by a number of Greek people who had gone on a pilgrimage to the Holy Land. Pyrgos, the capital of the district Elis, was the first area to be infected in Greece. There followed some more corona virus cases in Kavala, in Macedonia, the north part of Greece, and were detected to have been imported in the country, after a trip to China for professional purposes.

The Greek state was automatically alerted. It sensed quite correctly that we were facing an invisible enemy and that the Greek people needed protection. The Greek authorities made it clear right from the start that the protection of public health was their number one priority. The country had just come out of the austere fiscal measures that had been imposed on it for the last ten years. Nevertheless, it was now facing another fatal threat that nobody could imagine where it was going to lead. The state, in the face of the present government, had to act quickly and drastically.

The way the scenery was formed internationally was not encouraging. All countries were facing outbursts of cases, in some countries the number of deaths were increasing dangerously. However, the way the threat that this new pandemic has been posing, was dealt with by each country varied, depending on the moral and political values that each of them adhered to. In this sense, we have had instances of countries whose authorities gave priority to the common good of the community, i.e. the public health, at the expense of human rights and liberties. We thus watched on the TV World News pictures of the Chinese police who were dragging citizens on the ground in an attempt they made to convince them obey the social distancing rules, abandon their jobs, remain home and follow strict lockdown measures.

The other extreme has been presented by countries like Sweden, that has been following a completely different strategy. Sweden, unlike the other Scandinavian countries, imposed more moderate restrictions for the general public, did not shut down schools and educational institutions and preserved a certain degree of normality in the country.[4] As a consequence, the death toll mounted to 3.500 people and the infected cases to 32.000 (by the 18th May 2020), when in the other Scandinavian countries the deaths were only 200 (in Finland), 500 (in Denmark) and 200 (in Norway) by the same date.[5]

However, the particular model of herd-immunity that was implemented by the Swedish authorities has been widely criticized not only by foreign mass media but also by native health care providers.[6] The BBC interviewer Stephen Sacker asks Anders Tegnell, the Swedish state epidemiologist and architect of the Swedish model, how he feels about the deaths of 3.500 people, when most of them could have been prevented, if a different strategy had been followed.[7] Similarly, Maddy Savage, the BBC News Correspondent from Stockholm, reports that 48,9% of the deaths were care home residents to whom access to physicians and to hospitals was denied, once they got infected with the disease.[8] In the same report, Savage has a nurse revealing that

---

[4] Journalist Stephen Sacker interviews Swedish epidemiologist Anders Tegnell in BBC HARDtalk. https://www.bbc.co.uk/sounds/play/w3cszc1s (accessed 25 June 2020).

[5] Ibid.

[6] Journalist Stephen Sacker interviews Swedish epidemiologist Anders Tegnell in BBC HARDtalk. https://www.bbc.co.uk/sounds/play/w3cszc1s   See also, "Coronovirus: What's going wrong in Sweden's care homes?" by Maddy Savage, BBC News Correspondent in Stockholm,   https://www.bbc.com/news/world-europe-52704836 (accessed 25 June 2020).

[7] Journalist Stephen Sacker interviews Swedish epidemiologist Anders Tegnell in BBC HARDtalk. https://www.bbc.co.uk/sounds/play/w3cszc1s

[8] "Coronovirus: What's going wrong in Sweden's care homes?" by Maddy Savage, BBC News Correspondent in Stockholm,   https://www.bbc.com/news/world-europe-52704836

once infected, the elderly people were not given even oxygen, nor was an ambulance called, and that they were left on their own and helpless to die. As she puts it:

Most of the 3.698 people who have died from coronavirus in Sweden so far were over 70, despite the fact that the country said shielding risk groups was its top priority.[9]

The Greek authorities were very well aware of these two extremely opposite alternative courses of action. Wishing to protect all citizens, regardless of age, health condition, race and origin, and at the same time wishing to respect human rights and the laws of democracy, the Greek state struck the Aristotelian golden medium and produced a fairly comprehensible model, avoiding in this way the two extremes we have just seen.

The Greek state realized at once that this was a health issue, and mainly an issue that concerned public health – and only secondarily a political issue. As a consequence, politicians under the Prime minister sought the advice of the top epidemiologists of the country. A Committee of Expert Epidemiologists was automatically formed and Sotiris Tsiodras, Professor of the Medical School of the National and Kapodistrian University of Athens, was put at its head. This Committee of Experts advised on a daily basis the government and mainly the Prime minister and the Minister of Health (an orthopedist) about the medical facts and the details that concerned the new virus. Once the basic medical facts about the disease were understood, it became clear to the government that measures for the protection of the public had to be taken. This was undoubtedly a very delicate issue and had to be addressed with "phronesis" and sensitivity. Implementing measures of containment and social distancing in contemporary democratic societies, even under the pretext of protecting public health, may sound provocative and even totalitarian. Consequently, the Greek government produced a very well worked out plan. It included, if put roughly, the following steps.

1. The public was informed on a daily basis at a specific time through all the national TV channels by the President of the Expert Epidemiologists' Committee about the most recent developments and/or spread of the disease mainly nationally but also internationally. Professor Tsiodras explained in terms that could be understood by the general public, certain medical facts about the disease and put forward briefly the attempts that were made by national and international medical centers to develop a vaccine for the disease. By explaining the facts, he was at the same time pointing out certain guidelines that had to be respected by people and had to be implemented by the government. We had to protect ourselves and, of course, at the same time we had to protect the others. In other words, we had to protect each other. The notion of "individual responsibility" that each citizen had to show under the circumstances became very central during the first phases of the corona virus disease in the country. As it was pointed out, this was a burden that all citizens in the country were called to share, regardless of age, health condition, sex or race.

2. After the epidemiologist of the country Professor Tsiodras, Mr. Nikos Chardalias, the under-Secretary of the Ministry of Citizen Protection, announced the particular measures that had been taken by his Ministry in order to prevent the disease from spreading to more individuals, to more parts of the country. The measures were implemented gradually and very carefully, i.e. containment, social distancing, closing down schools and universities, closing down shops and businesses and staying home and/or working from home. The measures normally went to effect on the next day of their announcement. As one may imagine, the measures were very difficult to be kept, especially at the beginning. The first two or three days that they were implemented were not followed by everyone. In any case, the Greeks have had the reputation that

---

[9] Ibid.

they are "undisciplined". However, in this respect the police did a very good job. During the first two or three days each time some new measures were implemented, the police made recommendations to those citizens that did not respect them. After the third day, certain fines were imposed but these were only the exception. In the end, complete lockdown was imposed and going out was allowed only in very few cases, as these were specified by the measures taken: (a) for going to the hospital, physician or the chemist; (b) for going to the food stores; (c) for personal exercise or to exercise one's pet, or for certain exceptional other reasons, e.g. attending a funeral service. The Greek state was the first to ask citizens to send a free SMS to a national number, stating beforehand the reason for which they were going out – a practice that was later adopted by other countries.

3. In this very same daily medical update was also present the Secretary of the Ministry of Health Mr. Vassilis Kontozamanis, who received the word and spoke when questions about the National Health System (NHS) were raised. As already mentioned, Greece had just come out of measures of austerity that had been imposed by the ten years' memoranda. As a consequence, the main concern of the Experts' Committee and of the Ministry of Health was to support the NHS and not overload the intensive care units of hospitals. However, this had to be secured not in ways that would put at risk people's life and health, especially the life of those who were old, over 70 years old and suffered from chronic cardiac and other diseases. The Ministry of Health acted quickly and in a coordinated manner: first of all, it defined the hospitals in the country that would accept and treat only corona virus cases. Secondly, it increased the number of intensive care units in the public hospitals. Thirdly, it employed a number of intensive care units of private hospitals. Fourthly, there were donations with equipment for intensive care units from national benefactors and legacies. The Ministry of Health could report at the end of the corona virus lockdown that the NHS came out of the fight with the virus much stronger and much richer than it was at the beginning. Needless to say, of course, that at the end of each daily medical update all the three of them, Professor Tsiodras, under-Secretary of the Ministry of Citizen Protection and Secretary of the Ministry of Health answered all the questions that were put by journalists.

There is no doubt that the measures implemented were gradually endorsed by the Greek people. The government pursued a policy of democracy and transparency, educated the Greek citizens to show mutual respect to one another, and cultivated in them an ethos of empathy (sympathy, einfuhlung, in Greek ενσυναίσθηση). Such an ethos of course has not been built up in one day. Moreover, it has required a number of activities. First, it gave priority to the Committee of Experts who informed the general public on a daily basis. It is interesting to consider the values that were underlying Expert Immunologists' daily briefing. Apart from the strict medical facts and the statistical data, the way in which the Expert Immunologists talked expressed a concern for their fellow human beings, and their words were invested with the humanistic values that lie at the roots of the Greek civilization and thinking. Professor Tsiodras quite a few times has explained and underlined why and how we had to protect the elderly people, "our grand-fathers and mothers", as he usually called them. When the first covid-19 cases burst out in Rom or Immigrants camps in particular areas of the country, he did not hesitate to go personally to the affected areas, accompanied by Nikos Chardalias, the under-Secretary of the Ministry of Citizen Protection, and attempt to convince them why having tests for covid-19 were necessary for them and their safety, why they had to wear masques, keep social distancing and lockdown measures. At the beginning there were wild reactions, something which is understandable and half-expected, but thank to Professor Tsiodras' serious and responsible way of handling such a delicate issue, the reactions yielded at once. It was obvious to everyone, the immigrants included, that Tsiodras and, by and large, the Experts Committee and the Greek state treated everyone, in Tsiodras' words, as "brother", and in this sense surpassed the Millian principle of equality that claimed:

Everybody to count for one, and nobody for more than one.[10]

At the same time there has been the "staying home" ("Μένουμε σπίτι") campaign through the TV and the other mass media that encouraged a lot the policy of social distancing and the cultivation of the ethos of mutual respect and sympathy. (This very same campaign is still going on slightly modified and enriched as to read now: "staying home, keeping distances up to two meters, wearing masques in the public means of transport and in all places in which social distancing is difficult or impossible"). All the TV channels undertook a campaign during all these months of social distancing and self-confinement at home to show and convince the public why keeping these measures was for our own good and the good of our beloved persons.

Obviously, all these measures struck the right chord in the heart of the "undisciplined Greeks" who realized that, along with their autonomy and personal freedoms, they had to preserve public health at any cost, they had to exhibit responsibility for themselves and for the others. If there is something that the outburst of the covid-19 pandemic has thrown into sharp relief is the extent to which human beings depend on one another, or to use Alasdair MacIntyre's famous expression, how much of "a dependent rational animal" man is.[11]

As a consequence, they have undertaken this responsibility and tried their best to protect themselves and the others. The catchphrase that was thrown at the beginning of the pandemic crisis that each of us has to exhibit "individual responsibility" was further elaborated and transformed into "collective responsibility". The Greek people came to realize soon that their actions and total behaviour did not simply affect themselves and the narrow circle of their family and relatives but also the whole of society. In this way, they surpassed the narrow limits of individualist liberalism and showed concern for society and even the global community.

Conceptually speaking, this meant that they had stopped thinking and acting in terms of simple individual responsibility and autonomy. Deciding in an individualistic manner would have implied that each agent was only concerned for his own good, in this case his own health, and that he did not bother at all about what had happened or could have happened to others under the covid-19 pandemic circumstances. The individual autonomy notion, creation of the 18th century Enlightenment project, could not prove of much help now that a common good was under threat, the health of global community. This is why we had to -and we still have to- recourse to moral universal values. Individual autonomy on its own does not lead us anywhere. It simply restricts us to ourselves and our boundaries, my house, my field, my property. It is not concerned with the other nor with the others' good. In a sense, it cuts us off from the other. On the contrary, the kind of autonomy that operated during the covid-19 pandemic crisis in the case of Greek people was moral autonomy.

Moral autonomy has its roots in Immanuel Kant's Categorical Imperative and it has been further elaborated and worked out by the British philosopher Onora O'Neill.[12] As she points out,

---

[10] John Stuart Mill, *Utilitarianism*, chapter 5, p. 58 (quoting Bentham) in John Stuart Mill, *Utilitarianism, On Liberty and Considerations on Representative Government*, ed. by H.B. Acton, J.M. Dent – E.P. Dutton, London – New York 1972.

[11] From Alasdair MacIntyre's book, *Dependent Rational Animals. Why Human Beings Need the Virtues,* Duckworth (1999) 2009.

[12] Immanuel Kant, *Groundwork of the Metaphysics of Morals*, ed. by Mary Gregor, introd. by Christine M. Korsgaard, Cambridge University Press, Cambridge 1997. Onora O'Neill, *Autonomy and Trust in Bioethics*, Cambridge University Press, Cambridge 2002.

this is a "principled autonomy".[13] Contrary to individual autonomy which simply safeguards what I, the particular individual, wants in disregard of everybody else, moral autonomy operates in virtue of principles. The agent who thinks and acts in terms of moral autonomy is concerned with examining whether the rule of his action can become a universal law, i.e. can become universally accepted not only by him under these circumstances but also by anybody else similarly situated. In universalizing in this way the rule of his action, the agent is checking whether it can be adhered to by everybody who shares the same ends with him. This sharing of ends among people opens up the perspective of "kingdom of ends" to which all moral agents participate equally to the extent that they operate under universal-izable principles. But if acting on universal principles becomes a moral ethos, then it is entirely understandable why and how mutual trust is developed and cultivated among people.

Conclusion

In conclusion, in Greece people have succeeded, after a lot of efforts and the steady and continuous support of the state, to surpass what is standardly known as (narrow) individual autonomy, and to develop a sense of moral autonomy, something which in the end enhanced concern for the other, trust and solidarity among people in society under the hard circumstances of the COVID-19 Pandemic.

References

Kant 1997. Immanuel Kant, *Groundwork of the Metaphysics of Morals*, ed. by Mary Gregor, introd. by Christine M. Korsgaard, Cambridge University Press, Cambridge 1997.

MacIntyre 2009. Alasdair MacIntyre's book, *Dependent Rational Animals. Why Human Beings Need the Virtues,* Duckworth (1999) 2009.

Mill 1972. John Stuart Mill, *Utilitarianism*, chapter 5, p. 58 (quoting Bentham) in John Stuart Mill, *Utilitarianism, On Liberty and Considerations on Representative Government*, ed. by H.B. Acton, J.M. Dent – E.P. Dutton, London – New York 1972.

O'Neill 2002. Onora O'Neill, *Autonomy and Trust in Bioethics*, Cambridge University Press, Cambridge 2002.

Sacker 2020. Journalist Stephen Sacker interviews Swedish epidemiologist Anders Tegnell in BBC HARDtalk. https://www.bbc.co.uk/sounds/play/w3cszc1s (accessed 25 June 2020)

Savage 2020. "Coronovirus: What's going wrong in Sweden's care homes?" by Maddy Savage, BBC News Correspondent in Stockholm, https://www.bbc.com/news/world-europe-52704836 (accessed 25 June 2020)

Thucydides, *History of the Peloponnesian War*, Book 2, 52.

Eleni Kalokairinou is Professor of Philosophy, Ethics and Bioethics, Aristotle University of Thessaloniki, E-mail: ekalo@edlit.auth.gr.

---

[13] O'Neill, ibid., chapter 4.

The Technology Utilization and Social Background that led to the K-Quarantine

Jiwon Shim, Chung-Ang University, Korea

Juhee Eom, Yonsei University, Korea

Sun Geu Chae, Hanyang University, Korea

abstract
Abstract

We examine the current status of COVID-19 in South Korea and the social background: MERS Experience, Public Healthcare System, Digital Infrastructure, Preemptive Response, the use of Artificial Intelligence, Familiarity with Mask-Wearing, Relaxation of Infectious Disease Law System, Closeness of Public Administration) in which Korea was able to cope well with COVID-19

Key words

artificial intelligence, digital infrastructure, health crisis, human crisis, social crisis, social isolation, solidarity, wearing mask

1. Introduction

COVID-19 is changing our daily lives. Is it really? South Korea is coping with COVID-19 without restricting the entry and exit of other countries based on the existing MERS experience. Is it really? Some Western scholars criticized the dangers of violating individual liberty while taking a positive stance on the response of South Korea to combat COVID-19. Is their criticism just? We show the social meaning of wearing masks and contact tracing in South Korea through News and Twitter with text scraping methods. K- quarantine has been criticized for violating individual liberty in connection with public health, which is an important point of view. But we mention three things to the contrary: 1) The issue of individual liberty should be discussed in the concrete situation of infectious diseases, not abstract dimensions. 2) We would like to argue that in a Corona crisis, not only the discussion of the meaning of liberty violates individual liberty for public health, but also the discussion of how the meaning of individual liberty will relate to solidarity or the right to survive. 3) Today we are experiencing many crises due to COVID-19. But COVID-19 only reveals the crisis that our society already has, not its fundamental cause.

2. Status of COVID-19 in South Korea

After the first confirmation with the inflow of the virus from abroad on January 19, 2020, mass infection has occurred among religious groups and long-term care facilities in Daegu. After the mass infection, the government of South Korea raised its warning levels of infectious disease to 'serious' on February 23, 2020, releasing its policy of early isolation and treatment of potential COVID-19 patients with social distancing policy to stop further spread of the virus. With the preemptive measures and help of digital technology, confirmed cases of COVID-19 patients in South Korea dropped from 1,062 on March 1 to 46 new cases confirmed on July 5. (Kang 2020, KCDMH 2020)

3. Social and technical Backgrounds of South-Korea Regarding COVID-19

1) MERS Experience

Due to the experience and knowledge gained from the outbreak of 2015 MERS (Middle East Respiratory Syndrome) which killed around 38 people in the country, South Korea managed to reduce the number of new infections with COVID-19. During the MERS crisis, South Korea failed to recognize the importance of mass testing, resulting exposures of people in hospitals with the virus where people with disease visited to confirm that they are positive of the disease (Balilla 2020)

2) Public Healthcare System

Allocation proposals of medical resources including high-filtration N-95 masks in pandemic situations converge on four fundamental values: benefit maximization, equality, promotion and reward of instrumental value and finally prioritizing people in worse situations. During the early stages of COVID-19 crisis, filtration masks which help prevent the spread of disease became scarce among most of the countries including Korea. While other countries suffered from hoarding of medical supplies including face masks, Korean government distributed face masks by taking advantage of a well-established public healthcare system with "Mask purchase 5-day rotation system" to promote fair distribution of scarce supplies. (Emanuel et al. 2020)

3) Digital Infrastructure

With the development of rapid screening tactics, Korea took advantage of its highly developed digital infrastructure. Local and national governments released daily and frequent briefings of COVID-19 related information to both web and mobile services to increase civil awareness about the disease and provide essential information to help stop the spread of the virus. Also, Korean Center of Disease Control investigated the trace of the contact using interviews, mobile phone location tracking, credit card transaction history and surveillance cameras to track movements of confirmed COVID-19 cases, with support of automated contact tracing using big data. As described below, following the 2015 MERS outbreak, public disclosure provisions were added to the Infectious Disease Control and Prevention Act to easily share and take advantage of such information for contact tracing. Finally, digital mapping and alerts for confirmed cases and face mask distribution information made individuals easily identify such information with smart devices, and digital self-diagnosis and self-quarantine apps developed by the Ministry of Health and Welfare help monitoring of potential patients with ease. (Lee/Lee 2020)

4) Preemptive Response

A number of new problems related to the coronavirus, such as the nature of infectious diseases, problems of health inequality and the distribution of masks, fake news of coronavirus, have been brought about. Among them, Korea made excellent examples of Corona response, and among the various best practices, digital technology contributed a lot:

Case	description
Self-Diagnosis App (for management of immigrants)	Immigrants can self-diagnose COVID-19 symptoms, enabling fast management and response
Self-isolation safety protection app	Monitoring the health status of a self-isolated person if a person is suspected of having a COVID-19 infection via contact with infected person
Artificial Intelligence based Care Calls	Naver's AI system automatically calls the actively monitored person and the consultation results are sent to the official via email.
Mask purchase 5-day	In order to provide fair chance for purchasing the protective mask, days

rotation system	are assigned depending on the end of birth year
Mask notification app	The location of protective mask vendors, status of stocks, and arrival times are provided real-time, with the developed app taking advantage of public data.
Information Disclosure of Infected Person	emergency text messages are sent to mobile phones when disaster forecasts, alerts, notifications or emergency actions are needed
Self-isolation regime	Recommendation and support to self-contain non-inpatients who may be infected or spread by contact with infected patients
Triage Health Center (Drive-Through)	COVID-19 screening clinic installed in a separate place separate from medical institutions, suspicious patients are examined in their own vehicles
Community Treatment Center	Treatment of COVID-19 minor patients at national facilities or training centers of enterprises and public officials are deployed 24 hours.
Designated Public Relief Hospitals	separately designated medical institutions used by patients with other diseases

Table 1: Best practices of corona response in Korea.

5) The use of Artificial Intelligence in Combating COVID-19

Test-kit development: The stopping of the fast-spreading coronavirus requires fast development of the test kit. With the artificial intelligence based test-kit development, Korean life sciences company Seegene was able to develop COVID-19 testing kit in under three weeks.

Smart quarantine information system: The Korean Center of Disease Control quarantine information system gathers information of the inbound travelers from the Ministry of Justice, Ministry of Foreign Affairs, and also airlines and telephone communication service companies to enable health workers to have full information regarding the patient and use such data to identify and isolate the suspected coronavirus patient

Contact tracing: Also with the interviewed information, information of location data from the mobile phone, credit card transactions and CCTV footage is supplied to the officials to trace and test suspected COVID-19 patients, and the traced routes of the suspected patient are published to aware public to encourage others who believe that they might have been in contact with suspected person to seek out testing.

Enhancement of diagnosis efficiency and patent classification: With the help of artificial intelligence-based X-ray image diagnostic tools, faster diagnosis and classification of patients were made possible.

Use of mobile apps: Since the outbreak of the virus, numerous mobile apps for advising and responding to coronavirus have been developed. For example, mobile apps directing people with COVID-19 symptoms to the nearest available stations and chatbots automatically calling people requiring attention were deployed.

6) Familiarity with Mask-Wearing

In the early days of the COVID-19 outbreak, there was much controversy over whether wearing masks actually helped prevent epidemics. Especially in the West, where wearing a mask acts as a symbol of some illness, it has made it more difficult to try on a mask. On the other hand, wearing a mask is not a strange scene in Korea. The South Korean government made it mandatory to wear masks on May 26, 2020. In Korea, it is common to wear a mask to keep the cold from getting worse in the winter and to prevent the spread of cold to others. Also, as the yellow dust from China and fine dust became much more severe, it was common for many people, especially children, to wear masks even before the corona crisis. For this reason, many families even had a lot of masks in their homes before the corona crisis.

7) Relaxation of Infectious Disease Law System

The Infectious Disease Control and Prevention Act (hereinafter referred to as the Act) prevents the transmission of infections (Article 17 of the law) and epidemiological investigations (Article 18 of the Law), and the investigation of actual conditions in order to determine the status of the infectious diseases and the status of resistant bacteria. For this reason, the act established the legal basis for requesting the submission of personal information or data to targeted organizations, organizations or individuals (laws 18, 4 and 76-2). Data that can be collected include name, resident registration number, address, and telephone number with personal information as well as medical records, immigration records, personal location information or personal communication information with the request by the National Police Agency, etc. (Law 76 Article 2 Paragraph 1) Possible collection of the data includes credit card, debit card, prepaid card, transportation card Includes specifications, image information collected through image information processing equipment (Enforcement Decree Article 2-2), etc. The act states to prevent the collected data from being used for purposes other than infectious disease-related tasks and to destroy it immediately after the end of use (Law Article 76 (6)) and impose a notification obligation to the data subject (Law Article 76 (7)) In addition, there is a penalty clause (Article 79, 5 of the law) that imposes imprisonment for not more than two years or a fine not exceeding 20 million won in the event of violation of the obligation to prohibit the purpose of use and immediate destruction. In addition, it is necessary to disclose information that the public needs to know about the prevention activities such as the path of movement of patients with infectious diseases obtained from the collection of this big data, means of transportation, medical institutions, and contacts, so that the right to know of the people can be satisfied Paragraph 2, Article 34-2) If there is an objection to the disclosed matter, an objection can be made through the information and communication network, and if there is a good reason, necessary measures such as correcting the disclosed information may be taken. (Law Article 23-2, Paragraphs 2 and 3)

While specifying the right of the people to diagnose and treat infectious diseases and the country's obligation to pay for it, citizens are also imposed of obligations to cooperate in the prevention and management of infectious diseases (Articles 6, 3 and 4 of the Act) Since the government can identify places that are contaminated with infectious diseases from the collection of big data, it can take measures such as closing and disinfecting suspected contaminated places, and disposing and disinfecting suspected contaminated objects. (Act Article 47. Article 48) In order to prevent infectious diseases, measures such as blocking traffic, restricting meetings or meetings, or ordering school or academy to be closed or closed are also possible. (Article 49 of the Act) In addition, it is possible to compensate for the damage suffered by being quarantined or treated as an infectious disease (Article 6 (1) of the Act). This will allow protection of privacy, surveillance of infectious diseases and promotion of public health at the same time.

In this regard, the Act on Infectious Diseases provides a normative basis for countermeasures against the collection and misuse of big data, and a basis for limiting the basic rights of privacy and personal information and the legal basis for public health activities that protect the people's right to life, health and safety.

8) Closeness of Public Administration

Social services require specific reaching strategies for each individual, including a variety of service contents and features. Thus, service reachability should consider mobility, affordability, equality, comfortability and effectiveness. (Lee et al. 2006) In Korea, especially, public welfare services are being reformed to provide market-oriented services to increase reachability of public services to citizens, such as "Visiting Community Service" in which social welfare officers visit each individual to provide public services. (Kim 2018) Since controlling infectious disease requires public health authorities to raise community consciousness regarding the transmission mode(s) of the virus and distribute guidelines, social service reachability which affects information distribution is a critical aspect in disease control. (Lakshmi Priyadarsini/Suresh 2020)

4. Social Meaning of Mask-Wearing, Contact Tracing in South Korea

1) Selfish Mask-Wearing and Altruistic Mask-Wearing

There are various types of masks, including self-interest masks that can prevent infection from others, such as the N95 masks, and altruistic masks that are focused on preventing other people from getting infected. Of course, the boundary between altruistic and selfish masks is not very clear, and when it comes to infectious diseases, selfishness can also be altruistic, so the distinction is not very important. However, it would be meaningful to look at what purpose people consider more important when it comes to wearing masks.

To investigate the social meaning of mask-wearing in South Korea, news articles scraped from news aggregators, Google News, and texts from Twitter, one of the most popular social network services in Korea are analyzed using text analysis software. Total of 13202 twitter posts and 212 news articles were extracted from each source respectively using the keyword of "Corona" with "Mask" in Korean between the date of the first suspected COVID-19 case, Dec. 1. 2019. (WHO 2020) and Jun. 30. 2020. News articles from Google News are scrapped only using summaries of news due to limitations in scraping methods.

Extracted text data were analyzed using KoNLPy package (Park/Cho 2014) and NLTK (Bird et al. 2009) for news articles and Twitter texts respectively for extracting nouns from articles, and finally, Word Cloud based on frequent keywords were drawn as below.

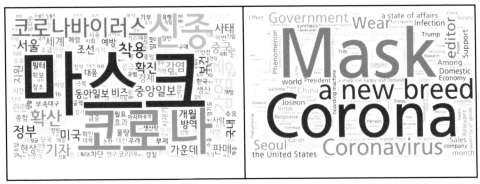

Figure 1: Word Cloud of Korean news articles about COVID-19 and the face mask (righthand: Word Cloud translated from Korean)

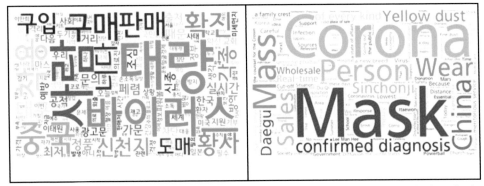

Figure 2: Word Cloud of Korean twitter posts about COVID-19 and the face mask (righthand: Word Cloud translated from Korean, duplicated due to translation were omitted)

According to the above results, while there are many objective facts in the news, such as patients, infections and symptoms, it can be assumed on Twitter that content about buying masks for individual interest or discussions about China are mainly taking place. Discussions on China in connection with the Corona virus need to be examined in more detail, but they also pose many ethical problems that could further lead to discrimination against Chinese and discrimination against Asians.

2) Double-Sided Meaning of Wearing a Mask

The wearing of face masks signals two aspects: stigma and virtue-signaling with the participation of a social distance movement. The example of stigma is as follows: "A friend of mine who lives in an apartment building tells me that when he's wearing a mask other people won't get in an elevator with him." Finally, example of virtue-signaling (wearing a mask to protect others) is as follows: "Someone else told me, 'I started to wear a mask when I go to the grocery store because other people stay away from me.'" In Western cultures, wearing a mask is often accompanied by a stigma effect because people wear a mask when they have a disease. In Korea, however, masks are 1) aimed at protecting themselves from viruses and 2) not to harm(spread of disease) others because they may have a potential virus. (Kluger 2020)

Compared to Western countries, mask wearing is well maintained in South Korea. However, the following criticism is also possible behind the relatively good wearing of masks in South Korea. Along with the international atmosphere of a medicalized society, medical care in South Korea is used not only for prevention or treatment but also for "active health concepts." Beyond a society that values health, it needs to consider the possibility of transition to a society that is obsessed with health. It should also be noted that there is a risk of virusing individual humans behind a well-established alternative to infectious diseases, such as wearing a mask. Wearing a mask for the purpose of protecting yourself or for the purpose of protecting others is to keep social distance from others. Behind these acts is the possibility of treating others as viruses rather than humans.

3) Contact Tracing and Surveillance

In order to search for the difference of conceptions regarding the technologies related to 'contact tracing' of COVID-19, news articles scraped from news aggregators are analyzed using network analysis software. News articles on topic "COVID contact tracing" in Korean news aggregator, NAVER news and "South Korea COVID contact tracing" in worldwide news aggregator, Google News are scraped using automated scraping software, and total of 3998 Korean news articles and 237 English news articles between the date of the first suspected COVID-19 case, Dec. 1. 2019. (WHO 2020) and Jun. 30. 2020 are scrapped. News articles from Google News are scrapped only using summaries of news due to limitations in scraping methods.

Extracted text data were analyzed using KoNLPy package (Park/Cho 2014) and NLTK (Bird et al. 2009) for Korean and English news articles respectively for extracting nouns from articles, and finally, Word Cloud based on frequent keywords were drawn as below.

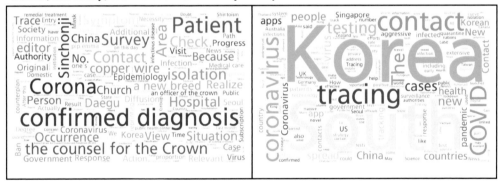

Figure 3: Word Cloud of news articles featuring "COVID contact tracking" (left, translated from Korean) and "South Korea COVID contact tracking"(right)

Although many public opinions around the world expressed a positive view that Korea responded well to the Korona crisis, at the same time, Korea was criticized for violating individual liberty regarding contact tracking. The infringement of individual liberty for public health certainly poses many ethical problems and no one will dispute the importance of the value of individual liberty. According to the above results, it can be seen that foreign articles mentioned concerns about the surveillance society in relation to information tracking. In contrast, as from the word cloud result above, it can be said that Korean news articles do not express concerns related to surveillance and privacy infringement in relation to contact tracking. The reason for this phenomenon may be attributed to Korea's social background, which favors newly developed technologies, circumstances where many technologies are already being used, and prefers active concepts regarding health. In order to solve the problem of coronavirus and infringement of privacy information, some research institutes and companies in Korea as well as in other countries have developed a technology to receive notification service when an individual is close to a confirmed person without disclosing the personal information. However, since the technical solution does not solve all of these problems. It is imperative to create a social atmosphere that recognizes the importance of the value of infringement of personal information.

But it is time for us to discuss the meaning of public health in 'the concrete situation of infectious diseases', not the abstract discourse of 'public health'. The issue of Korea's quarantine has been criticized a lot for violating individual freedom for public health. But it is within the community that the concept of freedom is realized. Although freedom is a priority value, it does not have absolute priority among various values. The question of how to maintain the concept of freedom itself in a society in the face of an epidemic crisis is not how much it violates the existing concept of freedom. The question is how the concept of freedom forms a relationship with the concept of solidarity or the right to live.

Also, it is Confucian culture that often appears when News from Western refers to Asian countries in connection with the Corona response. However, the characteristics of many Asian countries cannot be reduced to Confucianism, and each Asian country has different cultural characteristics. Have you seen Asian scholars explain by reducing it to Christian culture when discussing Western countries? In addition, Confucian culture does not exert much influence in the real life of Korean society today. Confucian culture cannot explain Korea.

5. Conclusion: our crisis is not based just in COVID-19

Many theorists note that our society is undergoing many changes due to the COVID-19. Of course it's true. But COVID-19 is not the cause of the crises we are experiencing now. However, COVID-19 only revealed the problems that our society had before. These examples include: The lonely deaths of elderly people living alone due to COVID-19; the difficulty of living as small merchants are encouraged by the Corona crisis; the burden of housewives having to pay for their children's education at home due to the closure of schools; the reduction in the number of female scholars' papers due to COVID-19; the risk of infection among female medical workers as medical devices, such as masks, are produced to the size of ordinary men; aversion against gays has increased since the news that there has been a confirmed case of COVID-19 infection in gay clubs in Korea. It can be seen that aversion against gays arose from contact tracing results, but these circumstances are results from people's perceptions against gay, not the direct result from contact tracing. COVID-19' crisis comes from the human crisis.

References

Ahn 2020. Ahn, S. M. Government's legitimacy, solidarity behind Korea's success battling COVID-19:

Balilla 2020. Balilla, J. Assessment of COVID-19 mass testing: the case of South Korea. Available at SSRN 3556346.

Bird et al. 2009. Bird, S., Klein, E., & Loper, E. Natural language processing with Python: analyzing text with the natural language toolkit. " O'Reilly Media, Inc.".

Emanuel et al. 2020. Emanuel, E. J., Persad, G., Upshur, R., Thome, B., Parker, M., Glickman,

A., ... & Phillips, J. P. Fair allocation of scarce medical resources in the time of COVID-19.

Griffiths 2020. Griffiths, J. Asia may have been right about coronavirus and face masks, and the rest of the world is coming around. https://edition.cnn.com/2020/04/01/asia/coronavirus-mask-messaging-intl-hnk/index.html (Accessed June 10, 2020)

Kang 2020. Kang, Y. J. South Korea's COVID-19 Infection Status: from the Perspective of Re-Positive after Viral Clearance by Negative Testing. Disaster Medicine and Public Health Preparedness, 1-7.

Kim 2018. Kim, S. Entrepreneurship and Consumerism in Korea"s Customized Welfare Services : Critical Study on the Market-originated Identities of Public Welfare Actors, Journal of Korean social welfare administration 20(4), 175-211

KCDMH 2020. Korean Central Disaster Management Headquarters. Coronavirus Disease-19, Republic of Korea. http://ncov.mohw.go.kr/en/

Kluger 2020. Kluger, J. The Ethics of Wearing (or Not Wearing) a Face Mask During the Coronavirus Epidemic. https://time.com/5815299/coronavirus-face-mask-ethics/ (Accessed Jun. 12, 2020)

Lakshmi Priyadarsini/Suresh 2020. Lakshmi Priyadarsini, S., & Suresh, M. Factors influencing the epidemiological characteristics of pandemic COVID 19: A TISM approach. International Journal of Healthcare Management, 13(2), 89-98.

Lee et al. 2006. Lee, B. J., Kim, Y. D., Kim, M. G., et al. A Study on Reorganization of Social Welfare Service Supply System. Presidential Committee on Social Inclusion

Lee/Lee 2020. Lee, D., & Lee, J. Testing on the Move South Korea's rapid response to the COVID-19 pandemic. Transportation Research Interdisciplinary Perspectives, 100111.

Park/Cho 2014. Park, E. L., & Cho, S. KoNLPy: Korean natural language processing in Python. In Proceedings of the 26th Annual Conference on Human & Cognitive Language Technology (2014, October, Vol. 6, pp. 133-136)

Sorman 2020. Sorman. http://www.koreaherald.com/view.php?ud=20200511000863 (Accessed Jun. 10. 2020)

WHO 2020. WHO. Coronavirus disease 2019 (COVID-19) Situation Report – 94. https://www.who.int/docs/default-source/coronaviruse/situation-reports/20200423-sitrep-94-COVID-19.pdf (Accessed Jul. 12. 2020)

Jiwon Shim is Research Professor in Humanities Research Institute at Chung-Ang University in Korea. She wrote her PhD dissertations on human enhancement at Muenster University in Germany, and leads an NRF-funded (National Research Foundation of Korea) project on issues of human enhancement, artificial intelligence, and medical ethics; g1dmpkr@gmail.com.

Juhee Eom is Research Professor in the Graduate School of Public Health at Yonsei University in Korea. She studied constitutional law, public law and bioethics at Yonsei University in Korea and leads an NRF-funded (National Research Foundation of Korea) project on neurolaw foundation construction in relation to emerging technology, neuroscience and ethics on legal perspectives; juheelight@gmail.com.

Sun Geu Chae is Research Engineer at the Industrial Engineering Department in Hanyang University, South Korea. His research interests include data mining based on machine learning and deep learning algorithms; itwavesu@gmail.com.

Corona Combat, Human Dignity and the Rights: Global Reflections and Indian Milieu - An Ethical Evaluation

Rishi Raj Kishore, Indian Society for Health Laws and Ethics, India

Abstract

COVID-19 is much more than a health crisis. Faced with no direct answer, the policy planners are resorting to improvised strategies such as home internment, lockdown and curfew leading to devastating social, economic and political consequences, with deep scars. In this paper I identify COVID-19 challenges, analyze the global strategies and the Indian response concerning Corona campaign to evaluate their ethical content. I conclude that corona combat reflects a cascade of hasty, fragmented and ill-conceived policies of an overburdened system, imperiling billions of lives and causing dehumanization of the poor and vulnerable, in utter disregard for human dignity and rights.

Key words

COVID-19, lockdown, poor, vulnerable, livelihood, starvation, ethics, human dignity, rights, economic recession, uncertainty, injustice

1. Introduction

Since 1 December 2019, when the first person fell ill due to the new virus in Wuhan,[1] the number of corona virus (COVID-19) cases have been growing continuously and, as on 13 June 2020, there are there are 7,651,175 confirmed cases of COVID-19 and over 425,869 deaths in 210 countries and territories around the world.[2] "As the coronavirus cases grew exponentially, the United States, in just six weeks, reported more COVID-19 fatalities than the persons killed in the Vietnam War."[3] An incredibly small organism of 125 nm diameter[4] has proven to be mightier than many missiles and bullets. World is gripped with utter helplessness as there is no drug to cure the virus nor is there any vaccine to prevent its spread. Faced with no direct answer, the policy planners are resorting to reactive and improvised strategies such as social distancing, isolation, quarantine, travel restrictions, home internment, lockdown and curfew in the hope of containing the disease. These methodologies, being practiced for more than two months, have generated unpalatable social impacts ranging from loss of business to loss of life due to starvation and suicide. The impacts, thus, appear to be as bad as the disease, perhaps even more unpleasant. "Worldwide, three quarters of informal workers are estimated to be severely impacted by lockdowns or are working in the hardest hit sectors."[5] In certain jurisdictions hun-

---

[1] Cohen, Jon (26 January 2020). "Wuhan seafood market may not be source of novel virus spreading globally". *Science*. https://www.sciencemag.org/news/2020/01/wuhan-seafood-market-may-not-be-source-novel-virus-spreading-globally, visited June 10, 2020.

[2] COVID-19 Dashboard by the Center for Systems Science and Engineering (CSSE) at Johns Hopkins University. https://www.arcgis.com/apps/opsdashboard/index.html#/bda7594740fd40299423467b48e9ecf6, visited June 13, 2020 .

[3] Xinhua Headlines: Challenges and opportunities in 100 days' fight against COVID-19 pandemic . Source: Xinhua| 2020-05-08   19:30:43|Editor: huaxia.   XINHUANET   http://www.xinhuanet.com/english/2020-05/08/c_139041041.htm, visited June 10, 2020.

[4] Fehr, A.R., and Perlman, S. 2015. Coronaviruses: An Overview of Their Replication and Pathogenesis. Methods in Molecular Biology. Nature Public Health Emergency Collection 2015; 1282: 1–23.   PMC436938523 https://www.ncbi.nlm.nih.gov/pmc/articles/PMC4369385/, visited June 10, 2020.

[5] Indhira Santos and Michael Weber. Supporting workers' transition to a new normal amid COVID-19. May 13, 2020. World Bank Blogs   https://blogs.worldbank.org/voices/supporting-workers-transition-new-normal-amid-covid-19, Visited June 10, 2020.

gry and exhausted migrant workers returning to their homes are dying on the highways and railways crushed under the wheels. The people who are already vulnerable and fragile cannot stand prolonged scarcities, deprivations and restrictions. With the passage of time, therefore, heterogeneous voices are emerging. On one hand are those who want to continue with drastic measures such as absolute lockdown, on the other hand are those who favour a subtle and humane approach keeping intact the normal activities of life and the interests of marginal and vulnerable sections of the society. "We are in uncharted territory."[6] Those who support the lockdown are perhaps haunted by the Justinian Plague of 541–542 AD claiming estimated 25–50 million lives during two centuries of recurrence[7][8][9], wishfully forgetting the grossly different scientific, socio-economic, political and demographic realities of today's world.

---

[6] COVID-19 pandemic. Humanity needs leadership and solidarity to defeat the coronavirus. United Nations Development Programme. https://www.undp.org/content/undp/en/home/coronavirus.html, visited June 10, 2020.

[7] An Empire's Pandemic. Los Angeles Times, May 6, 2002. https://www.ph.ucla.edu/epi/bioter/anempiresepidemic.html, visited June 10, 2020

[8] Rosen, William (2007). Justinian's Flea: Plague, Empire, and the Birth of Europe. New York City: Viking Adult. p. 3. ISBN 978-0-670-03855-8 ..

[9] "The Plague of Justinian". History Magazine. 11 (1): 9–12. 2009 https://www.scribd.com/document/350965798/Plague-of-Justinian) ,visited June 10, 2020.

The 13 May 2020 statement of Dr. Michael Ryan, World Health Organization Emergencies Chief, advising to be "realistic" as "this virus may become just another endemic virus in our communities, and this virus may never go away" is an eye-opener.[10] Since there is no sign of combating the virus in the near future it is imperative to candidly examine the validity of ongoing anti-corona strategies, particularly, in a realm where, "The richest 1% now have more wealth than the rest of the world combined."[11] In this paper I identify the challenges thrown by COVID-19 pandemic, analyze the global strategies and the Indian scenario in order to determine the ethical content of the continuing Corona crusade, on the touchstone of human dignity and rights. I conclude that corona combat policies are hasty, fragmented and ill-conceived, with no scientific basis, leading to devastating socio-economic and political consequences leading to dehumanization of the poor and vulnerable, reflecting utter disregard for human dignity and rights, and the world needs to be reopened at the earliest.

2. The Challenge

"The coronavirus COVID-19 pandemic is the defining global health crisis of our time and the greatest challenge we have faced since World War Two."[12] In a recent interview Dr. Anthony Fauci, director of the United States National Institute of Allergy and Infectious Disease and scientific face of America's COVID-19 response said, "I don't think there's a chance that this virus is just going to disappear. It's going to be around, and if given the opportunity, it will resurge."[13] On 12 May 2020, in his testimony to the US Senate he candidly admitted, "I am very careful and hopefully humble in knowing that I don't know everything about this disease"[14].

Because of its devastating characteristics COVID -19 pandemic has thrown a formidable challenge before the global community. Wide range of incubation period (2-14 days), which may extend up to 27 days;[15] initial asymptomatic course; widely varying symptoms – ranging from mild symptoms to severe illness;[16] common symptoms with other illnesses making it difficult to make the clinical diagnosis; easy spread through air or physical contact; propensity towards old and infirm; high risk in pre-existing conditions like cardiovascular disease, diabetes, chronic respiratory disease, hypertension and malignancies; and sudden and serious complica-

---

[10] COVID-19 could become endemic like HIV and may never go away: WHO expert Mike Ryan. Reuters May 14, 2020 11:39 AM IST. Firstpost. Wednesday, May 20, 2020https://www.firstpost.com/health/covid-19-could-become-endemic-like-hiv-and-may-never-go-away-who-expert-mike-ryan-8366961.html, visited June 10, 2020.

[11] An Economy For the 1%" " Deborah Hardoon (Deputy Head of Research, Oxfam GB), Sophia Ayele & Ricardo Fuentes-Nieva (Executive Director of Oxfam Mexico) How privilege and power in the economy drive extreme inequality and how this can be stopped. Publication date: 18 January 2016 OXFAM International https://www.oxfam.org/en/research/economy-1.

[12] COVID-19 pandemic. Humanity needs leadership and solidarity to defeat the coronavirus. United Nations Development Programme https://www.undp.org/content/undp/en/home/coronavirus.html, visited June 10, 2020.

[13] Nsikan Akpan and Victoria Jaggard Fauci: No scientific evidence the coronavirus was made in a Chinese lab Interview to National Geographic, published on May 4, 2020 . https://www.nationalgeographic.com/science/2020/05/anthony-fauci-no-scientific-evidence-the-coronavirus-was-made-in-a-chinese-lab-cvd/, visited June 10, 2020.

[14] Chris Cillizza. Anthony Fauci's quiet coronavirus rebellion. May 12, 2020. CNN politics https://edition.cnn.com/2020/05/12/politics/fauci-trump-coronavirus-senate-hearing/index.html, visited June 10, 2020.

[15] Worldometer. Coronavirus Incubation Period https://www.worldometers.info/coronavirus/coronavirus-incubation-period/, visited June 10, 2020.

[16] Worldometer. Coronavirus Symptoms (COVID-19) https://www.worldometers.info/coronavirus/coronavirus-symptoms/ (104), visited June 10, 2020.

tions requiring intensive care and hospitalization confront the healthcare professionals. "In addition, a very high proportion - around 80 per cent - of people develop very mild forms of the disease, which makes it difficult to identify and isolate cases quickly."[17] "Several factors make this new coronavirus particularly worrying. Being a new virus, there is no acquired immunity; as many as 35 candidate vaccines are currently in the study phase, but experts agree that no widely usable vaccine will be available for at least 12 to 18 months."[18]

"While a vaccine solution is still not in sight, the virus' spread remains largely uncertain."[19]

The above scenario is compounded by the absence of drug to cure the virus. In addition to distinct nature of the virus and the scientific unpreparedness, inadequate health delivery system, infrastructural constraints, unwillingness to sacrifice personal freedoms, financial limitations, economic repercussions, mass exodus of migrant workers, political conflict and displacement, lack of international solidarity and cooperation, and legal issues have created serious hurdles in the fight against the virus. Virus has also revived the dormant conflicts among the countries. China says that relations with the US are "on the brink of a new Cold War", fuelled in part by tensions over the pandemic. [20] While talking about the regional effect of the virus some believe that in certain areas such as " the Middle East—a region with no shortage of dangerous pre-existing conditions—it could be far worse"[21]. "In war-torn countries, COVID-19 represents a dramatic threat to life. Health systems have already been ravaged by violence, and the threat of further strain on health care from the corona virus is an enormous risk for communities."[22] The situation in certain African countries is miserable. "Wage earners who live hand to mouth had to decide between the possibility of dying from the virus and the certainty of dying from hunger." Trapped in their homes, and with their ability to earn money curtailed, Nigerians had started calling the Corona as "hunger virus".[23]

According to International Labour Organization, "As a result of the economic crisis created by the pandemic, almost 1.6 billion informal economy workers (representing the most vulnerable in the labour market), out of a worldwide total of two billion and a global workforce of 3.3 billion, have suffered massive damage to their capacity to earn a living."[24] The ILO Director-General Guy Ryder told a briefing, that "the jobs employment crisis and all of its consequences

---

[17] Coronavirus COVID-19 pandemic. Challenges in supporting COVID-19 response. Médecins Sans Frontières. 16 March 2020 https://www.msf.org/challenges-supporting-covid-19-response, visited June 10, 2020.

[18] Coronavirus COVID-19 pandemic. Challenges in supporting COVID-19 response. Médecins Sans Frontières. 16 March 2020 https://www.msf.org/challenges-supporting-covid-19-response, visited June 10, 2020.

[19] Xinhua Headlines: Challenges and opportunities in 100 days' fight against COVID-19 pandemic . Source: Xinhua| 2020-05-08   19:30:43|Editor: huaxia   .   XINHUANET   http://www.xinhuanet.com/english/2020-05/08/c_139041041.htm 669, visited June 10, 2020.

[20] China says virus pushing US ties to brink of new 'Cold War' The Times of India, New Delhi., May 25, 2020. p. 9.

[21] Ambassador Hesham Youssef . Six Challenges Facing a Fragile Middle East Amid Coronavirus. Unites States Institute of Peace. Wednesday, April 1, 2020 https://www.usip.org/publications/2020/04/six-challenges-facing-fragile-middle-east-amid-coronavirus, visited June 10, 2020.

[22] ICRC (International Committee of the Red Cross) COVID-19: ICRC global response to the coronavirus https://www.icrc.org/en/document/covid-19-coronavirus-pandemic-icrc#gs.6rcyfl , visited June 10, 2020.

[23] Láolú Senbanjo. African countries need to challenge the idea of a homogenous approach to COVID-19. May 16, 2020. QUARTZ AFRICA. https://qz.com/africa/1858008/africa-needs-to-challenge-the-homogenous-approach-to-covid-19/, visited June 10, 2020.

[24] COVID-19: Stimulating the economy and employment. ILO: As job losses escalate, nearly half of global workforce at risk of losing livelihoods Press release | 29 April 2020. International Labour Organization. https://www.ilo.org/global/about-the-ilo/newsroom/news/WCMS_743036/lang--en/index.htm, visited June 10, 2020.

is deepening by comparison with our estimates of 3 weeks ago." Ryder further said, "For millions of workers, no income means no food, no security and no future. Millions of businesses around the world are barely breathing," because they "have no savings or access to credit." According to him, these workers "are the real faces of the world of work. If we don't help them now, they will simply perish." Ryder added, "As the pandemic and the jobs crisis evolve, the need to protect the most vulnerable becomes even more urgent." [25]

"The COVID-19 outbreak is also a major education crisis' and about "1.2 billion students and youth across the planet are affected by school and university closures due to the COVID-19 outbreak." [26] For an average citizen, daily life has become inordinately arduous. "Goods and services are not readily available, and we're seeing price inflation as demand across the globe far exceeds the supply. Under normal circumstances, the global market regulates itself. But we are now in an unprecedented situation, where there is neither an automatic correction of the markets nor a global regulation in place to address market failures. And as COVID-19 is progressing very rapidly, new cases are being reported in many countries across the world, which makes the assessment of needs very difficult." [27]

---

[25] Stephanie Nebehay. Nearly half of global workforce risk losing livelihoods in pandemic - ILO Economic News. April 29, 2020. https://in.reuters.com/article/health-coronavirus-ilo/nearly-half-of-global-workforce-risk-losing-livelihoods-in-pandemic-ilo-idINKBN22B1LF, visited June 10, 2020.

[26] UNESCO. Global Education Coalition. COVID-19 Education Response. https://en.unesco.org/covid19/educationresponse/globalcoalition, visited June 10, 2020.

[27] Vinay Sharma. COVID-19 Challenges and Response: How procurement underpins the World Bank's response to the pandemic. World Bank Blogs. April 15, 2020. https://blogs.worldbank.org/voices/covid-19-challenges-and-response-how-procurement-underpins-world-banks-response-pandemic, visited June 10, 2020.

COVID-19 has thrown a daunting challenge before the policy planners. Disproportionate diversion of funds towards the corona combat has led to insufficient health coverage to non-Covid persons such as old and infirm, chronically ill and those requiring urgent interventions. In certain jurisdictions many hospitals have been exclusively reserved for Corona positive patients, denying care to non-Covid patients. Added to this, the health delivery system is confronted with the task of protecting their workers from the Corona infection. "After studying the health-care system response of various countries like Italy, Spain, Germany, UK and Korea we found that 20 per cent of infected patients are healthcare workers and this leads to a compound effect where these people can infect other patients and hence the number of patients increases while the healthcare workforce decrease. This is a double whammy to healthcare system."[28]

"Globally, the coronavirus shock is severe even compared to the Great Financial Crisis in 2007–08." because "Success in containing the virus comes at the price of slowing economic activity, no matter whether social distancing and reduced mobility are voluntary or enforced"[29] "It is difficult to imagine that the traumatic experiences of the pandemic will be forgotten quickly or disappear entirely over time. The human losses alone will remain strong reminders of the implications of change at the level of society and individuals".[30] While massive efforts are on to control the disease there is uncertainty about its future course and it appears a formidable challenges will continue to confront the world for many years to come.

Across the globe, COVID-19 has seriously disrupted other pressing human pursuits. "2020 is expected to be a pivotal year for climate change negotiations. Countries are to update their Nationally Determined Contributions (NDCs) and commit to more action-based efforts during the Conference of Parties (COP 26) in Glasgow later this year. However, with the global econ-omy predicted to go in recession, it seems likely that climate will again be put on the backburner — for now."[31]

In addition to aforesaid negative impacts, the world is confronted with various ethico-legal challenges in terms of human dignity, individual autonomy, privacy and rule of law, reflecting loss of equity, equality and transparency, as highlighted in the next part of this paper.

3. Global reflections

As on 13 June 2020, there are more than 7.65 million confirmed cases of COVID-19 and over 4 lacs deaths in 210 countries and territories around the world. The ten most affected coun-tries in terms of confirmed cases are the United States, Brazil, Russia, India, United Kingdom,

---

[28] Prem Sharma Corona virus is a global crisis and the biggest challenge we have faced in our life time. Health-world.com from The Economic Times https://blog.petrieflom.law.harvard.edu/2020/04/09/social-justice-covid19-law-coronavirus/.

[29] The IMF explains the economic lessons from China's fight against coronavirus. World Economic Forum, 21 Mar 2020. IMF Blog https://www.weforum.org/agenda/2020/03/imf-economic-lessons-from-china-fight-against-coronavirus, visited June 10, 2020.

[30] Rolf Alter. Challenges and Opportunities in the Post-COVID-19 World Regional Governance: An Opportunity for Regional Organizations? World Economic Forum. Insight Report Challenges and Opportunities in the Post-COVID-19 World. May 2020. p.12 http://www3.weforum.org/docs/WEF_Challenges_and_Opportunities_Post_COVID_19.pdf, visited June 10, 2020

[31] Parvathi Preethan/Nambi Appadurai/Shubham Gupta | With the global economy hit by Covid, climate issues may be put on the backburner. April 30, 2020 BusinessLine https://www.thehindubusinessline.com/opinion/with-the-global-economy-hit-by-covid-climate-issues-may-be-put-on-the-backburner/article31472214.ece#, visited Jun3 12, 2020..

Spain, Italy, Peru, France and Germany.[32]

National responses to the Covid -19 pandemic have been varied. The containment measures include social distancing, quarantine, isolation, ban of outdoor activities and total home confinement. Strategies reflect strict implementation by putting the areas under complete lockdown through statutory measures, including curfew and Incarceration. Steps include restriction on the entry of persons in to the country via the roads, air and sea, strict border control banning the movement of the people from one province to another inside the same country. All public activities have been brought to standstill by closure of educational institutions, Courts, administrative offices, markets, factories, transports, tourists spots, places of entertainment, recreation, concerts, marriage ceremonies, religious gatherings, cultural events, sporting events, political rallies, funeral services and all other social engagements. Draconian restrictions have been imposed to ensure that the people stay inside their homes.

According to BBC Reality Check Team's report dated 1 April 2020, Japan, which earlier banned entry to visitors from certain areas of China and South Korea, has now extended this to 21 European countries and Iran, and is telling arrivals from the US to go into quarantine for 14 days. Australia and New Zealand have banned entry to all foreigners, with Australia telling all citizens and residents who return to the country they must go into quarantine for two weeks. Singapore has done the same, stopping visitors entering and requiring all citizens, permanent and long-term residents to self-isolate at home for 14 days. And South Korea has said that anyone arriving from abroad, including their own citizens, will have to self-isolate for two weeks. The US has closed its northern border with Canada and is cracking down on people trying to cross illegally from Mexico. And China itself, where the COVID-19 outbreak started, has now banned all foreign visitors, concerned that new cases of the virus are starting to come from abroad. The EU sealed its external borders on 18 March to anyone from outside the bloc for at least 30 days.[33]

Opinion is fast emerging that, "Anti-lockdown protesters could have potentially contributed the spread of the coronavirus in the US as they often travelled for hundreds of kilometres , sometimes to different states , to attend rallies, according to an analysis of data gathered from location-tracing of the protesters cell phones."[34]

According to media reports of March and April 2020, more than 50 million people were in lockdown in the Philippines[35], about 59 million people were in lockdown in South Africa,[36] and 1.3 billion people were in lockdown in India.[37]

---

[32] Ibid 2, visited June 13, 2020..

[33] Coronavirus: What measures are countries taking to stop it? By Reality Check team BBC News, 1 April 2020. BBC News. https://www.bbc.com/news/world-51737226, visited June 10, 2020.

[34] Yashwant Raj. US Rallies may have spread virus, phone data suggests. Hindustan Times, New Delhi dated May 19, 2020. p. 7.

[35] "Philippines isolates hundreds of health workers as coronavirus cases rise in south-east Asia". The Guardian. 23 March 2020. https://www.theguardian.com/world/2020/mar/23/hundreds-of-filipino-health-workers-isolated-indonesia-thailand-malaysia-singapore-cambodia-myanmar-coronavirus-cases-rise-in-south-east-asia, visited June 10, 2020.

[36] Chutel L, Dahir AL (27 March 2020). "With Most Coronavirus Cases in Africa, South Africa Locks Down". The New York Times. https://www.nytimes.com/2020/03/27/world/africa/south-africa-coronavirus.html, visited June 10, 2020.

[37] Nair S (29 March 2020). "For a billion Indians, lockdown has not prevented tragedy". The Guardian. https://www.theguardian.com/world/commentisfree/2020/mar/29/india-lockdown-tragedy-healthcare-coronavirus-starvation-mumbai, visited March 31, 2020.

"The coronavirus landed in Latin America on February 26, when Brazil confirmed a case in São Paulo. Since then, governments across the region have taken an array of actions to protect their citizens and contain COVID-19's spread."[38] On march 19 2020, the Brazilian government restricted entry to foreigners at all land borders—excluding permanent residents, diplomats, or international organization officials, which was further strengthened on 27 March 2020 by closing of borders via air to all foreigners for 30 days, with commerce continuing as normal. On May 27, São Paulo state and city authorities announced a five-level plan to reopen commercial activity beginning June 1, 2020.[39]   On 31 May president **Jair Bolsonaro** and his U.S. counterpart **Donald Trump** issued a joint statement on May 31 saying they "stand in solidarity" and will "remain in close coordination" in their responses to the coronavirus pandemic."[40]

In Argentina, on May 8, the government announced a progressive reopening of the national quarantine, first announced March 20 while stricter measures continued in the metropolitan Buenos Aires region, the most affected part of the country and where roughly 32 percent of the population lives[41] Chile confirmed its first case on March 3, which involved a 33-year-old_male doctor who had travelled to Asia. On March 18, President **Sebastián Piñera** "declared a nationwide state of catastrophe as of March 19 for 90 days, following the government's Action Plan. This includes banning gatherings in public spaces, controlling the distribution of basic necessities, and limiting people's movement across cities and the country, all with the help of the Armed Forces."[42]

In Europe, "Since March 2020, more than 60 million people in Italy have experienced human rights restrictions that are unprecedented in the country's republican history." A state of emergency was declared for a period of six months and "a wealth of legal measures aimed at preventing and containing the spread of COVID-19" have been adopted by the Government", limiting "fundamental human rights (especially freedom of movement and of assembly and the right to privacy and to property)" and a total lockdown has been extended until 3 May 2020. "In order to deter non-compliance for futile reasons, maximum fines were raised for violations of the limitations on freedom of movement and assembly from €206 to €3,000, while breaching mandatory or fiduciary quarantine was qualified as "culpable spread of epidemics" punishable under art. 438 of the Criminal Code with imprisonment up to 12 years."[43] In Australia, "To help manage the pandemic, unprecedented powers were granted to the police. COVID-19-related fines and prison terms vary across the country and their enforcement is varied across groups in society. Penalties include fines of over $50,000 for corporations and fines and jail time for individuals."[44]

---

[38] Luisa Horwitz, Paola Nagovitch, Holly K. Sonneland, and Carin Zissis June 01, 2020 Where Is the Coronavirus in Latin America? AS/COA Americas Society/Council of the Americas https://www.as-coa.org/articles/where-coronavirus-latin-america, visited June 10, 2020.

[39] Ibid.

[40] Ibid.

[41] Ibid.

[42] Ibid.

[43] Stefania Negri. Anti-COVID Measures Restricting Civil Liberties in Italy: Issues of Legality and Legitimacy. May 12, 2020. Bioethics, Blog Symposia, Featured, Global Health, Global Responses to COVID-19: Rights, Democracy, and the Law, Health Law Policy, Human Rights, International, Public Health. https://blog.petrieflom.law.harvard.edu/2020/05/12/italy-global-responses-covid19/, visited June 10, 2020.

[44] Paul Harpur. COVID-19 in Australia: Protecting Public Health by Restricting Rights & Risking the Rule of Law. May 14, 2020 Blog Symposia, Global Health, Global Responses to COVID-19: Rights, Democracy, and the Law,

In the USA, the federal government publicly released its approach to COVID-19 testing on 28 January 2020. Estimates are that as of 12 April, nearly 300 million people, or about 90 per cent of the population, were under some form of lockdown in the United States.[45]

By the first week of April, 3.9 billion people— more than half of the world's population. were under some form of lockdown.[46]

While massive efforts are on to control the disease there is uncertainty about its future course. In a briefing on 13 May 2020, the World Health Organization Emergencies Chief, Dr. Michael Ryan said, "I think it is important we are realistic and I don't think anyone can predict when this disease will disappear," he added. "I think there are no promises in this and there are no dates. This disease may settle into a long-term problem, or it may not. Nothing can be said as of now." "It is important to put this on the table: this virus may become just another endemic virus in our communities, and this virus may never go away."[47] The statements belies the hope of an early relief.

On 19 May 2020, in the 73rd World Health Assembly, the delegates adopted a landmark resolution, co-sponsored by more than 130 countries, to bring the world together to fight the COVID-19 pandemic. The resolution calls for the intensification of efforts to control the pandemic, and for equitable access to and fair distribution of all essential health technologies and products to combat the virus. It also calls for an independent and comprehensive evaluation of the global response, including, but not limited to, WHO's performance. In his closing remarks the WHO Director-General Dr Tedros Adhanom Ghebreyesus said "COVID-19 has robbed us of people we love. It's robbed us of lives and livelihoods; it's shaken the foundations of our world; it threatens to tear at the fabric of international cooperation. But it's also reminded us that for all our differences, we are one human race, and we are stronger together."[48]

4. Indian milieu

The first case of COVID-19 was confirmed in India on 30 January 2020 in the state of Kerala when a university student returned to the state from Wuhan, China.[49] As the number of COVID-19 positive cases grew to 500 the Prime Minister Mr. Narendra Modi, on 19 March 2020, appealed to the nation to observe a Janata Curfew on 22 March 2020 for 14 hours, from 7 AM to 9 PM during which no citizen could step out or congregate and all markets and estab-

Health Law Policy, Human Rights, International, Public Health. https://blog.petrieflom.law.harvard.edu/2020/05/14/australia-global-responses-covid19/, visited June 10, 2020.

[45] "About 90% of Americans have been ordered to stay at home. This map shows which cities and states are under lockdown". Business Insider. 2 April 2020. https://www.businessinsider.in/science/news/almost-half-of-all-americans-have-been-ordered-to-stay-at-home-this-map-shows-which-cities-and-states-are-under-lockdown-/articleshow/74838246.cms.

[46] "Coronavirus: Half of humanity now on lockdown as 90 countries call for confinement". Euronews. 3 April 2020. https://www.euronews.com/2020/04/02/coronavirus-in-europe-spain-s-death-toll-hits-10-000-after-record-950-new-deaths-in-24-hou. visited June 10, 2020.

[47] COVID-19 could become endemic like HIV and may never go away: WHO expert Mike Ryan. Reuters May 14, 2020 11:39 AM IST. Firstpost. Wednesday, May 20, 2020https://www.firstpost.com/health/covid-19-could-become-endemic-like-hiv-and-may-never-go-away-who-expert-mike-ryan-8366961.html visited June 10, 2020.

[48] Historic health assembly ends with global commitment to COVID-19 response. World Health Organization. https://www.who.int/news-room/detail/19-05-2020-historic-health-assembly-ends-with-global-commitment-to-covid-19-response, visited June 10, 2020.

[49] Alex Ward. India's coronavirus lockdown and its looming crisis, explained. Mar 24, 2020 https://www.vox.com/2020/3/24/21190868/coronavirus-india-modi-lockdown-kashmir.

lishments except those dealing in essential goods and services were closed for the day. Public services, including the Railways and metro were also halted. The curfew was meticulously observed and people stayed inside their homes. Following this, on 24 March, the Prime Minister addressed the people again announcing a nationwide statutory lockdown from midnight of that day, for a period of 21 days. This lockdown was more vigorous and strict than the Janata Curfew imposed earlier, limiting the movement of country's more than 1.35 billion population. On 14 April, Prime Minister Mr. Narendra Modi extended the nationwide lockdown until 3 May. While addressing the nation he said, "India's fight against the Corona global pandemic is moving ahead with great strength and steadfastness. It is only because of your restraint, penance and sacrifice that, India has so far been able to avert the harm caused by corona to a large extent. You have endured immense suffering to save your country, save your India."[50]

On 1 May, the Government of India extended the nationwide lockdown further by two weeks until 17 May. The Government divided the entire nation into three zones – green, red and orange – with relaxations applied accordingly.[51] The policy envisaged that the districts with substantial numbers of positive cases would fall under the red zone. The coronavirus red zone will see no activity. The areas with limited number of cases in the past and with no surge in positive cases recently would be included under the orange zone. Only restricted activities such as limited public transport and farm product harvesting is expected to be allowed in orange zone. The districts with no corona virus positive cases would fall under the green zone.

On 17 May, nationwide lockdown was further extended till 31 May by the National Disaster Management Authority. "According to the guidelines for Lockdown 4.0, issued by the Ministry of Home Affairs (MHA), a number of activities will continue to remain prohibited throughout the country. They include all domestic and international commercial passenger flights and Metro rail services. Even running of schools, colleges, educational and training/coaching institutions; hotels, restaurants and other hospitality services will remain prohibited all across the country. All places of large public gatherings, including cinema halls, shopping malls, gymnasiums, entertainment parks, etc., will remain closed, as social, political, cultural and similar gatherings and other large congregations and access to religious places will remain prohibited."[52]

Indian scenario reflects the worst tragedy the country has faced since independence. However, it is inspiring to note that the Indian Prime Minister Mr. Narendra Modi directly turned to the masses. He has been consistently addressing the people through electronic media. He has personally made the announcements of the lockdowns, explaining to the people the compulsion for taking such harsh steps and praising them for their continued support, cooperation and fortitude. Besides, the Indian strategy reflects several other positive attributes namely: the decisions are being taken after close and continuous monitoring of the emerging situation; there is complete transparency in the decision making process; policies reflect open-mindedness, free of any dogma or fixation, candidly tuned to the pattern of virus spread and its effect; in view of the

---

[50] NDTV, Coronavirus: PM Modi's Full Speech On Extension Of COVID-19 Lockdown https://www.ndtv.com/india-news/coronavirus-pm-narendra-modi-full-speech-on-extension-of-covid-19-lockdown-2211390, visited on June 10, 2020

[51] Neeta Sharma, Sunil Prabhu, Edited by Deepshikha Ghosh. Lockdown For 2 More Weeks. What Will Be Different Now: 10 Points May 02, 2020 NDTV.com https://www.ndtv.com/india-news/nationwide-lockdown-over-coronavirus-extended-for-two-weeks-beyond-may-4-2221782, visited on May 4, 2020.

[52] Tribune News Service, New Delhi, May 17 Centre extends nationwide lockdown till May 31, new guidelines issued. 2020https://www.tribuneindia.com/news/nation/centre-extends-nationwide-lockdown-till-may-31-new-guidelines-issued-86042, visited on May 19, 2020.

federal structure of the country the policies are being evolved after effective consultation and concurrence of the state governments; decision are being taken with active participation of medical personnel, scientists, economists and administrators; the policies are being openly debated among all actors of the civil society in the electronic and print media; the healthcare infrastructure, particularly concerning the Corona combat, is being continuously enhanced and upgraded to meet the emerging challenge; the policies are independent and objective free from any religious, cultural, racial, regional, political or economic bias; policies are inclusive keeping intact the interests of all sections of the society; adequate arrangements within the resource constraints are being made to address the hardships faced by the poor, vulnerable and marginal sections of the society; non-governmental and voluntary organizations are being encouraged to help the people in need; and appropriate institutional access, including the judicial fora, is available for the ventilation of grievances in the event of injustice or undue hardship.

However, despite the sincere, robust and consistent efforts of the government and the people's participation under the dynamic leadership of Prime Minister Narendra Modi, the media reports are disquieting. Reservations are being expressed about the prolonged lockdown. As per the reports, many desperate journeys have ended in tragedies on the highways.

"Across India, lakhs of migrant workers, their livelihoods devastated by the nationwide lockdown to slow the spread of COVID-19, are walking hundreds of kilometers in an attempt to get back to their home villages. Approximately 120 of them have died in accidents along the way."[53] "Evicted by landlords, disowned by employers, asked by contractors to go back home, money running out—they had much in common to share."[54] In a country infested by poverty and unemployment where "millions of households sleep four or more people per room, making isolation and social distancing is difficult."[55] "The fundamental problem is that we are being ravaged not so much by Covid as our own lockdowns. The cure is proving worse than the disease. Lockdowns are killing enterprises, livelihoods and people on a massive scale" and "we have imposed terrible misery through draconian shutdowns."[56]

On 28 May 2020, the Supreme court of India taking sue motu notice of the plight of migrant workers made significant observations i.e., "we are at present concerned with the miseries and difficulties of the migrant workers in going to their native place and the difficulties with which they are faced."; "A large number of migrant workers are still seen proceeding on foot to different places."; "At present, looking into the difficulties and miseries of migrant workers, we are of the view that certain interim directions are required to be issued to be followed by the State Governments /Union Territories and the Central Government to redeem the immediate difficulties of the migrant workers." The apex Court, inter-alia, directed that, "No fare either by train or by bus shall be charged from any migrant workers"; "The migrant workers who are stranded at different places in the country shall be provided food free of cost by the concerned States / Union Territories"; and " the railways shall provide meal and water to the migrant wor-

---

[53] Sruthisagar Yamunan. As Supreme Court fails to protect migrant workers' rights, High Courts show the way. Scroll.in Tuesday, May 19th 2020. https://scroll.in/article/962214/as-supreme-court-fails-to-protect-migrant-workers-rights-high-courts-show-the-way.

[54] Abhijay Jha and Avishek Kumar Pandey. Migrant exodus: Leaving behind one crisis, heading into another. Times of India dated 17 May 2020, p. 3.

[55] Swaminathan S Anklesaria Aiyar. The speech Modi has not made but should. Times of India dated 17 May 2020, p. 14.

[56] Swaminathan S Anklesaria Aiyar. The speech Modi has not made but should. Times of India dated 17 May 2020, p. 14. 333.

kers and same facilities shall be extended when the migrant workers are transported by bus."[57]

A perception is growing that "A lockdown will never eliminate the infection ; it will just postpone it"[58] As on 13 June 2020, the total number of Covid cases recorded in the country crossed 308,916,[59]# with a total death toll of 8884.[60] Amidst mounting criticism against the stringent and prolonged lockdown the government is trying to justify its action on the plea that besides "showing the spread of the disease the lockdown allowed the government to line up resources in terms of health infrastructure and medical workers, increased medical supplies and gain experience in containment measures. It also shortened the wait for potential, drugs , vaccines and treatment besides stepping up research."[61]

With the passage of time, the Indian milieu is getting politically polarized. The opposition is blaming the government for their failure to contain the virus despite prolonged lockdown and the hardships faced by the people and the adverse impact on the country's economy. The government on the other hand is emphasizing their sincere, committed and effective campaign against the Corona virus, a daunting and unpredictable enemy and accusing the opposition not to encash a national calamity for unwarranted political mileage. However, the bottom line is that the people are sensitized about the virus and its virulence and the importance of preventive action. Also, the majority seems convinced with the inevitability of stringent measures taken by the government.

On 01 June 2020, after "over two months of lockdown, the government has now decided to open the economy in a phase-wise manner. Describing it as Unlock 1.0, the government has decided to open malls, hotels, places of worships and restaurants from June 8 with social distancing norms and other precautions. However, such establishments in containment zones shall remain shut till further orders. Private and government offices have also been opened with staggered timings and workforce. Night curfew – from 9 pm to 5 am – will remain enforce, the government said in its new lockdown 5 guidelines. "[62]

The government having realized the urgency of getting out of the lockdown has allowed a partial opening. The complete exit, although inevitable, is not easy. We are at the crossroads. The outcome seems uncertain. One has to wait and watch as the circumstances unfold themselves and define the future.

5. Ethical evaluation

Ethics is an intellectual enterprise founded on moral sensitivities and social imperatives. In a world divided by religious beliefs, cultural sensitivities, racial prejudices, economic disparities and political rivalries human dignity provides the most effective tool to determine the

---

[57] Supreme Court of India. A Record Of Proceedings suo motu Writ Petition (Civil) No(S). 6/2020 In Re : Problems And Miseries of Migrant Labourers with Writ Petition (Civil) Diary No(S). 11394/2020. Order dated 28-05-2020 https://main.sci.gov.in/supremecourt/2020/11706/11706_2020_34_24_22239_Order_28-May-2020.pdf.

[58] Chandra Bhushan. Breaking the Lockdown Chakravyuh. Times of India dated 18 May 2020, p.10.

[59] Livemint. Updated: 10 Jun 2020 Coronavirus update: COVID-19 cases in India cross 2.76 lakh; nearly 10,000 new cases in last 24 hours https://www.livemint.com/news/india/coronavirus-cases-in-india-cross-2-76-lakh-nearly-10-000-cases-in-last-24-hours-11591759131028.html, visited June 10, 2020.

[60] Ibid 2, visited June 13, 2020.

[61] Sushmi Dey. 'Lockdown prevented 37,000-78,000 deaths' The times of India, New Delhi dated May23, 2020, p.12

[62] Coronavirus (COVID-19) India Updates, Lockdown 5 News. Financial Express.   June 2, 2020 https://www.financialexpress.com/lifestyle/health/coronavirus-cases-in-india-covid-19-state-wise-tally-lockdown-5-unlock-1-live-updates-delhi-mumbai-maharashtra-corona-cases-vaccine-news/1977191/

moral content of human pursuits. Before I dwell further, it may be fruitful to understand the human dignity in its concrete form. The following portion of Universal Declaration of Human Rights, adopted by the United Nations in 1948 provides a candid notion of human dignity:

Preamble.

Whereas recognition of the ***inherent dignity*** and of the ***equal and inalienable rights*** of all members of the ***human family*** is the foundation of freedom, justice and peace in the world, *(emphasis added)*

Article 1.

"All human beings are born free and equal in ***dignity and rights***. They are endowed with ***reason and conscience*** and should act towards one another in a spirit of brotherhood." *(emphasis added)*

The above Declaration, very truthfully, prefixes **"inherent"** before the word **"dignity"** because dignity is not acquired or cultivated. It is an intrinsic human attribute. Also, the word **"foundation"** is very significant because it indicates that it is the human dignity that creates a just and humane world order. The existence of **"human family"** and the "**sprit of brotherhood"**, recognized in the above Declaration by the global community in 1948 was enshrined in the Indian cultural thought thousands of years ago, as reflected in the following verse (in *Sanskrit* language):

अयं निजः परो वेति गणना लघुचेतसाम्
उदार चरितानां तु वसुधैव कुटुम्बकम्

(Verse 137, Tantra 5, Panchatantra)

"That person is my own, and the other one is not my own is a thinking of

small-heartedness. For the generous ones the entire humanity is one family"

The words "dignity and rights" in the Universal Declaration clearly indicate that dignity and rights are two different propositions. Rights have political connotation indicating recognition of people's aspirations, expectations and privileges while dignity signifies an innate moral and intellectual content. Similarly, the words "reason and conscience" also make it clear that reason alone is not the sole human attribute, the conscience too is an intrinsic human characteristic. What is this conscience?

Homo sapiens is endowed with certain properties which are not present in any other creature. In the Indian cultural thought these properties are collectively recognized as *Dharma,* which is a Sanskrit term, with no synonym in English language. Thus, *Dharma* signifies the properties because of which Homo sapiens is known as human being. These properties may be many but ten of them can be easily identified namely, love, trust, righteousness, truthfulness, compassion, beneficence, tolerance, forgiveness, sacrifice, and reverence. These properties constitute human virtues that create awareness about good and bad. Thus, *Dharma* is the source of our entire moral enlightenment as human beings. This inherent moral content, unique to Homo sapiens, constitutes human dignity. For this reason the concept of human dignity is universal, not confined to regions, cultures, religions or races.

Since the war against Corona contemplates protection of the humanity as a whole it needs to be fought with due regard to prevailing global realities such as poverty, inequality, unemployment, illiteracy, superstition, religious dogma, cultural sensitivity, ethnic diversity, demographic heterogeneity, infrastructural insufficiency, economic constraint, life styles exclusivity , regional conflicts, political rivalry, legal ambiguity and above all the lack of scientific knowledge. Viewed in this context, the ongoing COVID-19 strategies reflect following ethical miscarriages:

1. The impact on the poor, unemployed and daily wage earners has been totally ignored. Strategies have snatched their jobs compelling them to return to their native places, hungry and exhausted, on foot, often being crushed under the wheels of running trucks and trains.

2. No thought has been given to the plight of vulnerable sections of the society such as poor, elderly, children, chronically ill, pregnant women, mentally or physically disabled.

3. The process is totally non-consensual, severely curtailing the individual autonomy and the right of self-determination.

4. Individual's privacy is being severely breached by tracking their movements and collection of personal profiles, including the details of their families and the status of their health

5. Persons found to be COVID-19 positive are being socially stigmatized and the disease is being linked to specific population or nationality.

6. The policies are dictatorial and vital stakeholders have not been consulted, severely jeopardizing their interests.

7. All democratic institutions such as executive, legislature, judiciary and the intelligentsia have abdicated their social responsibility as there is no perceptible effort on their part to intervene in the state's ill-conceived and anti-humanitarian policies.

8. The adverse economic impact of the measures has been totally forgotten, throwing the national economies into long-lasting recession and stagnation.

9. There has been no international dialogue among the countries although the policies are tuned to fight a virus which is a common enemy that does not recognize political boundaries.

10. There is no effective forum to ventilate the grievances in the event of victimization arising out of arbitrariness, highhandedness, subjectivity or abuse.

11. The policies are not grounded in sound scientific knowledge, empirical study or experience.

12. There is no time limit for continuance of the ongoing measures compelling the people to live in perpetual suspense and uncertainty.

13. People are on the mercy of chosen few, feeling throttled and voiceless, and their personhood has been reduced to nullity.

14. Deceased are not being buried/cremated according to their cultural and religious traditions, violating the dignity of the dead.

In a world where priorities in health range from safe drinking water to breast prosthesis, promises of biotechnology range from humanizing animals to creating new life forms, and the concerns of human rights range from the rights of the dead to the rights of the unborn, the art of policy making lies in equitably balancing the diverse and heterogeneous perspectives. Communities are made of individuals. No community goal can be achieved by ignoring the individual stakes. Current COVID-19 policies are a glaring example of misplaced priorities. Poor and helpless human beings are being used as a raw material in an attempt to combat the corona virus. In fact, the lockdown is eliminating the people, not the virus. In such a dire and desperate milieu several vital questions need to be answered, including the following:

(1) Is compulsory testing for the corona virus consistent with individual autonomy and the right of self-determination? (2) How to prioritize the medical care between the COVID-19 patients and the patients suffering from other diseases requiring urgent medical intervention? (3) Can the established procedures and ethical safeguards relating to biomedical research on human subjects be compromised in view of urgency to develop vaccines and drugs against corona virus? (4) Is it ethical to lock down the people in their homes for long periods under insanitary conditions denying them access to essential items of daily use and depriving them the care and comfort of their friends and relatives? (5) Is it fair to stop the persons from carrying on their professions, occupations and works, leading to loss of their livelihood? (6) Is it just to snatch the future from the persons who are in the process of developing and concretizing their goals, prospects and expectations by imposing restrictions on their legitimate pursuits? (7) Is it wise to close down educational institutions, administrative offices, legislative business, judicial fora and other allied activities for an indefinite period in the hypothetical hope of containing the spread of corona virus? (8) What is the dividing line between individual autonomy and social objective and in the event of conflict which one should prevail? (9) Can a strategy in disregard of structural and economic constraints of the society be ever successful to win over the menace of corona virus? (10) Is it ethical to discriminate on the basis of age and comorbidity in the matter of medical care of COVID-19 patients? (11) Why can't we learn to live with Corona virus when we have been living with the HIV, Hepatitis, cancer and many more diseases far more lethal, taking a toll of billions of lives? (12) Is it fair and equitable to spend disproportionately large portion of scarce healthcare resources on the Corona virus at the cost of other morbidities? (13) How to compensate those who died due to starvation, exhaustion and denial of medical care inside their homes and on the roads while returning to their homes due to loss of jobs and livelihood following the corona lockdown? (14) On whom and how to fix the responsibility for the chaos arising out of callous and creepy policies leading to loss of human lives and economic disaster.

It seems that the policy planners have not considered the above questions because their answers assume relevance only in respect of the poor and vulnerable sections of the society. However, this short-sightedness is counterproductive because the poor and vulnerable are not in minority. They constitute a big chunk of the global population, the exact number is difficult to estimate. Even when we talk of "extreme poverty" (people living on less than $1.90 a day) the figure as quoted on January 28, 2020 is as enormous as 10 percent of the world population i.e., 780 million people.[63]

The answers to the aforesaid questions are vitally important in order to evaluate the ethical validity of anti-corona strategies on the touch stone of human dignity and rights, which are intrinsic features of human identity, as per the aforesaid Universal Declaration of Human Rights. In this context, it may be fruitful to examine the Corona combat strategies in the light of International Health Regulations, adopted by the World Health Assembly, on 23 May 2005.[64]

These Regulations contain vital checks and balances to ensure that, while resorting to containment measures, the States do not infringe the rights of the people by subjecting them to unnecessary and excessive hardships. The relevant provisions of these Regulations may be ex-

---

[63] Lifewater Home / Blog / 9 World Poverty Statistics that Everyone Should Know. January 28, 2020 | Clean Water Poverty Cycle https://lifewater.org/blog/9-world-poverty-statistics-to-know-today/

[64] International Health Regulations (2005) https://apps.who.int/iris/bitstream/handle/10665/43883/9789241580410_eng.pdf;jsessionid=C3E277F071325C91F 63F0959C70B15BD?sequence=1, visited June 7, 2020.

cerpted as follows: Article 2 restricts the public health response to the international spread of disease in ways that "avoid unnecessary interference with international traffic". Article 3, Principles 1, subjects the implementation of these Regulations to "full respect for the dignity, human rights and fundamental freedoms of persons". Articles 6, 7 and 9 cast a duty on the States to notify the WHO "by the most efficient means" " all events which may constitute a public health emergency of international concern within its territory" "irrespective of origin or source" "within 24 hours of assessment" and "receipt of evidence of a public health risk identified outside their territory that may cause international disease spread, as manifested by exported or imported" Article 42 mandates that the Regulations shall be "applied in a transparent and non-discriminatory manner". Article 43 (1) instructs that the "measures shall not be more restrictive of international traffic and not more invasive or intrusive to persons than reasonably available alternatives that would achieve the appropriate level of health protection" Article 43 (2) lays down that while implementing the measures the States parties shall base their determination upon "scientific principles" and "available scientific evidence of a risk to human health".

The chronology of the Corona cognizance also needs to be examined in the context of abovesaid regulations: On 1 December 2019, the first person fell ill due to the new virus in Wuhan, China[65], on 31 December 2019 a "novel coronavirus was eventually identified"[66], on 30 January 2020 the World Health Organization declared the outbreak as a "Public Health Emergency of International Concern[67] and on 11 March, 2020 the WHO declared COVID-19 as a pandemic.[68] As such, the virus was declared as a pandemic after more than three months of its detection. The delay is thus clearly violative of the International Health Regulations. An earlier declaration would have obviously been helpful in checking the spread of the virus. Non-disclosure of information and stringent lockdown provisions imposed on the people are contrary to the letter and spirit of the said Regulations. "The COVID-19 epidemic bears witness to several direct IHR infractions, particularly Articles 6 and 7, governing reporting, and Article 43, regarding the implementation of protective measures."[69]

Despite the World Health Organization (WHO) Director General's recent remarks on COVID-19 emphasizing that "All countries must strike a fine balance between protecting health, minimizing economic and social disruption, and respecting human rights",[70] there are reports of gross human rights violations in several jurisdictions. "In a number of countries, governments have failed to uphold the right to freedom of expression, taking actions against journalists and healthcare workers. This ultimately limited effective communication about the

---

[65] Cohen, Jon (26 January 2020). "Wuhan seafood market may not be source of novel virus spreading globally". *Science.* https://www.sciencemag.org/news/2020/01/wuhan-seafood-market-may-not-be-source-novel-virus-spreading-globallyanuary 2020. visited June 2, 2020.

[66] WHO Timeline - COVID-19 dated 27 April, 2020 https://www.who.int/news-room/detail/27-04-2020-who-timeline---covid-19, visited June 8, 2020.

[67] World Health Organization Rolling updates on coronavirus disease (COVID-19) Updated 01 June 2020, visited June 8, 2020 https://www.who.int/emergencies/diseases/novel-coronavirus-2019/events-as-they-happen,

[68] WHO Timeline - COVID-19 dated 27 April, 2020 https://www.who.int/news-room/detail/27-04-2020-who-timeline---covid-19

[69] Lauren Tonti. The International Health Regulations: The Past and the Present, But What Future? Filed Under: Blog, Online Scholarship. Harvard International Law Journal. https://harvardilj.org/2020/04/the-international-health-regulations-the-past-and-the-present-but-what-future/

[70] WHO. Director General, Media Briefing, March 11. https://www.who.int/dg/speeches/detail/who-director-general-s-opening-remarks-at-the-media-briefing-on-covid-19---11-march-2020, visited June 8, 2020.

onset of the disease and undermined trust in government actions".[71]

The United Nations document of April 20 relating to COVID-19 and human rights provides a candid account of human rights violations on the altar of COVID-19 crusade.[72] The relevant portion of the said document is reproduced as below:

"Human rights are key in shaping the pandemic response, both for the public health emergency and the broader impact on people's lives and livelihoods. Human rights put people centre-stage. Responses that are shaped by and respect human rights result in better outcomes in beating the pandemic, ensuring healthcare for everyone and preserving human dignity. But they also focus our attention on who is suffering most, why, and what can be done about it. They prepare the ground now for emerging from this crisis with more equitable and sustainable societies, development and peace."

"Observing the crisis and its impact through a human rights lens puts a focus on how it is affecting people on the ground, particularly the most vulnerable among us, and what can be done about it now, and in the long term."

"The COVID-19 crisis has exacerbated the vulnerability of the least protected in society."

"Women and men, children, youth and older persons, refugees and migrants, the poor, people with disabilities, persons in detention, minorities, LGBTI people, among others, are all being affected differently."

"For more than 2.2 billion people in the world, washing their hands regularly is not an option because they have inadequate access to water. For 1.8 billion who are homeless or have inadequate, overcrowded housing, physical distancing is a pipe dream. Poverty itself is an enormous risk factor."

"Widespread closure of schools has interrupted the education of more than 1 billion children."

"Unfortunately, discrimination is rearing its ugly head in this crisis. All regions have seen incidents of discrimination, xenophobia, racism and attacks against people scapegoated for spreading the virus. In some countries, leaders have used labels like 'foreigner's disease' to describe COVID-19. There is mounting stigmatization of those infected by the virus."

A humane approach contemplates that in the event of conflict the interest of the weaker must prevail over the stronger. In this context, one finds solace and inspiration in the words of Mahatma, the father of Indian nation (Mohandas Karamchand Gandhi) who many decades ago wrote to a friend to clear his doubts. The text known as "Gandhi's Talisman"[73] runs as below:

"I will give you a talisman. Whenever you are in doubt, or when the self becomes too much with you, apply the following test. Recall the face of the poorest and the weakest man [woman] whom you may have seen, and ask yourself, if the step you contemplate is going to be of any use to him [her]. Will he [she] gain anything by it? Will it restore him [her] to a control over his [her] own life and destiny? In other words, will it lead to swaraj [freedom] for the hungry and spiritually starving millions?

---

[71] Human Rights Dimensions of COVID-19 Response. Human Rights Watch. March 19, 2020. https://www.hrw.org/news/2020/03/19/human-rights-dimensions-covid-19-response#_Toc35446578, visited May 8, 2020.

[72] "COVID-19 and Human Rights. We are all in this together. APRIL 2020. United Nations. https://unsdg.un.org/sites/default/files/2020-04/COVID-19-and-Human-Rights.pdf.

[73] Pyarelal. 1958. Mahatma Gandhi, The Last Phase, Volume II . Navajivan Publishing House, Ahmedabad, India. p. 65. https://Www.Gandhiheritageportal.Org/Ghp_Booksection_Detail/Ltu1lti=#Page/10/Mode/2up.

Then you will find your doubts and your self melt away."

The above mantra provides the surest pathway for taking decision and moving forward during the moments of ethical dilemma.

One cannot lose sight of the fact that malnutrition and communicable diseases are still the major killers in developing countries and the poverty-health nexus continues as ever before. In fact, Corona has laid bare a longstanding global passivity and inertia in the realm of healthcare. Even after the Corona viral explosion there is no concerted and unified global policy, reflecting lack of coordinating and holistic mindset. Corona combat policies must embrace both retrospectivity and prospectivity. Past needs to be scrutinized and future needs to be delineated. What should be the post-corona world like? The interests of future generations need to be protected. The policies therefore need to be wisely and meticulously evolved. Not only the theoretical but the real life situations assume importance during this pandemic. We ought to appreciate that the world is different from what it was during the earlier pandemics. We must reassure ourselves that blessed with modern medicine, advancing biotechnology and global interconnectedness we are in a winning position.

"Long after the heat and dust will settle down, and the earth will breathe at ease—unafraid to shed any death provoking virus—we might look back into this current pandemic as tragedy of unpardonable human errors."[74]

6. Conclusion

1. Contemporary world order is founded on human dignity, scientific promise and the rule of law. Corona crusade has contravened all the three values. It is violative of human dignity because it has snatched the livelihood from the poor and voiceless compelling them to starve; it is contrary to scientific promise because it has failed to achieve any breakthrough against the virus, and it is inconsistent with the rule of law because it is subjective, breeding inequality and injustice.

2. For many years, diseases have been an inevitable accompaniment of human life. World has faced several violent and virulent pandemics. But, COVID-19 has come at a time when the world is equipped with profound scientific knowledge and technological resource, capable of decoding and modifying the life at molecular level. Failure to win the virus in such a predominant milieu is disheartening and calls for deep introspection of our scientific pursuits and healthcare strategies.

3. While the honesty and sincerity of the current corona crusade seems beyond doubt it lacks wisdom and foresight, bringing to the fore fundamental flaws in our planning and performance. The negative reflections include host of strategic deficiencies and ethico-legal violations such as inequity, mal-prioritization of resources; neglect of primary healthcare, hasty and knee jerk reactions, ill-conceived economic policies, arbitrary decisions, and lack of international solidarity and cooperation.

4. In the statutory context, the corona combat policies are, per se, intrusive and invasive, violating the mandatory provisions as enshrined in the International Health Regulations (IHR) 2005, adopted by the World Health Assembly

5. Judged in terms of people's reaction, the corona crusade is a sad story of anguish and de-

---

[74] Shuvendu Sen. First edict for surviving corona: Cover your face. Ignoring simple healthcare principles cost America dearly. The Times of India dated June 6, 2020. p.12.

spair of countless individuals struck by economic disaster, lost livelihoods, starvation, forced internments, opacity, discrimination, breach of privacy, stigmatization, suspense and uncertainty.

6. There is no time limit for continuance of the ongoing measures compelling the people to live in perpetual suspense and uncertainty. A feeling is fast emerging that since there is no cure for the corona virus we have to learn to live with it as we have been living with influenza, HIV, malignancies and many other incurable diseases.

7. 7.78 billion people of this world are anxiously waiting for the auspicious moment when they will come out of the prevailing inhuman milieu and breath the earth's fresh air. The world needs to be reopened at the earliest. The key values such as human dignity, compassion, public health, civil liberty, equality, welfare of future generations and economic revival may set the criteria for reopening the world.

8. Following the un-lockdown, the corona combat needs to be carried forward with optimism, scientific rigor and spontaneity, with active participation of all sections of the society, with due regard to human dignity and rights.

In sum, despite clear intention and motive, today's corona crusade is a conundrum of surging corona infections, mounting death tolls, macabre crowds of starving workers and crippling economy. Judged on the touch stone of human dignity and human rights there are manifest miscarriages and several ethical questions remain unanswered.

References

Aiyar 2020. Swaminathan S Anklesaria Aiyar. The speech Modi has not made but should. Times of India dated 17 May 2020, p. 14.

Akpan et al. 2020. Nsikan Akpan and Victoria Jaggard Fauci: No scientific evidence the coronavirus was made in a Chinese lab. Interview to National Geographic, published on May 4, 2020 . https://www.nationalgeographic.com/science/2020/05/anthony-fauci-no-scientific-evidence-the-coronavirus-was-made-in-a-chinese-lab-cvd/, visited June 10, 2020

Alter 2020. Rolf Alter. Challenges and Opportunities in the Post-COVID-19 World Regional Governance: An Opportunity for Regional Organizations? World Economic Forum. Insight Report Challenges and Opportunities in the Post-COVID-19 World. May 2020. p.12 http://www3.weforum.org/docs/WEF_Challenges_and_Opportunities_Post_COVID_19.pdf, visited June 10, 2020

Anon. 2020a. "About 90% of Americans have been ordered to stay at home. This map shows which cities and states are under lockdown". Business Insider. 2 April 2020. https://www.businessinsider.in/science/news/almost-half-of-all-americans-have-been-ordered-to-stay-at-home-this-map-shows-which-cities-and-states-are-under-lockdown-/articleshow/74838246.cms

Anon. 2020b. "Coronavirus: Half of humanity now on lockdown as 90 countries call for confinement". Euronews. 3 April 2020. https://www.euronews.com/2020/04/02/coronavirus-in-europe-spain-s-death-toll-hits-10-000-after-record-950-new-deaths-in-24-hou. visited June 10, 2020

Anon. 2020c. "Philippines isolates hundreds of health workers as coronavirus cases rise in south-east Asia". The Guardian. 23 March 2020. https://www.theguardian.com/world/2020/mar/23/hundreds-of-filipino-health-workers-isolated-indonesia-thailand-malaysia-singapore-cambodia-myanmar-coronavirus-cases-rise-in-south-east-asia, visited June 10, 2020

Anon. 2020d. An Empire's Pandemic. Los Angeles Times, May 6, 2002. https://www.ph.ucla.edu/epi/bioter/anempiresepidemic.html, visited June 10, 2020

Anon. 2020e. China says virus pushing US ties to brink of new 'Cold War' The Times of India, New Delhi, May 25, 2020. p.9

Anon. 2020f. Coronavirus (COVID-19) India Updates, Lockdown 5 News. Financial Express. June 2, 2020 https://www.financialexpress.com/lifestyle/health/coronavirus-cases-in-india-covid-19-state-wise-tally-lockdown-5-unlock-1-live-updates-delhi-mumbai-maharashtra-corona-cases-vaccine-news/1977191/

Anon. 2020g. Coronavirus: What measures are countries taking to stop it? By Reality Check team BBC News, 1 April 2020. BBC News. https://www.bbc.com/news/world-51737226, visited June 10, 2020

Anon. 2020h. COVID-19 could become endemic like HIV and may never go away: WHO expert Mike Ryan. Reuters May 14, 2020 11:39 AM IST. Firstpost. Wednesday, May 20, 2020https://www.firstpost.com/health/covid-19-could-become-endemic-like-hiv-and-may-never-go-away-who-expert-mike-ryan-8366961.html visited June 10, 2020

Anon. 2020i. Historic health assembly ends with global commitment to COVID-19 response. World Health Organization. https://www.who.int/news-room/detail/19-05-2020-historic-health-assembly-ends-with-global-commitment-to-covid-19-response, visited June 10, 2020

Anon. 2020j. Livemint. Updated: 10 Jun 2020 Coronavirus update: COVID-19 cases in India cross 2.76 lakh; nearly 10,000 new cases in last 24 hours https://www.livemint.com/news/india/coronavirus-cases-in-india-cross-2-76-lakh-nearly-10-000-cases-in-last-24-hours-11591759131028.html, visited June 10, 2020

Anon. 2020k. NDTV, Coronavirus: PM Modi's Full Speech on Extension of COVID-19 Lockdown https://www.ndtv.com/india-news/coronavirus-pm-narendra-modi-full-speech-on-extension-of-covid-19-lockdown-2211390, visited on June 10, 2020

Anon. 2020l. Tribune News Service, New Delhi, May 17 Centre extends nationwide lockdown till May 31, new guidelines issued. 2020. https://www.tribuneindia.com/news/nation/centre-extends-nationwide-lockdown-till-may-31-new-guidelines-issued-86042, visited on May 19, 2020

Bhushan 2020. Chandra Bhushan. Breaking the Lockdown Chakravyuh. Times of India dated 18 May 2020, p. 10

Chutel 2020. Chutel L, Dahir AL (27 March 2020). "With Most Coronavirus Cases in Africa, South Africa Locks Down". The New York Times. https://www.nytimes.com/2020/03/27/world/africa/south-africa-coronavirus.html, visited June 10, 2020

Cillizza 2020. Chris Cillizza. Anthony Fauci's quiet coronavirus rebellion. May 12, 2020. CNN politics https://edition.cnn.com/2020/05/12/politics/fauci-trump-coronavirus-senate-hearing/index.html, visited June 10, 2020

Cohen 2020. Cohen, Jon (26 January 2020). "Wuhan seafood market may not be source of novel virus spreading globally". *Science*. https://www.sciencemag.org/news/2020/01/wuhan-seafood-market-may-not-be-source-novel-virus-spreading-globally, visited June 10, 2020 .

Cohen 2020. Cohen, Jon (26 January 2020). "Wuhan seafood market may not be source of novel virus spreading globally". Science. https://www.sciencemag.org/news/2020/01/wuhan-seafood-market-may-not-be-source-novel-virus-spreading-globallyanuary 2020. visited June 2, 2020

Dey 2020. Sushmi Dey. 'Lockdown prevented 37,000-78,000 deaths' The times of India, New Delhi dated May23, 2020, p.12

Fehr et al. 2015. Fehr, A.R., and Perlman, S. Coronaviruses: An Overview of Their Replication and Pathogenesis. Methods in Molecular Biology. Nature Public Health Emergency Collection 2015; 1282: 1–23. PMC436938523 https://www.ncbi.nlm.nih.gov/pmc/articles/PMC4369385/, visited June 10, 2020

Hardoon et al. 2016. Deborah Hardoon (Deputy Head of Research, Oxfam GB), Sophia Ayele & Ricardo Fuentes-Nieva (Executive Director of Oxfam Mexico). An Economy For the "1%". How privilege and power in the economy drive extreme inequality and how this can be stopped. Publication date: 18 January 2016 OXFAM International https://www.oxfam.org/en/research/economy-1

Harpur 2020. Paul Harpur. COVID-19 in Australia: Protecting Public Health by Restricting Rights & Risking the Rule of Law. May 14, 2020 Blog Symposia, Global Health, Global Responses to COVID-19: Rights, Democracy, and the Law, Health Law Policy, Human Rights, International, Public Health. https://blog.petrieflom.law.harvard.edu/2020/05/14/australia-global-responses-covid19/, visited June 10, 2020

Horwitz et al. 2020. Luisa Horwitz, Paola Nagovitch, Holly K. Sonneland, and Carin Zissis June 01, 2020 Where Is the Coronavirus in Latin America? AS/COA Americas Society/Council of the Americas https://www.as-coa.org/articles/where-coronavirus-latin-america, visited June 10, 2020

HRW 2020. Human Rights Dimensions of COVID-19 Response. Human Rights Watch. March 19, 2020 https://www.hrw.org/news/2020/03/19/human-rights-dimensions-covid-19-response#_Toc35446578, visited May 8, 2020

ICRC 2020. ICRC (International Committee of the Red Cross) COVID-19: ICRC global response to the coronavirus https://www.icrc.org/en/document/covid-19-coronavirus-pandemic-icrc#gs.6rcyfl, visited June 10, 2020

ILO 2020. COVID-19: Stimulating the economy and employment. ILO: As job losses escalate, nearly half of global workforce at risk of losing livelihoods Press release | 29 April 2020. International Labour Organization. https://www.ilo.org/global/about-the-ilo/newsroom/news/WCMS_743036/lang--en/index.htm, visited June 10, 2020

IMF 2020. World Economic Forum, 21 Mar 2020. IMF Blog https://www.weforum.org/agenda/2020/03/imf-economic-lessons-from-china-fight-against-coronavirus, visited June 10, 2020

Jha et al. 2020. Abhijay Jha and Avishek Kumar Pandey. Migrant exodus: Leaving behind one crisis, heading into another. Times of India dated 17 May 2020, p.3

JHU 2020. COVID-19 Dashboard by the Center for Systems Science and Engineering (CSSE) at Johns Hopkins University. https://www.arcgis.com/apps/opsdashboard/index.html#/bda7594740fd40299423467b48e9

ecf6, visited June 13, 2020

MSF 2020. Coronavirus COVID-19 pandemic. Challenges in supporting COVID-19 response. Médecins Sans Frontières. 16 March 2020   https://www.msf.org/challenges-supporting-covid-19-response, visited June 10, 2020

Nair 2020. Nair S (29 March 2020). "For a billion Indians, lockdown has not prevented trag-edy".   The   Guardian. https://www.theguardian.com/world/commentisfree/2020/mar/29/india-lockdown-tragedy-healthcare-coronavirus-starvation-mumbai, visited March 31, 2020

Nebehay 2020. Stephanie Nebehay. Nearly half of global workforce risk losing livelihoods in pandemic - ILO Economic News. April 29, 2020. https://in.reuters.com/article/health-coronavirus-ilo/nearly-half-of-global-workforce-risk-losing-livelihoods-in-pandemic-ilo-idINKBN22B1LF, visited June 10, 2020

Negri 2020. Stefania Negri. Anti-COVID Measures Restricting Civil Liberties in Italy: Issues of Legality and Legitimacy. May 12, 2020. Bioethics, Blog Symposia, Featured, Global Health, Global Responses to COVID-19: Rights, Democracy, and the Law, Health Law Policy,   Human   Rights,   International,   Public   Health. https://blog.petrieflom.law.harvard.edu/2020/05/12/italy-global-responses-covid19/, visited June 10, 2020

Parvathi et al. 2020. Parvathi Preethan/Nambi Appadurai/Shubham Gupta | With the global economy hit by Covid, climate issues may be put on the backburner. April 30, 2020 Busi-nessLine   https://www.thehindubusinessline.com/opinion/with-the-global-economy-hit-by-covid-climate-issues-may-be-put-on-the-backburner/article31472214.ece#, visited Jun3 12, 2020

Pyarelal 1958. Mahatma Gandhi, The Last Phase, Volume II . Navajivan Publishing House, Ahmedabad,   India.   p.   65 https://www.Gandhiheritageportal.org/Ghp_Booksection_Detail/Ltu1lti=#Page/10/Mode/2 up

Rosen 2007. Rosen, William. Justinian's Flea: Plague, Empire, and the Birth of Europe. New York City: Viking Adult. p. 3. ISBN 978-0-670-03855-8

Ryan 2020. COVID-19 could become endemic like HIV and may never go away: WHO expert Mike Ryan. Reuters May 14, 2020 11:39 AM IST. Firstpost. Wednesday, May 20, 2020https://www.firstpost.com/health/covid-19-could-become-endemic-like-hiv-and-may-never-go-away-who-expert-mike-ryan-8366961.html, visited June 10, 2020

Santos et al. 2020. Indhira Santos and Michael Weber. Supporting workers' transition to a new normal   amid   COVID-19.   May   13,   2020.   World   Bank   Blogs https://blogs.worldbank.org/voices/supporting-workers-transition-new-normal-amid-covid-19, Visited June 10, 2020

Sen 2020. Shuvendu Sen. First edict for surviving corona: Cover your face. Ignoring simple healthcare principles cost America dearly. The Times of India dated June 6, 2020. p.12

Senbanjo 2020. Láolú Senbanjo. African countries need to challenge the idea of a homogenous approach   to   COVID-19.   May   16,   2020.   QUARTZ   AFRICA. https://qz.com/africa/1858008/africa-needs-to-challenge-the-homogenous-approach-to-covid-19/, visited June 10, 2020

Sharma 2020. Vinay Sharma. COVID-19 Challenges and Response: How procurement underpins the World Bank's response to the pandemic. World Bank Blogs. April 15, 2020, https://blogs.worldbank.org/voices/covid-19-challenges-and-response-how-procurement-underpins-world-banks-response-pandemic, visited June 10, 2020. Prem Sharma Corona virus is a global crisis and the biggest challenge we have faced in our life time. Health-world.com from The Economic Times, https://blog.petrieflom.law.harvard.edu/2020/04/09/social-justice-covid19-law-coronavirus/

Sharma et al. 2020. Neeta Sharma, Sunil Prabhu, Edited by Deepshikha Ghosh. Lockdown For 2 More Weeks. What Will Be Different Now: 10 Points May 02, 2020 NDTV.com https://www.ndtv.com/india-news/nationwide-lockdown-over-coronavirus-extended-for-two-weeks-beyond-may-4-2221782, visited on May 4, 2020

Tonti 2020. Lauren Tonti. The International Health Regulations: The Past and the Present, But What Future? Filed Under: Blog, Online Scholarship. Harvard International Law Journal, https://harvardilj.org/2020/04/the-international-health-regulations-the-past-and-the-present-but-what-future/

UN 2020a. "COVID-19 and Human Rights. We are all in this together. APRIL 2020. United Nations, https://unsdg.un.org/sites/default/files/2020-04/COVID-19-and-Human-Rights.pdf

UN 2020b. COVID-19 pandemic. Humanity needs leadership and solidarity to defeat the coronavirus. United Nations Development Programme. https://www.undp.org/content/undp/en/home/coronavirus.html, visited June 10, 2020.

UNESCO 2020. Global Education Coalition. COVID-19 Education Response. https://en.unesco.org/covid19/educationresponse/globalcoalition, visited June 10, 2020.

Ward 2020. Alex Ward. India's coronavirus lockdown and its looming crisis, explained. Mar 24, 2020 https://www.vox.com/2020/3/24/21190868/coronavirus-india-modi-lockdown-kashmir

WHO 2020a. WHO Timeline - COVID-19 dated 27 April, 2020 https://www.who.int/news-room/detail/27-04-2020-who-timeline---covid-19, visited June 8, 2020

WHO 2020b. WHO. Director General, Media Briefing, March 11. https://www.who.int/dg/speeches/detail/who-director-general-s-opening-remarks-at-the-media-briefing-on-covid-19---11-march-2020, visited June 8, 2020

WHO 2020c. World Health Organization Rolling updates on coronavirus disease (COVID-19) Updated 01 June 2020, visited June 8, 2020 https://www.who.int/emergencies/diseases/novel-coronavirus-2019/events-as-they-happen,

Worldometer 2020. Worldometer. Coronavirus Incubation Period https://www.worldometers.info/coronavirus/coronavirus-incubation-period/, visited June 10, 2020

Xinhua 2020. Xinhua Headlines: Challenges and opportunities in 100 days' fight against COVID-19 pandemic . Source: Xinhua| 2020-05-08 19:30:43|Editor: huaxia . XIN-HUANET http://www.xinhuanet.com/english/2020-05/08/c_139041041.htm, visited June 10, 2020

Yamunan 2020. Sruthisagar Yamunan. As Supreme Court fails to protect migrant workers' rights, High Courts show the way. Scroll.in Tuesday, May 19th 2020, https://scroll.in/article/962214/as-supreme-court-fails-to-protect-migrant-workers-rights-high-courts-show-the-way

Yashwant 2020. Yashwant Raj. US Rallies may have spread virus, phone data suggests. Hindustan Times, New Delhi dated May 19, 2020. p. 7

Youssef 2020. Ambassador Hesham Youssef . Six Challenges Facing a Fragile Middle East Amid Coronavirus.   Unites States Institute of Peace.   Wednesday, April 1, 2020 https://www.usip.org/publications/2020/04/six-challenges-facing-fragile-middle-east-amid-coronavirus, visited June 10, 2020

Dr. **Rishi Raj Kishore** is an expert in both, Medicine and Law. He served the Ministry of Health, Government of India for nearly 35 years and was associated with the drafting of Indian Transplantation of Human Organs Act, 1994. In 1997, Dr. Kishore founded the Indian Society for Health Law and Ethics (ISHLE) of which he continues to be the President till date. In 2002, Dr. Kishore was appointed a Health Law and Bioethics Fellow in the Boston University School of Health Law, USA. He has been on the Board of Governors, World Association for Medical Law and has been the Chairman, International Committee on Organ Transplantation. He has also been a *rapporteur* for the World Health Organization. Subsequent to his retirement from the Ministry of Health in 2004, Dr. Kishore has been practicing as an advocate in the Supreme Court of India. Dr. Kishore has been working on a variety of issues in bioethics, health law and human rights such as organ transplantation, end of life, clinical trial on human subjects, assisted reproductive technologies, foetal rights, abortion, sex selection, stem cells, cloning, HIV/AIDS, DNA sampling, and human dignity. By now, he has presented nearly 100 papers in international conferences and several of his articles have appeared in leading international journals.

Controversy in Japan's testing policy against the novel coronavirus disease and the difficulties surrounding the fact

Yutaka Kato, Ishikawa Prefectural Nursing University, Japan

Abstract

Polymerase chain reaction (PCR) testing has been considered a key factor in the fight against coronavirus disease. However, wider use of the PCR test has been surrounded by controversy in Japan. Primarily based on existing literature, this article aims to shed some light on the question of whether it is ethically justifiable or desirable to advance or deter PCR testing. The contradictory views on testing were caused by partisanship, lack of data (because the virus was unknown), attitudes toward it, and anticipated behaviors of the general public (how [un]ethical they could be). Collecting information on the ethics of the public and creating greater educational opportunities for interaction between the government and the public may help people overcome the disagreements and fissures in society.

Key words

Competition, partisanship, PCR test, fact, public policy, zero risk

Introduction

The COVID-19 pandemic has been damaging multiple aspects of Japanese society, with nearly 1,000 confirmed deaths as of June 30, 2020.[1] As the number of newly confirmed cases begins to rise again, the country needs to take necessary measures. Testing has been considered a key factor in the fight against coronavirus disease. In particular, polymerase chain reaction (PCR) testing, which relies on a technique of multiplying copies of a specific DNA region of a pathogen to detect the infection (since the genetic material of the coronavirus is RNA, DNA is reverse-transcribed from the viral RNA), is used widely to test asymptomatic patients who may spread the virus. Some have been dubious as to whether the administration has adopted effective and consistent testing policies. Antibody tests have been used to determine the real infection transmission status and to assess the population with immunity to the virus. Considering the limited scope of this paper, the focus here is exclusively on PCR testing. Some do not believe the government has provided a sufficient number of PCR tests, with the number of tested cases much lower other countries.[2] Japan has focused on clusters and those who had close contact with confirmed cases have been the main target of the PCR test. However, wider use of the PCR test has been surrounded by controversy in the country.

Based on common sense, it is irrational to restrict the number of PCR tests, which is exemplified in a response to President Donald Trump given by Dr. Anthony Fauci, Director of the National Institute of Allergy and Infectious Diseases.[3] For political leaders, however, if the number of confirmed infection cases appears large, the risk of the administration being criticized increases, which is why the President of the United States had to provide excuses regarding the increased number of confirmed cases.[4] In Japan, there has been controversy about

---

[1] The current situation of infection is summarized at the Ministry of Health, Labour, and Welfare website https://www.mhlw.go.jp/stf/seisakunitsuite/bunya/newpage_00032.html.

[2] Ritchie, H. et al. "Coronavirus (COVID-19) Testing" Our World in Data. https://ourworldindata.org/coronavirus-testing

[3] CNN. "Trump wants to slow down coronavirus testing. Hear Fauci's response" https://www.youtube.com/watch?v=s9vzT-0hchw

[4] CNBC Television. "Pres. Donald Trump: Coronavirus 'testing is a double-edged sword' and driving up U.S. case numbers" https://www.youtube.com/watch?v=J56q43rb558

whether the implementation of PCR testing has been limited and whether this was justifiable.

Primarily based on existing literature, this article aims to shed some light on the question of whether it is ethically justifiable or desirable to advance or deter PCR testing.

Methods

This article is based on online resources, and media coverage related to the controversy on testing in Japan and aims to summarize the current state of affairs and the arguments surrounding COVID-19.

Findings

Conditions to be tested

Part of the basic information required for PCR testing is the list of conditions to be tested. On February 17th, the Ministry of Health, Labour and Welfare (MHLW) announced that four consecutive days of fever of 37.5 degrees or higher was among the conditions for receiving consultation and visiting a health institution.[5] In a typical case, those who met these conditions were advised to call a public health center, where phone calls were handled by public health nurses, which requires a separate qualification stipulated by the Act on Public Health Nurses, Midwives, and Nurses of Japan. Once hospitalized, those with mild symptoms must be tested negative twice to be discharged from the hospital. On March 1, the Novel Coronavirus Response Headquarters issued a document addressed to those in charge of public health in municipalities and instructed efforts to establish a system where, in case of an increased number of patients who needed to be hospitalized, asymptomatic patients or patients with mild symptoms could stay home in principle.[6] On April 6, Prime Minister Abe noted that the number of daily PCR cases would be doubled to 20,000 cases per day. However, the number of tested cases did not increase as expected. The government's official explanation for the limited number of PCR tests was that there was a shortage of manpower and equipment.[7]

The general public has been concerned about the possibility that the government intentionally limited the PCR testing, and many of those who needed to be tested might have been denied access to the test. On April 2, Seiji Osaka, a member of an opposition party, the Constitutional Democratic Party of Japan, voiced this concern and the prime minister answered that he would have the issue followed up. The reason behind this theory was that the greater number of confirmed cases of coronavirus infection contradicts the interests of the government. According to some, for example, the central government and the Tokyo Metropolitan government had an incentive to host the 2020 Olympic Games as scheduled, which would have been impossible if the pandemic raged in the country.

At an Upper House Budget Committee meeting on April 29th, Katsunobu Kato, Minister of

---

[5] An MHLW website for providing relevant information, available at https://www.mhlw.go.jp/stf/seisakunitsuite/bunya/0000121431_00094.html [in Japanese].

[6] The Novel Coronavirus Response Headquarters. "On transition of measures (surveillance, preventive measures against the infection spread, health care delivery system) in case the number of patients increases" March 1, 2020. https://www.mhlw.go.jp/content/000601816.pdf [in Japanese].

[7] In a press conference on May 4, the prime minister stated that the government was not unmotivated to increase the amount of PCR testing, but the process of testing was clogged due to labor shortage. Dr. Shigeru Omi, the vice-chair of the committee, stated that there was a historical delay in increasing the capacity of PCR testing. https://www.kantei.go.jp/jp/98_abe/statement/2020/0504kaiken.html [in Japanese].

Health, Labour and Welfare, denied that the condition of four consecutive days of fever of 37.5 °C or higher was among the conditions necessary to receive the PCR test, adding that it was simply misunderstood.[8] This remark evoked harsh criticism because the public and the media considered the government to have been irresponsible, using a deceptive way to restrict the eligibility for being tested, and government had tacitly accepted the alleged "misunderstanding." On April 10, the head of a public center in Saitama Prefecture admitted that they intentionally tightened the availability of the test so that the institution would not be overwhelmed.[9]

Testing in practice

The media coverage of celebrities who took (or did not take) the test attracted the attention of the general public and made them doubt the consistency of the testing policy. Some of them reported the results of the PCR tests on SNS. An example of inconsistency in the conditions to be tested was seen in the case of a professional baseball player, who reportedly tested positive in March.[10] He took the PCR test after he had recognized an impaired sense of taste. Some appreciated this news coverage because the possibility of a disturbed sense of taste due to coronavirus disease was not known at the time. Meanwhile, others expressed skepticism about the consistency of the conditions for receiving the PCR test because impaired taste alone did not fulfill the conditions publicized by the government. On the other hand, a well-known actress died of pneumonia caused by coronavirus on April 23.[11] She had fever on April 3rd but stayed at home as requested by the government. She was hospitalized on April 6th as her condition deteriorated but could not be saved. Inconsistency in the conditions to be tested has made the general public doubt the fairness and equality in access to PCR tests. Japan is an egalitarian country where people tend to think every person has equal access to health care,[12] thus inconsistency is a grave problem. In addition, the limited testing can lead some people to think that ordinary people could not take the test even when it was necessary because the government unjustifiably limited the availability of PCR testing.

Divided Evaluation and comparison with other countries

Japan's policy on PCR testing has attracted both praise and criticism domestically and internationally. For example, on May 25th, Tedros Adhanom Ghebreyesus, Director-General of the World Health Organization praised Japan. He presumably wished to laud Japan in to retain a money dispenser after the United States left. In contrast, The United States Embassy criticized Japan's policy by stating that "The Japanese Government's decision to not test broadly makes it difficult to accurately assess the COVID-19 prevalence rate."[13] *The Economist*'s unit rated Japan's coronavirus response "mediocre," ranking the country 13th out of 21 member states of the

---

[8] Prime Minister of Japan and His Cabinet https://japan.kantei.go.jp/98_abe/meibo/daijin/KATO_Katsunobu.html

[9] "A health center in Saitama City limited the number of virus tests due to shortage of hospital beds" *Jiji*. April 10, 2020. https://www.jiji.com/jc/article?k=2020041001135&g=soc [in Japanese].

[10] "Star pitcher for Hanshin Tigers tests positive for coronavirus" *The Asahi Shimbun*. March 27, 2020 http://www.asahi.com/ajw/articles/13250035

[11] Jiji. "Drama star Kumiko Okae, host of 'Hanamaru Market,' dies from coronavirus at 63" *The Japan Times*. April 24, 2020. https://www.japantimes.co.jp/news/2020/04/24/national/actress-kumiko-okae-dies-coronavirus/

[12] For example, a Japan Medical Association website states "Anybody can get medical care any time." (Japan Medical Association. "Prominent characteristics of Japan's medical insurance system." https://www.med.or.jp/people/info/kaifo/feature/)

[13] U.S. Mission Japan. "Health Alert – U.S. Embassy Tokyo" April 3, 2020. https://jp.usembassy.gov/health-alert-us-embassy-tokyo-april3-2020/.

Organization for Economic Cooperation and Development.[14]

To determine whether Japan has been a successful case or an example of failure, a comparison with other countries was attempted. Compared with the EU and the US, Japan appears to have been successful[15]. Meanwhile, critics of the administration's performance tend to refer to comparisons with other Asian countries, such as South Korea and Taiwan.[16] It is difficult to objectively determine which comparison is appropriate, considering the numerous factors involved. In addition, despite these attempts at comparison, it is impossible to specify the contribution of the testing policy of the government among the numerous other factors. For example, compared to neighboring countries, Japan has both advantages and disadvantages. Some other Asian countries can impose stricter coercion on their citizens. It would be difficult for Japanese society because of vehement concerns about or fear of the return of totalitarianism, and the advent of surveillance society. Further, Taiwan suffered from severe acute respiratory syndrome (SARS) in 2003 and South Korea the Middle East Respiratory Syndrome (MERS) in 2015, which better prepared these countries for the novel virus infection.

Views and positions on PCR testing

Japan does not have an agency that is equivalent to the United States' Centers for Disease Control and Prevention (CDC). From the utilitarian perspective or based on the principle of beneficence, experts in the field are the best people to make infection-related decisions. Accordingly, in Japan, instead of establishing a CDC, the administration established a committee of experts titled the Novel Coronavirus Expert Meeting, chaired by Takaji Wakita MD, PhD. In addition, the Cluster Intervention Group was established directly under the Novel Coronavirus Response Headquarters within the MHLW.[17] This cluster tracing policy was cited as a success in a WHO conference.[18]

This controversy has not been limited to committee members. Several public figures, including Nobel laureates, have emphasized the need to expand the testing. Among them was Harue Okada, Ph.D., arguably the most popular figure on mass media,[19] including tabloid shows.[20] She is a professor at Hakuoh University, who specializes in "infectious diseases, public health,

---

[14] The Economist. Intelligence Unit. "How well have OECD countries responded to the coronavirus crisis?" https://www.eiu.com/n/campaigns/oecd-countries-responded-to-the-coronavirus-crisis/

[15] Sposato, William. "Japan's Halfhearted Coronavirus Measures Are Working Anyway" *Foreign Policy.* May 14, 2020. https://foreignpolicy.com/2020/05/14/japan-coronavirus-pandemic-lockdown-testing/

[16] Kurashige, Atsuro. "A fiction that Japan has no problem as the people are disciplined: Japan's damage by the coronavirus is the worst in Asia" https://weekly-economist.mainichi.jp/articles/20200622/se1/00m/020/005000d [in Japanese]. The author is an editorial board member of the Mainichi Shimbun, which is considered liberal. Also, Makita, Hiroshi. "The reality posed by data is that Japan is the second worst among the three major failures in East Asia and Oceania." *Harbor Business Online.* June 10, 2020. https://hbol.jp/220596

[17] The organization chart surrounding the Cluster Intervention group is available at https://www.mhlw.go.jp/content/10906000/000599837.pdf [in Japanese].

[18] "Live on COVID-19 transmission with Dr Michael Ryan and Dr Maria Van Kerkhove" Streamed live on Jun 9, 2020. https://www.youtube.com/watch?v=7RcJ2yyNkUk

[19] In a survey conducted by Nihon Monitor (July 1, 2020. http://www.n-monitor.co.jp/2020/07/01/1690), in the first half of the year, Okada appeared in television the second most (267 times), the top of the list being Niki, Yoshihito, a physician at Showa University Hospital (https://www.showa-u.ac.jp/SUH/department/list/cid/) and a specialist in infectious respiratory diseases.

[20] Her statement is cited extensively at "Magazine Articles of the Month: Coronavirus Pandemic" Foreign Press Center Japan. March 23, 2020. https://fpcj.jp/en/j_views-en/magazine_articles-en/p=79736/.

and children's literature."[21] She has no license in the health care field. Another figure in the same position is Masahiro Kami, M.D. Ph.D., who leads a specified nonprofit corporation, Medical Governance Research Institute,[22] and has appeared on the mass media, including tabloid shows. Shinya Yamanaka, M.D. Ph.D., who was awarded the Nobel prize in Physiology or Medicine (2012) for discovering a method to reprogram mature cells and obtain pluripotent cells, publicized a website on the coronavirus (http://covid19-yamanaka.com/) to inform the general public. He has argued for expanding PCR testing. He may be well intentioned but he has interests as vice representative director of a foundation funded by Softbank Group, led by Masayoshi Son. Some argued that if these researchers are not experts in the relevant field, they should not be involved merely because they are Nobel laureates. Even if their voluntary involvement in the controversy is driven by good intentions, their authority and influence could be disproportionately massive.

Oppositions and rationales

Compared to the proponents of PCR testing, the opponents have been less high-profile and mostly anonymous.[23] Nevertheless, the opposition to the promotion of PCR testing cannot be ignored. For example, a television studio was reportedly deluged with protest calls after an expert argued for expanding PCR tests.[24] Whereas rationales for promoting the test seem self-explanatory, those against it will need clarification.

The primary reason for opposing the promotion of the test is the possibility of what they call the collapse of medical services,[25] a situation which the principle of non-maleficence, when collectively applied, will require us to avoid. Conversely, it was argued that limiting the availability of PCR testing would prevent collapse of medical services, resulting in a decreased number of deaths related to the coronavirus disease. Some opponents of the promotion of PCR testing ascribed the high mortality rate in countries, such as Italy, to hospitalization of patients with milder symptoms, crowding out patients with more serious symptoms. According to opponents, the collapse of medical services can occur when increasing the number of tests overwhelms health institutions. This is partly because conducting PCR tests requires a workforce of health workers. In addition, the crowd asking for PCR tests can gather in a small place, risking a further contagion. This concern is not necessarily imaginary. Reportedly, in 2009, many people visited outpatient wards and spent hours in waiting rooms.[26] In addition, if the test should be conducted where the prior probability (of Bayesian statistics) is substantially low, a large number of those tested false positives would have to be quarantined, which could overwhelm medi-

---

[21] Her detailed information is available at https://hakuoh.jp/pedagogy/119 [in Japanese].

[22] The official website is available at https://www.megri.or.jp/ [in Japanese].

[23] Nishimura, Hidekazu. "On the PCR controversy; from a physician conducting PCR tests to the voice requiring a drastic increase of testing. April 30, 2020 Nikkei Medical. https://medical.nikkeibp.co.jp/leaf/all/report/t344/202004/565349.html [in Japanese].

[24] "Dr. Otani, who argued for expanding PCR testing in "Morning show" and other shows, reveals about phone call attacks by Internet rightists. His clinic got yelled saying 'anti-Japanese'" July 3, 2020. *Litera.* https://litera.com/2020/07/post-5503.html [in Japanese]. "Morning show" is a popular TV show broadcast on TV Asahi every weekday morning. Okada appeared in this show frequently.

[25] There was a controversy whether collapse of medical services actually occurred, when the governor of Aichi Prefecture stated that medical services collapsed in Tokyo and Osaka and the governor of Osaka Prefecture expressed his objection.

[26] "MHLW considers abolishing fever outpatient departments in principle, downsizing the quarantine system." *The Asahi Shimbun Digital.* June 18, 2009. http://www.asahi.com/special/09015/TKY200906170346.html [in Japanese].

cal institutions. Moreover, some argue that false negatives can be problematic in that those tested false-negative may feel a false sense of security and spread the infection to people around them. If the virus has not yet propagated in samples, those who would eventually test positive may initially produce false negative results. Another concern is the discrimination observed against those tested positive.[27] Some have been concerned that if PCR test is conducted on a broader scale, those tested false positives can also face discrimination and their human rights can be compromised.[28]

Partisanship

An article on a news website described the controversy as based on threads on an internet forum.[29] This description is not completely valid. Measures taken against the pandemic can affect the public's view on which party to support. Opinion polls conducted by the mass media unanimously showed declining support ratings of the administration, which suggests that a certain percentage of former supporters have withdrawn their support. However, where detailed and comprehensible explanation to the public has been lacking, pre-existing (mis)trust in the administration could have affected the public's view. Though quantitative analysis is not attempted in this article, there seem to be cases of criticism and support based on partisanship. According to the *Cambridge Advanced Learner's Dictionary & Thesaurus*, partisanship is "the quality or action of strongly supporting a person, principle, or political party, often without considering or judging the matter very carefully."[30] In this article, the term partisanship refers to the argument for or against the expansion of PCR testing, which was closely linked to their typical criticisms against the opposing position. In the above case of Dr. Otani, it is stated that the internet rightists attacked the physician. It is noteworthy that the label of "anti-Japan" is used to criticize the opposition parties and critics of the Abe administration.[31] Meanwhile, there are leftist criticisms against the measures taken by the administration for abandoning the socially vulnerable.[32,33] The LDP is not monolithic or homogenous in terms of their political views, but rather a patchwork of individuals on a diverse continuum of political thoughts, including pro-China politicians. Nevertheless, another article linked the alleged failure of the administration to the administration's alleged xenophobia.[34] In these cases, the focus is not the pros and cons of

---

[27] In extreme cases, stones were thrown at the houses of those who had tested positive. "By any means unacceptable; human rights infringement including lapidation; Saga Bar Association issued a statement on discrimination against an infected person." May 27, 2020. https://www.saga-s.co.jp/articles/-/527447 [in Japanese].

[28] Osaki, Akiko. "Scientific and realistic strategies that allow Japan to overcome the second wave of the coronavirus." *Toyo Keizai Online.* June 19, 2020. " https://toyokeizai.net/articles/-/357530 [in Japanese].

[29] "Discussions both for and against the government measures against the coronavirus; pointing out the situation of 'Internet   rightists   versus   leftists.'"   March17,   2020   https://www.news-postseven.com/archives/20200317_1549237.html?DETAIL.

[30] https://dictionary.cambridge.org/dictionary/english/partisanship.

[31] For example, the CDPJ has been criticized for allegedly being quinslingistic. Article 4 of the CDJP Bylaw does not require Japanese nationality to become a member (partner) of the party; individuals of 18 years of age or older (including foreigners residing in Japan can join (https://cdp-japan.jp/about-cdp/byelaw [in Japanese]).

[32] Koga, Shigeaki. "The Abe administration's measure against the coronavirus abandoning the vulnerable." *Shukan Asahi.* March 3, 2020. https://dot.asahi.com/amp/wa/2020030200013.html [in Japanese]. The author is an ex-bureaucrat.

[33] Morinaka, Takaaki. "The novel coronavirus questions Japan and the World; a thought of abandoning the vulnerable." *The Akahata.* May 15, 2020 https://www.jcp.or.jp/akahata/aik20/2020-05-15/2020051501_03_1.html. The author is a professor at Waseda University.

[34] Tatsuru Uchida, The reasons some people still continue to support the do-nothing Abe Administration - urgent proposals by Tatsuru Uchida" April 9, 2020. *Shukan Bunshun.* https://bunshun.jp/articles/-/37140 [in Japanese].

expanding PCR tests, but the underlying political thoughts.

Unknown factors

With many unknown factors, people have varying levels of understanding about the infection. Yamanaka, afore-mentioned Nobel laureate, called the unknown factor that brought about Japan's relative success "factor X." For one thing, the effectiveness of wearing masks has been controversial. There is still little knowledge on antibodies or the acquisition of immunity against the corona virus. Dr. Hiroshi Nishiura, professor at Hokkaido University, who predicted the spread of infection based on a mathematical model, was criticized for using an inappropriate (too large) value as the basic reproduction number. At that time, the appropriate value was undetermined. Therefore, he simply used a value that is often used by experts. Finally, the political leaders and the health providers have been uncertain about how the public should behave in a pandemic situation. Despite these unknown factors, the government and society must take timely action.

Discussion

Partisanship

The literature searched and cited for this article often showed partisanship and connected evaluations of the measures taken against the disease with their evaluations of the administration. Although it is not necessarily the case that everyone involved in the controversy has a particular political position or is aware of their partisanship. However, equally, it is not the case that groups and societies of professionals are necessarily free from partisanship. For example, the Japan Medical Association has supported LDP, except for several occasions, whereas, individual members of groups and societies are usually not monolithic.

Although the political division is not as widespread and consistent as in countries such as the United States, there is a clear gap between those in favor of LDP and those who are not. This facetiousness or partisanship has apparently affected how some people view the policies taken by the Abe administration to fight the coronavirus disease. The Abe administration has been subject to harsh criticisms by the opposition parties and the media regarding a case where the administration allegedly favored Kake Gakuen (an educational corporation), and another case where public money was spent inviting people they selected to annual cherry blossom viewings in Shinjuku Gyoen National Park. They also criticized the administration for attempting to extend the retirement age for Hiromu Kurokawa, superintendent public prosecutor at the Tokyo High Public Prosecutors Office. The former Minister of Justice, appointed by Prime Minister Abe, and his wife were arrested for violating the Public Offices Election Act.. This criticism against the administration is translated into increased criticism of their policies concerning the coronavirus disease, including PCR testing. Despite all these scandals, Shinzo Abe has been in the office of Prime Minister for the longest term since the Meiji Constitution. His grandfather was Nobusuke Kishi (1896–1987), the 56th and 57the Prime Minister, who was arrested after World War II as a probable A-class war criminal but later discharged. His discharge was not sufficient for critics of the current administration, mainly liberals, to forget the horror and the tragedy of imperialism. His term is scheduled to end on September 2021. For his critics and the opposition parties, discrediting the administration in any aspect matters.

The roles of mass media

Related to partisanship, mass media has voiced problems about freedom of press and biased coverage. The current freedom of the press in Japan is equivocal. There is a discrepancy in the evaluation of the Japanese press between the rankings by Reporters Without Borders and the ranking by Freedom House. Further, biased coverage is a major concern. Other countries, such as the United States, have similar problems[35] but the media often make clear its political positions. In contrast, Article 4 of the Broadcast Act of Japan requires broadcast companies to be politically impartial.[36] However, the public does not consider the media impartial.[37] Japan's television companies (except NHK, which is a national broadcaster) are affiliated or in close relation with major newspaper publishers, which the public considers to be biased.[38] In terms of the coronavirus disease , media coverage has often been one-sided. Several tabloid TVs shows, in particular, apparently waged campaigns on the issue. In Japan, the massive influence of the existing mass media and the growing mistrust in those media seem to coexist.

Sound discussion

One of the aspects that has hampered the controversy from producing positive consequences is verbal attacks, sometimes related to partisanship. Reading articles in the mass media and comments the public leave for entries in major news websites, one is reminded that Japan is a country where people are not accustomed to debates and discussions, and arguments are often marred by strident verbal attacks and insults. To avoid this situation, it is essential to base arguments on data and facts. It is necessary for each person to become accustomed to non-emotional debating and exert more virtuous personality traits.

The truth and beyond

The proponents and opponents of expanding the PCR test criticized each other for not being based on data or distorting the facts.[39] It is often, however, difficult to decide what is fact and what is not. Thus, "fact check" has been attempted. A major portal website (https://hazarsd.yahoo.co.jp/article/20200207) is linked to two fact check websites.[40] For example, a private company, Eltes Co., Ltd., provides a list of cases of proliferated uncertain infor-

---

[35] "American views: Trust, media and democracy." *Knight Foundation.* https://knightfoundation.org/reports/american-views-trust-media-and-democracy/.

[36] The terrestrial television channels in Japan have been under oligopolistic control. The stipulations of the Broadcast Act of Japan and the licensing authority of Ministry of Internal Affairs and Communications have not allowed a new entry in the industry, which makes it more important that existing media maintain neutrality.

[37] Reuters Institute for the Study of Journalism "Digital News Report 2020" https://www.digitalnewsreport.org/survey/2020/japan-2020/

[38] Ibid.

[39] One example of an article by the opponents is this by Nakata, Hiromi. "Masahiro Kami, the emperor of hypocrisy, and Kentaro Iwata, the prince of hypocrisy; revealing lies surrounding COVID-19 by physicians appearing on TV shows." A blog entry within Jingu Gaien Minerva Clinic website. https://minerva-clinic.or.jp/blog/king-of-fake-lie-of-the-medical-doctors-on-air/ [in Japanese]. An example of an article by the proponent is this by Ida, Masato. "Unnatural citation of data in a blog by a physician spreading among those against expanding PCR testing; a lie that Japan has no excess mortality." *Harbor Business Online.* May 16, 2020. https://hbol.jp/219193 [in Japanese].

[40] Websites by a non-profit organization, FactChek Initiative Japan (FIJ) (https://fij.info/coronavirus-feature) and an independent media, In fact, which is affiliated with the FIJ (https://infact.press/category/factcheck/) .[in Japanese]

mation.[41] It is true that presenting uncertain information as confirmed information is unjustifiable. However, there may be cases where expressing views on speculations and doubts are worthwhile. In casual exchanges of information, the demarcation can sometimes be blurred. Some of the cases listed on the above website were mentioned in popular media.[42] As clearly noted in the FIJ website, if a statement is found not to be a fact, it simply means that it cannot be announced a fact as of the judgment. In the words of Dr. Varia Van Kerkhove, "Evidence is not static."[43] Of course, some will not be convinced because these websites can also be biased.

The above description of the divided evaluations may have reminded some of the term "post-truth" (adjective), which is explained as "relating to a situation in which people are more likely to accept an argument based on their emotions and beliefs, rather than one based on facts" and one of the example usages reads: "In this post-truth era, science is needed more than ever."[44] Science is necessary, but not sufficient.

It is necessary to avoid obvious misunderstandings, intentional malice, and harm to society. In addition, other wrong-guided values should not affect the argument. Although approval of drugs or expenditure of public funds can pose problems, as far as testing is concerned, with very few exceptions (including one case where it was pointed out that testing were restricted because an institution attempted to monopolize the data of test results) scientists voluntarily participated in the controversy, presumably without malevolent intention. Obviously, however, this is not the case where finding the "truth" or presenting scientific data can prevent disagreement and lead to one single conclusion. There must be cases and points where finding data can produce a cogent solution on which the scientific community agrees. Scientists, for example, can identify the strains of the virus that spread in a specific area. Nevertheless, even with the same data before one's eyes, the contradictory views among scientists on testing could arise from diverse views of lacking data (because the virus was unknown). If we take into consideration the societal situation and the economic elements, such as the anticipated behaviors of the general public, the (mis) trust in governmental performance, and the anticipated interaction between the two, providing such a single cogent answer seems unlikely.

Dealing with negative prospects

It is true that arguments presupposing ineffective policies and the folly of the public are meaningful as precaution. With such precaution, policies will be more sophisticated and foolproof. However, some negative responses, for example from the public, can be avoided. In this fight against the coronavirus disease, despite anticipated social panic that can lead to collapse of medical service, it is possible to find ways to avoid the panic of the general public. To deal with a large number of false positive cases, they could be quarantined elsewhere (e.g. hotels). In January, the administration revised the existing law and the coronavirus infection was deemed a

---

[41] https://eltes-solution.jp/202004-07/ [in Japanese].

[42] Nagata, Takeshi. "The Prime Minister, the Olympic Games and the virus." *The Nishinippon Shimbun.* March 1, 2020. https://www.nishinippon.co.jp/item/n/588314/ [in Japanese]. The author appeared as a panelist in an anti-Abe Administration rally held on September 17, 2016. (http://woman-action-network.s3-website-ap-northeast-1.amazonaws.com/uploads/event/f87ab560cad9990615b5101a4374cd75.pdf).

[43] "Live on COVID-19 transmission with Dr Michael Ryan and Dr Maria Van Kerkhove" Streamed live on Jun 9, 2020. https://www.youtube.com/watch?v=7RcJ2yyNkUk.

[44] An online entry from *the Cambridge Advanced Learner's Dictionary & Thesaurus* https://dictionary.cambridge.org/dictionary/english/post-truth.

"designated infectious disease," which required those tested positive to be hospitalized.[45] However, on April 6th, Prime Minister Abe stated that those with milder symptoms would be advised to recuperate at home in principle. Further, to avoid a situation where those tested false positive feel a false sense of security and spread the infection, the government and the professional community could provide information on the limitations of the PCR testing and the meaning of false positive/negative— information that had not been delivered to the general public through the mass media and other media as of June 30th. There is a compelling need for the government to create more opportunities for communication with the public.

There were also concerns about the risks of discrimination against those tested (false) positive. Nevertheless, measures can be taken to avoid harmful consequences. If necessary, it is even possible to criminalize discrimination.

Some concerns were based on anticipated panic and unethical behaviors of the public, such as the crowd beating a path to medical institutions to be tested. However, following the past catastrophes, Japanese citizens were often praised for their orderly conduct. In addition, it is possible to provide guidance and promote communication so that the public can behave appropriately. To prepare for the next resurgence of coronavirus disease, it is advisable to collect knowledge on how (un)ethical the general public could be with or without legal restraints, which can inform the government and the generations to come.

There is also a possibility that Japanese citizens will change their ethical attitudes. The general public of Japan has been described as being inclined to "zero risk," which refers to their tendency not to allow any risk; they reject, for example, genetically modified organisms. Living with the coronavirus disease may result in altered attitudes amongst people. In contrast, it may strengthen their passion for cleanliness. Data on people's views of the ethical aspects of social life are much needed.

In the face of the above difficulties surrounding data, fact, and "truth," efforts in education, involving scientific literacy and liberal arts can be promising. Scientific literacy is of course significant to enable better discussions related to health care. Liberal arts education should also be of highlighted because a fight against the emerging disease clearly requires consideration of multiple aspects of society. In this regard, Japan's future is not rosy, since most of the universities have relinquished liberal arts education.[46]

Conclusion

The government's testing policy has been inconsistent and leaves room for improvement. Opponents of the promotion of PCR testing also had reasons for their position. In a controversy on whether the government's performance has been successful, contrary evaluations were made depending on which countries were cited for comparison. The contradictory views on PCR testing were derived from partisanship, lack of data (because the virus was unknown), attitudes toward it, and anticipated behaviors of the general public (how [un]ethical they could be). Al-

---

[45] For example, a physician recommended establishing a system where asymptomatic patients and patients with mild symptoms need not to be hospitalized (Ishizaka, Tomoki and Igusa, Emi. "Collapse of medical services in Japan can still be prevented; Recommendations by Dr. Nobuhiko Okabe, Director General at Kawasaki City Institute for Public Health." Toyo Keizai Online. March 28, 2020. https://toyokeizai.net/articles/-/340470 [in Japanese].)

[46] The University of Tokyo, which has produced by far the largest number of highest-ranking bureaucrats, is one of the few education institutions where liberal arts education survived. It is true that liberal arts education in the past did not confer enough leverage to the ministers to get the nation through difficult times. But the future prospect is more dismal, if more people, including political leaders have only narrow academic backgrounds.

though unethical elements such as verbal attacks made meaningful discussions difficult, exercising virtuousness in debates can solve the problem. Collecting knowledge on how ethical the public can be will help people to fight the current pandemic and will also help future generations whenever they face emerging challenges. Despite the political rivalry between parties and their supporters, we have to construct a social milieu where this rivalry can constitute a competition for better consequences, materializing in a better society. Greater opportunities for interaction between the government and the public and better education may help people overcome the disagreements and fissures in society.

Yutaka Kato currently holds an associate professorship in the Department of Liberal Arts at Ishikawa Prefectural Nursing University and will be a professor at Shiga University of Medical Sciences in October 2020. His main research interests include comparative study of the ethical, legal, and social dimensions of healthcare. He received a Ph.D. in medical ethics from Osaka University after completing a master's degree in religious ethics at Yale University.

Ethical and Policy Issues in the Epidemic of Coronavirus in China

A Defense for Offensive Strategy against the Spread of Zoonosis

Ruipeng Lei, Huazhong University of Science and Technology, China

Renzong Qiu, Chinese Academy of Social Sciences and Renmin University of China, China

Abstract

The authors argue that the defensive strategy we have adopted so far in response to the epidemic is seriously flawed and recommend an offensive strategy. The offensive strategy is designed to make us in advance of the spread of zoonosis in the general population or already detected a few cases to take pre-emptive actions including tracing the source of zoonosis pathogens, studying the pathogen transmission between animals and its possible variations, exploring the possibility of the spread of the pathogen from animals to humans and its influencing factors, and trying to prevent the possible spillover of zoonosis from animals to humans. When the zoonosis starts to spillover to humans, all necessary public health interventions should be taken in advance including treating patients in isolation, tracing contacts, implementing quarantine and isolation measures in some local areas in order to prevent the spread of the disease from becoming an emergent outbreak even under uncertain condition.

Key words

zoonosis; defensive strategy; offensive strategy; spillover; surveillance

Foreword

Hegel says: "We learn from the history that we do not learn from the history". The recurrence of coronavirus epidemic in China proves his insight to be right.[1][1] The first half title of our paper is simulated with the title of a paper written by one of us in 2003 near the end of the SARS epidemic in China. This is the first paper to be published in the 6th issue of the journal of Studies in Dialectics of Nature.[2] We want to show that after SARS, although we have learned some lessons, but we have not fully learned the lessons that should be learned. In particular, we have reduced the support for the agency of disease prevention and control, taken discouraging measures to public hospitals, and forced public hospitals and their medical staff to make profits like state-owned enterprises, instead, encourage and promote private capitals to invest healthcare, or even enter into public hospitals as stockholder. If we had learned enough from SARS, the outbreak of COVID-19 could have been avoided. Even though the coronavirus is of a new type, it is a coronavirus, along with SARS and MERS, and was named by the International Committee on Taxonomy of Viruses (ICTV) as SARS-COV-2 on 11 February 2020.[3] We can see that the fight against SARS-COV-2 is basically the same as the fight against SARS, only the former is on a far much larger scale and much harder to deal with, but not "as no more severe as SARS," as some experts or Wuhan authorities say.[4]

---

[1] Georg　　　　　Wilhelm　　　　　Friedrich　　　　　Hegel　　　　　Quotes.
http://goodreads.com/authors/6188.Georg_Wilhelm_Friedlich_Hegel/quotes.

[2] Qiu, R. 2003. Ethical and policy issues raised by the SARS epidemic in China. Studies in Dialectics of Nature (6)1-5.

[3] WHO.　Naming　the　coronavirus　disease　(COVID-19)　and　the　virus　that　causes　it.
http://who.int/emergences/disease/noval-conoravirus-2019/technical-guidance/naming-the-conoravirus-disease-(covid-19)-and-the-virus-that-cause-it.

[4] Lei, R. & Qiu, R. 2020. Report from China: Ethical questions on the response to the coronavirus, Bioethics Forum, The Hastings Center, January 31. https://www.thehastingscenter.org/report-from-china-ethical-questions-on-the-response-to-the-coronavirus/　.

Preparedness for the Outbreaks of the Zoonosis

Many people, especially some policy makers, have the wrong idea that diseases will naturally decrease and disappear as we industrialize, modernize, and urbanize the country, as we develop science, technology, and medicine. This is a big mistake. In the 2003 article mentioned the Swiss American medical historian pointed out in his book, Civilization and Disease[5] that the civilization is a factor of diseases, Civilization may help us control some diseases, but the civilization produced a variety of factors that cause much more diseases which are more complicated, widely spread, and even more fatal than before, for it provides human beings with much more opportunities to expose new physical, chemical and biological pathogens which is unknown by human beings. In human history, as a whole, many more people have died from diseases than from wars.[6] The most dangerous diseases to human health and life are zoonosis, which are diseases and infections naturally transmitted from animal hosts to humans, and then from humans to humans. Animal-based infections have long been recognized as important categories of emerging diseases that are incubated in animal reservoirs which provide new sources of infection for human beings throughout evolutionary history. There are two different mechanisms for the outbreak of zoonotic diseases: some pathogens originated in animals but have evolved primarily or exclusively to infect humans and have adapted to human-to-human transmission after crossing the species barrier from animals to humans. The others require continued reintroduction from animal reservoirs and have never become epidemic in humans on their own. Many of the former pathogens are ancient and originated in domestic animals, such as measles, which originated in cattle, and smallpox, which originated in the pox virus of camels or cattle. The most recent zoonotic diseases, including HIV-1 and HIV-2, are new human diseases that cross the species barrier from primates to humans. SARS, which originated as an zoonotic disease, has adapted to spread from humans to humans.[7]

What we need to see is that the changes in the environment, in the intrinsic biology of the pathogens themselves, and in the extrinsic biology caused by technological and industrial development are increasing the opportunities for the possible generation and transmission of zoonotic diseases among humans. The emergence of zoonotic diseases in the human body goes through two stages: (1) human contact with the infectious agent and (2) cross-species transmission of the infectious agent. There are also two stages of transition: (3) sustained human-to-human transmission and (4) genetic adaptation to human hosts. Phase (4) is not necessary for the emergence of many zoonotic diseases in humans, but it is a prerequisite for the outbreak of a pathogen in humans. Now we understand the pathogenesis of zoonotic disease include: the evolution have occurred in zoonotic virus, so they can survive in wild animal hosts; after crossing the species barrier they spread into taxonomically different hosts, and start causing pathological process of the disease; and through repeated infections in the species as secondary host (such as humans) produce morbidity and mortality on a mass scale, and become a national, regional or global health problems to humankind. During the process first the zoonotic pathogen has

---

[5] Sigerist 1943. Sigerist, H. Civilization and Disease. Chapter 1: Civilization as a factor in the genesis of disease. Ithaca and London: Cornell University Press, 7-41.

[6] Zou et al. 2013. Zou, Z., Liang, Z., Yang, X. The fight between humankind and epidemic. Baidu Library. https://wenku.baidu.com/view/b169d2445a8102d276a22f83.html.

[7] Cleaveland 2007. Cleaveland, S., Haydon, D., Taylor, L. Overviews of pathogen emergence: Which pathogens emerge, when and why? in Childs, J., Mackenzie, J., Richt, J. (eds.) 2007. Wildlife and Emerging Zoonotic Diseases: The Biology, Circumstances and Consequences of Cross-Species Transmission. Springer-Verlag Berlin Heidelberg, 85-111.

adapted to its host reservoirs (HRs), expanded at a large geographic scale, and already widely disseminated locally. And historical factors have changed and blurred traditional patterns of species distribution, then increase the chances of virus-carrying HRs mixing with susceptible secondary hosts (HSs). Current historical conditions provide unprecedented opportunities for these viruses and hosts to expand into new ecological environment. Over the last 20 years virus-infected HRs and HSs rapidly shift the sites in at an accelerated pace, it heralds a major turn in how zoonotic viruses pose a public health threat to humans.[8]

These factors that alter the emerging course of zoonotic diseases include: non-biological factors (such as climate change and El Nino) that alter the potential for contact between HR and HS populations or vectors, and increase the opportunity for spillover; some zoonotic viruses have inherent biological and evolutionary factors that enhance their ability to cross species barriers; in recent years external biological interactions such as infected or implicitly infected individuals in HR or host vector (HV) species have played a particularly important role in zoonotic disease outbreaks due to natural or human-induced site migration. The most important factors that greatly increase the scale and scope of zoonotic diseases are all human factors. The rapid growth of the human population and the farming modes of modern agriculture prompted human migration into the hinderland of ecosystems with high biodiversity, turning large amounts of these areas into arable land and pasture. Commercial farming practices move into open spaces in forest habitats, mixing humans and livestock with local animal populations and also with any zoonotic pathogens. Over the past 50 years, huge number of people have migrated to cities, forcing many to live on the fringe areas of large cities (shanty towns), poor sanitation and water shortages have been closely linked to outbreaks of diseases caused by vector-borne pathogens. Changes around cities in land use change the area and quality of wildlife habitats, increase the potential for human-animal-vector interactions, and allow many wildlife species to act as reservoirs for different pathogens, leading to outbreaks of zoonotic pathogens related to bats. Strengthening social interaction through the construction of roads, railways and airports is the most influential human factor driving the expansion of the epidemic. Wildlife breeding, poaching and national and international wildlife trafficking networks consuming wild animals, using them for medicinal purposes or using their body parts as decorations provide a wide range of opportunities for the contact of new host carrying zoonotic viruses with humans. The widespread use of needles for injection, immunotherapy, organ transplantation, especially future xenotransplantation, and blood transfusions have also contributed greatly to the spread of zoonotic pathogens in modern medicine.[9] We have to remember that since 1994, the world has seen eight major outbreaks that have been caused by different bat-borne viruses including Hendra virus in 1994, Nipah virus in 1998, Marburg in 1998/2004, SARS in 2002, MERS in 2012, Ebola in 2014, and SARS-Cov-2/COVID-19 in late 2019.[10] It shows that our target of preventing and controlling zoonotic diseases has to be focused at the viruses which use the bats as host reservoirs, coronaviruses in particular.

The normative conclusion that draws from the account above is that we need to always prepare for the next pandemic of zoonotic disease and the one after the next pandemic. The

---

[8] Childs et al. 2007. Childs, J., Richt, A., Mackenzie, J. 2007 Introduction: Conceptualizing and partitioning the emergence process of zoonotic viruses from wildlife to humans, in Childs J, Mackenzie J, Richt J. (eds.) 2007. Wildlife and Emerging Zoonotic Diseases: The Biology, Circumstances and Consequences of Cross-Species Transmission, Springer-Verlag Berlin Heidelberg, 1–31.

[9] Childs et al. 2007.

[10] Qiu 2020. Qiu, J. How China's "Bat Woman" hunted down viruses from SARS to the new coronavirus, Scientific Americans, March 11, 2020. https://www.scientificamerican.com/article/how-chinas-bat-woman-hunted-down-viruses-from-sars-to-the-new-coro-navirus1/.

pandemic of an emerging zoonotic disease, whether mild, moderate or severe, affects a large proportion of the population and requires a coordinated response across many sectors within a country for months or even years, as well as coordination and cooperation among countries at the international level. Any country is therefore required to build in advance material, scientific-technological, financial, and human resources preparedness for the next possible pandemic on the basis of experiences and lessons learned from past pandemics despite the condition being uncertain.

Preparedness for the next pandemic can be justified ethically. In one of the Confucian classics, The Book of Rites, it is said that "Forethought leads to success, and unpreparedness leads to failure." Let alone such major problems as public health emergencies and pandemics of zoonotic diseases which affect millions of million people! If we were well-prepared in advance, the zoonotic pathogens might have not spilled over into humans, and even if they did, they might have been confined in local area without leading to an outbreak with hundreds, thousands, or even tens thousands (such as in USA these days) of additional cases every day! The pandemic of zoonotic diseases always brings about tremendous physical, mental, social, economic harms or damages to individuals, their family and society, the country, and the world as a whole! If all countries have the preparedness to the possible pandemic, it would be possible to avoid or at least reduce the catastrophic impacts on individuals, families, society, country and the world, and greatly benefit all parties. It is understandable, therefore, why World Health Organization has twice warned countries to have preparedness for a global pandemic. Unfortunately, the focus that WHO suggested is on moderate avian flu, but not on devastating coronavirus.[11]

But in our view, the key question that is not addressed in the WHO document on pandemic preparedness and other relevant literature is what strategy we should adopt in the pandemic preparedness. Looking at the situation of each country, what is used is a defensive strategy (reactive strategy or conservative strategy). We would like to propose another strategy, namely, an offensive strategy, a proactionary or pre-emptive strategy. For the sake of space, we will discuss only two parts of this strategy, namely, prevention and control of the spillover of zoonotic viruses from animal hosts to humans; and the prevention and control of the outbreak of zoonotic viruses-caused disease in humans after transmitting to humans.[12]

Prevent and Control the Spillover of Pathogens from Animals to Humans

Before discussing the prevention and control of spillover of infectious source from animals to humans, let's take a look at the work of a woman scientist Zhengli Shi known as "Batwoman".[13]

Dr. Zhengli Shi, a researcher at the Wuhan Institute of Virology, Chinese Academy of Science, has been tracking the SARS-causing virus for 16 years since the end of SARS epidemic, and has identified dozens of deadly SARS-like viruses which host reservoir is horseshoe bats. She tracked them down to their cave and took blood and swab samples from the bats. In 2004, she was part of an international team of researchers who collected blood, saliva, urine, feces and

---

[11] WHO 2007. WHO. A Strategic Framework for Emergency Preparedness.
https://www.who.int/ihr/publications/9789241511827/en/.

[12] WHO 2017. WHO. Regional Office for Europe. Guide to Revision of National Pandemic Influenza Preparedness Plans. 2017. https://www.ecdc.europa.eu/en/seasonal-influenza/preparedness/influenza-pandemic-preparedness-plans.

[13] Qiu 2020.

swabs from bats at a cave where there is a bat colony near Nanning City, the capital of Guangxi province. In one week, they explored 30 caves but saw only a dozen bats. When she was about to give up, a laboratory gave her a diagnostic kit to test antibodies in SARS patients. Tests found that samples from three species of horseshoe bat contained antibodies against the SARS virus. Shi's team used antibody tests to reduce the site and bat species, and ended up in a bat cave on the outskirts of Kunming City, the capital of Yunnan Province. Over the next five years they did intensive sampling at different seasons. Hundreds of bat-carrying coronaviruses, most of them harmless but dozens of them in the same population as SARS, were found to have an incredible genetic diversity.

In 2013, they found a coronavirus strain from horseshit bats that shared 97% of the genome sequence with the one which uses civets as intermediate host found in Guangdong Province. The discovery ended a decade-long search for natural reservoirs for the SARS coronavirus. In many bat habitats, including bat caves near Kunming, a constant mix of viruses creates huge opportunities for the emergence of dangerous new pathogens. In October 2015, Shi's team collected blood samples from 200 residents who live four villages near Kunming suburb, and detected 6 villagers, or nearly 3% of the people carry the SARS coronavirus (from bats) antibodies, but none of them have processed wild animals or reported the symptoms of SARS pneumonia or other pneumonia-like symptoms. On December 30, 2019, Shi was asked by the Director of the Institute to study a new type of coronavirus which have been found in the samples from two in-patients with unidentified pneumonia by Wuhan City Center for Prevention and Control of diseases. If the findings of unidentified pneumonia being caused by a new coronavirus are confirmed, then the new pathogen may pose a serious threat to public health, because it belongs to the same family with the virus living in bats that caused SARS epidemic. On January 7, 2020 her team determined that the new virus has indeed caused illness in these patients. The genome sequence of the virus is 96% homologous to the coronavirus found in Yunnan horseshoe bats. Shi's research suggests that wildlife trade and consumption are only part of the problem. Although the outbreak in Wuhan is the eighth caused by a bat-transmitted virus in the past 26 years, the problem is not the animals themselves, but our human contact with them. Since 70 percent of emerging infectious diseases transmitted by animals come from wildlife, we should find all these viruses in wildlife around the world and conduct better diagnostic tests. So, whether it is SARS or a new coronavirus, what we have found is just the tip of the iceberg. As many as 5,000 coronavirus strains are waiting to be discovered around the world. Dr. Shi is planning a nationwide project to systematically sample the viruses from bat caves to a much greater extent and intensity than her team has previously attempted. "Bat-borne coronaviruses will cause more outbreaks and we have to find them before they find us," she said.[14]

Dr. Shi's work is a paradigm for the offensive strategy that we suggest to prevent and control spillover effects of cross-species transmission. Her work suggests:

♦ The past rampant SARS and present pandemic of SARS-COVID-2 are both the tip of the iceberg. If we cannot run faster than the virus, that is, if we cannot take effective measures to cutting off of the contact between animals and humans before the virus cross the protective screen to contact humans, then the next spillover to humans and outbreak of coronavirus transmission in humans would be unavoidable. So the implementation of Preventing First is a moral imperative.

♦ To implement the prevention-oriented policy, we should trace the source to the host reservoirs (HR) of the coronavirus. We must follow the exemplar of Dr. Shi to conduct a general

---

[14] Qiu 2020.

survey of all bat caves that may be infected with coronavirus and take samples for testing.

♦ It is very likely that as host reservoirs the bats may have close contact with other wild animals and make the latter become secondary host (HS) or other intermediate host (HI, intermediate host), by natural (such as shrinking wildlife habitats) or social (hunting, transportation, processing for wild animals) factors, and genetic changes in viruses themselves might happen during their transmission from one wild animal to the other, so we must study all these possible changes including the contact between different wild animals, and the transmission of the viruses between secondary hosts and other intermediate hosts as well as genetic change of the viruses themselves during the transmission between animals..

♦ There is little chance of infection with coronavirus due to direct human contact with bats in their caves, but there may be more wild animals exposed to the secondary host. Biological and non-biological factors that promote the transmission of the virus to humans across the species barrier should be studied. This is a basic study to prevent the recurrence of coronavirus-causing disease outbreak. To put it in a nutshell, it is to build a wildlife-based surveillance system. But establishing such a surveillance system would require the country to invest a large amount of resources, need to do hard research work, which cannot bring about quick profits. It should not conceive a mentality of *ji gong jin li* (seeking quick success and instant profits) to approach to such a fundamental infrastructure building.

The concept of cross-species transmission (spillover). The term cross-species transmission (spillover) refers to the ability of an alien virus to complete the virus cycle once it enters an individual in the HS population, including (1) the ability to adsorb, penetrate, and detach or separate from the virus coat; (2) Transcriptional transformation and replication; and (3) assemble and release.[15] What we need to focus on now is to establish and strengthen the wildlife-based surveillance of virus transmission between animal species in order to prevent wildlife coronavirus from entering individuals in humans. Different from monitoring which is usually to observe or watch at a fixed site (such as police monitoring at the suspected), surveillance is the act of observing a particular threat in a particular area, accompanied by the collection of data. What we used to do for zoonotic diseases was post-spillover and human-based surveillance. This surveillance is necessary for treating patients and taking further measures to prevent or reduce the increase in cases, but cannot prevent cases of transmission from wild animals to humans or spillover. The prevention of pathogen spilling over from the second host animal (HSs) or intermediate host (HIs) to humans is only possible through our in-depth study and understanding of the ecological context and biological interaction of pathogens within the HRs.

The animal-based surveillance for zoonotic diseases would bring about huge benefits to individuals, family, society and country as a whole: (1) Once we understand the characteristics of zoonotic diseases the country with necessary public health infrastructure could immediately launch or establish systematic surveillance to systematically collect the data on possible infecting humans and causing disease at regional and national levels; (2) Early warning of zoonotic diseases that may spread to humans could be issued so that other parts of the country or other countries could respond timely; (3) To enable timely state intervention to prevent spillovers. In fact, global animal-based surveillance system has been established for poultry and livestock for influenza, but has not yet been extended to wild waterfowl and shorefowl HRs, although the latter are essential.

Our current approach to controlling zoonotic diseases ignores the research into the ecology of wildlife and the maintenance and transmission of pathogens, and therefore ignores the possi-

---

[15] Childs et al. 2007.

bility of blocking their transmission before they spill over into humans. The fundamental reason is that our prevention and control adopt a defensive strategy focusing only on human HS. Our advice is to turn the defensive strategy to offensive, that is, turn our efforts to the nest of zoonotic diseases, host reservoirs of zoonotic viruses. The offensive strategy enables us to get the information and data on the maintenance and transmission cycle of zoonotic viruses in wildlife HRs after the investigation and study, and then take appropriate interventions through the destruction of maintenance and transmission cycle of zoonotic viruses in their HRs so as to prevent or significantly reduce the transmission across species or spillover of zoonotic pathogens to infecting humans. However, the bias towards the approach of human-based surveillance and post-spillover treatment of people infected with the virus has been institutionalized, and decisive decision by policymakers is needed to reverse this approach and invest more resources in wildlife-based offensive strategies.[16][17]

The fundamental goal of offensive strategies is to prevent contact between wild animals and human beings. The establishment of an insurmountable barrier between these two different species is of primary and great importance. However, it is important to note that the custom of eating wild animals for thousands of years is not going to be reversed overnight, and that education needs to be accompanied by a series of administrative and legal measures (including help for wildlife workers to switch jobs) to prevent the trade and consumption of wild animals from becoming a highly profitable underground industry. Other measures need to be complemented, such as a ban on hunting and the need to relocate people from villages near bat caves to safer places.

Prevent and Control the Outbreak of Zoonotic Diseases in Humans

The first part of our proposed offensive strategy for preventing and controlling the spillover of zoonotic viruses into humans is to establish or improve wildlife-based surveillance systems to prevent the spillover of these viruses across the species barrier into humans; the second part is to prevent and control the outbreak of zoonotic diseases in humans when spillover prevention fails. An outbreak here refers to a sudden increase in the number of people suffering from a disease in a certain place at a certain moment. Zoonotic disease suddenly appears in the human population has three stages: (1) the transmission from animal hosts to human samplers (high-risky individuals who are susceptible to new virus infection); (2) the spread from samplers to spreaders (individuals in new host population who have high potential to transmit new virus), and (3) the spread from the spreaders to the general population.[18] Based on the above, we can contain the outbreak by controlling the spread of the virus from a few samplers to spreaders at stages 2or from spreaders to the general population at stage 3. Such control is possible only on the basis of two fundamental interventions: full disclosure and transparency of information and the early implementation of public health intervention such as contact tracing, physical distancing, quarantine/isolation, of which full disclosure and transparency of information is the precondition. If information about the spread of infection or disease is incomplete and opaque, the iso-

---

[16] Childs 2007. Childs, J. Pre-spillover prevention of emerging zoonotic diseases: What are the targets and what are the tools? In Childs, J., Mackenzie, J., Richt J. (eds.) Wildlife and Emerging Zoonotic Diseases: The Biology, Circumstances and Consequences of Cross-Species Transmission. Springer-Verlag Berlin Heidelberg, 2007, 389–443.

[17] Ellis 2007. Ellis, K. Health officials should be watchful of zoonotic diseases: Experts advise proactive public health monitoring for zoonotic diseases. Infectious Disease News. July. https://www.healio.com/infectious-disease/emerging-diseases/news/print/infectious-disease-news/%7B5e8423bc-fafd-4faf-b579-16211fbc5253%7D/health-officials-should-be-watchful-of-zoonotic-diseases.

[18] Cleaveland et al. 2007.

lation or interruption of human contact with the virus is an empty word.

Leaving aside the accountability, let's see whether the outbreak of the novel coronavirus disease that began in Wuhan (and may have begun elsewhere as well) could have been prevented or not. We believe that this outbreak could have been avoided if, instead of a conservative, reactive or defensive strategy, we had adopted an offensive, proactionary, or pre-emptive strategy.

The success of preventing and controlling an epidemic depends on the joint efforts of policy-makers, medical and public health professionals and the public, and the appropriateness and effectiveness of such efforts depends on the timely availability of information/data on ever changing transmission of the virus from animals to humans and humans to humans shared by the three parties. If information is incomplete and opaque after the virus has spilled over to humans, it is difficult to contain the transmission of the disease caused by the virus in a certain range, and the result is the outbreak of the disease caused by the virus being inevitable. We think at least from December 2019 to January 20, 2020 Wuhan health agency collected the necessary information on the epidemic not timely, developed a undue high standard for the disease report, deliberately lower the number of reported cases, refused to report complete information to the Expert Team sent by the central government, intentionally played down the seriousness of the disease, and made the public lacking of vigilance to the epidemic. Especially the local government did not promote the public and healthcare professionals to take the necessary protective measures, instead, they suppressed the reporting of the epidemic information by medical staff in hospitals, and ignored the fact of human –to-human transmission, and still organize large-scale conferences the participants of which came from all over Hubei Province, or approved large-scale commercial activities, As a result, asymptomatic or mildly infected people attending these large gatherings spread the virus to Wuhan City and other parts of Hubei Province, and further to other parts of the country.[19] In view of what happened like the above, people have reason to ask: Do we have delayed Wuhan's fight against the coronavirus epidemic for 43 days?[20] Forty-three days should be sufficient to take strong and effective measures to prevent scattered cases that have spilled over into humans from spreading to the whole city and forming an outbreak based on real information and data. However, the success in controlling the pre-outbreak status at early stage of the transmission depends on which strategy we adopt.

---

[19] Liu 2020. Liu, M. An interview with admonished doctor: I am to remind everyone of precaution. Network of New Beijing Daily. January 31, 2020. http://www.bjnews.com.cn/feature/2020/01/31/682076.html. Lei et al. 2020. Lei, R. & Qiu, R. Chinese bioethicists: Silencing doctor impeded early control. Bioethics Forum, The Hastings Center, February 13. https://www.thehastingscenter.org/coronavirus-doctor-whistleblower/ Gao 2020. Gao, Y. Rashomon on contact history of Southern Seafood Market: The puzzling "double standard" of Wuhan Municipal Health Commission. Caixin Network. February 19, 2020. http://www.caixin.com/2020-02-19/101517544.html
Chronicle of Novel Coronavirus Pneumonia (December 2019-January 20, 2020). Caixin Network. 2020-01-20. http://www.caixin.com/健康
Xu 2020. Xu, B., Chen, R., Wang, S., et al. Special Report: After January 6, the puzzle of zero newly increased case. China Business Network. January 20, 2020. https://m.yicai.com/news/100485217.html?clicktime=1580776530
Lei et al. 2019. Lei, R. & Qiu, R. Report from China: Ethical questions on the response to the coronavirus. Bioethics Forum. The Hastings Center. January 31. http://www.thehastingscenter.org/report-from-china-ethical-questions-to-the-coronavirus
Liu, Z. 2019. On current pneumonia epidemic，the bulletin of Wuhan Health Commission appeared. Science and Technology Daily, December 31. http://www.stdaily.com/02/hubei/2019-12/31/content_849442.shtml

[20] Ji 2020. Ji, D. It is who delayed the fight against Wuhan pneumonia for 43 days? February 3, 2020. http://www.blog.wenxuecity.com/myblog.

We believe that a complete grasp of epidemic information/data is a prerequisite for successful containment of the initial spillover into the pre-outbreak state, but not the key. The key is which strategy we take: conservative, defensive or pre-emptive, offensive? We believe that an offensive approach is more likely to succeed, especially in the face of new virus attacks and uncertainty about the development of the epidemic. It is reported[21] that the conservative strategy to deal with the spread of coronavirus recommended by the second expert team is based on the following reasons: "human-to-human" has long been inferred, but no obvious phenomenon of human-to-human transmission has been found", "the possibility of limited human-to-human transmission cannot be ruled out", etc. These remarks raise the following question: It is important to say that human to human transmission has been inferred leaving aside the fact that "human-to-human" has been occurred since December or early January 2019. In the face of a new virus attack, we lack information and data, thus we have to make the decision without sufficient evidences. But there is insufficient evidence to support not only the possible offensive strategy, but also the conservative and cautious strategy recommended by the expert team. In fact, decision makers did make decision under an uncertain condition. In making decision under uncertain condition, we need to rely on reason, experience and logical reasoning in addition to the evidence base. If the reason were to be relied upon, wouldn't it be more reasonable for us to assume (accept it as true but it has not been proven so far) that "human-to-human" would be transmitted even if the expert team had no evidence at hand? For humankind have already had the painful experiences of two coronavirus epidemics, both of which have "human-to-human" transmission in the cases of SARS and MERS. Coronaviruses do not belong to the category of viruses in which humans must come into contact with a second or intermediate host each time. There is no evidence and no reason to assert that the virus would not spread from human to human. More importantly, under uncertain condition, which is the better decision to make: a conservative decision or a proactionary one? That should be based on the ethical principle of taking the lesser of two evils in the context of a moral dilemma.

An offensive strategy in uncertain condition (in short, "better to isolate a lot of people than to let one infected person go") can be justified ethically. SARS was labelled as an unidentified pneumonia at the beginning, and its intermediate host was wild animal. Foreign countries also have rich successful experiences to follow. Snow's success in controlling cholera in Britain in the 19th century did not come about until the source of the infection had been identified. This offensive or pre-emptive strategy is temporary and can be mitigated or tightened as the epidemic eases or escalated. The ethical justification for this offensive strategy is as follows:

From the perspective of consequences, such a strategy is likely to limit the epidemic to a certain area of Wuhan (such as Hankou area, a part of Wuhan), or at most to Wuhan City, without spilling out of Wuhan. Of course, all over Hubei Province should pay attention to the detection, treatment and isolation of patients with respiratory symptoms, as well as the strict inspection of wildlife markets and restaurants. In a sense, this is an early and local "lockdown". Because the only effective way to control the spread of coronavirus is contact tracing and isolation.

One of the ethically defensible conditions of public health ethics for restricting individual liberty is the minimization of infringement on individual liberty. If strict prevention and control

---

[21] Yu, Q. & Li, S. 2020. Exclusive interview with an expert who are in the Second Expert Team dispatched by National Health Commission: Why the human-to-human transmission is not found? Financial Magazine February 26. http://news.sina.com.cn/c/2020-02-26/doc-3imxxstf4577244.shtml
Xu 2020. Xu, W. Exclusive response: Early inference on "human-to-human" transmission, reasons for conservative conclusion. New Beijing Daily Network. January 31. http://www.bjnews.com.cn/news/2020/01/31/682224.html

measures had been taken sooner, the actual intensity and scale of restrictions on freedom would surely have been much smaller. This, of course, would have caused public alarm sooner. But again, the panic was much smaller and less intense than it is now, especially in such countries where the people are disgustful at any restrictive interventions, even wearing face masks and keep physical distancing. Therefore, the key to adopting this strategy is to explain to the public its necessity and temporality with the help of administrative and legal measures such as wearing face mask and keep physical distancing should be mandatory, but not voluntary. .

An offensive prevention and control strategy would certainly have less impact on the national economy and people's lives than conservative strategies. Because the result of a conservative strategy (including the lax of restrictive measures too early) would be that you end up with a much more offensive and massive restriction, and with much greater costs and impacts.

As a result, it is possible to end up with no outbreak and only a few scattered cases. This outcome is not the failure of the offensive strategy, but its success. This is characteristic of public health. If there were a smallpox epidemic in a neighboring country, we would all have to be stayed at home and be vaccinated against smallpox, and the result is: we would all be safe. This does not imply that smallpox vaccination and restriction is a waste of effort. Although the offensive strategy requires a certain amount of human resources, material resources and even financial resources, and may cause some losses for national and individual/family economy, however, the strategy with stronger countermeasures, "the lesser of two evils", obviously brings much less losses than the strategy with weaker countermeasures. So public health professionals are unsung heroes.[22]

References

Childs 2007. Childs, J. Pre-spillover prevention of emerging zoonotic diseases: What are the targets and what are the tools? In Childs, J., Mackenzie, J., Richt J. (eds.) 2007 Wildlife and Emerging Zoonotic Diseases: The Biology, Circumstances and Consequences of Cross-Species Transmission. Springer-Verlag Berlin Heidelberg, 2007, 389–443.

Childs et al. 2007. Childs, J., Richt, A., Mackenzie, J. Introduction: Conceptualizing and partitioning the emergence process of zoonotic viruses from wildlife to humans, in Childs J, Mackenzie J, Richt J. (eds.) Wildlife and Emerging Zoonotic Diseases: The Biology, Circumstances and Consequences of Cross-Species Transmission, Springer-Verlag Berlin Heidelberg 2007, 1–31.

Chronicle 2020. Chronicle of Novel Coronavirus Pneumonia (December 2019-January 20, 2020). Caixin Network. 2020-01-20. http://www.caixin.com/健康

Cleaveland 2007. Cleaveland, S., Haydon, D., Taylor, L. Overviews of pathogen emergence: Which pathogens emerge, when and why? Childs, J., Mackenzie, J., Richt, J. (eds.). Wildlife and Emerging Zoonotic Diseases: The Biology, Circumstances and Consequences of Cross-Species Transmission. Springer-Verlag Berlin Heidelberg 2007, 85-111.

Ellis 2007. Ellis, K. Health officials should be watchful of zoonotic diseases: Experts advise proactive public health monitoring for zoonotic diseases. Infectious Disease News. July.

---

[22] Yu et al. 2020.
 Li 2020. Li, Y. An interview with Qiu, R.: Rather radical, even if it is a false alarm. Health Newspaper. February 7, 2020.
 Lei et al. 2020. Lei, R. & Qiu, R. A strategy to prevent and control zoonoses?, Hastings Center Report 50(3): 73-74.

https://www.healio.com/infectious-disease/emerging-diseases/news/print/infectious-disease-news/%7B5e8423bc-fafd-4faf-b579-16211fbc5253%7D/health-officials-should-be-watchful-of-zoonotic-diseases

Gao 2020. Gao, Y. Rashomon on contact history of Southern Seafood Market: The puzzling "double standard" of Wuhan Municipal Health Commission. Caixin Network. February 19, 2020. http://www.caixin.com/2020-02-19/101517544.html.

Ji 2020. Ji, D. It is who delayed the fight against Wuhan pneumonia for 43 days? February 3, 2020. http://www.blog.wenxuecity.com/myblog.

Lei et al. 2019. Lei, R. & Qiu, R. Report from China: Ethical questions on the response to the coronavirus. Bioethics Forum. The Hastings Center. January 31, 2019. http://www.thehastingscenter.org/report-from-china-ethical-questions-to-the-coronavirus

Lei et al. 2020. Lei, R. & Qiu, R. A strategy to prevent and control zoonoses?, Hastings Center Report 50(2020)3:73-74.

Lei et al. 2020. Lei, R. & Qiu, R. Chinese bioethicists: Silencing doctor impeded early control. Bioethics Forum, The Hastings Center, February 13. https://www.thehastingscenter.org/coronavirus-doctor-whistleblower/.

Lei et al. 2020. Lei, R. & Qiu, R. Report from China: Ethical questions on the response to the coronavirus, Bioethics Forum, The Hastings Center, January 31, 2020. https://www.thehastingscenter.org/report-from-china-ethical-questions-on-the-response-to-the-coronavirus/

Li 2020. Li, Y. An interview with Qiu, R.: Rather radical, even if it is a false alarm. Health Newspaper. February 7, 2020.

Liu 2019. Liu, Z. On current pneumonia epidemic, the bulletin of Wuhan Health Commission appeared. Science and Technology Daily, December 31, 2019. http://www.stdaily.com/02/hubei/2019-12/31/content_849442.shtml

Liu 2020. Liu, M. An interview with admonished doctor: I am to remind everyone of precaution. Network of New Beijing Daily. January 31, 2020. http://www.bjnews.com.cn/feature/2020/01/31/682076.html.

Qiu 2003. Qiu, R. Ethical and policy issues raised by the SARS epidemic in China. Studies in Dialectics of Nature (6)1-5.

Qiu 2020. Qiu, J. How China's "Bat Woman" hunted down viruses from SARS to the new coronavirus, Scientific Americans, March 11, 2020. https://www.scientificamerican.com/article/how-chinas-bat-woman-hunted-down-viruses-from-sars-to-the-new-coro-navirus1/.

Sigerist 1943. Sigerist, H. Civilization and Disease. Chapter 1: Civilization as a factor in the genesis of disease. Ithaca and London: Cornell University Press 1943, 7-41.

WHO 2007. WHO. A Strategic Framework for Emergency Preparedness. https://www.who.int/ihr/publications/9789241511827/en/

WHO 2017. WHO. Regional Office for Europe. Guide to Revision of National Pandemic Influenza Preparedness Plans, 2017. https://www.ecdc.europa.eu/en/seasonal-influenza/preparedness/influenza-pandemic-preparedness-plans

WHO 2020. WHO. Naming the coronavirus disease (COVID-19) and the virus that causes it. http://who.int/emergences/diseass/noval-conoravirus-2019/technical-guidance/naming-the-conoravirus-disease-(covid-19)-and-the-virus-that-cause-it

Xu 2020. Xu, W. Exclusive response: Early inference on "human-to-human" transmission, reasons for conservative conclusion. New Beijing Daily Network. January 31, 2020. http://www.bjnews.com.cn/news/2020/01/31/682224.html

Xu et al. 2020. Xu, B., Chen, R., Wang, S., et al. Special Report: After January 6, the puzzle of zero newly increased case.   China Business Network.   January   20,   2020. https://m.yicai.com/news/100485217.html?clicktime=1580776530

Yu et al. 2020. Yu, Q. & Li, S. Exclusive interview with an expert who are in the Second Expert Team dispatched by National Health Commission: Why the human-to-human transmission is not found? Financial Magazine February 26, 2020. http://news.sina.com.cn/c/2020-02-26/doc-3imxxstf4577244.shtml

Zou et al. 2013. Zou, Z., Liang, Z., Yang, X. The fight between humankind and epidemic. Baidu Library 2013. https://wenku.baidu.com/view/b169d2445a8102d276a22f83.html

Ruipeng Lei, PhD, works at the Department of Philosophy, Centre for Bioethics, Huazhong University of Science and Technology, Wuhan, China. Contact E-Mail: lxp73615@163.com.

Renzong Qiu works at the Institute of Philosophy, Chinese Academy of Social Sciences; and the Institute of Bioethics, Centre for Ethics and Moral Studies, Renmin University of China. Contact E-Mail: qiurenzong@hotmail.com.

Infectious diseases bear Philosophy

Kiyokazu Nakatomi, Chiba Prefectural Matsuo High School, Japan

Abstract

Regarding infectious diseases and philosophy, the 'illness of Athens' is famous, when Socrates was 40 years old. A quarter of the population of Athens died. Before the wonders of nature, humans are powerless and nothing as Pascal also said. Socrates experienced and learned nothingness from this situation in military service, so he seized and explained ignorance. His theory led to Plato, Aristotle and the heyday of Greek philosophy. The tribulation of an infectious disease gave birth to philosophy. The corona virus is a crisis of the human race in the world but this is a sign of a new philosophy.

Keywords

corona infectious virus (COVID-19), pandemic, illness of Athens, Thucydides , Ebola, Socrates, nothingness, benevolence of Confucius and philia of Aristotle, principle of nothingness and love, Biocosmological Association

Contents

1. Metaphysical consideration of the corona virus
2. Corona virus ravages
3. Reason for expansion to the world
4. Infectious Diseases of Athens and Socrates
5. Benevolence of Confucius and Philia of Aristotle

Conclusion

1. Metaphysical consideration of the corona virus

The corona virus epidemic that occurred on December 2019 spread to the world in an instant. The probable origin location is Wuhan (武漢), one of the most populous cities in central China. The population is 10.89 million. About 30 million people live in this metropolitan area. It is three times as big as Tokyo in Japan. A virus occurred in the seafood market (Huan Seafood Wholesale Market). In the past, in the case of SARS (Severe Acute Respiratory Syndrome), researchers were sent from the United States to the Wuhan Virus Research Institute of the Chinese Academy of Sciences and a quick response was made. France also supported this institute. However, this time, the United States and China were in conflict. The communications lacked among the United States, France and China. The United States did not send researchers until mid-February. Until that time China rejected them. The information was limited to China.

A corona virus is not a living being. However, it has RNA or DNA and is surrounded by protein. It is thus a mass of nucleic acids and proteins. However, when it enters a living organism, it proliferates like a living organism and causes various adverse effects on humans. In other words, it usually becomes a matter but when it comes into life, it becomes like a life form. If one says that it is matter, it is matter. If one says that it is life, it is life. It is something that goes beyond both. This cannot be explained by the conventional dichotomy of matter or life. The following is a metaphysical consideration. It can be explained by using the logic of Absolute Nothingness. If one says that it is, it exists. If one says that it is not, it does not exist. One says nothing. As it is beyond the expression of the words, one calls it nothingness. It requires the development of cosmology. I have already preached the Creation of the universe from nothingness[1]. Before the Creation, there is nothing. The universe occurred from the fluctuation of nothingness (shaking nothingness). The Big Bang took place and the expansion of the universe began. The energy that generates this Big Bang and propels the expanding universe is the flow of life, a way of ancient China and nothingness beyond the expressions that I say. It is the flow of life and energy flowing to the world and the universe. It is compatible with the energy concept of the organic worldview claimed by the Biocosmological Association[2]. From this concept, vacuum energy, dark matter, and dark energy are proposed by physics. This energy is filled in the world and the universe. Physics has confirmed that there are atoms, quarks, neutrinos, and so on. Since the Big Bang about 13.8 billion years ago, astronomical bodies, galaxies, solar systems, earth, and life have been formed. A virus is generated by this energy and the flow of life. It has appeared about 500 million years ago, so it is much older than humankind. A matter is generated from the resistance of energy but one can say that a virus is an intermediate state or existence between this flow of life and matter. Conversely, matter or life is a clearly limited expression. There are various such viruses. It cannot be extinct because it is in the flow of energy. It is easy to understand if you think this way. It exists everywhere and is latent. In terms of physics, virtual particle[3] corresponds. Though it is not, suddenly it exists. It appears at one time, then suddenly disappears. It looks like a ghost. A corona virus is a matter. In some situations it grows like a living organism. However, although it disappears under some circumstances, it will occur again in response to changes in temperature and ecosystem.

It infects and affects various living beings and humans. That is life-threatening. Various infectious diseases have existed in history and human races have managed to survive. Fortunately, it was the blessings of heaven that were peaceful without infectious diseases. It is a threat since the Spanish influenza: 1918 flu pandemic (1918-1920) ,100 years ago.

---

[1] Creation from nothingness, *"Philosophy of nothingness and love"*, Chapter 3, Nothingness in the Bible, Hokuju Company, Tokyo, 2002, p. 117, English version, Lambert Academic Publishing, Saarbrücken, 2016, pp. 169-170, 'The Synthesis of the theory of relativity and quantum theory' *Elixir International Journal, Elixir Condensed Matter Phys. 85 ,*Poland, 2015.

[2] Biocosmological Assocoation, Chief editor is Konstantin S. Khroutski (Veliky Novgorod, Russia). As he is philosopher and medicine, his study field is wide. Since, many various and creative papers are published in the articles *"Biocosmology-Neo-Aristotelism"*. The characteristics of the society are close to those of my philosophy.

[3] Virtual particle. This particle is not directly observed in the experiment. But this is confined in the intermediate process of reaction and disappears.

[4] Obama care: Patient Protection and Affordable Care Act (2010) by Barack Obama

[5] Dr. Xiao Botao is professor of South China University of Technology. He studied in Harvard University. Kensaku Tokito, The full impact translation of 'Erase Corona paper' of missing Chinese researcher will be published. https://gendai.ismedia.jp/articles/-/71310   Cf. Prof. Naoki Saito (斎藤直樹 Yamanashi Prefectural University), 'The mystery on the origins of new corona virus), e-Discourse *"Hundred Schools of Thought Contend (百家争鳴)"*, The Council on East Asian Community (CEAC), Tokyo, 2020-04-02, http://www.ceac.jp/j/index.html

[6] "Philosophy of Nothingness and Love", Chapter 4, Nothingness in ancient Greece, p.147-148, English version, Lambert Academic Publishing, Saarbrücken, 2016, pp.211-212

[7] *"Mystery of Oedipus"*, Atsuhiko Yoshida, Seidosha, Tokyo, p.216,1995

[8] Saitama Medical University, the curriculum bulletin, No.8, p.15-25 2000-03-31

[9] Thucydides, *"History of the Pelopponnesian War"*, *"Great Books of the World : Herodotus and Thucydides"* Chuōkōronsha, Tokyo, 1970, p. 366.

[3] Virtual particle. This particle is not directly observed in the experiment. But this is confined in the intermediate process of reaction and disappears.

2. Corona virus ravages

Dr. Li Wenliang (李文亮), who first discovered the corona virus, contacted his colleagues, but just before the Communist Party's convention, the Chinese police punished him and his colleagues as disordered persons. He was forced to sign a reflection document that he was detained with his colleagues and sent hoax information. Meanwhile, the virus spread. It can be said that the virus leaked from the ditch of the US-China conflict. The virus has no symptoms upon infection and has an incubation period of 2 weeks. After that, fever of 37.5 degrees continued for 5 days and suddenly a high fever came out, which made it difficult to breathe and led to death. The incubation period of 2 weeks is apt to be difficult to distinguish. The Chinese authorities officially admitted it on January 20 and Wuhan City closed the city on January 23. But it was too late. Wuhan is a central city in southern China with many people scattered in rural areas and in the world. The Chinese are now a globalized nation and have advanced all over the world. In Japan, the Diamond Princess suddenly stopped at the port of Yokohama. The captain of the Diamond Princess asked for help but Japan couldn't get the passengers off immediately because of the incubation period of 2 weeks. About 3,700 people were trapped aboard the ship. A super-sized luxury cruise ship backfired. On the other hand, China blocked the city with its national power. It banned the departure and entry of the country and left about 7,000 dead. Xi Jinping has declared that "Victory of the Communist Party of China ". After that, relief supplies have been sent to many countries.

On the other hand, it was the United States that suffered the conflict. The United States offered to provide virus samples but China refused it. It is deadly when fighting for the moment. Atlanta in the United States has the strongest infectious research institute in the world, the Centers for Disease Control and Prevention (CDC). However, if one cannot analyze the virus, one cannot take measures. American researchers entered China in mid-February on behalf of the WHO. Trump didn't understand what this situation meant. He relied on the strongest and most reassured CDC and actually resisted the advice of experts. The Democratic Party demanded anti-virus measures but Trump dismissed them as "Democratic conspiracy". It was until March 13th that the measures were delayed and the emergency started.

This virus doubled in speed in a few days. Exponentially increasing, the infections reached tens of thousands in a week. Thus, in overpopulated New York, 20,000 people died by April 19th. With Italy and France, the funeral is too late. Europe is also miserable. Although there is a habit of dense and close contact and a habit of not wearing a mask, the infection spreads explosively because infected persons cannot be identified. Especially in Italy where there are many elderly people, the death total was high and the next are France and Spain. People are sparse and main cities became ghost towns like the Champs Elysees in France and Main Street in New York. Only Korea, Taiwan and Vietnam have succeeded in containing the virus.

Japan also has 910 deaths but hospitals are full in the Tokyo metropolitan area and medical treatment is on the verge of collapse. Abe administration had ordered hospital consolidation due to financial difficulties. Many hospitals have disappeared because of low profits. This is the same for schools and education. This is the result of pursuing profits. The nurses are not well treated and cannot continue their activity for a long time. There are cases in which people quit when they have children. This also applies to nurseries and caregivers. Currently, Japan has a shortage of doctors and nurses but if the employment conditions are improved, it will be solved a little. In short, since Japan is trying to do it cheaply, Japan is starting to suffer. The same is true for Russia which saw a sharp increase of cases in April. According to recent TV news in Japan, the number of doctors and nurses has been reduced to about 130,000 in a few years. In Japan the number of PCR (polymerase chain reaction) tests prepared is too small to test as expected. Why can drive-through inspection be done in Korea and not in Japan? The point is that the Japanese government can't do things without equipment. The number of artificial respirators is half of that of Italy. The intensive care unit is barely present in a general hospital. It seems that the artificial respirators and the intensive care units are usually kept at the minimum use frequency. At present, the prime minister hurriedly placed an order of them with a private company. In order to cover this lack of treatment resources, two masks were planned to be distributed to each family. Until now, the budget for medical care and education has been cut down to cover the shortage of a mask. At the surface it protects the health of the people but it only covers the failure of budget reduction policies. The expenditure was 3.8 hundred million Euros. Although he praised the economic effect as Abenomics, he has been ironic about Abenomask as a cover mask. Today, nifty Japanese housewives are making their own family masks (washable and reusable). Before the disposable mask, we used to wash a gauze mask and use it several times. The traditional symbolic expression is "MOTTAINAI" that Prof. Wangari Muta Maathai, who received the Nobel Peace Prize, shouted to the world for moderation. It was better to give priority to the medical field and distribute protective clothing and masks to medical personnel rather than giving it to each family. Deadly, defective products are found in the distributed masks. Mold and hairs are present on these masks! Such a mask cannot be used with confidence. 70% of the people are not happy. Japanese schools are closed from March 2nd to May 31st. Students who cannot go to school smolder at home and have conflicts with their parents.

3. Reason for expansion to the world

At the previous SARS outbreak, cooperation between the United States and China provided an early initial response. So it did not spread to the world. But this time it didn't occur. There is a US-China conflict. President Trump's "America First" was the slogan of the administration. It is about rebuilding a strong American economy and military. It was China that stood there. China surpassed Japan and became the second largest power in the world. There are various ethnic groups in the country. To control them, the leader always needs an enemy outside. He turns domestic contradictions Overseas, Japan and America. Naturally, China also states "China First" against America First. Naturally, there will be a conflict. The confrontation appeared in economic and trade confrontation and explicit, tariff setting and export / import controls were performed. Among them, Trump was hostile to China and implemented a budget cut for health care. The famous universal health insurance Obama Care[4] was abolished. That slam has suspended the temporary staffing at the National Institute of Infection in Atlanta and China.

---

[4] Obama care: Patient Protection and Affordable Care Act (2010) by Barack Obama

[5] Dr. Xiao Botao is the professor of South China University of Technology. He studied in Harvard University. Kensaku Tokito, The full impact translation of 'Erase Corona paper' of missing Chinese researcher will be published. https://gendai.ismedia.jp/articles/-/71310 Cf. Prof. Naoki Saito (斎藤直樹 Yamanashi Prefectural University), 'The mystery on the origins of new corona virus), e-Discourse "Hundred Schools of Thought Contend (百家争鳴)", The Council on East Asian Community (CEAC), Tokyo, 2020-04-02, http://www.ceac.jp/j/index.html

[6] "Philosophy of Nothingness and Love", Chapter 4, Nothingness in ancient Greece, p.147-148, English version, Lambert Academic Publishing, Saarbrücken, 2016, pp.211-212

[7] "Mystery of Oedipus", Atsuhiko Yoshida, Seidosha, Tokyo, p.216,1995

[8] Saitama Medical University, the curriculum bulletin, No.8, p.15-25 2000-03-31

[9] Thucydides, "History of the Peloponnesian War", "Great Books of the World : Herodotus and Thucydides" Chuōkōronsha, Tokyo, 1970, p.366

[10] The first publication of this paper was Voice of Intellectual Man - An International Journal, Year 2011, Volume-1, Issue-2 (July–December), India, Lucknow University.

At one time, researchers from the United States were stationed at the Wuhan Virus Research Institute of the Chinese Academy of Sciences and engaged in joint research. However, Trump has stopped dispatching the researchers. Only Chinese were in the laboratory but they began to study new bat viruses to show their level of research (possibly converted to military weapons). It is suspected to be the corona virus of this time. The corona virus leaked from the laboratory, spread to the animal market and the virus spread. The report is 'The possible origins of 2019-n-CoV coronavirus' by Prof. Xiao Botao (肖波涛)[5]. At that time, bats were not sold in the seafood market. There is another virus institute (the Wuhan Center for Disease Control Prevention) near the seafood market. The Center is situated 280m from the market. In that center, there were about 600 bats. Sometimes researchers were hurled by bats in the process of the experiment of bat virus. Then the researchers were infected and went to the seafood market. Simultaneously corona virus spread. This is the contents of the paper of Prof. Xiao Botao. It was published on the site of Research Gate 6 February 2020. But this paper was erased on the site soon and Prof. Xiao Botao is currently missing. The Chinese government and Oxford Academy have denied this fact. Up to this point, it is still under investigation but there is decisive failure.

It was the event of punishment of several doctors who discovered infected persons in mid-December 2019. They detected that the virus was abnormal and dangerous like SARS. Dr. Ai Fen (艾芬, director of the emergency department at Wuhan Central Hospital), Dr. Li Wenliang (same hospital, Ophthalmology) and 6 other persons were dismissed. Dr. Li later became infected and died in February. The scene with the ventilator was broadcast overseas on TV. Dr. Ai Fen later wrote a note about the situation but disappeared and her note remained unknown. Though her note was erased suddenly some editors of other countries reposted it.

On January 2: From the hospital's inspection section (communist party discipline committee's administrative committee section), she received a call. What was said:

"Why do you throw a hoax and cause trouble?" The executive continued. "When you get back, don't tell hoax to all over 200 staff in the emergency department. Don't do it on Weibo (Chinese popular chat appli) or short email. Speak directly or call. But don't tell anyone about pneumonia. Don't even say to your husband... "

"I was stunned. I was not just blamed for my negligence in my work. It was as if the brilliant development of Wuhan City had been defeated by myself. I was in despair."

"*Wuhan Chinese Female Doctor's Note*" Bungeishunjū May issue 2020 and Bunshun Online: https://news.yahoo.co.jp/articles/439a6418a1ace5d82c375c87575d6e639ce1de03

What the author would like to insist on here is the big mistake of the authorities who dis-

---

[5] Dr. Xiao Botao is a professor of South China University of Technology. He studied in Harvard University. Kensaku Tokito, The full impact translation of 'Erase Corona paper' of missing Chinese researcher will be published. https://gendai.ismedia.jp/articles/-/71310 Cf. Prof. Naoki Saito (斎藤直樹 Yamanashi Prefectural University), 'The mystery on the origins of new corona virus), e-Discourse "*Hundred Schools of Thought Contend (百家爭鳴)*", The Council on East Asian Community (CEAC), Tokyo, 2020-04-02, http://www.ceac.jp/j/index.html

[6] "Philosophy of Nothingness and Love", Chapter 4, Nothingness in ancient Greece, p.147-148, English version, Lambert Academic Publishing, Saarbrücken, 2016, pp.211-212

[7] "*Mystery of Oedipus*", Atsuhiko Yoshida, Seidosha, Tokyo, p.216,1995

[8] Saitama Medical University, the curriculum bulletin, No.8, p.15-25 2000-03-31

[9] Thucydides, "*History of the Pelopponesian War*", "*Great Books of the World : Herodotus and Thucydides*" Chuōkōronsha, Tokyo, 1970, p.366

[10] The first publication of this paper was *Voice of Intellectual Man - An International Journal,* Year 2011, Volume-1, Issue-2 (July–December), India, Lucknow University.

guised the fact revealed by the doctors and punished them. Though the doctors reported the outbreak of the corona virus, the authorities regarded it as a hoax. The responsibility is of course that of the national constitution. It is a system that prioritizes security of communism rather than the truth. Injustice of concealment caused an outrageous world pandemic and tragedy. Chinese supreme leadership should apologize to the world.

Originally, China produced and respects Holy Sages like Confucius in the philosophical world. Personally, I have a lot of excellent Chinese friends and cannot imagine this from such a relationship. In 2018, the World Congress of Philosophy was held at the Beijing University. China has become a leading country in the world of philosophical circles. The president of the Biocosmological Association is Dr. Xiaoting Liu, the professor of Beijing Normal University. I visited there twice and many researchers welcomed me with respect. There is a prestigious Confucius Academy on this campus and it was truly a hospitality with Confucius kernels. The fact that China has given a good impression on us does not lead us to think about concealment of the truth. For Chinese leaders, it may be a small stain or mistake.

However, the opponent was an enemy of the micro world called corona virus. Earthquakes and tsunamis are macro threats. Chinese leaders were unwilling to threaten the micro world. From our perspective, even a small hole is a huge hole from a microscopic virus. The micro / macro analysis method comes from Aristotle. It has opened up academic fields by exerting its power in biology for micro analysis and astronomy for macro analysis. A large amount of viruses was released to the world from the hole. The city of Wuhan was locked from January 23. But the virus had already spread to the world in about a month. Japan holds the Sapporo Snow Festival which gathers 2.5 million people every year. In anticipation of this event, Chinese tourists were coming to Japan before January 23. So in Japan, apart from a luxury liner, the virus was widespread in Hokkaido. The Governor of Hokkaido announced a state of emergency in early February. People were restricted from going out. The first wave ended but the second wave hit in April. Tokyo was on the verge of medical collapse in mid-April. The United States has been hit by that largest deal. President Trump says he will seek damages from China. China has shown that it has succeeded in containing the virus "Victory of the Communist Party of China" and is providing masks, protective clothing and medical equipment to many countries. However, this is the actual shadow mask. This concealment should be honestly admitted to be dishonest and apology should be made to the world. After the Second World War, have not China and South Korea strongly urged Japan to apologize for their war responsibilities? And the missing doctor, Ai Fein and Prof. Li Xiao Botao should be brought to the public. Though Ai Fen posted a Video on her Weibo allowed in mid-April, it suggested that she had some restrict degree of freedom and her face was hidden with a mask. Missing further magnifies the suspicion that they have hidden because their writings are not convenient. In this way, the cause of the corona virus this time is the injustice of concealment and the outflow of virus from the ditch of the US-China conflict. I wrote this paper to keep this fact. Injustice should be most disliked by Confucius humanists. It should be noted that the confrontation between powerful nations causes war and causes illness. This has been repeated over time. It is taken up in my book "*Philosophy of nothingness and love*"[6]. A quarter of Athens citizens were killed.

[6] "*Philosophy of Nothingness and Love*", Chapter 4, Nothingness in ancient Greece, p.147-148, English version, Lambert Academic Publishing, Saarbrücken, 2016, pp. 211-212.

[7] "*Mystery of Oedipus*", Atsuhiko Yoshida, Seidosha, Tokyo, p.216,1995

[8] Saitama Medical University, the curriculum bulletin, No.8, p.15-25 2000-03-31

[9] Thucydides, "*History of the Peloponnesian War*", "*Great Books of the World : Herodotus and Thucydides*" Chuōkōronsha, Tokyo, 1970, p.366

4. Infectious Diseases of Athens and Socrates

Conflicts between powerful nations produced war. In Socrates' era powerful nations were Athens and Sparta. Athens was a democratic politics and Sparta was a military power. The conflict opposed the Delian League of Athens to the Peloponnesian League of Sparta. This conflict reminds us of the modern American-China confrontation. This conflict started with an economic conflict. The Peloponnesian War between Athens and Sparta lasted 27 years. Athens was a trading nation with a good navy and had an advantage over sea control. Spartans were superior with the Army. However, the predominance of this sea control became an unexpected minus. It was that the control of various countries was good but from that, they contracted an infectious disease. Starting from Ethiopia, the infectious disease entered Athens via Egypt and Libya. It is also said to have invaded parts of the Persian territory. In order to counter Spartan, which was strong in land battles, Pericles had a strong castle wall, so they took on the battle in the castle. But it backfired[7]. Infected people had a high fever, vomiting, severe seizures, and bleeding. A quarter of the population of Athens died. There are various theories about this infectious disease, plague, red fever, measles, etc. According to the paper of Hiroshi Saito[8], a researcher at Saitama Medical University 'Is the disease in Athens Marburg disease or Ebola fever?', it seems that the disease is Marburg virus or Ebola hemorrhagic fever. The deciding factor is a high fatality rate of 25%, high fever, bleeding and the outbreak area in Africa. According to Thucydides, the disease in Athens is from Ethiopia, the Ebola in the 20th century is in Congo. Both are Africa. Infectious diseases are timeless. Infectious diseases were widespread during the Peloponnesian War. Athens was in danger of death. In an army, over 1,000 out of 4,000 have died. Correspondingly, one-fourth of Athens' citizens died, so the medical system collapsed, the funerals could not be done in time and the corpses fell on the streets and piled up like garbage. Birds and animals that ate human flesh did not approach the corpses which have not been buried yet, otherwise they ate it and died[9], and raptors disappeared. Public order deteriorated, order was disturbed. Morality was lost, Athenians experienced darkness and nothingness.

Socrates lived in such an era. In order to reestablish order, morality, and way of life to a devastated country, he preached wisdom of ignorance (awareness of nothingness), match between knowledge and action and unity of happiness and virtue. This spirit is succeeded by Plato and blooms in Aristotle. It is the establishment of Greek philosophy. Philosophy was born not only by intellectual curiosity but also by the spirit and passion of rebuilding the nation. The lesson from Socrates is, moreover, the courage that does not fear death and the passion of friendship that helps a young friend who went missing on the battlefield. The attitude of Socrates is inherited by Plato and Aristotle. Especially, it is justice of Aristotle and Philia (friendship). At this point, I used to discuss 'Benevolence of Confucius and Philia of Aristotle' (included in my next book)[10]. Just the current virus problem originating in China overlaps with justice and friendship. Infectious diseases link Chinese and Greek philosophies. Both Confucius and Aristotle were honest in truth.

---

[10] The first publication of this paper was *Voice of Intellectual Man - An International Journal,* Year 2011, Volume-1, Issue-2 (July–December), India, Lucknow University.

[7] *"Mystery of Oedipus"*, Atsuhiko Yoshida, Seidosha, Tokyo, p. 216, 1995.

[8] Saitama Medical University, the curriculum bulletin, No.8, p.15-25 2000-03-31.

[9] Thucydides, *"History of the Pelopponnesian War"*, *"Great Books of the World : Herodotus and Thucydides"* Chuōkōronsha, Tokyo, 1970, p. 366.

[10] The first publication of this paper was *Voice of Intellectual Man - An International Journal,* Year 2011, Volume-1, Issue-2 (July–December), India, Lucknow University.

5. Benevolence of Confucius and Philia of Aristotle

A huge tsunami, caused by the Great East Japan Earthquake, occurred in 2011 swallowing many cities and killing 22,000 people. In addition, the tsunami caused a power outage at the Fukushima nuclear power plant and shut down the reactor cooling system. A nuclear reactor with heat had a steam explosion. The recovery is still pending. This is the paper I wrote for that crisis. I quoted this when Japan was once badly damaged by the Great East Japan Earthquake but at that time people from 130 countries helped. Where roads and railroads were cut off by the tsunami, American aircraft carrier and destroyers came offshore the Sanriku region where laid the damaged cities and carried necessary supplies by helicopters. This was called Operation Tomodachi (Friend) and was considered by President Obama at the time.

This kind of friendship assistance struck the Japanese heart. There, Aristotle's Philia (友愛, yūai), that wishes the best of the other and Confucius's human brothers (仁, jin) realized. Now is the global crisis. Every country is in a difficult situation. Japan, the United States, and Europe are suffering. However, we Japanese do not want to immerse ourselves in our pains but to recall the help and benefits that we once received from the world. Further we hope to encourage and cooperate with the people of the world. So I took up this report. The summary of this report is introduced.

Benevolence of Confucius and Philia of Aristotle

Through the difficulties of the huge earthquake and tsunami in Japan

Summary of the report: The huge earthquake and Tsunami assaulted Japan on March 11, 2011. The Great East Japan Earthquake, at it is known today, destroyed several cities immediately and devastated a quarter of the Japanese land. The damage in Japan is similar to the Great Kantō Earthquake (1923) and the destruction of World War II. Still more, nuclear plants lost their cooling equipment systems and as a result hydrogen explosions occurred. These are the triple catastrophes. We the Japanese people are facing a desperate crisis. But many countries support us, Japan. The rescue-teams and assistance from over 130 countries gave us a big encouragement and hope. How highly the civilization and sciences do develop, they are powerlessness against the might of nature. Some of the strongest embankments in the world that were 10 metres high were immediately wiped out by a tsunami tidal wave of up to 40 metres high. We have the emotion of fear for nature and we recognize the powerlessness and nothingness of human beings. But we helped and supported each other in these times of hardship. Rescue and encouragement are hope and light in the darkness. We learn that though the sciences develop highly, we need benevolence and philia (friendship). Infra I wish to expound on these hardships.

"New Horizon of Sciences by the Principle of Nothingness and Love" (Lambert Academic Publishing, 2012, p.188)

Conclusion

The damage of the corona virus continues still now. With the exception of China, South Korea and Taiwan, all countries are under the state of emergency. The shops are closed in the downtown areas and the schools are closed. Even during consecutive holidays, one is in a situation of waiting at home. Human beings are in danger of being threatened by the invisible corona virus. One cannot start by just worrying about this crisis. Looking back on history, a new philosophy is born in crisis. Socrates lived in the hardships of war and epidemic fever. Citizens of

Athens also encountered darkness and nothingness. However, in this encounter Socrates preached philosophy with endless passion for (infinite) wisdom, courage that does not fear death, respect for daimonion (the voice of the divine spirit), and love for the people of Athens. It conforms to the principle of nothingness and love that continues to nothingness → infinity → eternity → god (transcendent-being) → love. This was inherited from Plato and Aristotle. Aristotle also experienced nothingness as the lack of his parents as an orphan. Then he questioned the infinite and eternal nature and the world. He experienced the organic continuity of himself and the universe, and he intuited the god (transcendent-being). That is theōria as happiness. However, this happiness continues to the world peace not only by the individual but also by Philia who wishes the best for the other person. Confucius who preached benevolence (Jin) also experienced the lack of parents as an orphan and sought infinite, eternal learning and truth. It was Heaven (transcendent-being) that he encountered after that. The teaching of Confucius is the practice of benevolence and love in heaven. Socrates, Aristotle and Confucius are also synthesized by my principle of nothingness and love. This is the new horizon of philosophy. From there, what can be done towards this modern hardship is to humbly pray for the transcendent-being and for early recovery and peace. And it is the transmission of philosophy that overcomes the upcoming US-China confrontation by world cooperation.

References

Ai 2020. Ai, Fen (艾芬). "Wuhan Chinese Female Doctor's Note" Bungeishunjū May issue 2020 and Bunshun (URL: https://news.yahoo.co.jp/articles/439a6418a1ace5d82c375c87575d6e639ce1de03)

Aikawa 1997. Aikawa, Masamichi, Nagakura, Koichi: "*Modern Infectious Diseases*" Iwanami Shoten, 1997

Aristotle 1934. Aristotle. *Nicomachean Ethics,* translated by H.Rackham, The Loeb Classical Library, Harvard University Press, 1934

Aristotle 1935. Aristotle. *Metaphysics,* I & II volumes. Trans. by Hugh Tredennick & G. Cyril Armstrong, Loeb Classical Library, 1935.

Aristotle 1957. Aristotle. *The Physics,* I & II volumes. Trans. by Philip H. Wicksteed & Francis M. Conford, William Heinemann LTD Harvard University Press, 1957.

Aristotle 1959. Aristotle. *Metaphysics,* I & II volumes. Trans. by Takashi Ide, Iwanamibunko, Tokyo, 1959.

Aristotle 1968-1973. Aristotle. *Aristotle Complete Works*, old version 17 volumes, Translated and edited by Takashi Ide, Iwanamihoten, Tokyo, 1968–1973.

Aristotle 1976. Aristotle. *Aristoteles*, Great Books of the World, Translated and edited by Michitarō Tanaka, Chuōkōronsha, Tokyo, 1976.

Hinuma 1986. Hinuma, Yorio: "*New Story of Virus*" Chuko Shinsho, Tokyo, 1986

Nakatomi 2002. Nakatomi, Kiyokazu (中富清和): *Philosophy of Nothingness and Love(無と愛の哲学)*, Hokuju Company, Japanese original version, Tokyo, 2002.

Nakatomi 201. Nakatomi, Kiyokazu (中富清和): *Philosophy of Nothingness and Love,* Lambert Academic Publishing, Saarbrücken, English version, 2016.

Nakatomi 2012. Nakatomi, Kiyokazu (中富清和): *New Horizon of Sciences by the Principle of Nothingness and Love,* Lambert Academic Publishing, Saarbrücken, English version, 2012.

Nakatomi 2015. Nakatomi, Kiyokazu (中富清和): 'The Synthesis of the theory of relativity and quantum theory' *Elixir International Journal, Elixir Condensed Matter Phys. 85,* Poland, 2015

Okada 2004. Okada, Harue: "*Human race versus Infectious Diseases*", Iwanami Shoten, Tokyo, 2004

Pagels 1984. Pagels, Heinz R.: The Cosmic Code: quantum Physics as Language of Nature (Simon & Schuster, New York, 1982) Japanese translation title: The ultimate of a material. Translated by Eiichi Kuroboshi, Chijinshokan. Tokyo, 1984

Saito 2000. Saito, Hiroshi , 'Is the disease in Athens Marburg disease or Ebola fever?' Saitama Medical University, the curriculum bulletin, No.8, 2000-03-31

Saito 2020. Saito, Naoki, 'The mystery on the origins of new corona virus', e-Discourse "*Hundred Schools of Thought Contend (百家争鳴)*", The Council on East Asian Community (CEAC), Tokyo, 2020-04-02, http://www.ceac.jp/j/index.html

Thucydides 1970. Thucydides: "History of the Pelopponnesian War", "Great Books of the World: Herodotus and Thucydides" Chuōkōronsha, Tokyo, 1970

VIM 2011. *Voice of Intellectual Man - An International Journal,* Year 2011, Volume-1, Issue-2 (July–December), India, Lucknow University.

Xiao 2020. Xiao Botao (肖波涛), 'The possible origins of 2019-n-CoV coronavirus'

Yoshida 1995. Yoshida, Atsuhiko: "*Mystery of Oedipus*", Seidosha, Tokyo, p. 216, 1995

Kiyokazu Nakatomi was born in August 10, 1955 in Hakodate City, Hokkaido, Japan. He studied politics and economics at Meiji University, Tokyo and now he works at Chiba Prefectural Matsuo High School as a social study and ethics teacher. Also he is the author of "*Philosophy of Nothingness and Love*" (2002 Japan, 2016 Germany) and "*New Horizon of Sciences by the Principle of Nothingness and Love*" (2012 Germany). Nakatomi is a member of the Philosophical society of Japan, the Japanese Association for Comparative Philosophy, la Société franco-japonaise de philosophie, the World Congress of Philosophy and the Biocosmological Association. His papers are published in 10 languages in 16 countries.

Some of the basic and inspiring principles of his philosophy are as follows: in his book, to establish "the principle of nothingness and love", he researched the subject of 'nothingness' throughout all ages and civilizations and noted that 'nothingness' leads to infinity ~ eternity ~ the transcendent-Being which is God, and to love - a continuing process.

By this principle, he could establish a bridge of philosophy between East and West and synthesize the Asian and European philosophies.

It creates a road of world philosophy and a new horizon of sciences.

The Moment of Dao: Despair, Joy, and Resilience in the Time of Global Pandemic 2020

Robin R. Wang, Loyola Marymount University, USA

Abstract

Our life has been disrupted by sheltering in place for months, and there is no end to the pandemic in sight but amounts of uncertainty, agitation, stress, worry, and anxieties. How bad is the despair of lockdown? How sad is the absence of joy when our habituated travel stops? and how hard is it to live through this new normal? This pandemic manifests an existential tension between "things that cannot be avoided" (無可奈何 *wuke naihe*) and "following the desires of your heart" (随心所欲 *suixin suoyu*). Thus Convid-19 crisis offers a splendid opportunity to learn about the Dao. This moment of Dao compels us to combine the critical perspective of the Daoist version of life with the worldly immersion of ordinary living that continues to matter.

Key words

Chinese Culture, Connectivity, Daoism, Despair, Inevitable, Hope, Nourishing, Joy, Resilience, Wander.

> *"The difference between hope and despair is a different way of telling stories from the same facts"* (Alain de Botton)

Harmful viruses are nothing new. Human beings have been living with all kinds of microbes, those deadly companions, since the very beginning (Crawford, 2009,10). However, COVID-19 marks the first global crisis in human history that devastates at a deep level. This virus is no longer the problem of a specific person, region, or culture. Its indiscriminate nature strikes without regard to the social, economic, or even moral worth of the individuals affected, signifying that we all are in this together. The pandemic offers us a splendid opportunity to learn about the Dao. It is the moment of Dao, which is at the core of this moment of perspective, polarity, and paradox that continually stun. This pregnant moment compels us to combine the critical perspective of the Daoist version of life with the worldly immersion of ordinary living that continues to matter.

Our life has been disrupted by sheltering in place for months, and there is no end to the pandemic in sight but amounts of uncertainty, agitation, stress, worry, and anxieties. This is an existential tension between "things that cannot be avoided" (無 可 奈 何 *wuke naihe*) and "following the desires of your heart" (随心所欲 *suixin suoyu*). The situation Zhuangzi calls "inevitable" (*budeyi* 不得已) (*Zhuangzi*, Chapter 4). Zhuangzi claims, "Knowing something you can do nothing about but resting (安 *an*) in *ming* 命(trajectory, allotment, destiny) is the ultimate power (*zhide* 至德)" (*Zhuangzi*, Chapter 4). Here, Zhuangzi emphasizes recognizing the "contingency" (*youdai* 有待) of life and accepting the *ming* (allotment) rather than seeking an unattainable ideal of "control" (*zhi* 治). However, this complex global dynamic demands our ability to thrive in ambiguous and feebly defined situations. How bad is the despair of lockdown? How sad is the absence of joy when our habituated travel stops, and how hard is it to live through this new normal? These questions scale up over our daily life in response to our needs for a basic mental and physical copping tool.

This essay turns to the *Zhuangzi* for inspiration and solution. In *Zhuangzi* Chapter Four, we read, "Let yourself be carried along by things (*chengwu* 乘物) so that the heart/mind wanders freely (*youxin* 游心). Hand it all over to the unavoidable (不得已 *budeji*), so as to nourish what is central within you (*yangzhong* 养中). That is the most you can do." This position encompasses three specific modes of comportment: being carried along by things(*chengwu)*; letting the heart/mind wander(*youxin)*, and nourishing what is central within you (*yangzhong*). This essay will unfold these three aspects by clarifying "being carried along by things" in light of despair; appreciating "letting the heart/mind wander" through finding the ultimate source of joy; and aiming at human flourishing through "nourishing the center"! This essay is not an attempt to prove a point but an evocation or a vision that might bring out a composed mind comprehending human flourishing during this COVID-19 crisis.

1. Connectivity: The Link Between Despair and Hope

Epidemics are nothing new in Chinese history. The word *yi* 疫 (epidemic) is different than the word *bing* 病(illness). The *Shuowen jiezi* says, "Epidemic means that all people have a disease" 疫为民皆疾也. Among the many disasters in the Eastern Han and Three Kingdome period (25AD -280 AD), epidemics had about every 25 years and was the most severe impacts. With the dreadful experience of epidemic, people desperately envisioned a protective web. Two very influential grassroot movements often seen as marking the beginning of Daoist religious lineages, Great Peace (*Taiping* 太平) and Celestial Masters (*Tianshi Dao* 天師), emerged in that period, and they became the powerful allies in the fight against epidemics and the Han government. According to *Post Han History* (*Hou Hanshu*), Zhang Jiao, 张角 the founder of the Dao of Great Peace, prescribed medicinal herbs and drew *fu* 符 (talisman/charms)[1] for the curing of diseases; it states, "Patients healed quite well. People believed in it."[2] Drawing *fu* is the way to seek for cosmic help to make the sense of this tragic human life.

It is the similar with the case of Zhang Daoling, 张道凌, founder of the Celestial Masters that was also called Dao of Five Buckets of Rice (五斗米道 *Wudoumi Dao*).[3] That was because people paid five buckets of rice after being treated by the practitioners and recovering from the sickness.

These movements under the name of Dao addressed people's deepest needs to stay alive, to confront their urgent perplexity, to relieve the pain, to offer healing remedies to the sick, and to bring the community out of its difficult conditions. The Daoist text the *Classics of Great Peace* (太平经 *Tai Ping Jing*) discusses the Daoist art of healing as an integration of three historical practices: The Arts of Shamanism 巫术, the Arts of Healing 医术, and the Arts of *Yangsheng* 养生术. Freedom from disease, physiological signs of well-being, and avoidance of death appear as the consistent issues that Daoists cared about. There is no surprise that many Daoists were also famous and celebrated Chinese physicians who discovered many effective methods for treating or eliminating epidemics in Chinese history.

Zhuangzi's important notion of "letting be carried by things" or "riding with events and things" (*chengwu*) reveals that life is marked by contingency and the scope of human control is limited. This underlying assumption is the tenet of connectivity and relationality. Human beings are intrinsically connected with nature, other people, and all the myriad things. This con-

---

[1] The term *fu* is most readily translated as "talisman," but it can also be translated as "charm." During the Han dynasty, a *fu* was an agreement or contract between people. *Fu* states that an action needed to be taken, and it as an order of performance. This intention of a *fu* was retained in Daoist practice, but the contract was refocused between humans and numinous powers. So, a talisman is a kind of performance contract. *Fu* are used to bind demonic spirits and cure disease, protect sacred spaces, and transmit blessings.

[2] 《后汉书》张角 "符水咒说以疗病，病者顾愈，百姓信向之"。

[3] They were also known as the Yellow Turbans who envisioned a new era of Great Peace and rebelled in the 180s.

nectivity bears on nature as the wellspring of therapeutic healing. A consistent feature of the Daoist way is to deal with fear and despair in the human condition by going back to nature.

A striking phenomenon of this Daoist practice is its fascinating attraction to mountains, caves, rivers and oceans. Daoists are well-known for their love of natural places where they develop their creativity as well as pursue the techniques of longevity. Many stories of 仙人 *xianren* (semi-legendary humans who live in mountains) tell about their lives and accomplishments in mountains. One famous collection is by Ge Hong 葛洪 (283–343), *Traditions of Divine Transcendents* 神仙传, in which he writes, "All those who compound elixirs in cultivating the Dao, avoiding disorder to live in hiding, go into the mountains. But if one does not know the methods of going into the mountains, he will encounter misfortune and injury" (凡為道合藥及避亂隱居者莫不入山然不知入山法者多遇禍害). Mountain dwelling practices were developed into Daoist geographical places called "Heaven-reaching grottoes" (洞天 *dongtian*) and "blessed grounds" (福地 *fudi)* where practitioners underwent bio-spiritual transformations that rendered them into immortals (*xian*) or Perfected Person. Sima Chengzhen 司马承祯 (647–735) consolidated the lore about these grotto-heavens and blessed places into 10 major grotto-heavens, 36 minor grotto-heavens, and 72 blissful places, and provided details of their names, locations, and the numinous spirits associated with them. (Littlejohn, 2019, 99-100)

Why did Daoists want to dwell in mountains and what is special about their particular manner of doing it? Mountain dwelling is simply the best way to experience the rhythm of nature. One ought to take account of the specific hour, day, month, season, and year; pay special attention to other numerous natural conditions, such as snakes, poisonous insects and other creatures, and poisonous growths. Yet mountains also offer various medicines, pills, and potions for human survive. In the cave, seekers of the Dao enter into the space of quietude and stillness as if re-entering the mother's womb, and with a mind emptied of human destructions and paradigms, able to move in emptiness. Many Daoist temples have always been built on the mountains, far from the crowed city dwellings.

Subsequently, an exit strategy for anxiety, insecurity, and melancholy in human world at difficult times like the present is to attune or align with nature as something greater, comforting and easy to access. The link between the cyclic pattern of nature and the patterns of human existence is also the link between despair and hope. If one can truly appreciate the natural and inevitable flow of things, like the seasonal changes, then one can gain insight and hope for life, and thereby infuse the human mind and human perception with a greater energy flow to image, integrate and prosper. This vision is rooted in one important Daoist commitment: human well-being depends on the planetary world from which humans can possibly "get" or "attain" (得 *de*) the Dao. This Daoist dedication supports the contemporary call to redefine human being as a planetary being.

To guide humans to heed nature's voice and to direct their attention to trust the flow of nature is a gift to ourselves. It endows human beings with a cosmic dimension and captures the passion behind dashed hopes to turn them toward transformative change through which they can be ultimately realized. Zhuangzi teaches us that humans as co-existing with nature rather than existing in a bubble, can embellish the deep sense of interconnectivity. We should acquire the ability to communicate with, or become citizens of, the cosmos at large.

2. Heavenly Wander: The Ultimate Source of Joy

Our first real-time global pandemic has broken the inertia of old ways by forcing everyone to stay at home. Social distancing and lockdowns have shifted our living conditions beyond what we have ever experienced. This poses the very question of our own mental and spiritual immunity and the source of our joy in daily life. Can we still go through life with joy? While joy is relational and derives from the interaction among oneself, external things, and natural events, how is it possible to cultivate a deeper sense of joy while social distancing and being locked down at home? Of all the pressing challenges emanating from the COVID-19 crisis, one of the foremost is that of restoring the capacity for finding joy in life. And joy brings deeper, richer satisfactions than the fleeting emotions or despair.

Zhuangzi fashions a 游 *you*, a "wandering," to deepen one's existential rootedness within the world. *You* is one of the most significant philosophical positions in Zhuangzi's teachings and the key to open his inscrutable world. *You* as wandering is an indispensable part of Zhuangzi's critical mindset, playful attitude, and primary manner of being in the world. The title of the first chapter of the *Zhuangzi* is 逍遥游 "Xiaoyao You" (Free and Easy Wandering), a phrase that is used 113 times throughout the text. The original meaning of *you* referred to the flow of the flag or the flow of water, but it took on a more complex and stimulating signification. Wang Fuzhi 王夫之 (1619-1692) explains Zhuangzi's *you* as a state of being where "things all exist on a pair and are interdependent. *You* is the manifestation of this link and interaction…all the myriad things are bound to *you* and nothing but *you*." (Wang 1964, 1). The values of human experience as well as the optimal conditions for human life are inseparable from this *you*-ing reality. This *you* is not simply transforming with things and embodying the cosmic flow, but it is also the source of joy (*le*) in life. It is the most reasonable and valuable way to exist and respond to the world.

You as the source of joy emerges from three sources: 外游 *waiyou*, "external wandering" or *you*-ing in the natural landscape, as seen in the modern expression 游山玩水 *youshan wanshui*. It is an enjoyable experience to wander freely in the mountains or play in the water, or even to go on a sightseeing tour. Wandering in nature can provide a wide range enjoyment, however this is only "dependent *you*" as short-lived enjoyment rooted in external things that will quickly pass.

Another *you* is 內游 *neiyou*, the internal wandering through one's own heart/mind. This *you* is rooted in one's own internal horizon and the ability to perform inner observation. Wandering in one's heart/mind does not rely on external things, external stimulations or sensory input. This *you*-ing is a self-sufficient loop of *you* heart/mind. Zhuangzi defines that "the wandering of the heart/mind is the gestalt of *de* (potency or power)" (游心于德之和). This vantage point on *you* is a significant source of internal joy, and one does not need to physically go to the mountains or the ocean in order to experience a joy. One can adapt the current circumstance to find joy within despite physical limitations and other constrains. This is the transformation of the source of joy from external sources to a self-sufficient fountain. The pandemic has instantly turned our home into an office, a daycare center, a school, a restaurant, a concert hall and even a gym. We are confined in very limited physical spaces and require a special adaptive ability to make it joyful.

Third, *you* is the *you*-ing Dao (游道 *youdao*) where *you*-ing in eternity is unlimited. This *you* "does not depend on things," more importantly "it flows with Heaven and follow the Dao" and it "brings the ultimate beauty and the ultimate joy." Heavenly joy is using the heart/mind as a mirror to reflect and embody all things. (*Zhuangzi, Tiandao*)

Zhuangzi explains this in a dialogue between Confucius and Laozi. "Confucius asked, 'What is *you*?' Laozi replied, 'If one gets it, they have the ultimate beauty and joy. One who can get ultimate beauty and wander in ultimate joy is the ultimate person." (*Zhuangzi, Tianzifang*)

This heavenly *you* is consistent with Zhuangzi's grand project to lift up human being to the realm of total freedom. As such, this *you* is also "the wanderer of picked perfection." (*Zhuangzi* 天运). The vision of Heavenly joy has also clarifies a vital issue of choice and behavior, namely involving adaptation. Adaptation is about accepting a particular situation as it occurs and deciding for and by oneself the course of action that suits the situation best. This is a movement or transformation from the understanding of phenomenal reality to epistemological equanimity. Such this equanimity gives a person the prospect approaching the phenomenal world with ease.

3. Nourishing Life: A Resilient Processual Practice and Life Style

The global pandemic deconstructs not only the judgement of 'I have to do it this way" but also demands innovatively a "stay at home" new normal to live by. It compels us to examine those ingrained assumptions and become humbler. The resilient person from Daoist perspective will be able to make this transition smoothly from those ingrained past ways of doing things to resourcefully discovering a less familiar path to walk on.

The pertinent question is whether the global pandemic experience will fruitfully merge with a long-term vision of life and livelihood? Are we all waiting to go back to those old normal or are we undergoing a different future? The pandemic manifests that life is not all about assembly and manufacture. This brings a binary context: attunement vs. production. Does human life entail the attunement to nature and cosmos or is it simply about productivity?

It is worth pointing out that when one faces the unavoidable condition, Zhuangzi teaches to "respond" 感 *gan* with a way or strategy. The perfected person(真人 *zhenren*) will not solidify the condition but rather optimize it. This is the *de* of *zhenren*. This is why later Daoists took as a credo, "My allotted life span resides with me; it does not reside with Heaven." Daoist resilience is what gives people the psychological strength to handle with stress and hardship. It is the mental reservoir of power that people can rely on in times of need without falling apart.

Yet this is not only a mental strength but taking an action in day to day life. For Zhuangzi under the condition of the "inevitable" (*budeyi* 不得已) one can make the "nourishing what is central within you" (养中 *yangzhong*) as a circadian routine. There are different ways to interpret the concept of nourishment the center *yangzhong*, which can be seen in three practices: cultivating the heart/mind (养心 *yangxin*); harnessing *qi* energy (养气 *yangqi*); and the penetrating the central meridian (养督 *yangdu*). These are protective measures for contending with unescapable living conditions that express the multifaced characters of resilience.

The term *yang* 養 (to nourish) is a key Daoist concept and has a special position in Chinese thought. Philosophical works, self-cultivation manuals, canonical medical writings, transcendence writings, and scriptural Daoist texts all pay attention to this concept and its related practices. It emphasized the nourishing of the vital principle (*yangsheng* 養生), the nourishing of the body (*yangxing* 養形), the nourishing of inner nature (*yangxing* 養性 or *yangshen* 養身), the nourishing of aspiration (*yangzhi* 養志), the nourishing of the spirit (*yangxin* 養心), and the nourishing of the vital spirits (*yangshen* 養神). *Yang* signifies a process of cultivation that also includes a variety of health regiments. It engaged health as a quantitative object that could be stored in the body and as a processual goal rather than a conceptual object. It consists of adopting a way of daily life regulated by physico-mental-emotional hygienic standards.

The first aspect of *yangzhong* is *yangxin* "nourishing the heart/mind" to make it tranquil 靜

, calm 安, stable 定, aligned 正, orderly 治, complete, and concentrated 摶. This state of the heart/mind is attained through 坐忘 *zuowang* "sit and forget" and 心齋 *xinzhai* "the fasting of mind/heart." In Chapter two, Zhuangzi nicely describes *zuowang* and *xinzhai*, both of which lead to the inhibition of automatization or, as psychologists call it today, emotion regulation. Neurologically, this is the core process of *zuowang*. In other words, rather than a dismantling of consciousness, the practice involves a conscious reprogramming and refinement of mental reactions.

The second aspect of *yangzhong* is *yangqi* "nourishing *qi*." Zhuangzi mentions an important term in *qi* regulation, *tuna* 吐納 "to spit out and take in [*qi*]" or, more precisely, *tugu naxin* 吐古納新 "to spit out the old and take in the new [*qi*]." This guiding and refining the flow of vital energy or vital breath (*qi*) within the human organism *qi* treatment brings the mind and body out of an "agitated and impure" (*dongzhuo* 動濁) state to one that is more "still and clear (*jingqing* 靜清)" (Kohn 2009, 80). One approaches oneness with nature or embodying the Dao by filling the body with the cosmic *qi*. These sorts of *qi* cultivation practices deconstruct a lingering mind-body dualism, freeing the body—the carnal and somatic aspects of our lived embodiment—to choose, think, and possess its own wisdom.

The third aspect of *yangzhong* is *yangdu*. In Chapter 3, Zhuangzi mentions the central meridian (督 *du*), where he writes that humans amplify their life by "maintaining our bodies to keep the life in them intact, to nourish those near and dear to us, and to fully live out our years" (*Zhuangzi* Chapter 2) Zhuangzi seeks to convert temporary equanimity into a sustainable daily lifestyle by way of a macrobiotic hygiene practice. This involves experiencing the world through the totality of our existence, not just the mind, in the language of the body that thrives on reality.

Typically, early Daoist texts discuss this transformation of the body and its energies in the rhetoric of longevity 壽 (*shou*) or long life 長生 (*changsheng*), terms referring to the transformed body's ability to endure change and the passage of time without letting the energies of the body disperse. Such a discourse reveals that long life never constituted a separate and isolated soteriological goal in itself; rather, it translates into daily life practice to become a lifestyle. Only a body that was at the height of vitality could embody the Dao, and the vital body was more than enough to endow a longevity. This circle of maintenance and rejuvenation of the body's vitality is articulated in *Huangdi Neijing*. As to the question why people are short lived, Xi Bo says that those who only just know the Dao are able to enjoy the longevity of 100 years because they can do these things: "model yin-yang, synchronizing with cosmic numbers, regulate food and drink, standardize sleep routines, and not arbitrarily laboring; therefore, physical form and spirit can be amalgamated."

The most common methods for dealing with daily life events and ordinary decision-making involved calendars, action patterns and ordered behavior. They made clear the value of simple routines in proper diet, plentiful sleep and peaceful emotions.

We all hope that global scientists and political leaders around world will be able to unite as they come up with the most effective way to handle this global pandemic. In the meantime, we cannot just docilely wait for a change to come. We ought to turn to the world with a dose of self-vigilance, which Zhuangzi called "being watchful over oneself" (*shenqidu* 慎其獨). The pandemic has shove us to contend with the bare facts of life as we try to get by in whatever way we can, cooking your own meals, cleaning your house, and cutting your own peculiar hair. This is the simplicity of life! The pause is constructive and gives us a chance to reflect on the plain things in our life and our existence with discernment and clarity. More importantly, it calls us to live simply and joyfully. Could our character be strong like a soccer ball: kicked all directions in the day, it will still be round at night? This is Zhuangzi's axis of Dao (*Daoshu*)道枢.

Zhuangzi takes as an epistemological stance that sees through dichotomy to polarity, through the superficial to the subtle, from the manifold to the pluralistic, and he does this by privileging the concrete over the abstract. For example, if someone thought that lipstick will give her confidence in public, then wearing a face mask in public will impose her to find other sources of confidence. Zhuangzi cultivates a human ability to turn an apparently unfortunate situation into a fertile ground for planting a new kind of the fruit of life. In Daoist teachings, only understanding or having a proper perspective is not good enough or merely sufficient condition. The physical and mental *yang* (nourishing) must be in a place, which points to a physical regiment to follow, because this is the way to lead a Daoist life.

Conclusion

Though so much remains unclear in these rapidly evolving days, what is clear is that the COVID-19 pandemic is the "great accelerator" that suddenly moved us from the continuity of the past into a new era. This essay takes this moment of variance as a sudden emergence of new insight to grasp the Dao. Pandemic brings the world to a Dao moment in which we can learn, appreciate, and practice Dao. This essay has developed three bases for the construction of a new trajectory with which to validate Zhuangzi's way to manage existential conflict and tension. The COVID-19 pandemic is the "great accelerator" that suddenly moved us from the continuity of the past into a new era. This essay has developed three bases for the construction of a new trajectory with which to articulate Zhuangzi's way to manage existential conflict and tension. The scope of pandemic that affects everyone will inevitably also bring changes that impact everyone. Humans around world all will involve trade-offs between constituencies of the past and the future, among contending interests and contesting worldviews. This essay end with Zhuangzi's advice: "Let your mind wander in simplicity; blend your vital energy (*qi*) with the boundless silence, following the natural flow of each thing without your own bias. Then all under Heaven will be in order." This guides the unforeseen and unavoidable as conditions of possibility, of new dimensions and of being in this world. The reality of how things are and what they become always determines the way how we deal with them, taking advantage of those conditions rather than letting them become limitations.

References

Camany 2002. Campany, Robert Ford. To Live as Long as Heaven and Earth: A Translation and Study of Ge Hong's Traditions of Divine Transcendents. (University of California Press)

Crawford 2009. Crawford, Dorothy. *Deadly Companions: How Microbes Shaped Our History*, Oxford University Press.

Kohn 2010. Kohn, Livia. Sitting in Oblivion: The Heart of Daoist Meditation translated, Three Pines.

Littlejohn 2019. Littlejohn, Ronny. *Historical Dictionary of Daoism (Historical Dictionaries of Religions, Philosophies, and Movements Series*, Rowman Littlefield.

Nylan 2001. Nylan, Michael "On the Politics of Pleasure" *Asia Major* , 2001, Vol. 14, No. 1 pp. 73-124, Academia Sinica.

Wang 1964. Wang Fuzhi 王夫之著，王孝鱼点校，庄子解[M].中华书局，1964年10月版

Ziporyn 2009. Ziporyn, Brook. Translation: *Zhuangzi The Essential Writings with Selections from Traditional Commentaries*, translated by Brook Ziporyn, (Hackett)

Robin R. Wang is Professor of Philosophy at Loyola Marymount University, Los Angeles and The Berggruen fellow (2016-17) at The Center for Advanced Study in the Behavioral Sciences (CASBS), Stanford University. Her teaching and research center on Chinese and Comparative Philosophy, particularly on Daoist Philosophy, Women and Gender in Chinese culture and tradition. She is the author of *Yinyang: The Way of Heaven and Earth in Chinese Thought and Culture* (Cambridge University Press 2012) and editor of *Chinese Philosophy in an Era of Globalization*, (SUNY Press 2004) and *Images of Women in Chinese Thought and Culture: Writings from the Pre-Qin Period to the Song Dynasty* (Hackett 2003). She was the President of *Society for Asian and Comparative Philosophy* (2016-18). Contact: robin.wang@lmu.edu.

Communitarianism, Liberalism and Confucianism

Yuli Liu, Party School of the Central Committee of Communist Party of China, China

Abstract

Comparing with the constitutive self in new liberalism, the self in Confucianism is a role-carrying and inter-related self who lives in the five relationships. In order to adjust these relationships and to achieve harmony in the society, *li* were set up to make the relationships stable and the emphasis was laid on the duty and virtue demanded of the parties concerned in each relationship. Confucians emphasize the primacy of virtues over rights, the primacy of the common good over rational self-interest, which is echoed by communitarianism in the west.This will help us to understand why China has performed effectively to implement containment measures during the Corona pandemic period.

Key Words

Confucianism,common good, self, harmony

During the Corona pandemic period, China has acted effectively to implement containment measures. The Chinese people also performed very differently from that of the western countries who claim individual freedom and the 'so-called' human rights. Why did the Chinese response to the government's calls and obey the regulations so easily? In order to answer this question, it is necessary to understand Confucianism, the ruling school which has influenced China for more than two thousands years. In so doing, it would be easy for the westerners to understand Confucianism by comparing it with communitarianism and new liberalism in western philosophy.

I. The Challenges to Liberalism from Communitarianism

Communitarianism[1] is a political and ethical theory which gives the priority of the common good to individual rights and emphasises the importance of the social, historical, cultural and communal contexts in human being's moral life. It came into being in the movement challenging John Rawls's new liberalism at the beginning of the 1980s. Rawls abandoned the then-ruling theory of utilitarianism and erected his own in the tradition of contract theories and Kantian liberalism. Moreover, Rawls's theory bypassed the heretofore heavily discussed questions of political obligation and the state, and raised the issue of distributive justice, as well as --- indirectly--- the welfare state. It was a theory that put the issue of rights on the agenda and was constructed in individual terms.[2]

The challenges from communitarianism to liberalism result from two aspects: on the one hand, Ralws's liberalism offers an ethics based on the ideas of justice centring around the concepts of rational rights and practical principles which excludes a good foundation of morality. Liberals are said by communitarians to be only concerned about the issues of moral facts, while ignoring the foundation on which morals are based; only concerned about the importance of 'the

---

[1] Although Communitarianism is a contemporary political theory, the term 'community' is not new in political thought. In fact it goes back to Greek philosophy, to Aristotle's works, through Cicero and the Roman community of law and common interests, St. Augustine's community of emotional ties, Thomas Aquinas's idea of the community as a body politic, Edmund Burke's well-known concept of the community as a partnership 'not only between the living, but between those who are living, those who are dead, and those who are to be born', and the works of Rousseau in France and Hegel in Germany. (See Avineri, Shlomo. and de- Shalit, Avner. (ed.), *Communitarianism and Liberalism*, Oxford, Oxford University Press, 1992, p. 1.)

[2] Avineri, Shlomo. and de- Shalit, Avner. (ed.), *Communitarianism and Liberalism*, Oxford, Oxford University Press, 1992, p. 1.

basic structure of the society' in protecting individual rights, while ignoring the need to limit individual rights and behaviours, and ignoring the importance of individual's obligations in realising the common good of the social community. This leads them to be keen on the institution of moral rules, rather than exploring the intrinsic virtue of the moral subject.

On the other hand, Rawls was blinded by the unlimited free individual, an antecedently-individuated self, or a subject of possession, thus ruling out the conception of a 'constitutive self', the possibility of 'inter-subjective' forms of self-understanding, and the commonality embodied in the 'constitutive self'. This inevitably leads them to an antecedent individualism.

Michael J. Sandel writes in his Liberals and the Limits of Justice: 'If utilitarianism fails to take seriously our distinctness, justice as fairness fails to take seriously our commonality. In regarding the bounds of the self as prior, fixed once and for all, it relegates our commonality to an aspect of the good, and regulates the good to a mere contingency, a product of indiscriminate wants and desires 'not relevant from a moral standpoint''. [3]Since 'justice as fairness' is the core conception (keystone) of Rawls's liberal political philosophy, Sandel's critique of the conception is in fact the critique to the foundation of Rawls's new liberal ethics. As he argues, traditional utilitarianism fails to take seriously our distinctness, which gives its theory of the good a bad name of non-individual teleology; while in order to give priority to individual rights, Rawls's liberal ethics fails to take seriously our commonality and unity. So he only 'wins for deontology a false victory'.[4] Let alone that Rawls's liberalism fails to have an insight into the foundation on which individual agents cultivate their moral obligations ------the psychological and emotional elements and intrinsic virtue, its understanding of self is obviously one-sided. In other words, the notion of the self in Ralws's liberalism is a self of possession, rather than a self with ends. That is, the question they are concerned with is the possession of the individual---'what is mine', rather than the identity of the individual---'what is me'. According to Sandel, this is one of the most important reasons why Rawls cannot erect a 'constitutive conception of community' in his new liberal ethics.[5]

Other communitarians also attack liberalism from different aspects. Alasdair MacIntyre, basing on Aristotle and Aquinas's political ethics and virtue theory, argued that liberalism was not able to give an intrinsic virtue foundation on which justice ethics could base; Charles Taylor, following Hegel's historical philosophy, regarded liberalism ethics as 'atomism', which exposed its nature of individualism. Migel.Walzer, providing a conception of 'membership', argued that community has an important impact and influence on individual's moral life.

In short, the debates between communitarianism and liberalism focus on two questions: Should ethics be based on the right or the good? Should ethics value individual person or a group of persons in the community (Should it give priority to individual or community)? The former leads to the difference in types of ethical theories; the latter leads to disagreement in the priority given to individual or community. Liberal ethics, giving priority to a rational foundation for individual rights, seeks an ethic of justice and rules or an ethics of obligation; while communitarian ethics, based on the common good of the community, seeks a moral axiology aiming at the good of community or an ethics of virtue based on personal virtues. The relationship of Confucianism and communitarianism lies in the fact that Confucianism is an ethics of virtue aiming at the common good of the community---the common good of family or the common good of state.

---

[3] Sandel, Michael J., *Liberals and the Limits of Justice*, Cambridge, Cambridge University Press, 1982, pp.174.

[4] Ibid.

[5] Ibid., p. 55.

II. The Role-carrying Self in Confucianism

'Confucianism' is a western term. It is said to be the equivalent of the Chinese term *Ju Jia* which means the school of Literati. The western term does not suggest, as the Chinese term does, that followers of this School were scholars as well as thinkers; they were the teachers of ancient classics and thus were the inheritors of ancient culture legacy. This is the reason why this school always carried on the orthodox tradition of the Chinese society, and for more than two thousand years its teaching was recognized by the State as the official philosophy both in education and in daily life.

There are three great thinkers in the Confucian School: Confucius (551-479 B.C.), Mencius or *Mengzi* (371-289 B.C.) and *Xunzi* (298-238B.C.). Confucius, the founder of he School, was primarily a moral teacher who set up a new standard of human values and a new ethical code to improve the conduct of life of his contemporary and later generations. He digested and synthesized the cultural achievements of the past and of his time and re-evaluated and re-interpreted them within the framework of his philosophy. The central theme of his teachings is a perfect development of personality and a proper standardization and adjustment of human relations with a view to the attainment of the supreme good, which is a parallel to communitarianism.

In order to have a thorough understanding of the thoughts and systems of Confucianism, it is better to start with the concept of self in Confucianism. Unlike a purely rational, rights-claiming, autonomous individual in western liberal ethics, the self in Confucianism is a role-carrying and interrelated individual, which is described vividly by Henry Rosemont, JR. as following:

For the early Confucians there would not have been much of me to be seen in isolation, to be considered abstractly: I am the totality of roles I live in relation to specific others. Moreover, these roles are interconnected in that the relations in which I stand to some people affect directly the relations in which I stand to others, such that it would be misleading to say that I play or perform these roles; on the contrary, for Confucius I am my roles. Taken collectively, these roles weave, for each of us, a unique pattern of personal identity, such that if my roles change, others will of necessity change also, literally making me a different person...

Further, my role as father, for example, is not merely a one-one relation to my daughters. In the first place, it has a significant bearing on my role as husband, just as the role of mother bears significantly on my wife's role as wife. Second, I am 'Samantha's father' not only to Samantha but also to her friends, and, someday, her husband's and her husband's parents as well. And Samantha's role as sister is determined in part by my role as father.

Going beyond the family, if I should become a widower, both my male and female friends would see me, respond to me, and interact with me, somewhat differently than they do now. A bachelor friend of mine, for instance, might invite me as a widower to accompany him on a three-month cruise, but he would not invite me as long as I was a husband.[6]

It can be seen from the above that the individual is always considered as person-in-society in Confucianism, existing in a network of relations. Mencius, the second sage of Confucianism, pointed out five human relations (*wulun*) in the book of Mencius: (1) father and son, (2) ruler and subordinate, (3) husband and wife, (4) brother and brother, and (5) friend and friend. In or-

---

[6] Henry Rosemont, JR., 'Classical Confucian and Contemporary Feminist Perspectives on the Self: Some Parallels and Their Implications', *Culture and Self*, Allen, Douglas. (ed.), Colorado, Westview Press, 1997, pp.71.

der to adjust these relationships, rules of conduct in the name of *li*[7] were set up to make the relationships stable and the emphasis was laid on the duty and obligation demanded of the parties concerned in each relationship and base on right ideal. Hence it is taught that the ideal ruler is benevolent, the ideal minister, loyal; the ideal father is compassionate, the ideal son filial; the ideal elder brother is kind, the ideal younger brother respectful; the ideal husband is righteous, the ideal wife submissive; the ideal friend is faithful.[8] If every person can abide by the rules of conduct (*Li*) and carry out the obligations suitable to his status, there will be peace in society.

In order to help people to carry out the obligations in practice, Confucius recommended what he called the "rectification of names". By which he meant that an act should correspond to its name. If one is a father or a son, one should live up to the relationships which the name implies. Confucius said: " when the father is father, the son is son, the elder brother is elder brother, the husband is husband, and the wife is wife, then the family is in proper order. When all families are in proper order, all will be right with the world."[9]This means, each name not only has a prescribed set of obligations, but also reflects a status. For example, that a son should be filial to his parent is not only an obligation. Performance of filial piety is the acid test by which a son can know that he is fulfilling his own life's role. In other words, the son fulfills it, not solely for the sake of the parent, but because this is what he owes to his own moral integrity. By this act, he proves to himself, as well as to others, that his claims to true manhood have validity.[10]

III. The Importance of Performing *Li* in Achieving Harmony in Confucian Ethics

Confucius said, "In carrying out *li*, harmony (*he*) is to be cherished." [11] Here the harmony (*he*) is not only meant to be in harmonious relationship with others in the society but also meant to be in harmony with oneself so that one can perform *li* with a peaceful state of mind. Thus the function of *li* is twofold: the self-realisation of individual man and the consequent harmonization of a society--- a community of men. So it is very important for everyone in the society to act according to *li*.

What is needed emphasis here is that *li* (rules of conduct) is not arbitrary. Confucius taught that the importance of *li* exists in that it is what is in harmony with universal order (the way of *Tian*) and based on human nature. Only thus could it successfully execute its function as a means of social control.

According to Confucianism, the way of heaven is harmony. *The Doctrine of the Mean* (*zhongyong*) teaches that "equilibrium is the great foundation of the world, and harmony its universal path. When equilibrium and harmony are realized to the highest degree, heaven and earth

---

[7] *Li* is a concept pregnant with ethico-religious connotations. The mere fact that it has been rendered as 'ceremony', 'ritual', 'rites', 'propriety', 'rules of propriety', 'good custom', 'decorum', 'good form', and a host of other ideas including that of nature law suggests the scope of its implications. Etymologically, the ideograph *li* symbolize a sacrificial act. As Wing-tsit Chan has pointed out, it originally meant 'a religious sacrifice'. Whether we focus on its original meaning of sacrifice or its derivative meaning of propriety, *li* implies the existence of an 'other'. To dwell on *li*, therefore, is not to remain isolated. On the contrary, it necessarily involves a relationship or a process by which a relationship comes into being. Thus, to relate oneself to another is the underlying structure of *li*. See Tu, Wei-ming, Li as process of humanization, in *Philosophy East and West*.

[8] *Liji, Liyun, the work of Mencius, Tengwengong.*

[9] The Yi King, in: Legge, James. (trans.), *The Scared Books of the East*, Vol. 16, Oxford, Claredon Press, 1899, p. 240.

[10] Hummel, Arthur W., 'The Art of Social Relation in China', *Philosophy East and West*, vol. 10, 1960-61, p. 14.

[11] *Analects*, I:12.

will attain their proper order and all things will flourish."[12] Confucius also said: "Does Heaven say anything? The four seasons run their course and all things are produced. Does Heaven say anything?" [13]What Confucius means is, although Heaven does not speak to man in a literal sense, we can know from the manifestation of the work of Heaven that there exist an objective order. The way of Heaven embodies a cosmic pattern --- a pattern which is an organic whole and in which everything is related to everything else. To be out of the relation is to be a non-entity.

The way of man and the way of Heaven are correlated with each other. Just as Mencius said, "Those who followed the way of *Tian* will be preserved, and those who act contrary to the way of *Tian* will perish". [14] So *Li* was made by sage-kings to guide conduct. Thereby would men perfectly order society and thereby would they be in proper accord with the cosmos. As the *Li Ji* (*Li Chi*) says, "It was by these rules that the ancient kings sought to represent the ways of Heaven and to regulate the feelings of men." [15]*Analects* also said, "Among the functions of propriety *(li)* the most valuable is that it established harmony. The excellence of the ways of ancient sage kings consists of this. It is the guiding principle of all things great and small."[16]

Li also has its origin in human nature. This is the reason why *li* can successfully regulate the feelings of men. According to Confucianism, human nature is originally good. All men, Mencius maintains, possess the four beginnings of humanity (*Jen*), righteousness (*Yi*), propriety (*Li*) and wisdom (*zhi*). The reason why man should have these four beginnings and his nature should consequently good, is that nature is what heaven have given to us. So Mencius said, "Man's innate ability is the ability possessed by him that is not acquired through learning. Man's innate knowledge is the knowledge is the knowledge possessed by him that is not the result of reflective thinking. Every child knows enough to love his parents, and when he is grown up he knows enough to respect his elder brothers. The love for one's parents is really humanity and the respect for one's elders is really righteousness---all that is necessary is to have these natural feelings applied to all men." [17] So if you let people follow their feelings (original nature), they will be able to do good. This is what is meant by saying that human nature is good. If man does evil, it is not the fault of his nature endowment. The feeling of commiseration is found in all men. For example, here is a man who suddenly notices a child about fall into a well. Invariably he will feel a sense of alarm and compassion. And this is not for the purpose of gaining the favour of the child's parents, or seeking the approbation of his neighbors and friends, or for fear of blame should be fail to rescue it. Thus we see that no man is without a sense of right and wrong. The sense of compassion is the beginning of humanity; the sense of shame is the beginning of righteousness; the sense of courtesy is the beginning of propriety, the sense of right and wrong is the beginning of wisdom. Every man has these four beginnings, just as he has four limbs. So it is said that the virtues of humanity (*Jen*), righteousness (*Yi*), propriety (*Li*), wisdom (*Zhi*) are not drilled into us from outside. We originally have them with us. They are rooted in

---

[12] The Doctrine of the Mean, in Chan, Wing-tsit. (ed. and trans.), *A Source Book of Chinese Philosophy*, Princeton, Princeton University Press, 1963, p. 98.

[13] *Analects,* 17:19.

[14] *The Book of Mencius*, IV.a.7.

[15] VII.1, 4. Legge, James. (trans.), *The Sacred Books of China: The Texts of Confucianism, Part III: The Li Ki, Sacred Books of the East*, Vol. 27, Oxford, The Clarendon Press, 1885, pp.367.

[16] *Analects,* 1:12, in: Chan, Wing-tsit (ed. and trans.), *A Source Book of Chinese Philosophy*, Princeton, Princeton University Press, 1963, pp.21.

[17] *The Book of Mencius*, VII A: 15, in: Wm. Theodore de Bary, (ed.), *Sources of Chinese Tradition*, New York, Columbia University Press, 1960,Vol.1, pp.91-92.

human nature. When the people keep their normal nature they will love excellent virtue. The ceremonial or rituals are there to express and strengthen the natural human inclinations, thus to make man keep a harmony mood in oneself: a thoroughgoing harmony among his thoughts, words, and actions.

It seems that *li* (propriety) is very closed to rules---rules governing ritual behaviour or moral choice. But *li* requires more than just the application of established rules. An important element in *li* has to be humanity (*Jen*). The man of true propriety (*li*) has to be basically human- ity. Just as Confucius said, "If a man is not humane (*Jen*), what has he to do with ceremonies (*li*)? If he is not humane, what has he to do with music?" [18] Indeed, for a Confucianist, propriety (*li*) without humanity (*Jen*) is empty. Confucius said, "to master oneself and return to *li* is hu- manity". [19] To master oneself and return to propriety is to cultivate one's personal virtues ac- cording to the Way. Although abiding by the rules of conduct *(li)* in practice helps a person to be a sage------a person with virtues of humanity (*Jen*), righteousness (*yi*), wisdom (zhi) and so on, the essence or the spirit of *li* has to be humanity (*Jen*). *Jen* is a centre theme of Confucian ethics.

So basically Confucian ethics is an ethics of virtue, rather than an ethics of rule. Based on the idea that the way of heaven is harmony, Confucian ethics aimed at a peaceful and harmoni- ous society in which each person related to others. In order to keep the harmonious relationship to others, it is essential for each person to act according to *Li*. This is the right way to live one's life because *li* not only reflected the way of heaven, but also had its origin in human nature. What is needed emphasis is that one has to perform *li* with correct attitude. For example, when performing a sacrifice, one has to feel reverence for the spirits, when carrying out the rites of mourning, one was to feel grief for the decreased. In serving his lord, a minister was to be re- spectable; in governing his people, a ruler was to be benevolence. Without this emotional com- ponent, according with ritual becomes a hollow performance. That means the most important thing is that the person performing *li* has to be a virtuous person. So how to cultivate a person to be a person with the virtue of *Jen*---a sage king became a centre theme of Confucian ethics. That is the reason why Confucianism is regarded as a virtue ethics aiming at the common good of the community.

In sum, the society that Confucians aim to build is not one that is an aggregate of self- interested claimers, but one composed of virtuous individuals who live in harmonious relation- ships with other members of a community. For Confucianism, a genuine sense of freedom can be found in a virtuous and spontaneous conformity to community norms that one believes to be worthy of following. In contrast to the liberal emphasis in individual rights, Confucian commu- nitarianism gives a central place to the concepts of virtues------qualities necessary for one's suc- cessful contribution to the good that is common to all members of a community. In the eyes of Confucians, the liberal view of freedom is an impoverished one, since it provides only a nega- tive sense of liberty without an aspiration for the good life. Confucius, if living in our time, would agree with Sandel in saying that the liberal view of freedom is "thin" and "devoid of in-

---

[18] *Analects*, 3:3, in: Chan, Wing-tsit (ed. and trans.), *A Source Book of Chinese Philosophy*, Princeton, Princeton University Press, 1963, pp.24. According to Confucianism, although rites and music perform different functions, both serve the purpose of shaping the individual character and of establishing a harmonious man-to –man relation- ship, thus help to secure social harmony and order. The book of Rites XVII.i.23 said, " Music is an echo of the harmony between heaven and earth; ceremonies reflect the orderly distinctions in the operations of heaven and earth. From that harmony all things receive their beings; to those orderly distinctions they owe the differences be- tween them. Music has its origin from heaven." (Legge, pp 100.)

[19] *Analects*, 12:1, in: Chan, Wing-tsit (ed. and trans.), *A Source Book of Chinese Philosophy*, Princeton, Princeton University Press, 1963, pp.38.

herent meaning." [20] Confucius would also join MacIntyre in saying that the liberal self is disembodied from "narrative history," lacking "character" and "social identity." [21] Thus, Confucians emphasize the primacy of virtues over rights, the primacy of the common good over rational self-interest, which is echoed by communitarianism in the west. The coincide will not only helps us to reconsider the theme of ethics and enrich contemporary western ethics to provide us ultimate concern, but also help us to avoid the bad effects in practice raised by new liberalism, and other ethical theories as well, because of its ignorance of the common good.

Liu, Yuli is a Professor in traditional Chinese Ethics at the Department of Philosophy, the Party School of the Central Committee of C.P.C. She graduated from Renmin University of China with Master's Degree in 1997 and got her PhD in Philosophy at the University of HULL, UK in 2002. She was a post-doctoral fellow in the National University of Singapore in 2003. She was also invited to be a visiting scholar at Yale University and the University of Trinity St. David Wales. In 2015, 2016 and 2017, she was invited to give speeches in the World Peace Convention in the UNESCO.

---

[20] Sandel, Michael J., *Liberals and the Limits of Justice*, Cambridge, Cambridge University Press, 1982, pp.175. See also Lee, Seung-hwan, 'Liberal Rights or/and Confucian Virtues?' , *Philosophy East and West*, vol. 46, Num.3, July 1996, pp. 367.

[21] MacIntyre, Alasdair, *After Virtue*, London, Duckworth, 1981, Chap.6.

Bioethics and Pandemics
in the Modern World: COVID-19

Farida Tansykovna Nezhmetdinova, Kazan State Agrarian University, Russia

Marina Elisovna Guryleva, Kazan State Medical University, Russia

Abstract

The current epidemic has suddenly and radically destroyed all ideas about the norm, not only in medical practice, but also in society. This was particularly acute for the health system, doctors, and the distribution of life-support therapy in the context of limited resources and the absence of a known treatment Protocol. One of the main bioethical dilemmas of the coronavirus epidemic is the confrontation between public health ethics, which is expressed in the fair distribution of limited resources and orientation to public safety, and patient-specific clinical ethics. After all, the COVID-19 pandemic puts health workers in tragic situations they have never experienced. And if there are not enough health care workers, ventilators, or hospital beds, it is often necessary to classify patients and prioritize them to determine who will get (or will not get) what care and where. Another important issue was the issue of digital control of citizens who must reduce their freedoms for the sake of the health of other citizens. Many people are afraid that the current situation will allow them to manipulate citizens in the future. There is also a problem of responsibility of politicians and authorized organizations for the health of not only the population of their country, but also the entire planet Earth. These and other issues today require bioethical expertise.

Key words

bioethics, pandemic, COVID-19, ethical principles, health, medicine, justice, health

Today, in the XXI century, we can state that our civilization is faced with a whole complex of global problems: the problem of preserving peace on Earth, the environment, the food problem, population, overcoming the poverty of most of humanity, problems of health and quality of life. As a result, there are large-scale problems that are waiting to be solved, and the place of bioethics in this context is not the last. The COVID-19 pandemic has become particularly important in updating and implementing the principles of bioethics.

A little historical retrospect should help to understand why it is so important to use the experience of bioethics in the situation in which the world found itself in the conditions of the COVID-19 pandemic. In 1971, the book "bridge to the future" by V. R. Potter was published (Potter 1971). In it, he introduces the concept of "bioethics", defining it as "a new field of knowledge that combines biological knowledge with knowledge of the system of human and moral values .... I took bio to represent biological knowledge, the science of living systems, and I took ethics to represent knowledge of value systems of human morality." (Potter 1971). According to Potter, the creation of a new discipline of bioethics was to build a bridge between two concepts: science and human nature. In this work, Potter prioritized the problem, namely, the problem of survival in the modern world. However, in his other work "global bioethics", Potter formulated his concept based on the close connection of bioethical theory with environmental ethics. Here Potter continues to develop the idea of close interaction of ethics with ecology, medicine, science, focusing on the ethics of survival and the ethics of global (Potter 1988:72).

German theologian and Pastor Fritz Jar (1895-1953), who, as the scientist Hans Martin Sass rightly notes, was called the father of the ethics of biological research, proposed the term bioethics (Bio-Ethik) in 1926, where the main thing is the sacredness of life. Jar recognizes the interaction between self-care and caring for others, replacing the dignity of respect for the law with the dignity of compassion for all "living growth factors", i.e., both for life and for all its forms (Sass 2013:126-129).

The emergence of modern bioethics was the result of global changes both at the level of deep transformation and achievements in modern science, and as a consequence of the globalization process, expressed in the speed of its development, as well as in the increasing influence of the importance of mutual activities of the international community to solve global problems.

The high degree of potential and real danger of the achievements of modern biotechnologies, prevention and prevention of their use without prior humanitarian expertise has assigned a special socio-regulatory status to bioethics. Today, bioethics is the science of searching, evaluating and selecting criteria for moral attitude to the living (definition F. N.) (Nezhmetdinova 2013:548-550).

The range of issues covered by bioethics is striking in its diversity, but all of them are united by the priority of such universal values as life, health, well-being, and justice. Another characteristic feature of bioethics is its interdisciplinary nature, when representatives of medicine, law, philosophy, biology, and representatives of various religious denominations participate equally in bioethical discussions.

There is a consensus in the international community on the basic principles of bioethics, which are reflected in various declarations and recommendations. They are most fully reflected in the document "universal Declaration on bioethics and human rights" (UNESCO, 2005). These include, first of all:

Human dignity and human rights

Good and harm

Autonomy and individual responsibility

Informed consent

Persons who do not have the legal capacity to give consent

Recognition of human vulnerability and respect for the integrity of the individual

Privacy and confidentiality

Equality, equity and equity

Non-discrimination and stigmatization

Respect for cultural diversity and pluralism

Solidarity and cooperation

Social responsibility and health

Sharing benefits

Protection of future generations

Protection of the environment, biosphere and biodiversity

However, many of the principles of bioethics in the context of the COVID-19 pandemic have faced serious challenges. Representatives of various professional groups, doctors, philosophers, and journalists were quick to claim that bioethics "failed" the COVID-19 exam (Harter 2020).

Whether this is so, we will try to briefly consider in this article. However, it is important to note that a serious analysis is still ahead. The reasoning presented below is a first impression and an attempt to understand what is happening.

AIDS, SARS, Ebola, and finally COVID-19-severe infectious diseases and accompanying social experiments are firmly embedded in human life. The current epidemic has suddenly and radically destroyed all ideas about the norm, not only in medical practice, but also in society. This particularly affected doctors and the distribution of life-support therapy in conditions of limited resources and the absence of a known treatment Protocol. One of the main bioethical dilemmas of the coronavirus epidemic is the confrontation between public health ethics, which is expressed in the fair distribution of limited resources and orientation to public safety, and patient-specific clinical ethics. The doctor acts using the "rule of salvation" - to help everyone with all available means. After all, the COVID-19 pandemic has put health care workers in more tragic situations than they have ever faced. And if there are not enough health care workers, ventilators, or hospital beds, it is often necessary to classify patients and prioritize them to determine who will get (or will not get) what care and where. Who to treat: a young person without education, a driver or pizza delivery man — or a world-famous figure of science or culture, who can continue to bring great benefits to humanity? How do you decide who to save, who to provide artificial respiration, and who to doom to death? The moral duty of a doctor, as it is usually understood, is to each individual: to do whatever is necessary to heal him. This is a one-on-one relationship. But when there are hundreds and thousands of patients, as during wars and epidemics, another extreme ethics begins to operate, which seems monstrous from the point of view of ordinary moral norms.

Of course, over the past decades, when faced with epidemics that can be considered as emergencies, the public, and especially the medical community, has responded actively from the point of view of ethics. Thus, according to the principles developed at the social justice and flu Convention held in Bellagio, Italy, in July 2006, the interests of vulnerable populations and individuals should be of primary importance in planning and responding to avian flu outbreaks or flu pandemics. The Convention was organized by Johns Hopkins University with the participation of the Rockefeller Foundation.

A working group of the joint center for bioethics at the University of Toronto identified the following key ethical issues that should be taken into account when planning responses to the pandemic:

➢ the obligation of health workers to provide medical services during an outbreak of an infectious disease;

restriction of freedom in the interests of public health through measures such as quarantine;

determination of priorities, including the allocation of scarce resources such as vaccines and antiviral drugs;

guidance on global management, such as recommendations for tourists.

The following are recognized as the most important values in planning the response to the pandemic: personal freedom, protection of society from possible harm, proportionality, privacy, responsibility to provide health services, interaction, equality, trust, solidarity and good governance.

Only adherence to these moral principles and their inclusion in the complex of sanitary-epidemic, medical, economic, legal, administrative and social technologies can ensure success and prevent unjustified risks for all population groups (Kubar 2020).

Bioethics in recent decades has mainly focused on modern biomedical technologies: cloning, genetic engineering, and assisted reproductive technologies. Recently, bioethical understanding of end-to-end technologies has been added to them: robotics, artificial intelligence, virtual and augmented reality, the Internet and social media. Without disputing the importance of ethical expertise of these technologies, we must admit that bioethics was not ready for COVID-19. The pandemic has put health workers in tragic situations that they have never experienced (Kubar 2020).

There is a lot of bioethics in discussions about providing quality medical care. First of all, the governments of many countries in 2020 hastily introduced after the Chinese authorities medical and social protocols based on utilitarian ethics – to conduct radical selection in intensive care units (ICU), to refuse to provide a number of medical services that can be delayed (Sándor 2020).

Ethics textbooks contain numerous philosophical dilemmas that question the morality of constantly applying utilitarian calculus to human lives. One of the most widely known was developed by the British philosopher Philippa Foot and is an unmanageable trolley, rushing towards five people, tied to the rails (Foot 1967). By switching the arrow, you can move the trolley to another track and save these five lives, but the cart will kill one person who is also tied to the rails on this track. What are your actions? Based solely on the mathematical outcome of the choice, many will probably consider it right to step in and sacrifice one human life to save five others.

But both in this dilemma and in real life, shouldn't we also take other values into account.

The Nuffield Council for bioethics in the UK is considered the world's Premier research centre for bioethics, and even it does not have a standard ethical approach or guidelines to follow for working groups set up in critical situations. They follow different ethical principles in different reports. In other words, each time a small group is created that makes decisions on the scale of "life and death" and develops some "ethical compass" for a specific situation. In mid-March of this year, the Italian society of anesthesia, analgesia, resuscitation and intensive care (SIAARTI) issued recommendations for the distribution of intensive care to patients with COVID-19. This includes, in the worst case, compliance with the "right of first" principle when there is no longer an ICU (SIAARTI 2020).

The Hungarian medical chamber has released a series of utilitarian selection guidelines that focus on saving more lives and giving priority to patients with a higher chance of survival. The Russian Government did the same.

There are examples of attempts to follow a consultative path, to establish a dialogue between the Government and the public on issues of action during the epidemic. For example, in the US, a coalition of 50 bioethics experts from various practical and academic institutions has been established in Chicago to discuss bioethics issues (Chicago bioethics coalition COVID-19 (CBC) on March 20, 2020). They hold weekly meetings and exchange plans via video link: 1) distribution of beds, ventilator units and ECMO, 2) policies and committees for triage of patients, 3) policies for visitors, 4) distribution of the antiviral drug Remdesivir, and 5) distribution of the vaccine. The group sought to become a public resource for making tough medical and public health decisions that can and should be made (Klugman 2020).

The main goal of the coalition is social justice, encouraging coordinated efforts to ensure that health resource allocation plans do not differ depending on the hospital, but instead use a regional approach. The CBC tried to participate in the issues of reallocation of resources of medical personnel in medical institutions, resuscitation equipment, etc., which proved difficult to implement due to the heterogeneity of medical centers, religious and secular health systems, public hospitals, their resistance to the adoption of standard policies and the sharing of resources. The group's failure to coordinate the efforts of institutions in various health and social care systems raised questions about the role and place of bioethicists during the pandemic (Klugman 2020).

COVID-19 tests the limits of how seriously the field of bioethics takes the principle of justice. On the one hand, excellent work has been done on the ground to raise questions and discuss the nuances of how best to allocate limited resources. Questions about what principles should guide possible sorting decisions have become the new norm of conversation. Principles including "first come, first served, ""life cycle, ""lottery, "" doctor's judgment," "short-or long-term survival forecast," "maximizing life expectancy," and "instrumental value to others" dominated, but each religious and enclave group had its own priorities.

Therefore, in mid-March, both the Hastings Center and the Nuffield Council on bioethics issued ethical guidelines for responding to COVID-19 (Hastings 2020). According to the Nuffield report, public health measures must be evidence-based and proportionate, minimize coercion and intrusion into human lives, and treat people equally in terms of morals. Moreover, the purpose of interventions, as well as the scientific knowledge, values, and judgments on which they are based, must be communicated to the public.

Then, on April 14, 2020, the Council of Europe's bioethics Committee stated that even with limited resources, access to health care should be fair (DH-BIO 2020). In addition, medical criteria should be applied to prevent discrimination against vulnerable groups, such as people with disabilities, the elderly, refugees and migrants.

Many believe that doctors are not reflective, they just don't have the luxury of time to really reflect and think about anything other than medical reasons, when in the middle of the night, you must decide which of two patients gets a ventilator and who later turns out to be palliative care where death is an expected outcome, and therefore easy to make decisions "do not resuscitate" patients COVID-19, through the prism of health indicators (Harter 2020).

However, this is not the case. According to a number of American doctors, today, during the coronavirus epidemic, hospitals should create multidisciplinary teams, following the example of existing in Oncology and well-established ones, for psychological support of doctors. And the authors created such a team at Foch hospital in France to support professionals - a new organization that:

organizes information from public health physicians (and epidemiologists) and academic recommendations to guide action in a new situation.

holds meetings of clinicians representing all disciplines involved in this revision of therapeutic practices in favor of basic transdisciplinary thinking.

brings together all available scientific specialists (biologists, sociologists, anthropologists, philosophers, lawyers) to develop a reasoned and legitimate decision, taken with full responsibility by medical professionals.

The main goal of this team is to help physicians resolve the contradictions they observe between their clinical practice and the standards set by good clinical practice under normal conditions (Stoeklé 2020).

This approach is also supported by the French national ethics Committee (CCNE) initiative to create "ethical support cells" to help clinicians in cases of complex medical decisions. Developing this approach may be vital in the context of COVID-19 and possible future epidemics.

We should not discard the basic bioethical principles in the COVID-19 panic, the Committee believes. Only by maintaining the doctor-patient relationship and our commitment to society as a whole can we guarantee that the heroic efforts of medical professionals will not be wasted, and the moral integrity of participants will be preserved. After all, when the pandemic is over, we will still have to look into each other's eyes, not just at the screen (Haseltine 2020).

Questions regarding the treatment of patients uninfected with CAVID-19 are even more complex. For example, the Hungarian government has ordered the country's hospitals to release up to 60% of their beds to accommodate patients with COVID-19, patients with other pathologies are essentially left without medical care and become vulnerable. In such conditions, there is almost no help for COPD patients. Unfortunately, many countries have the same situation.

Ambiguous statistical information raised issues of its reliability and revealed different approaches to recording cases and deaths in different countries from COVID-19. Despite the recommendations of who, the world's largest megacities take into account the death rate of their residents from coronavirus in different ways. Such conclusions can be drawn from the study of the Boston Consulting Group (BCG)" Moscow and other megacities and countries in the fight against the pandemic", which evaluated the practice of 16 major cities in the world, including Moscow, Berlin, new York, London, Madrid, Stockholm, Tokyo and Beijing, in terms of collecting data on victims of the pandemic (BCG 2020). Overall, there are three key approaches to recording and reporting COVID-19 fatalities. In the first case, those who died from COVID-19 as the main cause of death form a separate group. So from the BCG sample do Singapore, London and Beijing, and did Moscow until April 2020, when it switched to the second approach. In the second case, cases from the first group are presented together with cases where there is COVID-19, but this is not the main cause of death. Deaths due to obvious external causes, such as injuries, with confirmed COVID-19 are not included in this group. Thus, the data form 13 cities from the BCG sample, i.e. the majority. Finally, eight cities also estimate mortality based on monthly data on the number of deaths, which allows for estimates of supermortality during the epidemic. As for publishing these data, BCG claims that most cities publish data on deaths among all patients with both the primary and concomitant diagnosis of COVID-19. Only Moscow provides a breakdown of the number of deaths by all groups, analysts say. Based on BCG data, it can be assumed that it is not yet possible to conduct a full international comparison of the effectiveness of different cities in the fight against coronavirus.

A separate issue was the search for a life-saving vaccine. Many countries are now involved in this process, including Russia. Here, too, bioethical problems arise. Starting with accelerated clinical research procedures, ending with the question of how this vaccination will be carried out. Just remember the scandal in the Philippines after dozens of children who were vaccinated against Dengue fever died there in 2017 and 2018. The only dengue vaccine available on the market was Dengvaxia produced by the French company Sanofi Pasteur. Sanofi Pasteur admitted that their product may put young children at risk.

The COVID-19 epidemic is not the first in the history of mankind. Only at the beginning of the 21st century, we have experienced an attack of avian, swine flu, SARS, and in social circles, many times and widely discussed issues of ethics, law, and health organization that arise in the life of society. Therefore, measures to prepare for pandemics that will haunt humanity in the future must be based on ethical values:

➢ the decisions made must be reasonable,
➢ open and transparent,
➢ comprehensive,
➢ clear to all,
➢ sensitive and accountable.

Planning and response strategies in the areas of health, epidemiology, and veterinary medicine should involve civil society, religious groups, and the private sector. Any measures should take into account the interests of the most vulnerable groups of the population. The most important values in planning the response to the pandemic are:

➤ personal freedom,

➤ protecting the public from possible harm,

➤ proportionality of actions,

➤ privacy,

➤ obligation to provide medical service (WHO 2016).

Russia, like other countries of the world, has taken competent and serious measures that have significantly reduced the consequences of the cjvid-19 pandemic. At the same time, certain ethical problems also arose here:

1) In state policy, when conducting anti-epidemic measures, there is a restriction of personal freedoms of citizens, which are enshrined in the Constitution of the Russian Federation (article 2) and are the highest value of humanity (Constitution 2001). Such violation of the rights of citizens is justified for the purpose of protecting public safety, while the restriction of freedoms cannot be unreasonably strict and must be limited to the extent necessary to ensure the safety of others or entail a violation of international obligations of the state, or be associated with discrimination on any grounds.

Although the President of the Russian Federation during the period of COVID-19 disease did not declare quarantine measures, nevertheless, the restrictions imposed on the territory of the state imply the responsibility of citizens under quarantine – administrative and even criminal responsibility for non-compliance with the isolation regime, infection with the virus of others (FSIN 2016). The procedure for applying these regulatory rules was determined by the fact that the who declared a coronavirus pandemic on March 11, 2020, and the entry into force of the who international health regulations (JCB 2005).

2) In the context of pandemic coronavirus-2019 ethical challenges associated with the disclosure of private information about cases (violation of the right to confidentiality, right to privacy, protection of personal data) (FL 2017), availability of medical care in resource-limited settings and, therefore, their distribution (FL 2019a). Legal norms regulating the specifics of informed consent and medical confidentiality in special situations of medical care are enshrined in a number of legislative acts. (FL 2019b).

3) The fact that doctors of all levels need to perform their professional duties in conditions of immediate threat to their health and the health of their loved ones is also difficult from an ethical point of view. In FZ "About bases of health protection of citizens in Russian Federation" Chapter 9 "Medical workers and pharmaceutical workers, medical organizations" (FL 2019c) stipulates the constitutional right of every person "...to work in conditions meeting safety requirements..." (point 3, article 37 of the Constitution) (Constitution 2001). When providing medical care under COVID19, these conditions are not feasible, which gives grounds for special protection of physicians and encouragement of their work, which was done (Decree of the Government of the Russian Federation under COVID-19 (FL 2019d).

4) In the context of an epidemic, society, represented by health care managers responsible for decision-making, faces the need for strict regulation of restrictive measures, taking into ac-

count all the data on the risk/benefit ratio (FL 2019e). It should be carried out with active inter-action with the population to truthfully and fully inform citizens about the state of Affairs and the feasibility of the measures (FL 2019f).

The result will depend on the effectiveness of interaction: the population's compliance with the regulations and the fact that citizens trust their actions. This trust will be established only if these restrictions are supported by measures of social protection of the population and high quality of medical care, the latter is extremely difficult in the absence of knowledge and experi-ence of not only domestic but also world medicine in the treatment of a new infection.

It is currently not possible to assess the adequacy of restrictive and punitive measures. This takes time, as was the case with the influenza A(H1N1) pandemic that swept the world in 2009. Then the analysis of the conducted restrictive measures was carried out 2 years later and con-firmed the expediency of the measures and the justification of violations of the rights of indi-viduals (CDC 2007).

In this article, we have focused on healthcare. Of course, there are still many issues that need scientific analysis and public discussion.

For example, another important problem in the context of the pandemic was the control of citizens who had to reduce their freedom for the sake of the health of other citizens. Following who recommendations, many countries have introduced universal testing, isolation, and other social distancing measures that restrict individuals' physical interaction. However, there are many differences between countries in the way these measures are applied: some impose a state of emergency, while others manage to tighten border controls

A new specific role of digital technologies was revealed, which demonstrated a wide pos-sibility of their application. On the one hand, many people today have a fear that the current situation will allow manipulating citizens in the future. However, they quickly and promptly regulate the safety of citizens in public places. On the other hand, there is a lot of false informa-tion and news on the Internet. There was even such a term as infomdemia. The Internet itself is not the cause of misinformation, but it helps spread rumors and lies faster and further than ever before. But at the same time, it is an important tool for governments, health authorities, and sci-entists to quickly disseminate important information to the General public. The Web Foundation has published a policy brief (Covid Policy Brief Misinformation_Public) with recommendations for governments, companies, and citizens to promote accurate information, free expression, and open knowledge. They are based on international human rights standards, emphasizing the need for a detailed approach to balancing public health and safety with the right to freedom of ex-pression and privacy (https://docs.google.com/document/d/1XwcQDtr_aSYbL7mU2biLt9cqwT zZdoDEIia5knO2on0/edit).

Also, individual professional groups (doctors, entrepreneurs, officials) were extremely vul-nerable in the new medicalized reality. These groups and ordinary citizens were obviously" guilty» in the bioethical and legal sense in their actions and decisions. This includes (not) im-plementing emergency / extraordinary government measures, (not) performing professional du-ties, and deviating from numerous and confusing emergency rules. The situation has shown that the health and life of others depends on the actions of each of us.

It is obvious that there is also a problem of responsibility of politicians and authorized or-ganizations, such as the world health organization, for the health of not only the population of their country, but also the entire planet Earth. These and other issues today require bioethical expertise.

Planning and preparing responses to a pandemic of infectious diseases should be based on proven scientific methods and public health principles. Discussions on ethical issues and value priorities, with particular attention to the needs and rights of economically and socially vulnerable groups, should be held before a health crisis erupts. The COVID-19 pandemic has shown that health systems need better training to address the complex ethical issues that arise quickly during a crisis.

Preparations for a pandemic should be based on a broad approach to ethical values. The absence of a pre-agreed ethical framework leads to loss of trust, loss of morale, fear, and misinformation.

References

BCG 2020. The Boston Consulting Group (BCG) «Москва и другие мегаполисы и страны в борьбе с пандемией». https://ria.ru/20200623/1573337024.html

CDC 2007. Ethical guidelines in pandemic influenza, prepared by ethics subcommittee of the advisory committee to the director. CDC February 15, 2007. URL: http://www.cdc.gov/od/science/phec/panFlu-Ethic-Guidelines.pdf

Constitution 2001. Constitution (Basic law) of the Russian Federation. Moscow, 2001. 39 p.; On protection of the population and territories from emergencies of natural and technogenic character: Federal law of 21.12.1994 No. 68 (ed. from 03.07.2019), On technical regulation: Federal law of 27.12.2002 No. 184-FZ (ed. from 28.11.2018).

Constitution 2001. Constitution (Basic law) of the Russian Federation. Moscow, 2001. 39 p.

DH-BIO 2020. DH-BIO Statement on human rights considerations relevant to the COVID-19 pandemic https://rm.coe.int/inf-2020-2-statement-covid19-e/16809e2785

FL 2017. On personal data: Federal law of 27.07.2006 No. 152-FZ (ed. from 31.12.2017), On immunoprophylaxis of infectious diseases: Federal law of 17.09.1998 N 157-FZ (ed. from 28.11.2018)

FL 2019a. On protection of the population and territories from emergencies of natural and technogenic character: Federal law of 21.12.1994 No. 68 (ed. from 03.07.2019)

FL 2019b. On the introduction of additional sanitary and anti-epidemic (preventive) measures aimed at preventing the emergence and spread of a new coronovirus infection (COVID-19): Resolution of the Federal penitentiary service (FSIN) of Russia], On isolation, medical examinations (or) medical supervision, hospitalization: Resolution of the Federal service for supervision of consumer protection and human welfare Saint Petersburg No. 78-03-09/722020] the circulation of medicines: Federal law of 12.04.2010 No. 61-FZ (ed. from 27.12.2019)

FL 2019c. On the circulation of medicines: Federal law of 12.04.2010 No. 61-FZ (ed. from 27.12.2019)

FL 2019d. On the bases of tourist activity in the Russian Federation: Federal law of 24.11.1996 No 132-FZ (ed. from 02.12.2019)

FL 2019f. On the circulation of medicines: Federal law of 12.04.2010 No. 61-FZ (ed. from 27.12.2019)

FL 2919e. On information, information technologies and information protection: Federal law of 27.07.2006 No. 149FZ (ed. from 02.12.2019)

Foot 1967. Foot, Philippa "The Problem of Abortion and the Doctrine of the Double Effect."

Oxford Review. 1967. Vol. 5:5-15.

FSIN 2016. On the introduction of additional sanitary and anti-epidemic (preventive) measures aimed at preventing the emergence and spread of a new coronovirus infection (COVID-19): Resolution of the Federal penitentiary service (FSIN) of Russia, On the state of emergency: Federal constitutional law of 30.05.2001 No. 3-FKZ (ed. from 03.07.2016)

Harter 2020. Thomas D. Harter, Mary E. Homan. *Forgotten communities: what bioethics should learn from COVID-19.* (URL: http://www.bioethics.net/2020/06/forgotten-communities-what-bioethics-should-learn-from-covid-19/)

Haseltine 2020. William A. Haseltine. What AIDS Taught Us About Fighting Pandemics https://www.project-syndicate.org/onpoint/what-aids-taught-us-about-fighting-pandemics-by-william-a-haseltine-2020-05?barrier=accesspaylog

Hastings 2020. *Ethical Framework for Health Care Institutions Responding to Novel Coronavirus   SARS-CoV-2   (COVID-19)*   https://www.thehastingscenter.org/wp-content/uploads/HastingsCenterCovidFramework2020.pdf

JCB 2005. Stand on Guard for Thee. Ethical considerations in preparedness planning for pandemic influenza. A report of the University of Toronto Joint Centre for Bioethics. November 2005. URL: http://www.jointcentreforbioethics.ca/people/documents/upshur_stand_guard.pdf

Klugman 2020. Craig Klugman, Kelly Michelson, Kayhan Parsi. *Local Bioethicists Respond to the Pandemic: The Birth of the COVID-19 Chicago Bioethics Coalition (CBC)* http://www.bioethics.net/2020/06/local-bioethicists-respond-to-the-pandemic-the-birth-of-the-covid-19-chicago-bioethics-coalition-cbc/

Kubar 2020. O. I. Kubar. "Ethical commentary on COVID-19." *Russian Journal of Infection and Immunity* (2020) vol. 10, no. 2, pp. 287–294. https://doi.org/10.15789/2220-7619-ECO-1447

Nezhmetdinova 2013. F. Nezhmetdinova. "Global challenges and globalization of bioethics." *Croat Med J.* (2013)54:548-550. doi: 10.3325/cmj.2013.54.83

Potter 1971. Potter, Van Rensselaer. *Bioethics: Bridge to the future*. Englewood Cliffs, N/J.: Prentice-Hall, 1971. 340 p.

Potter 1988. Potter, Van Rensselaer. *Global bioethics*. Michigan State University Press, 1988.

Sándor 2020. Judit Sándor. *Bioethics for the Pandemic.* https://www.project-syndicate.org/commentary/bioethics-principles-for-covid19-response-by-judit-sandor-2020-05?barrier=accesspaylog

Sass 2013. Hans-Martin Sass. Postscript. Fritz Jar. Essays in Bioethics 1924-1948. 2013.

SIAARTI 2020. *Clinical Ethics Recommendations for the Allocation of Intensive Care Treatments in exceptional, resource-limited circumstances* - Version n. 1 posted on March, 16th – 2020 http://www.siaarti.it/SiteAssets/News/COVID19%20-%20documenti%20SIAARTI/SIAARTI%20-%20COVID-19%20-%20Clinical%20Ethics%20Reccomendations.pdf.

Stoeklé 2020. Henri-Corto Stoeklé, Asmahane Benmaziane, Philippe Beuzeboc, Christian Hervé. COVID-19: The Need for "Emergency Multidisplinary Team Meetings" http://www.bioethics.net/2020/05/covid-19-the-need-for-emergency-multidisplinary-team-meetings/

UNESCO 2005. Universal Declaration on bioethics and human rights (UNESCO, 2005).

https://www.un.org/ru/documents/decl_conv/declarations/bioethics_and_hr.shtml

WHO 2016. World Health Organization. Guidance for managing ethical issues in infectious disease outbreaks. World Health Organization. https://apps.who.int/iris/handle/10665/250580

F. T. **Nezhmetdinova**, Kazan State Agrarian University, Russia, e-mail: nadgmi@mail.ru

Sustainable COVID-19 Response Measures: An Ethical Imperative for Enhancing Core Human Capabilities

Leonardo D. de Castro, University of the Philippines Diliman, Philippines

Jeanette Yasol-Naval, University of the Philippines Diliman, Philippines

Abstract

COVID-19 has caught individuals and many countries by surprise. With its high transmissibility rate and potential for severe destruction, it has obliged governments to rush emergency measures if only to survive until the pandemic fades away. COVID-19 response measures have been effective if they are able to help people attain capabilities required for human flourishing, although only temporarily. Using the framework of Martha Nussbaum's core human capabilities, we observe that response measures have had to address chronic capability deficits rather than deficits that only materialized because of the pandemic. There is an ethical imperative for sustainable measures that can enhance human capabilities beyond the duration of the current pandemic and ensure readiness for future disasters and emergencies.

Key words

COVID-19, core human capabilities, pandemic ethics, Nussbaum, corona virus,

1. Introduction – the importance of a personal perspective

This effort to examine the problems brought about by the COVID-19 pandemic starts by trying to understand specific issues from the perspective of individual human beings whose diminished capabilities have been brought to public focus by recent events. It is important to look at the impact of SARS-CoV-2 using the lens of particular individuals because societal response has to be sensitive to the uniqueness and variability of human experiences. The medical symptoms, sufferings and fears that have to be addressed are experiences of concrete and specific human beings. The hunger and starvation that society is confronted with are felt by individuals around us who have been deprived of essential goods and services.

In contrast, government response tends to focus on conventional parameters centered on economic indicators and accumulated health statistics. This is often seen as the logical way to go since the success or failure of governmental efforts has to be measurable. Otherwise, it will be difficult to determine whether these efforts have attained their objectives or not. Governments have to be able to show, for example, that the number of people testing positive for the corona virus is going down, that the number of patients dying of COVID-19 is no longer increasing, that business establishments are reopening, or that more people are getting employed again. That is government's task. But that is not all of it. What the government accomplishes in terms of aggregated statistics must be felt at the level of individual human experiences.

In this paper we proceed by highlighting cases of individuals and communities touched by the pandemic. We explore the use of Martha Nussbaum's capabilities approach (Nussbaum 2001, Nussbaum 2008, Nussbaum 2011) in assessing the nature, significance and effectivity of COVID-19 response measures. We examine how the cases reflect pre-existing limitations on human capabilities, thereby magnifying the impact of the pandemic on individuals and communities. Conversely, we observe how the impact of the pandemic magnifies the limitations on human capabilities, thereby hampering human flourishing. In the end, we emphasize the need to see the corona virus pandemic not as a stand-alone emergency but as a phenomenon that exists within the context of societies hamstrung by the presence of vulnerabilities that need to be addressed in order to promote human flourishing.

2. Vulnerable individuals, vulnerable populations

We start with the story of Ramon, a 39-year-old Filipino male, who was working as a minimum wage private security guard when the pandemic struck. Ramon lives in a depressed housing community about 12 kilometers away from the place where he used to work. When the operation of public transportation was suspended in accordance with quarantine regulations, Ramon decided to live temporarily in a tiny guardhouse in his place of work. However, he developed presumptive COVID-19 symptoms so he decided to go home. His employers tried to help him but soon realized how complicated the problem was.

Ramon's dwelling is only slightly bigger than the tiny guardhouse that was his temporary shelter. He shares with his mother and sister a rented space with a floor area equal to that of four medium sized cars. A curtain serves as the only partition so there was no way for him to be safely isolated from the rest of his family. The employers explained to him that if he went home he could transmit the virus (if he truly carried it) to his elderly mother, who could then be severely affected. Ramon understood the risk. He was also afraid because they do not have running water where his family lives. They have to collect water from a public faucet about half a kilometer away. More importantly, he was afraid of the stigma that his family would have had to endure. Theirs is a very densely populated neighborhood and everybody knows what is happening everywhere in their barangay (village). Clearly, going home would not have been a very good option for Ramon.

The employers then phoned the community office to ask if they could refer Ramon to health authorities. One of the community officers said they would call an ambulance to fetch Ramon and bring him to a hospital. After several follow up calls and further promises, no ambulance came. The officers explained that the only ambulance they had was still responding to earlier calls. The employers also phoned a local government office to ask if Ramon could be admitted to one of the temporary isolation facilities that were being set up to accommodate patients who could no longer be admitted to hospitals. The official at the other end of the hotline explained that since Ramon's symptoms were apparently mild, he could not be accepted. He had to go home for self-quarantine—stay in an isolated room at home to avoid passing the virus on to other members of the family. This was obviously going to be impossible for Ramon because there is not enough space at home to do that.

The temporary isolation facilities were being built for people like Ramon but at that point he could not be accommodated—the isolation facilities were filled to capacity. Thus, even if he was worried about the risk to his mother, Ramon decided to go home. His employers started to phone the community office again to ask if an ambulance could come for him but he rejected the idea. He said his family was going to suffer if people knew he arrived home in an ambulance. Over his employers' objections, and feeling weak and in pain, Ramon walked two and a half hours to get home. After resting overnight, Ramon went with his mother to the barangay office to ask if he could be referred to a doctor. They were prevented from getting near the office by a barricade and told that if they had any questions or concerns they had to get in touch by phone first—person to person contact with the officials was prohibited. As they were getting ready to go back home, they learned from a neighbor that patients were being referred to a government hospital about two kilometers from their place. They walked to the hospital and were finally able to see a doctor who assured them that Ramon's symptoms indicated a stress disorder and not COVID-19.

At this point, it is tempting to say that the story had a happy ending after all. But that is just one side of the truth. It is understandable if one's reading of Ramon's story focuses on medical symptoms. The immediate context in which the story took place suggests this approach. Faced with the deadly threat of SARS-CoV-2, Ramon's employers wanted to make sure that he got medical attention. In the middle of a pandemic, that was obviously the most important thing for them to do. However, the fact that so many factors were getting in the way of Ramon's being seen by a doctor alerts us to a host of other "symptoms" that were very intimately related to his predicament. In the pandemic context, village officials themselves did not have sufficient and accurate information about the public health situation, health care resources were inadequate, the sole ambulance was overbooked, emergency response resources were being overwhelmed by the overflowing demand, and safe isolation facilities were not enough.

An examination of these "symptoms" tells us that the failure to deal adequately with Ramon's issues was not a result of the corona virus but of a virus of a social kind. The community could not cope with Ramon's issues because it was seriously hampered by a lack of human capabilities that we should expect individuals and communities to possess. Ramon himself was similarly hampered. As a result, he was confused and unsure of what to do. The only option he was left with was to go home. Under normal circumstances, that should have meant going back to a place where he could feel safe and secure. But things were not normal. Worse, things were never normal for Ramon and his family. Home was never a place where they could feel safe and secure because of their economic circumstances and the political situation had imposed severe limitations on the exercise of human capabilities that are essential for human flourishing.

3. Human capabilities – a key to understanding pandemic issues from a personal perspective

The story of Ramon encapsulates various problems that vulnerable people in the Philippines have experienced as a result of the pandemic. With slight variations, the story is repeated many times over involving other people who continue to be similarly situated. Each story is a narrative showing how limitations on human capabilities are magnifying the impact of the pandemic and how the pandemic is magnifying the limitations on human capabilities.

Martha Nussbaum's "capabilities approach" to comparative quality-of-life assessment provides a framework for theorizing about basic social justice that we consider essential for evaluating the significance and effectiveness of COVID-19 response measures. At its most basic, the approach holds that when comparing societies and their efforts to promote social justice, the key question to be answered is, "What is each person able to do and to be?" (Nussbaum 2011: 18) It takes the position that each person must be treated as an end, which effectively means that we should be concerned not just about the total or average well-being of the collection of individuals in society but also about the opportunities available to every single person. This is necessary because the approach is focused on choice or freedom. And this is important for understanding the reaction of individuals like Ramon to COVID-19 response measures and the impact that these are making at the level of individual experiences. In the midst of the pandemic, we are understandably concerned about the total or average well-being of society in general but we also have to be simultaneously concerned about opportunities available or withheld from every single person, especially if they are like Ramon, whose pre-existing vulnerabilities have been imposed on him already for a long time.

Nussbaum highlights the need for societies to promote crucial goods consisting of a set of opportunities, or substantial freedoms, which people then may or may not exercise in their actions, depending on their free choice. Thus, the capabilities approach gives due prominence to people's own powers of self-definition as it regards them as ends in themselves. The approach also gives importance to pluralism of values. Hence, the capability achievements that are central for each differ in quality and in quantity. Human capabilities cannot be reduced to a single numerical scale – we have to understand the person-specific nature of capability. The concern with entrenched social injustice and inequality, particularly with issues resulting from discrimination or marginalization, is something that is integral to our effort to assess the significance and effectiveness of COVID-19 response measures. We readily see how marginalization has worked in the case of Ramon and we appreciate how the capabilities approach of Nussbaum ascribes an urgent task to government and public policy, in general "to improve the quality of life for all people, as defined by their capabilities." (Nussbaum 2011: 18)

Nussbaum's capability theory takes off from the approach to quality of life assessment developed by Amartya Sen in the field of economics. Sen's approach has become influential and institutionalized because of the publication of *Human Development Reports* by the United Nations Development Program (UNDP). Nusbaum's approach differs because of the primary emphasis given to the central capabilities and the idea of a threshold level of capabilities, that may serve as the foundation of basic political principles for constitutional guarantees.

"Sen has focused on the role of capabilities in demarcating the space within which quality of life assessments are made; I use the idea in a more exigent way as a foundation for basic political principles that should underwrite constitutional guarantees." (Nussbaum 2001:70)

Nussbaum comes up with a list of central capabilities that may be endorsed for political purposes by people with differing views on what constitutes a complete and good life. According to her, the list is an outcome of years of cross-cultural discussions and, borrowing from Rawls, a type of overlapping consensus among people with varying views of human life. She insists that the justification still gravitates around the intuitive conception of a truly human functioning and what it entails. However, Nussbaum directs our attention to capabilities or opportunities for functioning rather than actual functions, so that people still retain space to pursue their favored functions:

"It is very important to notice that the view I defend makes capability, not actual functioning, the appropriate political goal. Thus, a just society offers people the opportunity to vote, but it does not require them to vote. … A just society offers people freedom of religion, but it does not dragoon all citizens into mandatory religious functioning, which would be violative of the commitments of the atheist, the agnostic, or whoever does not share the sort of religion that the state has chosen." (Nussbaum 2008: 8)

Nussbaum further claims that "For this purpose, [the list] isolates those human capabilities that can be convincingly argued to be of central importance in any human life, whatever else the person pursues or chooses. The central capabilities are not just instrumental to further pursuits: they are held to have value in themselves, in making the life that includes them fully human." (Nussbaum 2001: 74) She recognizes that the list of central capabilities is flexible, partial, and not a comprehensive conception of the good, and since it is based on the intuitive conception of human functioning and capability, it may also demand continued reflection and testing against the most secure of our intuitions. (Nussbaum 2001)

The capability approach presupposes that there are functions supported by the central capabilities that play a central role in living a life truly worthy of human dignity. The approach advances a society that treats each person as worthy of regard. This fosters an environment that gives individuals the choice to flourish and thus facilitate a truly human functioning, after having developed the basic capabilities. This is where her idea of threshold becomes important. To allow an individual to live humanly is to place one within a certain level of capability that does not fall beneath the threshold of that area, where one is not enabled to live in a truly human way. Although Nussbaum admits that "the threshold level of each of the central capabilities will need more precise determination, as citizens work toward a consensus for political purposes." (Nussbaum 2001: 77) Nonetheless, the ultimate political goal in this approach is always the promotion of the capabilities of each person, and to guarantee that they don't fall beneath the threshold.

The list of Central Human Functional Capabilities includes the promotion of the capabilities for Life, Bodily Health, Bodily Integrity, Senses, Imagination and Thought, Emotions, Practical Reason, Affiliation, Play, Control over One's Environment and to be able to live with Other Species. Among these capabilities, practical reason and affiliation are considered to be of special importance by Nussbaum, since they both organize and permeate in all the other capabilities without necessarily being ends to which other capabilities can be reduced. (Nussbaum 2001)

In the application of the capability approach to our analysis of the COVID-19 response measures, it is vital to consider that this approach starts on the premise that certain human capabilities like the ones enumerated exert a moral claim that they should be developed. Nussbaum recommends that they should be thought of "as claims to a chance for functioning, claims that give rise to correlated social and political duties." (Nussbaum 2001: 84) This calls for the clarification of her three types of capabilities, which are necessary for our analysis – basic, internal and combined capabilities. Basic capabilities, sometimes referred to as the untrained capabilities, are the innate capabilities that may be developed into more advance capabilities, and a ground of moral concern. They are so fundamental that sometimes they are ready to function like seeing or hearing. However, Nussbaum says they may be too rudimentary and cannot be directly converted into functioning. Examples of these are the capabilities of a newborn child for reason, or for love and gratitude.

Second are the internal capabilities which are the trained capabilities or the developed states of the person, and may be sufficient conditions for the exercise of necessary functions. These capabilities are said to be developed through time or through bodily maturity or with support from the surrounding environment. The capability for play, for example, is developed when there is available space that makes possible the engagement of the child with others or the provision of any recreational tool. She also cites how the internal capabilities for religious freedom or freedom of speech may already be there at some point, for the person to use.

Third are the combined capabilities which Nussbaum defines as internal capabilities that are combined with suitable external conditions for the exercise of the functions (Nussbaum 2001) An individual with internal capability to exercise freedom of expression, but is not allowed to do so by a repressive political system, only has internal capability, but not the combined capability. It is therefore, important to emphasize that for Nussbaum, the list must be understood as a list of combined capabilities. "To realize one of the items on the list for citizens of a nation, entails not only promoting appropriate development of their internal powers, but also preparing the environment so that it is favorable for the exercise of practical reason and the other major functions." (Nussbaum 2001: 85) The political goal of the capability approach, therefore, calls on the government, considered to be the basic structure of the society, to promote the combined capabilities by providing the necessary conditions for a minimally decent human life.

4. Core capabilities in the context of the pandemic: Indispensable trade-offs

The significance of Ramon's story can be better understood when we read related narratives of people living in communities with severely crowded living spaces. For example, there is an account of a village in Manila where compact structures made of scrap materials serve as living quarters for hundreds of families. The emergency lockdown came as a huge surprise and it left many of the residents without means of earning a living. (Sabalza & Reyes-Guerrero 2020) Many of them were engaged in daily wage jobs as factory hands, public utility vehicle drivers, department storekeepers, waiters, or utility workers in establishments that suddenly were forced to close. Many depended on the informal economy as drivers of tricycles (motorcycles fitted with sidecars to ferry passengers), sidewalk vendors, market stall assistants, or casual workers of one kind or another.

Before long, some of the residents, in an effort to salvage some capabilities, started to pawn or sell items such as cellphones or watches to have a little money to spend. Others managed to deal with their hunger by collecting discarded vegetables at the markets. (Sabalza & Reyes-Guerrero 2020) Drivers of public utility jeepneys slept inside their vehicles. A few of them started begging for money. Clearly, the effort to salvage some core capabilities was causing underprivileged victims of the pandemic to sacrifice their dignity. What was taking place then was an ironic vicious cycle – in order to salvage some core capabilities necessary to maintain their dignity, they had to sacrifice their dignity in the process.

Many vulnerable people continue to feel that they are inextricably caught in the jaws of another dilemma. They are effectively being made to choose between staying at home to observe quarantine and minimize risks from the virus and on the other hand, going outside to try and find ways of mitigating their hunger. People caught in such a trap became the subject of controversy when residents of an informal settlement were persuaded to wander away from their quarantine area by unconfirmed news that aid was being distributed to needy people a short distance outside. Publicly expressing outrage when they discovered the news to be fake, twenty-one of them were then arrested by authorities who charged them with violating quarantine regulations and promptly put them in jail. (Talabong 2020) Once again, we see in this narrative how vulnerable people succumbed to a temptation to try undignified ways of restoring core capabilities but failed. As a result they suffered even greater indignity and lost more capabilities because of the firm but highly inconsiderate implementation of the law. The residents were also subjected to public insults by authorities whose single-minded focus on minimizing the risk of spreading the virus could not be tempered even by the desperate cries of people severely dispossessed of their most basic capabilities.

Even when relief goods and financial aid are made available to capacitate communities to stand a better chance against the impact of the pandemic, disadvantaged people's core capabilities remain compromised. At least three elderly men in separate provinces in the country died of stroke while waiting to get their cash aid from the government's Social Amelioration Program (SAP). An 84-year old man from Bacolod City was reported to have been going back and forth to the cash aid distribution center even when he was already told to return only when the cash was already available for release. Still, he lined up early together with many others, until he succumbed to the elements and died, his body enfeebled by old age and illness. (Masculino 2020)

This was another case where the provision of opportunities that should aid bodily health to promote life exacted a conflicting trade-off involving the very capability that was being advanced. What needs to be recognized, however, are the other capability deficits that relate to this dilemma. Part of the core capabilities that must be recognized and promoted is the individual's capability to use his senses to imagine, think and reason. Nussbaum suggests that to be able to actualize this in a manner appropriate for humans, adequate access to education or literacy is necessary. People who flock to relief and aid distribution centers, or continue with their mobility despite the lockdown, may be lacking in awareness of how contagious and dangerous the virus is, and so may be downplaying the danger of the coronavirus. Access to vital information about the disease may not be readily available to them or the means to basic education must have been neglected. Hence, the resulting capability deficit. Nussbaum likewise emphasized the unique importance of practical reason. This makes for a thinking being, the very pursuit of which enables one to be truly human and not just a mere machine or a cog. This capability appears to have been suppressed because of the precarious situation of these socially vulnerable groups.

When the lockdown was imposed, access to food became insecure. Work was suspended and casual jobs were terminated. With no income or savings, and with curtailed mobility, people were made to depend on insufficient relief goods and aid like the SAP. During the strictest levels of quarantine, there was no opportunity to exercise freedom of choice or to do critical reflection on the implication of one's actions, much less to plan for one's life. The need for sustenance hampered the function of choice and practical reason. It is worth noting that for Nussbaum, the core capabilities are all considered to be of central importance and the needs cannot be fulfilled by promoting one capability while disregarding another, or having it pushed below the threshold.

The emphatic message coming from the authorities to the public was that in the context of the pandemic, people had to be willing to accept trade-offs of core capabilities in order to deal with the threat of the virus. But, as the stories above illustrate, vulnerable populations were not just having to give up some capabilities in order to gain others; they were actually losing more and more while gaining very little, if anything at all, in return. Matters were made worse for vulnerable and marginalized groups whose capabilities were further decimated by the lack, or misleading nature of information, about the risk of disease. Long before the virus came knocking at informal settlers' doors, people were forced to disregard emerging symptoms of any diseases because they could not afford to go for medical treatment. Fevers were brushed aside as something no one dies from as many residents had been used to facing it in their daily lives. Body aches and coughs could not worry residents living in the midst of food shortages, overcrowding and poor sanitation together with neighbors engaged in drug-fueled petty crime. It comes as no surprise that "restrictions have not stopped runny-nosed children from playing tag in the slum's labyrinth of alleyways, as parents shout halfhearted admonitions to stay away from one another." (Gutierrez 2020)

5. Quarantine and the loss of human capabilities

At the very start of the quarantine period, the police officer in charge of Metro Manila announced that quarantine orders should be taken seriously by everybody. The police regional director issued a stern warning that violators of community quarantine orders were going to be arrested. (Gonzales 2020) His office announced that those arrested were going to face a case for violation of Article 151 of the Revised Penal Code on Resistance and Disobedience to a Person in Authority as well as "other laws that will apply to other possible violations." (Gonzales 2020)

Thus was the stage set for the deployment of police officers to implement the law at checkpoints set up at many locations throughout the country. Their presence was strongly felt in many areas in Metropolitan Manila. In some communities, people felt uneasy because they had learned to associate the visibility of soldiers and police with extra judicial killings of people reported, or mistaken to be drug users or sellers as they asked: "Is that coronavirus for real? Maybe they're just saying that to make us afraid, so that we would follow their orders about staying inside." (Sabalza and Reyes-Guerrero 2020) To them, police presence represented further threats to their enjoyment of core human capabilities. The virus was perceived as a distraction that aggravated long-standing issues of injustice.

After three months, a total of 177,540 persons were reported to have been accosted by state officials for defying quarantine protocols. A total of 52,535 were detained, although it is not clear if all of them were actually issued formal arrest orders. (Tupas 2020) The official reasoning given by the Department of Justice for the restriction of movement is based on the provisions of the Mandatory Reporting of Notifiable Diseases and Health Events of Public Health Concern Act: there is no "curtailment of one's right to mobility" because such a right "yields to the safety of the community at large." (Lagrimas 2020) This formulation is paradoxical in that yielding to the safety of the community at large precisely involves the curtailment of the right to mobility. In any case, curtailment of the right to mobility is truly what the law intends and it is difficult to quarrel with the validity of such a law in the face of the magnitude of the pandemic now prevailing. What the paradoxical formulation captures is the bewilderment of the vulnerable populations that are most adversely affected as well as of the officials themselves whose task is to explain. For those who have not been stricken by COVID-19, the virus and its impact have remained invisible. On the other hand, the hunger resulting from the disadvantaged people's failure to make a living has been felt intensely. In fact, many of them have experienced it for a protracted period already. A survey done by the Social Weather Stations showed that an estimated 8.8% or a total of 2.1 million Filipino families experienced self-reported hunger in December 2019. (SWS 2020) Hence, such a huge number of Filipino families were already experiencing the lack of corresponding capabilities even before the onset of the pandemic. Realizing this, one should easily realize why so many people also could not fully comprehend the reasons for their being prevented from breaching quarantine regulations.

Quite simply, the people concerned had to find ways of making money. They were not very successful in this effort before the pandemic came and certainly they would have failed miserably if they remained at home. A confirmation of the need go out and find food actually came in the form of a more recent survey by Social Weather Stations showing that the number of Filipinos who reported having experienced hunger increased to an estimated 16.7%, or a total of 4.2 million households two months after quarantine started. Also significant was the finding that the diminished capability in terms of responding to hunger was directly related to diminished capability related to educational attainment: "Hunger was higher among those who had fewer years of formal schooling: it was 21.1% among non-elementary graduates and 24.4% among elementary graduates, compared to 16.5% among high school graduates and 6.9% among college graduates." (SWS 2020). Once more, we see an iteration of the way pre-existing capability deficits aggravate the impact of the pandemic and how the pandemic aggravates the situation insofar as the attainment of core capabilities is concerned.

For health authorities, as well as for people who are economically better situated, the story of the pandemic is the story of the spread of the virus. For those who are experiencing hunger, the main issue is the loss of human capabilities needed for living a life of dignity. It is a loss that they have suffered even before the onset of the current pandemic. Any response to the pandemic, to be successful, must do something about this loss at the same time.

6. Imprisonment in the context of COVID-19

The reference above to quarantine violators being detained takes on added significance in the context of the pandemic because of the situation in Philippine prisons. As soon as the pandemic was felt to threaten the country, security measures were reported by the Philippine Bureau of corrections. Visits were curtailed and presents from outside to inmates were thoroughly screened. However, in the highly corrupt environment of Philippine prisons, no preventive measures could be strict enough.

We are told of the story of a boy (let's call him Eddie) who was disowned by his family for being gay. Accused of shouting in public and carrying a concealed knife, he was arrested when he was only 15 years old. In order to ensure his detention, the arresting officers put down a date of birth to indicate that he was no longer a legal minor. After spending two months at the Manila City Jail, his status as a minor was established through a dental examination. Yet, after spending almost two years more as a detainee, there still was no indication that he was going to be released at the time when the story was written. Eddie had spent more time in prison as a pretrial detainee than he would have had to spend had he been already convicted of the alleged crime. (Almendral 2019)

Although the news story was published before the pandemic, it describes the kind of person entrapped in the country's prisons with severely diminished capabilities and subjected to further threats of capability-sapping experiences because of the pandemic. Eddie was actually detained at a facility where 518 men were squeezed into a space meant only for 170. Like Eddie, many of the men were pre-trial detainees, meaning that they were not yet convicted of any crimes but therefore were being unjustly deprived of core capabilities because the courts were too slow to dispatch cases. (Almendral 2019)

Following 21 quarantine violators who were arrested in Quezon City, reporters cite the testimony of the detainees' lawyer that her clients were treated carelessly. According to her, the only health precaution taken by the police was the use of a thermal scanner. The new detainees were not tested for SARS-CoV-2 before being left together with other inmates. They were not made to undergo a 14-day quarantine. The 16 men were crammed in a 3x4-meter cell while the 5 women were made to share a cell with other female detainees. According to the lawyer: "At night, the inmates slept side-by-side on the same cold floor. They didn't have easy access to toilets, making frequent handwashing difficult. The jail did not provide rubbing alcohol, masks or soap, although some donors sent some supplies." (See 2020)

People were not surprised when it became apparent later on that COVID-19 was spreading through the country's prisons. Inmates as well as Bureau of Corrections personnel were affected. (Cabalza 2020, Lagrimas 2020b) In response, the Supreme Court of the Philippines reminded the trial courts of the need effectively to implement existing policies laid down by the Constitution, specifically with reference to laws and the rules respecting the right of the accused to bail and to speedy trial. Although the Supreme Court had clearly laid down the policy prior to the onslaught of the virus, it saw the need to speed up the efforts to decongest jails and humanize the conditions of detained persons pending the hearing of their cases. (Navallo 2020a) It gave due course to appeals for release coming from relatives and advocates for persons deprived of liberty. It also was mindful of the growing risk of the contagious coronavirus disease while held in the country's overcrowded jail facilities. Thus it allowed reduced bail and release on own recognizance for poor inmates. (Navallo 2020b) In its explanation, the Supreme Court recognized the removal of such barriers to core capabilities as a constitutional right. It also gave due regard to the prisoner's pecuniary circumstances especially during the period of public health emergency. (Navallo 2020b)

Such a response to problems facing persons deprived of liberty during pandemic times supports the observation that the concerns being raised preceded the existence of the public health emergency. The unfair suppression of human capabilities has existed for a long time. The circumstances have been aggravated by the pandemic and the impact of the pandemic has been aggravated by the preexisting conditions. This is why an effort to address the related concerns arising from the pandemic can only be truly successful if it restores unfair restrictions on human capabilities. A narrow focus on the corona virus cannot lead to a sustained solution.

7. Human capabilities in relation to specific COVID-19 response measures

In the Philippines, a number of policies were immediately implemented after the first case was recorded, namely, the Enhanced Community Quarantine (ECQ) and social distancing protocols to prevent contagion, the provision of financial assistance through the Social Amelioration Program (SAP) to address economic concerns corollary to the implementation of the ECQ, the augmentation of health care services and facilities, and others. It is possible to examine how all of these measures are aligned with the promotion of a number of capabilities in the list. Protection against the virus and its high transmissibility promotes the capacity to have good health which subsequently promotes our capacity to be able live life to the end of its normal length and not to die prematurely. The declaration of the ECQ affirms our commitment to respect our capacity to establish affiliation as we recognize that the virus is not just one man's concern but everyone's. It has provided conditions that promote concern and compassion towards other human beings, as we were provided the opportunity not to be carriers of the virus to protect others, as well as ourselves. At the same time, ECQ resulted in conditions that may not exactly favor the development of the other internal capabilities. It has prevented people from moving freely from place to place which has affected the development of bodily integrity. As people were confined to their homes, ECQ threatened the economic productivity of daily wage earners because it prevented them from doing work. This has threatened the ability to promote bodily health as it requires adequate nourishment that could not be provided due to the lack of income during the quarantine period. Ultimately, this exacts its toll on the promotion of life.

The government tried to address these deficits by providing financial assistance through the SAP. But this also backfired as people who deserved to receive the SAP were forced to gather in covered courts or in front of barangay (village) halls without regard for social distancing. The activity exposed people to the dangers of contagion. (Lalu 2020) Many were humiliated as they had to beg on national media because they were not given the support, and some died because of heatstroke as they were waiting for hours in line to get their SAP. (Timtim and Lauro 2020) Needy people were arrested as they staged political expressions of their dismay over what they felt was utter disregard of their basic needs. They resisted the violation of their practical reason and capacity to participate in political exercises regarding policies that concern their basic sustenance. (Peralta-Malonzo 2020) The government efforts still placed people impacted by the COVID crisis without the capability to promote health and life. How could the ECQ, as it required people to stay at home to protect themselves, be able to provide conditions for living a life worthy of human dignity when people are homeless, or are staying in structures that do not provide adequate shelter? SAP addresses temporary loss of jobs during the ECQ, but many had been jobless even before the pandemic.

The public health crisis resulted in various forms of discrimination against COVID-19 and other patients and their families, as well as healthcare workers and other frontliners. There were traumatic experiences of mothers denied of proper childbirth in hospitals. They were forced to deliver their babies in less than decent places. This blighted their capacity for emotional development as they suffered anxiety and neglect. Some of them even died after being turned down by several hospitals. (Ong Ki 2020) Thus, they were denied practical reason to choose how to be taken care of in a manner that further promotes their life, health and self-respect. Similar stories of COVID-19 patients who were refused admission to health institutions, illustrate abhorrent capability deficits. Issues of infringement of bodily integrity surfaced as suspected COVID-19 individuals were harassed by their neighbors and evicted from their apartments. They fell victim to assault and overwhelming fear and anxiety. While interventions were made by local government units to address this kind of discrimination, the phenomenon may be traced to undeveloped internal capabilities due to lack of external support in the form of adequate education or poor access to information. Healthcare workers and other frontliners exercised practical reason in choosing to promote central human functional capabilities to live, be healthy, enjoy emotional development, and establish affiliation through care and concern for others. But they were sometimes denied conditions necessary to exercise their combined capabilities. They suffered humiliation and direct threats to their lives and security as hundreds of assaults against them were recorded during the Enhanced Community Quarantine. (Reuters 2020) The cases of discrimination that continue during this time of public health crisis manifest a lack of appropriate support for the development of both internal and combined human capabilities.

In this regard, COVID-19 response measures have failed to place people above the Nussbaum threshold that would enable them to develop their capabilities that would let them function if they choose to, in ways worthy of human dignity. Such measures have not provided the social and material support for the development of their internal capabilities nor the environment that is favorable for the exercise of practical reason and the other major functions. Somehow, some of the capability deficits were temporarily addressed through ECQ, SAP and improvement of health care system, and the measures enabled most of us to be able to live a healthy life, and be allowed to enjoy affiliation and exercise of care and compassion to others. Concomitant issues, however, came up as people refuse to follow social distancing protocols, choose to still get out of their homes, and some even became agents of discrimination. Maybe because the development of the basic capacity for practical reason was left out. These issues point therefore to chronic capability deficits that pre-dated the pandemic. To be able to admit people within the threshold of capabilities that are necessary to live a truly human life, it is imperative that we all work towards enhancing these capabilities.

8. Enhancing capabilities through COVID-19 response measures

Not very far from the Philippines, long-standing vulnerabilities of migrant workers in Singapore were exposed by the impact of the pandemic. Singapore was looked up to by neighbors as one of the countries that were well prepared for a pandemic. Having learned important lessons from its experience with SARS, the country had detailed and well thought out protocols for dealing with another pandemic. After the pandemic reached Singapore, the World Health Organization praised the country's aggressive contact tracing that enable quick identification and isolation of new cases. Clusters of cases were promptly shut down. Most of the economy and many schools remained open. (Beaubien 2020)

But, as this paper has emphasized, the current epidemic is about much more than the virus. Focusing energy on the task at hand is important in dealing with an emergency of this magnitude. However, focusing on the virus alone could be distracting because the task at hand could be much bigger on some of the fronts where we have to do battle.

It did not take long before new cases spiked in the country and Singapore rose to the top of the list of countries with the most coronavirus cases in Southeast Asia. This was highly surprising considering that its population of less than 6 million is so small compared to almost 110 million of the Philippines and 275 million of Indonesia. The surge of infections was linked to tightly packed dormitories where migrant workers resided: "Around 300,000 low-wage workers, mostly from South Asia, work in Singapore in construction and maintenance. Most of them live together in huge dormitory complexes on the outskirts of the city they've helped build." (Tan & Illmer 2020) The migrant workers accounted for 90% of Singapore's total cases. (Toh 2020)

The initial response was targeted isolation and quarantine. (Aw 2020) With some variation, it was similar to response to outbreaks in crowded communities in countries like the Philippines and India. Thousands of healthy workers were evacuated to floating dormitories, sports halls and vacant public housing buildings in an attempt to minimize the risk of infection. In some isolation dormitories, areas were marked for isolation so workers were confined to their rooms and meals were delivered to them. Isolation and quarantine of this kind, of course, is a temporary measure. It is a way of hanging on while waiting for things to improve before the situation could return to how it was before the onset of the pandemic. It recognizes that the virus is causing havoc but it does not do anything to remove the restrictions on human capabilities arising from the crowded living conditions. BBC quotes the observation by the non-profit organization called Transient Workers Count Too that "keeping … [the workers] in such living conditions creates systemic vulnerabilities waiting to erupt … even with smaller-scale disease outbreaks like tuberculosis" and that they "are beginning to have a sense that they are just kept there and are waiting to get the virus." (Tan & Illmer 2020) Isolation and quarantine were not addressing the root cause of the problem and could not be a sustainable solution.

Fortunately, the response seems to be going beyond these interim measures. Trade associations and ethnic chambers of commerce have highlighted the important role of migrant workers in keeping Singapore's economy strong, noting that "they have enabled Singapore to continue developing as a good home and a good place to do business," and that "given Singapore's limited workforce, we would not be able to stay competitive in certain sectors otherwise if not for migrant workers." (Lim 2020a) They have also warned of repercussions should there be a reduction in the number of migrant workers. (Co 2020) The Singapore Indian Chamber of Commerce and Industry called migrant workers the backbone of Singapore's construction, marine shipyard, and process sectors, emphasizing it was crucial to take care of them. (Lim 2020a)

The recognition of migrant workers' worth would count for nothing if it did not lead to sustained measures restoring the vulnerable population's core capabilities beyond the period of the pandemic. A further sign of the recognition is that numerous contributions have been flowing directly to improve the current conditions of the workers and their families. (Toh, Wen Li & Tan, Sue-Ann 2020) Authorities have also been looking beyond the short term to build less dense housing facilities. Housing meant for the short and medium terms includes fitting out several unused state properties, as well as temporary on-site housing so that all workers involved in a project could be housed together. It has been reported that for the long-term, 11 purpose-built dormitories will be built in the next two years that can accommodate close to 60,000 workers. (Lim 2020b) We have yet to see how things will work out in the end but National Development Minister Lawrence Wong, co-chair of a multi-ministry task force handling the COVID-19 outbreak, has been quoted as saying that "We really need to appreciate the contributions of all that our migrant workers have been doing... and we welcome them as part of our community. And this is an important part of how we can also learn from this whole experience and become a more inclusive society." (Lim 2020b) In practical terms, quick build dormitories that will be completed at the end of the year will eventually be replaced by new purpose-built dormitories, that can fit up to 100,000 workers in the long term. (Goh 2020)

There are a number of things that we wanted to focus on by exploring the response to the problems of Singapore's migrant workers in the context of the pandemic. One is the recognition of the value – even indispensability – of migrant workers for the progress of Singapore. It involves an acknowledgement of the sacrifice that these foreign workers are making for the rest of Singapore society and, as a result, that the country owes migrant workers a debt of gratitude that translates into a commitment to improved human capabilities when the pandemic is over. (Ng 2020) Thus, there is the acceptance that the solution to the problems have to be sustainable beyond the period of the pandemic. Third is the existence of concrete plans for sustaining the response. Implicit in these factors is the understanding that the problems for which solutions are being sought go beyond the virus. For, it is not solely the virus that has given rise to the magnitude of the pandemic. To reiterate, the restriction on human capabilities is the central component. The attitude of Singapore's authorities recognizes this. This is the kind of attitude that we think is essential for a COVID-19 response that can upgrade readiness even for the next pandemic.

9. Conclusion

It is not difficult to understand why COVID-19 response measures initiated by the government have been characterized by rigidity and paternalism. Caught by surprise because of the pandemic's swift and stealthy transmission in addition to the possibility of severe consequences, authorities have felt the need to respond quickly while also presuming that the urgency left no time to consult the people who could have been most adversely affected. Like many other governments elsewhere, Philippine authorities proceeded by telling individuals and communities what to do, with minimal, if any consultations. Yet, as we have learned from recent experiences, inputs from the governed – especially from vulnerable and marginalized groups – constitute invaluable insights that show how measures can succeed or fail. Many leaders make the mistaken assumption that in times of emergency they have to act rigidly and without waiting for time-consuming consultations. They do not realize that it is precisely during times of extreme emergencies that the interests of the vulnerable and marginalized can be easily overlooked.

One ought to recognize that local communities are in the best position to "provide insight into stigma and structural barriers; and they are well placed to work with others from their communities to devise collective responses. Such community participation matters because unpopular measures risk low compliance. With communities on side, we are far more likely—together—to come up with innovative, tailored solutions that meet the full range of needs of our diverse populations." (Marston 2020: 1676) Indeed, tailored solutions are what we need. That is what local communities have been clamoring for—solutions that are sensitive to the core capabilities they have lost and are asking to be restored.

In order to achieve these core capabilities that will help people pursue a flourishing life amid or beyond the pandemic, opportunities need to be put in place. We have known them for decades but neglected in favor of what is seen to be a better measure of growth and progress for the population. People must be allowed political and material control over their environment. They must enjoy political liberties that will enable them to participate effectively in choices that govern their lives. They need material control so that they can have fair access to decent employment. These capabilities, while distinctly important in themselves, will also provide opportunities necessary for them to have adequate food on the table, decent housing and other basic needs for bodily health. The government must focus on providing suitable external conditions essential for the exercise of these functions such as universal health care coverage. Access to meaningful education is likewise imperative if people are to be able to imagine, think and reason in a truly human way concerning the meaning of their lives during or beyond this pandemic. Institutions should promote fair and compassionate policies, and not rules or laws that are too rigid and paternalistic. This is to encourage people to establish meaningful relationships and safe communities. This will serve as social basis of self-respect and non-humiliation, so that everyone can be treated as dignified human beings. Underlying all of these is the provision for the full exercise of practical reason that will enable people to practice freedom of choice to make decisions and plans on what for them would constitute quality existence. Policies must be crafted to address pre-existing vulnerabilities imposed on marginalized sectors so that the government is can advance sufficient social bases for these capabilities.

We know the capabilities that people must have but which they have not been able to achieve. We have known these for decades. They must have all of these things as a matter of right and not merely as a matter of privilege or of random acts of charity. As ends in themselves, they must have the opportunity to examine the ideas and the structures that have created endemic injustice and suffering and identify new ideas and new structures that should be put in their place. The chance to improve one's life rests on having core capabilities consistent with our common humanity and dignity. We have to organize our society to achieve the necessary conditions for human flourishing.

What we find ourselves having to address during this public health emergency are chronic human capability deficits rather than deficits that only materialized because of the pandemic. Hence the core capabilities have to be provided not only during the emergency period but even beyond the duration of the current pandemic. This is the only way to proceed if we are to be truly prepared for future pandemics or disasters.

References

Almendral, Aurora 2020. Where 518 inmates sleep in space for 170, and gangs hold it together. The Indian Express [URL: https://indianexpress.com/article/world/where-518-inmates-sleep-in-space-for-170-and-gangs-hold-it-together-5527889/, visited June 14, 2020]

Aw, Cheng Wei 2020. Parliament: More than 32,000 healthy foreign workers moved into temporary accommodation. The Straits Times. [URL: https://www.straitstimes.com/politics/parliament-more-than-32000-healthy-foreign-workers-moved-into-temporary-accommodation, visited June 14, 2020]

Beaubien 2020. Singapore Was A Shining Star In COVID-19 Control — Until It Wasn't. NPR. [URL: https://www.npr.org/sections/goatsandsoda/2020/05/03/849135036/singapore-was-a-shining-star-in-covid-control-until-it-wasnt, visited June 14, 2020]

Cabalza, Dexter 2020. 161 inmates has COVID-19; 6 die– BuCor. Philippine Daily Inquirer. [URL: https://newsinfo.inquirer.net/1282125/161-inmates-has-covid-19-6-die-bucor, visited June 14, 2020]

Co, Cindy 2020. Reducing migrant worker population will affect Singapore's competitive edge, lead to higher costs: Industry groups. Channel News Asia. [URL: https://www.channelnewsasia.com/news/singapore/reducing-migrant-worker-affect-singapore-economy-higher-costs-12774646, visited June 14, 2020]

Dutta, Mohan J. 2020 Structural constraints, voice infrastructures, and mental health among low-wage migrant workers in Singapore: Solutions for addressing COVID 19. Centre for

Culture-Centred Approach to Research and Evolution. [URL: https://www.massey.ac.nz/~wwcare/wp-content/uploads/2020/04/CARE-White-Paper-Issue-8-April-2020.pdf, visited June 14, 2020]

Goh, Timothy 2020. Former Serangoon JC and Innova JC among 36 properties to be converted into temporary housing for foreign workers. The Straits Times. [URL: https://www.straitstimes.com/singapore/former-serangoon-jc-and-innova-jc-among-36-properties-to-be-converted-into-tempo-rary?utm_source=emarsys&utm_medium=email&utm_campaign=ST_Newsletter_AM&utm_term=Former+Serangoon+JC+and+Innova+JC+among+36+properties+to+be+converted+into+temporary+housing+for+foreign+workers&utm_content=02%2F06%2F2020, visited June 14, 2020]

Gonzales, Cathrine 2020. Sinas: Cops will arrest unruly individuals defying community quarantine. Inquirer.net [URL: https://newsinfo.inquirer.net/1241389/sinas-cops-will-arrest-unruly-individuals-defying-community-quarantine, visited June 14, 2020]

Gutierrez, Jason 2020. 'Will We Die Hungry?' A Teeming Manila Slum Chafes Under Lockdown. The New York Times. [URL: https://www.nytimes.com/2020/04/15/world/asia/manila-coronavirus-lockdown-slum.html, visited June 14, 2020]

Lagrimas, Nicole Anne C 2020°. Violators of quarantine can be arrested, even without serious resistance — DOJ. GMA News [URL: https://www.gmanetwork.com/news/news/nation/730131/violators-of-quarantine-can-be-arrested-even-without-serious-resistance-doj/story/, visited June 14, 2020]

Lagrimas, Nicole Anne C 2020b. BuCor reports 222 COVID-19 cases, 10 deaths among inmates. GMA News [URL: https://www.gmanetwork.com/news/news/metro/741219/bucor-reports-222-covid-19-cases-10-deaths-among-inmates/story/, visited June 14, 2020]

Lalu, Gabriel 2020. Lucena residents slam long lines, lack of social distancing in aid distribution. INQUIRER.NET [https://newsinfo.inquirer.net/1266272/lucena-residents-slam-lack-of-physical-distancing-long-lines-in-sap-disbursement, visited June 8, 2020]

Lim, Min Zhang 2020a. Coronavirus: Migrant workers important to S'pore economy, say business and trade groups in response to calls to limit numbers. The Straits Times. [URL: https://www.straitstimes.com/singapore/business-and-trade-groups-underline-importance-of-migrant-workers-to-singapore-economy, visited June 14, 2020]

Lim, Min Zhang 2020b. Govt to build 11 dorms in next 2 years; temporary spaces for 60,000 workers ready by year-end. The Straits Times. [URL: https://www.straitstimes.com/singapore/11-dorms-to-be-built-by-govt-in-next-2-years-for-100000-workers-temporary-spaces-for-60000, visited June 14, 2020]

Marston, Cicely Renedo, Alicia & Miles, Sam 2020. Community participation is crucial in a pandemic. The Lancet. (395)10238 1676-1678.

Masculino, Glazyl 2020. Elderly man in Bacolod dies while waiting in line for SAP benefit. Manila Bulletin [https://news.mb.com.ph/2020/05/03/elderly-man-in-bacolod-dies-while-waiting-in-line-for-sap-benefit/, visited June 14, 2020]

Navallo, Mike 2020a. Amid COVID-19 pandemic, SC reminds judges to implement jail decongestion measures. ABS-CBN News. [URL: https://news.abs-cbn.com/news/04/20/20/amid-covid-19-pandemic-sc-reminds-judges-to-implement-jail-decongestion-measures,   visited June 14, 2020]

Navallo, Mike 2020b. SC allows reduced bail, release on recognizance for poor detainees during COVID-19 crisis. ABS-CBN News. [URL: https://news.abs-cbn.com/news/04/30/20/sc-allows-reduced-bail-release-on-recognizance-for-poor-detainees-during-covid-19-crisis, visited June 14, 2020]

Ng, Jun Sung 2020. The Big Read: Solving Singapore's foreign workers problem requires serious soul searching, from top to bottom. Channel News Asia. [URL: https://www.channelnewsasia.com/news/singapore/coronavirus-covid-19-foreign-workers-big-read-dormitories-12718880?cid=h3_referral_inarticlelinks_24082018_cna, visited June 14, 2020]

Nussbaum, Martha (2001). Women and Human Development: The Capabilities Approach. Cambridge: Cambridge University Press.

Nussbaum, Martha (2008). Human Dignity and Bioethics : Essays Commissioned by the President's   Council   on   Bioethics   [URL   : https://bioethicsarchive.georgetown.edu/pcbe/reports/human_dignity/chapter14.html,   visited May 29, 2020.]

Nussbaum, Martha (2011). Creating capabilities: the human development approach. Cambridge, Massachusetts and London, England, 2011.

Ong Ki, Czarina Nicole 2020. CHR calls out medical facilities for refusing patients. Manila Bulletin [https://news.mb.com.ph/2020/04/29/chr-calls-out-medical-facilities-for-refusing-patients/, visited June 8, 2020]

Peralta-Malonzo, Third Anne 2020. Villagers protest, demand release of promised aid. Sunstar [URL: https://ph.news.yahoo.com/villagers-protest-demand-release-promised-065000286.html, visited June 8, 2020]

Reuters 2020. COVID-19: Philippines health care workers suffer abuse, stigma. New Straits Times [URL: https://www.nst.com.my/world/world/2020/03/579698/covid-19-philippines-health-care-workers-suffer-abuse-stigma, visited June 8, 2020]

Sabalza, Bernadette and Reyes-Guerrero, Gerlene (2020). .Hard choices in Slip Zero, Barangay 20, Tondo, Manila. Rappler [URL: https://www.rappler.com/move-ph/ispeak/260754-analysis-hard-choices-slip-zero-tondo-manila, visited June 14, 2020]

See, Aie Balagtas 2020. Philippine Jails are a COVID-19 Time Bomb. Philippine Center for Investigative Journalism. [URL: https://pcij.org/article/4087/philippine-jails-are-a-covid-19-time-bomb, visited June 14, 2020]

SWS 2020. Social Weather Stations. May 4-10, 2020 COVID-19 Mobile Phone Survey – Report   No.   2:   Hunger   among   families   doubles   to   16.7%.   [URL: https://www.sws.org.ph/swsmain/artcldisppage/?artcsyscode=ART-20200521200121,   visited June 14, 2020]

Timtim, Alven Marie and Lauro, Paul 2020. Man waiting to claim his SAP cash dies of heatstroke. Cebu Daily News [URL: https://newsinfo.inquirer.net/1266272/lucena-residents-slam-lack-of-physical-distancing-long-lines-in-sap-disbursement, visited June 8, 2020]

Talabong, Rambo (2020). Quezon City residents demanding help amid lockdown arrested by police.   Rappler   [URL: https://www.rappler.com/nation/256628-residents-quezon-city-protesting-help-coronavirus-lockdown-arrested-by-police-april-1-2020,   visited   June   14,

2020]

Tan, Yvette & Illmer, Andreas 2020. Coronavirus: Singapore spike reveals scale of migrant worker infections. BBC News. [URL: https://www.bbc.com/news/world-asia-52320289, visited June 14, 2020]

Toh, Wen Li & Tan, Sue-Ann 2020. Businesses affected due to COVID-19, but bosses step up to help foreign workers. The Straits Times. [URL: https://www.straitstimes.com/singapore/businesses-affected-but-bosses-step-up-to-help-foreign-workers, visited June 14, 2020]

Toh, Yong Chuan 2020. Rethink mega dorms beyond COVID-19 outbreak. The Straits Times. [URL: https://www.straitstimes.com/opinion/rethink-mega-dorms-beyond-covid-19-outbreak, visited June 14, 2020]

Prof. Leonardo d. de Castro, Ph.D. - Professorial Lecturer, Department of Philosophy, University of the Philippines Diliman, Quezon City. He chairs the Philippine Health Research Ethics Board and is a member of the National Ethics Committee. He has been lecturing for UNESCO's Ethics Teacher Training Course. He has served as Senior Research Fellow at the National University of Singapore, Editor-in-Chief of the Asian Bioethics Review, Vice President of the UNESCO International Bioethics Committee, President of the Asian Bioethics Association, and Centennial Professor at the University of the Philippines. His research interests include research ethics, transplant ethics, ethics of migration, bioethics teaching and Pilosopiyang Pilipino. Decastro.bioethics@gmail.com.

Jeanette L. Yasol-Naval, Ph.D. - Professor at the Department of Philosophy, College of Social Sciences and Philosophy (CSSP), University of the Philippines, Diliman. She has served as the Chairperson of the Department of Philosophy and is currently the Director of the UP Padayon Public Service Office under the Office of the Vice President for Public Affairs, UP System. She has completed two Postdoctoral Research Fellowships at Kobe University, Japan where she worked in the areas Environmental Ethics and Philosophy of Food. Her current researches include emerging animal ethics in disaster and epistemological, ethical and political discourses in gastronomy. Contact : jlyasolnaval@up.edu.ph.

Personal Data and COVID-19

Márcia Santana Fernandes, Hospital de Clínicas de Porto Alegre, Brazil

José Roberto Goldim, Hospital de Clínicas de Porto Alegre, Brazil

Abstract

COVID-19 changed the year 2020. It is one of the greatest challenges that reaffirm the need to preserve the values of democracy, human rights and fundamental rights. Sharing and using personal data is essential for epidemiological research, for health assistance and for public policies design. Our aim is to discuss the limits of sharing personal data in a pandemic context. Flexibility in sharing personal data in contexts of emergency may involve a chain of actions and events justifiable for reasons of public health and public interest, but for this to happen safely, considering the slippery slope argument, these actions must have the guarantee of fundamental and personality rights as a barrier.

Key words

COVID-19; personal health data; confidentiality; data sharing; bioethics.

1. Introduction

Sars-CoV-2 virus change the year 2020. COVID-19, coronavirus pandemic, is a milestone in human history. It is one of the greatest challenges that reaffirms the need to preserve the values of democracy, human rights, fundamental rights and rights of personality. World Health Organization (WHO) declared COVID-19 as a Public Health Emergency of International Importance (ESPII), on March 11, 2020. [1] Since then, more than 27 million persons was contaminated and more than 880 thousand deaths occurs all around the world.[2]

COVID-19 pandemic imposes multiple challenges and impacts to social and private life. The premise inherent to planning and implementing public policies to effectively confront pandemics concerns collecting, using, and sharing data and information. In different areas of life, countless measures have been taken daily to minimize negative effects on people's health.

In order to understand this unexpected situation, many basic and health research efforts have been made. For example, the search for a Sars-CoV-2 vaccine is one of the greatest efforts in science history.

On the other hand, many personal information is shared in unusual manners, as telemedicine, video calls to inform families about patient health status and professionals' rounds. New communication media was included in health scenario with minor previous reflections about technical, psychological, social and ethical issues.

One of the main justification to share sensitive data and personal information is the development of epidemiological, observational and experimental research in order to learn about COVID-19 pandemic focus on the world society good. But, it's important to preserve human rights through the guaranty of privacy and to informational self-determination.

The collection, storage, use, treatment, sharing and disposal of personal data and sensitive

---

[1] World Health Organization, 'International Heath Regulations' [2005] https://www.who.int/ihr/publications/9789241580496/en/.

[2] See the information on website Johns Hopkins University Coronavirus Resource Center https://coronavirus.jhu.edu/map.html.

personal data, are the basis to establishment of national and international public policies. These methods include new informational technologies that add value to the data collected. Tools to manage information aggregation and dissemination, broadens the horizons of theoretical and empirical knowledge in the area of public health and epidemiology, with a directed and declared purpose. [3]

However, we must reflect about the limits of sharing of personal data in emergency situations, such as the COVID-19 pandemic. This reflection must include issues related to personal and relational privacy, measures to protect personal data and respect to informational self-determination.

2. COVID-19, Data Sharing and Research

The high level of contagion and the uncertainty about COVID-19 is aggravated by lack of scientific information; vaccines or medicines that can treat infected patients or prevent contagion on populational level. The emergency imposed by the new coronavirus demand responsible research to find answers and adequate alternatives.

It is essential that the scientific community seek qualified data and information to conduct research projects in order to understand the virus and the disease. Research community made an important effort in order to achieve new knowledges. Scientists, all around the world, are researching many different issues related to COVID-19 and Sars-CoV-2.[4] It is important to balance between the urgency and the health necessities associated to scientific, ethical, legal and social issues.

2.1 Public Interest and trust

Public interest and trust are at the centre of reflection in the context of the pandemic. Public interest is the justified motivation to defend public health and to combat a global health crisis. In this respect, public interest must be underpinned by good administration and a balance of private and collective interests, in the light of fundamental rights and proportionality. The interdisciplinary character is inherent to the notion of public interest, and this notion must be flexible in order to contemplate a specific situation and, from that, to establish the composition of its content and its scope.[5]

Public interest, require, at least, two aspects related to collect and share personal data to be consider, in the concrete situation of the COVID-19 pandemic: First, scientific knowledge must be the rational criterion to motivate measures, proposals and possible solutions, including the collection of data and information and second, to disseminate information the governments have to consider its scientific recognition, as well as the political, governmental and general communication actions must be guide by principles of morality and transparency.

The proportionality between combating the pandemic and limiting the collection and use of

---

[3]   Jürgen Mittelstrass, 'The Loss of Knowledge in the Information Age', in Erik de Corte and Jens Erik Fenstad (eds), *From Information to Knowledge, from Knowledge to Wisdom: Challenges and Changes Facing Higher Education in the Digital Age* (Portland Press 2010).

[4]   See the information on website Clinicaltrials <https://clinicaltrials.gov/ct2/results/map?cond=COVID-19&map=>

[5]   Fernandes, M S. 'Slippery Slope: The Tracking of Personal Data and Covid-19', Work in press, 2020.

personal data, therefore, must be based on sampling and relevance of personal data, in order to support epidemiological studies of significance with regard to statistics, ethics and good scientific practices, so as to ensure legal certainty.

The principle of trust lies at the basis of social relations, whether these are public or private. In turn, the principle of the protection of trust is presented in the individual dimension, or in the subjective aspect of legal security. This principle depends on the exercise of trust, with concrete indication of the breach of expectations in law or clear demonstration of the requirements for its demonstration.

From the philosophical perspective, trust is a central element in human relations, whether interpersonal or between individuals and the state, involving trust in institutions and their representatives. It is a fact that the relationship between the democratic state and individuals is already born out of the assumption of the supremacy of the interests of the public administration, which must guide its actions in the obligation of constitutional principles of morality, impersonality and legal security.

The principle of trust, articulated with the principle of good faith, must ensure legitimate expectations for the administrators. The state administration must look after the common interest and act by means of proportional and justifiable acts, maintaining a uniform and coherent performance, even in situations of emergency a "state of trust" must stablished.

However, a "state of trust" is not presented merely by the disclosure of data and information, but must be underpinned by an intelligible narrative. As O'Neill understands, trust cannot be confused with the mere disclosure or transparency of information and accountability.[6] So, acts of collecting, storing, processing and using personal data on a massive scale, performed by the state or by private companies, with the justification that they do so in order to protect the public health in pandemic situations, cannot serve to promote the control of individuals and populations and the repression of freedoms. Similarly, attempts to reduce communication to mere disclosure and visions of informed consent which lack justification or consistency do not support trust in individuals or institutions.

The data used in studies and research must be controlled and justified, meet scientific and ethical standards, be feasible, abide by good practice requirements, and whenever possible, be pre-established, declared and accepted by participants. Control over the collection, storage, use and disposal of data and personal information has to be done both in relation to the justification conferred by a public interest in the storage of data, and in relation to the justification of the transmission of the content to third parties.

Informational self-determination is crucial in this scenario in order to establish the dividing line between individual benefit or abuse.[7] There is absolutely no reason to use massive databases of personal data collected via cell phones, electronic bracelets, drones, cameras or other means, if they neither advance projections of COVID-19 nor contribute to manage the pandemic. The surveillance and contact tracing contrast with the principle of motivation.

---

[6] Onora O'Neill, 'Accountability, trust and informed consent in medical practice and research' [2004] 4(3) Clinical Medicine.´

[7] Maria Claudia Cachapuz, *Intimidade e Vida Privada no Novo Código Civil Brasileiro: Uma leitura orientada no Discurso Jurídico* (Sergio Antonio Fabris Editor 2006).

The principle of motivation, on the other hand, should be perceived from the perspective of the administrator and not in the perspective of individuals. It requires that broad administrative acts, as well as political acts, be proposed and enunciated for reasons of fact and law, including the justification of the decision-making process, with a clear, timely and congruent narrative.[8]

2.2 Epidemiological research

Epidemiology is responsible to develop methods and concepts to identify health determinants and disease; to describe health states in populations, endemics and pandemics; to investigate disease outbreaks; to compare groups; to find new types of problems; and to use, with increasing degrees of complexity, the concepts of bias, confusion and interaction and epidemiological approaches to causal inference to improve medical assistance.[9]

All epidemiological research must comply with scientific, ethical and legal standards and guidelines, as well as with the responsibility of researchers, institutions and health authorities to ensure the integrity of studies and the proper use of data. The prior evaluation of projects by Ethics in Research Committees (RECs) is a regular requirement for the publication of results and aims to support accountability to the scientific and academic community, as well as to society and research development agencies.

Thus, the collection, storage, systematization and use of health data and information enable the global increase of knowledge in the health area, both in terms of individual patient care, population health and global health. Data and information collected for epidemiological purposes should be collected from individuals considering statistically significant samples, in order to demonstrate the impacts that diseases have or whether practices related to personal care and health influence and/or are causative of diseases or health promoters. And, the purpose and justification for the use of personal and sensitive data and information must be associated with concrete actions in favour of individuals and society, whether they concern sanitary, epidemiological, clinical or biobanking measures.

In this context, the principle of trust is essential in the relationship between researchers and research participants, and consultation, proper information and participants' expression through informed consent formalizing their interest in participating is also essential and must guarantee confidentiality and anonimization of the data.

In association with the direct collection of data and personal information from research participants are the Internet, communication and information technologies and systems (ICTs), artificial intelligence, machine learning and big data. These technologies enable an expansion in the collection of personal data and information, allowing the interconnection of data and information in the health area, generated by different independent sources.

The interaction of data and information in health provides an innovative perspective with unpredictable results, whether this data is dispersed or concentrated, available in health systems, electronic medical records, clinical studies, epidemiological studies, disidentified databases, social media or personal applications for storing health data. In this sense, a positive example is

---

[8] Eduardo Brigidi Mello, 'O Princípio da Expectativa Legítima e a exposição de motivos das Medidas Provisórias' [2006] 66 Revista Tributária e de Finanças Públicas 173.

[9] Alfredo Morabia, *History of Epidemiologic Methods and Concepts* (Springer 2004).

the technology involved in the real-time dashboards for the COVID-19 pandemic, containing the number of contaminated and deceased people worldwide in real time. Concrete examples are the dashboards produced by Johns Hopkins University, the World Health Organization and the Chinese Centre for Disease Control (CDC). The objective of these dashboards is to promote reliable information and user-friendly access for governments, scientists, researchers and the general public and to integrate data from various public and/or available sources, such as government data, scientific data and social media data. However, these data are de-identified, i.e., they are not presented in an identified or identifiable manner.[10]

2.3 Clinical research

In clinical research, data can be collected directly from patients or in databases. These two approaches demands many ethical issues.

Consent process is one of the most important issue related to clinical research. Patients must agree to participate in a research project. COVID-19, because of contagion risk, introduces new ways to obtain valid authorization from patients, like video calls and internet consent process. These ways are not new, but the disseminated use of them are.

The great research pressure for COVID-19 has been in the area of vaccines. The U.S. government has held a meeting with vaccine manufacturers in the United States, United Kingdom, France and Germany. The goal of the meeting was to accelerate vaccine production and processing. The desire is for a new vaccine in a matter of months.

Research into new drugs or new indications for existing drugs for use in VOCID-19 has also been an important demand.

The methodological and ethical issue is that any drug or vaccine research must follow steps that are already established to ensure safety, tolerability and efficacy of a product. The preclinical phase should give minimum safety for its first use in humans. In the clinical phase three phases of studies are necessary. Phase 1 involves a small number of people in order to verify mainly the safety. In phase 2 it increases the number of participating patients and aims at the safety and tolerability of the product being tested. Finally, phase 3 adds an even larger number of patients and aims to verify the efficacy, besides continuing to evaluate safety and tolerability.

On average, a new drug or vaccine has a duration of 11 years between the beginning of pre-clinical research and the end of phase 3 studies.

The political and social pressure to have results in a very short period of time in order to transpose this new knowledge generated by research to patient care also impacts the evaluation by Research Ethics Committees and Regulatory Agencies. This can lead to some important ethical and regulatory problems. The elimination of steps involving research on animal models and human beings may add unnecessary risks to research participants and users of these products.

A human research project should only be initiated after its evaluation and approval by a Research Ethics Committee. Committees can make a faster assessment in emergency situations

---

[10] Ensheng Dong and Hongru Du and Lauren Gardner, 'An interactive web-based dashboard to track COVID-19 in real time' [2020] Thelancet <www.thelancet.com/infection> <https://doi.org/10.1016/S1473-3099(20)30120-1> accessed 15 May 2020.

like this. The difficulty is to have access to information that will ensure the safety of research participants. It is worth remembering that in research on human beings an evaluation of the proportion of the risk associated with it with the potential benefit can and should be made. However, collective benefit can never supplant the individual safety of each participant.

This evaluation depends on information that was generated by other projects previously carried out. The sequence of pre-clinical and clinical studies is what allows us to generate data on the safety, tolerability and efficacy of new products for the health area.

The fastest evaluation of research projects has been called fast-track. This modality of evaluation arose due to the demands of organized groups of patients with HIV in the early 1990s.

With the shortening of research deadlines, projects may be submitted to the evaluation of Research Ethics Committees without a set of sufficient information to ensure the safety of participants. Political and social pressure for the production of a vaccine may predominate over the individual safety of the participants in these researches. The stages and phases of research may be carried out in parallel and not in sequence, as would be recommended.

Operation Warp Speed (OWS), a partnership between the Department of Health and Human Services (HHS), the Department of Defense (DOD) and numerous private companies, was created to accelerate the development of vaccines, drugs and diagnostic methods for OVID-19. This agreement was established on May 15, 2020. The goal was to have Phase 3 studies started between July and November 2020 to obtain results by July and 2020 for eight different vaccines.[11]

In September, 4th, nine phase 3 vaccine trials were recruiting thousands of research subjects and other 38 trials in phase 1 or 2 was approved to be executed too. It's important to notice that three vaccines, one from Russia and two from China was approved for limited use in large populations.[12]

Other clinical research studies involving new and old drugs was executed too. Some of them testing directly on patients and others using clinical information from assistance medical records.

All these studies have challenges In personal records protections. Many editors and all the regulatory agencies demand access to research data collected. In some cases, these informations are presented deidentificated, in others don't. Even deidentificated, many informations could be reversed and reidentification of data is possible. In the vast majority of cases, only aggregate data is needed, but all individual data are requested.

Many COVID-19 research papers was retracted. Many of them related to fraud. The most impressive was a group of four papers, published in renown medical journals, that used a large health databased that was impossible to audit, after the publication.[13] The reason presented by

---

[11] Slaoui M, Hepburn M. Developing Safe and Effective Covid Vaccines — Operation Warp Speed's Strategy and Approach. N Engl J Med [Internet]. 2020 Aug 26;382(21):NEJMp2027405.

[12] Corum J, Grady D, Wee S-L, Zimmer C. Coronavirus Vaccine Tracker. New York Times [Internet]. 2020; Available from: https://www.nytimes.com/interactive/2020/science/coronavirus-vaccine-tracker.html

[13] Mehra MR, Ruschitzka F, Patel AN. Retraction—Hydroxychloroquine or chloroquine with or without a macrolide for treatment of COVID-19: a multinational registry analysis (The Lancet, (S0140673620311806),

the database owner company is the protection of personal data. To perform an audit is different to expose persons by their data. This database fraud generates huge problems, because many governments use the results to make health public policies.[14]

3. COVID-19, Data Sharing and Heath Care

Health care demands and depends on data. Health data is considered as sensitive data in many legal documents. COVID-19 patients, due to the contamination of the disease, had to be kept isolated from other patients in the hospital. For the same reason, their relatives could not make visits or have contacts with them. Health professionals also had to adopt numerous precautionary measures, with the use of individual protection equipment, as a manner to prevent themselves from being contaminated with the virus.

This isolation of the patients led to the need to plan and implement new ways of making communication between professionals, patients and family members.

3.1 Health Records

Hospitals, especially, had to adapt quickly to the restrictions imposed by the high contamination rate of COVID-19. Many information systems used only in hospitals' closed internal networks had to be made available to health professionals who could be performing their activities remotely.

The challenge was to maintain the security measures in place with this new degree of information sharing.

All the patients' personal information started to travel through external networks, demanding security strategies never thought before, but now necessary.

The answers were the most diverse. Many of them using resources available on the Internet free of charge, others that demanded the generation of new software developed in the institutions themselves. The solutions obtained, at least with the knowledge available up to the present moment, have allowed to give good security to this data.

The greatest challenge was to maintain the quality of the information and the safety associated with it, as well as the legal standards on the treatment and distribution of health information, even during a global health emergency.

Another important issue was to keep family members informed about the patients without direct contact either with the patient or the health professional. Many forms of contact were used, most using conventional applications available for making video calls. It was a great challenge for health professionals to adapt to give this information in a different way. It is worth remembering that even the patients' death communications started to be given in this way.

Telemedicine

(10.1016/S0140-6736(20)31180-6)). Lancet [Internet]. 2020;395(10240):1820. Available from: http://dx.doi.org/10.1016/S0140-6736(20)31324-6.

[14] Patel AN, Desai SS, Grainger DW, Mehra MR. Usefulness of Ivermectin in COVID-19 Illness. SSRN Electron J [Internet]. 2020;1–13. Available from: https://ssrn.com/abstract=3580524

Communications systems, such as videoconferencing and e-mail, in accordance with the Tel Aviv Declaration, allow doctors from various specialties to consult colleagues and patients more frequently and maintain excellent results in these consultations (Art. 2). The principles dictated in this declaration have the primary function of providing a first frame of reference for the proper use of telemedicine.[15]

Therefore, telemedicine should, at all times, seek to reduce distances by providing support for health care of quality and expanding access, resources and scientific information. It is relevant to highlight that the data and information used are personal data from patients, therefore, their use must be authorized and there must be specific assistance protocols for this type of care, as well as proper registration in electronic records.[16]

The emergency of the COVID-19 pandemic stimulated the use of telemedicine in many countries. In Brazil, Ordinance 467/2020, issued by the Ministry of Health when former health minister Luiz Henrique Mandetta was in office, regulated telemedicine on a temporary basis, enabling assistance, information, guidance and referral of patients in isolation, telemonitoring, psychoeducation and teleinterconsultation, in addition to guidance to the public and interested people.[17]

The characteristic that particularly distinguishes Brazilian telemedicine from any other remote care network, among others, is the prohibition of virtual meetings between doctor and patient. The current Code of Medical Ethics, established by Resolution CFM 2217/2018, maintained, in the caput of Article 37, the prohibition that physicians prescribe treatment or other procedures without direct examination of the patient, except in cases of urgency or emergency where the impossibility to perform it can be proven.[18]

However, the Federal Council of Medicine (CFM) followed the determination of the Ministry of Health, which, through Ordinance 467/2020[19] and Official Letter 1756/2020[20], authorized, during the period of the COVID-19 pandemic, in items 6, 7 and 8, teleorientation (so that physicians could remotely provide guidance and refer patients in isolation); telemonitoring (an act performed under medical orientation and supervision for remote monitoring or validity of health and/or disease parameters) and teleinterconsultation (exclusively for the exchange of information and opinions among doctors, for diagnostic or therapeutic assistance).

In Brazil, it was essential to have the previous experience of the Telehealth Center associ-

---

[15] Ibid.

[16] Botrugno C and Goldim JR and Fernandes M S, 'The telehealth Brasil networks: A socially engaged technological system' [2019] 6 (1) Latin American Journal Telehealth

[17] Ministério da Saúde do Brasil, Portaria 467 de 20 de março de 2020 <http://www.planalto.gov.br/CCIVIL_03/Portaria/PRT/Portaria%20n%C2%BA%20467-20-ms.htm#:~:text=PORTARIA%20N%C2%BA%20467%2C%20DE%2020,import%C3%A2ncia%20internacional%20previstas%20no%20art.>

[18] Botrugno C and Goldim JR and Fernandes M S, 'The telehealth Brasil networks: A socially engaged technological system' [2019] 6 (1) Latin American Journal Telehealth

[19] Ministério da Saúde do Brasil, Portaria 467 de 20 de março de 2020 <http://www.planalto.gov.br/CCIVIL_03/Portaria/PRT/Portaria%20n%C2%BA%20467-20-ms.htm#:~:text=PORTARIA%20N%C2%BA%20467%2C%20DE%2020,import%C3%A2ncia%20internacional%20previstas%20no%20art.>

[20] Conselho Federal de Medicina, 'Oficio de Telemedicina 1756', [2020] < https://portal.cfm.org.br/images/PDF/2020_oficio_telemedicina.pdf>

ated with the Hospital de Clínicas de Porto Alegre and the Federal University of Rio Grande do Sul. This experience enabled communication between professionals, and between professionals and patients, to be effective more quickly. Many forms of remote care were made available, including one that provides mental health support to health professionals who assist COVID-19 patients.[21]

One of the factors that contributed significantly to the preservation of sensitive information throughout the COVID-19 pandemic was the historic tradition of health professionals in terms of confidentiality. The duty of confidentiality is central to the training and practices of health professionals. This characteristic contributes to the incorporation of new means of recording and transmitting data more effectively.

Thus, the use of personal data in epidemiological studies, as well as in the practice of telemedicine, has a guarantee for privacy rights and safeguards an effective protection of personal data. In these scenarios, duties and responsibilities are imposed on behalf of individuals.

COVID-19:Contact Tracing, Personal Data Tracking and Surveillance of Citizens

In response to the COVID-19 outbreak, according to data published by Woodhams, there are currently 47 contact tracing applications being used in 28 countries; alternative digital tracking measures are active in 35 countries; physical surveillance technologies are being used in 11 countries; censorship related to COVID-19 has been imposed by 18 governments; and Internet disruptions continue in 3 countries despite the pandemic.[22]

Tracking measures to minimize the risks of contagion during the pandemic is use by many countries. Woodhams points out that, out of the 47 tracking applications running worldwide because of COVID-19, 24 applications (51%) contain Google and Facebook tracking, 11 (23%) have no privacy policies; 25 (53%) do not reveal how long they will store user data; and 28 (60%) do not have publicly stated measures of anonymity. These numbers highlight that contact tracing applications pose risks to the safety privacy rights and protection of personal and sensitive data.[23]

This context can lead a slippery slope situation.[24] The grey zone presented in the situation of contact tracing applications because, depending on the way they are produced, elaborated and used, they can go beyond the purpose of public health protection and pandemic control to a point of control, enforcement and abusive restrictions of freedoms.[25]

The prevention of contamination of COVID-19 was carried out using individual and collective measures such as quarantine, isolation and confinement. The most effective preventive approach to block the spread of a contagious disease is to reduce interpersonal contacts. These

---

[21] Botrugno C and Goldim JR and Fernandes M S, 'The telehealth Brasil networks: A socially engaged technological system' [2019] 6 (1) Latin American Journal Telehealth

[22] Samuel Woodhams, 'COVID-19 Digital Rights Tracker' (*TOP10VPMA*, 20 March 2020) <www.top10vpn.com/research/investigations/covid-19-digital-rights-tracker/> accessed 20 May 2020.

[23] Geolocation is a type of device tracking that works by locating geographic coordinates, thus allowing to track people and trace the contacts they have had

[24] Frederick Schauer, 'Slippery slope' [1985] 99 (2) Harvard Law Review 361.See also: Douglas Walton, 'The Basic Slippery Slope Argument' [2015] Vol. 35 (3) Informal Logic 273.

[25] Fernandes, M S. 'Slippery Slope: The Tracking of Personal Data and Covid-19', Work in press, 2020.

are complex measures at both individual and collective levels. [26]

Isolation traditionally occurs at the individual level. A contaminated individual is kept away from living with others as a way to prevent the spread of the disease. This was the measure adopted in hospitals in relation to the patients and the units that attend them.

Quarantine is a collective measure to isolate a group of potentially contaminated people. It is a historically adopted measure. The group of people remains distant from other members of society for as long as the disease is in its contaminating phase.[27]

Confinement is the prevention of large populations from moving or having activities. Many countries have taken this confinement as a voluntary and supportive activity, others have made it mandatory, with important restrictions on mobility in cities. This type of restriction has been called lockdown. The strategy of lockdown is to reduce the number of new cases and thus reduce the impact on health systems.[28]

Contact tracing is being used with the help of communication and information technologies, as well as geolocation.[29]

The contact tracing is being developed by mobile applications, i.e. an application software that works on smart devices, namely smartphones, generally designed for comprehensive and specific interaction with online resources, that handle proximity data and other contextual information collected by various sensors present in any smart device, and that are able to exchange information through various network interfaces with other connected devices.

However, must be considered, in mobile applications contact tracing's scenario, the precariousness of accessibility to applications, inaccuracy of information and possible stigmatization of people, which contrast with the motivation to defend public health – with regard both to the operating system and telephone model.

As defined in the EU Recommendation 2020/518/2020, item 12, tracking measures should mainly serve three general purposes: i) informing and advising citizens and facilitating medical follow-up for people with symptoms, often with the help of a self-testing questionnaire; (ii) alerting people who have been in the proximity of an infected person to interrupt infection chains and prevent the reoccurrence of infections during the reopening phase; and (iii) monitoring and enforcing the quarantine of infected persons, possibly in combination with features that assess their health status during the quarantine period.[30]

However, countries in the European Union have been unable to establish a single standard

---

[26] José Roberto Goldim, 'COVID-19 e Integridade na Pesquisa' (*Bioética Complexa*, 6 June 2020) <https://bioeticacomplexa.blogspot.com/> accessed 30 June 2020.

[27] José Roberto Goldim, 'COVID-19: Isolamento Quarentena e Confinamento' (*Bioética Complexa e COVID-19*, 26 February 2020) <https://bioeticacomplexa.blogspot.com/2020/02/> accessed 20 May 2020

[28] Ibid.

[29] Commission, 'Recommendation (EU) 2020/518 of 8 April 2020 on a common Union toolbox for the use of technology and data to combat and exit from the COVID-19 crisis, in particular concerning mobile applications and the use of anonymised mobility data C/2020/3300', <http://data.europa.eu/eli/reco/2020/518/oj>

[30] Commission, 'Recommendation (EU) 2020/518 of 8 April 2020 on a common Union toolbox for the use of technology and data to combat and exit from the COVID-19 crisis, in particular concerning mobile applications and the use of anonymised mobility data C/2020/3300', <http://data.europa.eu/eli/reco/2020/518/oj>

despite the General Data Protection Regulation.[31,32] Brazil is using geolocation technology, which is normally used by companies in sectors such as retail, to reach and involve users safely without the need to share personal information. This technology was developed by the start-up inLoco.[33]

Digital interventions to provide sensitive personal data come at a price related to the potential threat to privacy, equality and justice. Tracing apps for COVID-19 can serve as tools to create permanent rather than temporary personal data records; to interfere in social movements and interactions and overshadow informational self-determination, exposing people to a situation of uncertainty and risk in which they have little or no control, as Morley, Cowls, Taddeo and Floridi point out in the article Ethical guidelines for COVID-19 tracing apps.[34]

According to Woodhams, during this pandemic many countries are 'legitimizing' many different control measures and practices with the support of ICTs and social media.[35] State control and surveillance systems, formerly performed through physical means, are now possible use powerfull ICTs tools to do vigilance of citizens and control of their movement. Historically, this type the surveillance is use to undemocratic and tyrannical regimes.

As Kuo's headline in The Guardian points out, it may be that the "new normal" in China, which is an 'excessive coronavirus public monitoring', using different forms of surveillance with the justification to combat the pandemic, will be here to stay.[36] China has been widely reported in the media as the country with the initial focus of the pandemic and recognized as having the most sophisticated surveillance system in the world.

The lack of consideration for good practices, ethics and national or international legal standards (such as human rights), combined with deviations from aims and purposes, could undermine confidence in governments and in measures suggested by public health services to address COVID-19. So, can't be normal, in any circumstance undermine protection of human rights, of the fundamental right to privacy and of the protection of personal data.[37]

---

[31] Regulation (EU) 2016/679 of the European Parliament and of the Council of 27 April 2016 'General Data Protection Regulation', <http://data.europa.eu/eli/reg/2016/679/oj>

[32] See the information on website Politics, 'Telekom teilt Daten über Bewegungsströme von Handynutzern mit RKI' (18th March 2020) < https://www.welt.de/politik/deutschland/article206624141/Coronavirus-Telekom-teilt-Bewegungsstroeme-von-Handynutzern-mit-RKI.html> accessed 26 June 2020.

[33] See the information on website inLoco, 'Controle à COVID-19 respeitando a privacidade individual' <www.inloco.com.br/covid-19?__hstc=227211714.293a2716b954c4011059e764f045a483.1593030417559.1593030417559.1593030417559.1 &__hssc=227211714.1.1593030417559&__hsfp=2239244108&hsCtaTracking=5a87f305-e68e-49be-b04c-f3afec6d948c%7C91d9a390-f6a7-4e9e-abc0-b26f84f1d519> accessed 26 June 2020.

[34] Jessica Morley and others, 'Ethical guidelines for COVID-19 tracing apps. Comment' [2020] <https://www.nature.com/articles/d41586-020-01578-0> accessed 15 June 2020

[35] Samuel Woodhams, 'COVID-19 Digital Rights Tracker' (*TOP10VPMA*, 20 March 2020) <www.top10vpn.com/research/investigations/covid-19-digital-rights-tracker/> accessed 20 May 2020. (emphasis added)

[36] Lily Kuo, 'The new normal: China's excessive coronavirus public monitoring could be here to stay' The Guardian, 9 March 2020 <www.theguardian.com/world/2020/mar/09/the-new-normal-chinas-excessive-coronavirus-public-monitoring-could-be-here-to-stay> accessed 26 June 2020.

[37] Ibid.

4. Final Considerations

In response to the central questions in this article, Iit's possible to say that the limit for sharing personal data in situations of emergency, such as the COVID-19 pandemic, must be backed up by objective, temporally fixed and scientifically grounded justifications to establish the balance between the public interest and the private interest.

The various circumstances and situations involved in COVID-19, and the rights involved in the protection of privacy rights and informational self-determination, show that a certain flexibilization of the limit of personal data sharing is justifiable in situations of epidemiological research and clinical research for the development of health technologies, such as drugs and vaccines, and for health care. These situations are supported by rules of law, deontology and good practices. They are also submitted to the scrutiny of the scientific community, committees of ethics in research, and professional bodies, and are consented when they meet the imposed standards.

Contact tracing, personal data tracking and surveillance, on the contrary, do not serve the public interest. The public policies responsible for dealing with the emergency situation of COVID-19 should avoid not only reaching the point of no return, but also reaching the grey zone, i.e. they should avoid or at least backtrack practices such as those evidenced in 28 countries.

Emergency situations do not in themselves justify the indiscriminate suppression or even minimization of human rights, fundamental rights and personality rights. The administration's power of discretion is not absolute; it must be framed by the principles of proportionality, purpose, morality and transparency.

Finally, flexibility in sharing personal data in contexts of urgency and emergency may involve a chain of actions and events justifiable for reasons of public health and public interest, but for this to happen safely, considering the slippery slope argument, these actions must have the guarantee of fundamental and personality rights as a barrier.

References

Botrugno C and Goldim JR and Fernandes M S, 'The telehealth Brasil networks: A socially engaged technological system' [2019] 6 (1) Latin American Journal Telehealth

Commission, 'Recommendation (EU) 2020/518 of 8 April 2020 on a common Union toolbox for the use of technology and data to combat and exit from the COVID-19 crisis, in particular concerning mobile applications and the use of anonymised mobility data C/2020/3300', <http://data.europa.eu/eli/reco/2020/518/oj>

Conselho Federal de Medicina, 'Oficio de Telemedicina 1756', [2020] < https://portal.cfm.org.br/images/PDF/2020_oficio_telemedicina.pdf>

Corum J, Grady D, Wee S-L, Zimmer C. Coronavirus Vaccine Tracker. New York Times [Internet]. 2020; Available from: https://www.nytimes.com/interactive/2020/science/coronavirus-vaccine-tracker.html

Eduardo Brigidi Mello, 'O Princípio da Expectativa Legítima e a exposição de motivos das Medidas Provisórias' [2006] 66 Revista Tributária e de Finanças Públicas 173.

Ensheng Dong and Hongru Du and Lauren Gardner, 'An interactive web-based dashboard to track COVID-19 in real time' [2020] Thelancet <www.thelancet.com/infection>

<https://doi.org/10.1016/S1473-3099(20)30120-1> accessed 15 May 2020.

Fernandes, M S. 'Slippery Slope: The Tracking of Personal Data and COVID-19', Work in press, 2020.

Frederick Schauer, 'Slippery slope' [1985] 99 (2) Harvard Law Review 361.See also: Douglas Walton, 'The Basic Slippery Slope Argument' [2015] Vol. 35 (3) Informal Logic 273.

Jessica Morley and others, 'Ethical guidelines for COVID-19 tracing apps. Comment' [2020] <https://www.nature.com/articles/d41586-020-01578-0> accessed 15 June 2020

José Roberto Goldim, 'COVID-19 e Integridade na Pesquisa' (*Bioética Complexa,* 6 June 2020) <https://bioeticacomplexa.blogspot.com/> accessed 30 June 2020.

José Roberto Goldim, 'COVID-19: Isolamento Quarentena e Confinamento' (*Bioética Complexa e COVID-19,* 26 February 2020) <https://bioeticacomplexa.blogspot.com/2020/02/> accessed 20 May 2020

Jürgen Mittelstrass, 'The Loss of Knowledge in the Information Age', in Erik de Corte and Jens Erik Fenstad (eds), *From Information to Knowledge, from Knowledge to Wisdom: Challenges and Changes Facing Higher Education in the Digital Age* (Portland Press 2010).

Lily Kuo, 'The new normal: China's excessive coronavirus public monitoring could be here to stay' *The Guardian*, 9 March 2020 <www.theguardian.com/world/2020/mar/09/the-new-normal-chinas-excessive-coronavirus-public-monitoring-could-be-here-to-stay> accessed 26 June 2020.

Maria Claudia Cachapuz, *Intimidade e Vida Privada no Novo Código Civil Brasileiro: Uma leitura orientada no Discurso Jurídico* (Sergio Antonio Fabris Editor 2006).

Mehra MR, Ruschitzka F, Patel AN. Retraction—Hydroxychloroquine or chloroquine with or without a macrolide for treatment of COVID-19: a multinational registry analysis (The Lancet, (S0140673620311806), (10.1016/S0140-6736(20)31180-6)). Lancet [Internet]. 2020;395(10240):1820. Available from: http://dx.doi.org/10.1016/S0140-6736(20)31324-6

Ministério da Saúde do Brasil, Portaria 467 de 20 de março de 2020 <http://www.planalto.gov.br/CCIVIL_03/Portaria/PRT/Portaria%20n%C2%BA%20467-20-ms.htm#:~:text=PORTARIA%20N%C2%BA%20467%2C%20DE%2020,import%C3%A2ncia%20internacional%20previstas%20no%20art.>

Ministério da Saúde do Brasil, Portaria 467 de 20 de março de 2020 <http://www.planalto.gov.br/CCIVIL_03/Portaria/PRT/Portaria%20n%C2%BA%20467-20-ms.htm#:~:text=PORTARIA%20N%C2%BA%20467%2C%20DE%2020,import%C3%A2ncia%20internacional%20previstas%20no%20art.>

Morabia A., *History of Epidemiologic Methods and Concepts* (Springer 2004).

Onora O'Neill, 'Accountability, trust and informed consent in medical practice and research' [2004] 4(3) Clinical Medicine.´

Patel AN, Desai SS, Grainger DW, Mehra MR. Usefulness of Ivermectin in COVID-19 Illness. SSRN Electron J [Internet]. 2020;1–13. Available from: https://ssrn.com/abstract=3580524

Regulation (EU) 2016/679 of the European Parliament and of the Council of 27 April 2016 'General Data Protection Regulation', <http://data.europa.eu/eli/reg/2016/679/oj>

Samuel Woodhams, 'COVID-19 Digital Rights Tracker' (*TOP10VPMA*, 20 March 2020) <www.top10vpn.com/research/investigations/covid-19-digital-rights-tracker/> accessed 20 May 2020.

Slaoui M, Hepburn M. Developing Safe and Effective Covid Vaccines — Operation Warp Speed's Strategy and Approach. N Engl J Med [Internet]. 2020 Aug 26;382(21):NEJMp2027405.

Telekom teilt Daten über Bewegungsströme von Handynutzern mit RKI' (18th March 2020) https://www.welt.de/politik/deutschland/article206624141/Coronavirus-Telekom-teilt-Bewegungsstroeme-von-Handynutzern-mit-RKI.html

World Health Organization, 'International Heath Regulations' [2005] https://www.who.int/ihr/publications/9789241580496/en/

Márcia Santana Fernandes -Brazil. PhD in Law (UFRGS) and Post-Doctorate in Medicine in Medical Sciences (UFRGS). Professor of the Professional Master in Clinical Research of the Hospital de Clínicas de Porto Alegre (HCPA) and Associate Researcher of the Bioethics and Ethics in Science Research Laboratory (LAPEBEC/HCPA). Collaborating Professor at PPGD-PUCRS. Professor at Feevale University. Associate and member of the board of the Institute for Cultural Studies (IEC). Fellow of the Digital Society Inititiave, University of Zurich. CV: http://lattes.cnpq.br/2132565174726788

José Roberto Goldim - Brazil. PhD in Medicine: Medical Clinic at the Federal University of Rio Grande do Sul (UFRGS). Master in Education (UFRGS) and Biologist. Biologist at Hospital de Clínicas de Porto Alegre (HCPA) and head of the Bioethics Service at the Hospital. He is a Collaborating Professor at UFRGS School of Medicine, being responsible for the disciplines of Bioethics at PPG in Medicine: Medical Sciences/UFRGS and Supervising Professor at Master's and Doctorate level at this same PPG. Associate Professor at PUCRS Medical School, in charge of Bioethics and Gerontology discipline at PPG in Biomedical Gerontology/PUCRS and Supervising Professor at Master's and Doctorate level. He coordinates the Bioethics Research Group - Interinstitutional Bioethics Nucleus, existing since 1998, with a line of research on Bioethics and Complexity. He is the researcher responsible for the Bioethics and Ethics in Science Research Laboratory of the Experimental Research Center of HCPA. In 2017 he received the Fritz Jahr International Award for Research and Promotion of European Bioethics. Fellow of the Digital Society Inititiave, University of Zurich. CV http://lattes.cnpq.br/0485816067416121.

A Shift in Economic Paradigms – The Newmality

Christian Buschmann, Frankfurt School of Finance & Management, Germany

Abstract

The COVID-19 pandemic caused a sudden halt in economic activities. Namely, this pandemic caused a, mostly, government-driven simultaneous demand and supply shock to the developed economies. This shock caused most companies to adjust their business models towards a new economic reality, e.g., paying tribute to extensive sanitary rules or a shift in consumption behaviour. It's the paper's goal to gauge the potential social and economic consequence of this economic paradigm shift: More government spending and a larger focus on system-relevant parts of the economy with an assumed backward shift from the tertiary sector to the secondary sector within the economies.

Key words

Corona Crisis, COVID-19, Economic Development, Globalisation

1. Introduction

Pandemics are of episodic nature: they have a beginning and they do have an end. Quite likely, this leads to the fallacy that after the epidemic, both the economy and the society is back to normal. After national lock downs were imposed in most countries in Europe, economies and societies are, indeed, back to somehow normal. But this normal is, as the normal after most crises, a new normal, a "newmality".

After the health crisis is almost left behind in Europe, this article will shed light onto the potential economic and social consequences of this crisis. Based on the experience of the COVID-19 crisis run up and the lock down, this article will discuss the change in working behaviour, a change in consumption, regionalisation of production as well as the winners and losers of the crisis. This article is less driven by theory or a vast data set which supports the author's line of argumentation. In fact this article is a summary of anecdotal evidence which was either collected from the press or observed by the author in person.

In the following sections, we will describe how the pandemic changed the people's social and economic behaviour but also how assumed to be carved-in-stone processes and thinking were abandoned to meet real necessities. To do this the article is organised as followed: the next section give a brief overview how the crisis came into being and what the economic consequences of this crisis are on a macroeconomic level. The third section will leave the macroeconomic sphere and will go to a case by case level while discussing changing working behaviour, changes in consumption, regionalisation of production. and the winners of this process. Finally, Section 4 will conclude this article.

2. The COVID-19 Pandemic and Economic Development

Within just a few weeks, the rapid spread of the novel coronavirus has plunged the world economy into a deep recession.[1] The impact of COVID-19 has been profound and global. The virus is the largest threat to public health since the 1918 Spanish life pandemic.[2] In contrast to the pandemic a hundred years ago, protecting humans lives and allowing health care systems to cope with the outbreak required isolation, lock downs, and widespread closures of businesses to slow the spread of the virus. A mammoth task in today's globally connected economy. Hence,

---

[1] See Bundesbank (2020), p.12.

[2] See Ferguson et al. (2020), p. 1.

this sanitary crisis therefore had a severe impact onto economic activity on global, regional, local level.[3]

The outbreak of COVID-19 differs markedly from past triggers of economic crises like 2008/09 financial crisis or the 2011/2012 sovereign debt crisis in Europe. Infections effectively reduce workforces (labour supply) and imposed quarantines, regional lockdowns, and social distancing had instant adverse effects on sectors that rely on social interactions (travel, hospitality, entertainment, and tourism). The closures of workplaces disrupted supply chains and lower productivity. At the same time, putting workforces on short hours or even laying parts of the work force heightened uncertainty and forced people to reduce consumption. But since consumption was also reduced due to the forced closure of non-essential part of the economy, a de facto shutdown of a significant portion of the economy was the result. These domestic disruptions, not matter they occurred in Asia, Europe, or in the North America, spilled over to trading partners through trade and global production, and caused adverse macroeconomic effects on a global level.[4]

The sudden materialization of extensive disruptions to economic activity forced to reprice traded assets and liabilities by incorporating this economic uncertainty. Hence, the initial shock amplifies through channels familiar from past severe downturns and crises. The rising unemployment in many increases the risk of widespread defaults among borrowers and banks started to worry that consumers and firms will not be able to repay.[5] In fact, the far-reaching measures imposed in many countries to contain the spread of the virus have weighed heavily on economic activity.[6]

3. A Shift in Paradigms

3.1 Run up of the crisis

The world as we knew, a world which worked as 2019 did is, by now, part of history. The pandemic caused a re-organisation of business activities around the globe. When threat of COVID-19 became more and severe, driven by the obligation to take of their work force, companies acted in two steps. First, companies decided to bar their employees from any kind of business travel, either true business-related trips or visiting industry conferences. As consequence, even before official lock downs were in place, many events had to be cancelled simply because no one either willing or allowed to attend. As second step was to split the companies' workforces, wherever possible, into two or more groups and teams. In making sure that both groups do not mingle, employers tried to mitigate the health threat to their employees. Even before official lock downs were in place, both measures hit the parts of the tertiary sector industries which rely on social interactions. Since the service industry was even more hit when lock downs were imposed, we will therefore discuss the spill over effects of working from home (henceforth: WFH) in the following section.

In large cities, e.g., Frankfurt am Main, Paris, London, or New York City, working from home features several benefits for employees. For example, there is no need to get up very early to commute to the office where one is working. For the related service industries, however, exactly this is a economic disaster. Coffee shops, either run by large corporations, like *Starbrucks*,

---

[3] See International Monetary Fund (2020), p. 1.
[4] See International Monetary Fund (2020), p. 2.
[5] See International Monetary Fund (2020), p. 3.
[6] See Bundesbank (2020), p.12.

or small businesses, which mainly rely on office staff as a customer base, were largely hit by declining turnover due to the absence of their customers. The very same happened to other small businesses, such as delis or laundries. Being at home, there was no need for a takeaway lunch or a freshly ironed business shirt any more.

When governments decided to lock down their countries this initial effect, customers staying away, was even reinforced: When the lock downs were imposed all hospitality places (restaurants, bars, hotels), non-food shops, schools, universities, places of worship and cultural places such as theatres or museums were force to closed. While the corporate precautionary measures only had limited effects to a whole economy, this was un-precedent demand shock to each and every economy as a whole.

In addition to this, one point which is nearly omitted in the current discussion of the economic consequences of the COVID-19 pandemic is that many manufacturing companies needed to reduce their production way before non-manufacturing companies, e.g., financial services companies, law firms, consultancies, sent their workforce into the home office or put their workforce on short hours. The reason for this was that China locked down about two months before the rest of the world did likewise. As a consequence, due to lack of supply materials, many manufacturing companies were forced to reduce their production and to put their work force on short time. Even now, after most of the lock downs were lifted, many manufacturing companies are still working shorts hours.

3.2 Economic Newmality

The new normal, the "Newmality", took shape as soon as the lock down was lifted. In following sections, we will describe the assumed changes in people's working behaviour, the assumed change in consumption behaviour, how production processes will change, and why large technology companies, "big tech", will emerge from this crisis stronger than before.

Change in working behaviour

Over the last couple of months, most of office employees who normally go or commute to work each and every day were forced to spend their work time at home. Even though the lock downs were set aside, many companies are still in the WHF mode. This is simply driven by the motivation not to expose workforces to a still existing health threat. Some companies either plan to return to the office after the summer holidays or in late 2020. But what does this mean for future's working behaviour?

During the lock down companies were and are still part of an unparalleled experiment: During a short period of time they were forced to send people into the home office and to set up a virtual organisations. Meetings were not held in person any more but by the use of telephone conferences, skype, webex, zoom, and other technologies. Reportings, like monthly management reporting, quarter-end, and even annual reportings were performed from the home office. Even board meeting, either management or supervisors, and annual share holders meetings (if allowed) were held virtually via one of the aforementioned technology platforms.

All this leads to question how to organise a business operations properly in the future. Even though set up was in the greatest hurry and without a proper testing beforehand, the preliminary evidence of this experiment demonstrates that the almost virtual organisation is possible – at least from an organisational / the employer's perspective. Employees, however, benefit on the one hand from not being required to commute (long) distances to their work places. On the other hand, they need to organise the commonly accepted infrastructure, e.g., coffee shops, delis, and small restaurants by themselves. Combining this, gives office employees a previously unknown degree of freedom. They can organise their work around their private life and not hitherto the other way around.

However, this developed into a sheer disaster for transportation companies like airlines, railway companies, or municipality-owned public transportation companies. While railway companies and local public transportation companies lost their frequent commuters, airlines lost their most profitable and therefore valuable customers: Business travellers. With the emergence of COVID-19 crisis, companies were reluctant to let their employees travel. With lock down business travel came to a complete hold. Here, while commuting is likely to start again after the lock downs were lifted, it is somehow questionable whether companies allow their employers themselves to travel again. For two reasons: First, companies still have impose precautionary measure to guarantee the wellbeing of their employees and second during the lock down business prevails by the use of modern technologies.

Change in Consumption

During the lock down social life was reduced to the absolute minimum. Often, only shops with a food license were allowed to open. In some countries in Europe, e.g., Germany, restaurants were allow to open to delivery and for take away. All other kind of retailers, no matter they are located on High Street or Main Street, were not allowed to open. As previously mentioned, any kind of cultural activity, theatres, cinemas, museums, were prohibited. Gyms were closed, too. While in countries like Germany, people were allowed to do sports outside or go for a walk, countries like France, Italy and Spain enforced hard lockdown so people were only allowed to leave their homes to buy food in their local supermarket. So what does this mean for consumption?

Over the last years, there was often the call for slowing down social life. Social media put a enormous pressure, especially on young people, to compete with each other by posting the latest events in their life on one of the social media platforms. All this came to a sudden hold when government imposed the lock downs. People were forced to stay at home and often home are not instagramable as the places to be in the city you live. But not only social media community were forced to stay at home, but also the families and merely everyone because there was no place to go with the kids on the weekend. Being forced to be at home for such "long"period of time is likely to change the mindset of many people and they are asking what part of consumption is important and what part is not.

Being forced to stay at home and being responsible for your own kind of infrastructure and personal well being demands for answers. Consumption-wise it is the choice of buying the newest it-bag and watch or buying proper kitchen equipment or new home office furniture - a proper home office can even exceed the costs of the latest high street it-watch. All this might lead to an increasing demand for home goods, furniture and, as the basis of this, a shifting demand in property itself. Apartments with less than three rooms / two bed rooms might be unattractive for future tenants simply because they need a room serving as an office – working from home from a kitchen or dinner table might be cumbersome at some time. So land lords needs to adjust their business model to meet the future demand of their customers / tenants.

But not only local land lords ay review their business model. Formally tourist hot spots might to re-think their business model as well. Recently, there was a documentary about Venice on the German-French television channel *arte*. In this documentary the mayor of Venice stated that the business model of his city failed. Simply because Venice was and is over-reliant onto tourism. Walking through the city, he told the camera team that the lock down forced the businesses and the municipality of the city to rethink what they are currently doing. The city is, according to his words, just a large stage what people think Venice is. He came to the conclusion that this is not a proper and future-orientated business model (it is actually not too far away from the one of Las Vegas) and that the city of Venice need to shift it business model towards a more sustainable one; one which can exist even when there are no crowds shuffling in from mega-ocean liners.

Regionalisation

Another business wise re-thinking might occur in the production industry. Focusing on office worker alone is only one side of the story. As indicated beforehand, the secondary sector of the economy, production, was not less affected by the health crisis. When the COVID-19 virus initially spread across Asia, factories were forced to close down their production; causing a shortage of supply for their customers, mostly European and North American companies. This was mainly due to global supply changes. Due to this shortage of supply, factories were force to put their work force on short time simply.

This example demonstrated the dependence of Western manufacturing on Asian, mostly Chinese, companies regarding prefabrication. Even if the COVID-19 virus had remained a regional phenomenon, it would still had have affected Western manufacturers in the same way: no prefabricated goods. Reducing the dependence from other parts of world, manufacturing companies, might choose supplying companies which are in the same regions as they are. For example, a Western European small medium sized enterprise (SME) would benefit if the parts of the production are much cheaper Eastern European countries such Bulgaria or Romania.

Having these supplies regionally organised rather than globally, these companies would benefit from regionally organised supply chains. This regionalisation does not mean de-globalisation but the creation of regional production and supply chains which can be controlled more easily than global chains.

Big Technology

In contrast to other major pandemics like the Spanish Flue a century ago, modern technologies, predominantly the internet-based ones, helped to compress the health crisis in the very beginning. Half a century or even twenty years ago it would not have been possible to have entire companies working from home. Recently, there was an interview with the CEO of Deutsche Bank, Christian Siewers, in the papers. During the interview Mr. Siewers recognised that around sixty thousand of the nearly ninety thousand employees of Deutsche Bank were working from home and the bank was still functioning. An astonishing moment for the CEO of one of Europe's largest banks.

This was only possible because today companies have the necessary technologies at hand to create the aforementioned virtual companies. While previously, the work took place in dedicated places, e.g., a towering corporate head quarter, management reportings, weekly team meetings were now held via webex, zoom, skype, and other applications. But not only office-related work found its way into the internet, for many retailing companies, the point of sale also shifted from main street and high street into "web street".

While established retailers distrustful eyed on shopping platforms, such as *ebay* or he behemoth *amazon*, these very platforms, of course together with other more individual platforms, turned out to be the last resort of selling goods to customers during the lock down. In the United States, for example, *amazon* hired an additional work force of more than hundred thousand people to meet customer demand and also shifted it process in a way that daily supply of goods and food is ensured. The internet giant saw a chance in the crisis to directly attack retailers like *Walmart* by delivering goods and food to the places where people lived.

During this time, however, there was often the claim "Don't buy on *amazon*, buy local.". But what if local shops needed cash flow and couldn't wait until the lock down is lifted? Of course, large retail chains already had a competitive advantage toward smaller companies and local shops when the crisis emerged. However, these smaller companies and local shops quickly closed the gap and launched their own online shops or used ebay to sell their products to their customers.

But not only retailers used web-based technologies to generate revenues. Restaurant did as well. During the lock down in Germany, restaurants were only allowed to open for take away and delivery. This fact was often advertised on social media like *facebook* and / or *instragam* under the slogan "We are with you.", pretending that these restaurants are still there and servicing their guests with their favourite meals – as *amazon* did with food in general. This was, in fact, a well-placed marketing stunt. Instead of "We are with you.", the slogan should have been called "Don't forget about us.". But it does no fail its purpose: Bored from being at with their own poor cooking skills, people ordered and as soon as the desired dish arrived at home they posted it on their social media accounts and linked the respective restaurant to it. This restaurant again reposted its customers post and so the word was spread. But what is the lesson on from this?

Crises are always driving innovation and consolidation: Even though social media was used by large firms to advertise their products or the life style of their products, this marketing channel was discovered by local shops and restaurants in broader scale to actively advertise their products in collaboration with their customers. It is hard to imagine that this will go away after four months of successful implementation. So local businesses shifted towards the large platform because it was their only chance to advertise and sell their products. At the same time the large tech companies, all of them cash-rich, invested heavily in their research and development, for example, zoom's best characteristics were quickly copied by *google* or *Microsoft*. But big tech companies also used their cash research to expand their business into the classic food and grocery business.

4. Conclusion

Pandemics are of episodic nature: they have a beginning and they do have an end. This leads to the fallacy that after the epidemic, everything is back to normal. This article showed that we are quite likely transformed new normal, as we call it "newmality". This newmality will be shaped by the experiences made by companies and individuals during the lock down and shifted economic behaviour resulted from.

Regarding working behaviour, this results in more digitalised processes in companies, in less centralised work spaces; the home office will remain even after the sanitary crisis is over. Consumption will shift back goods-based consumption for, e.g., home goods, and away from event-based consumption such as holidays or visit to restaurants. At the same time, production will be regionalised again. All this will be supported by even bigger technology companies which made the decentralisation of work place or web-based retailing possible.

All this will be accompanied by the disappearance of two types of companies. First, companies which were not able to withstand the lock down and the reduced economic activities. And second, companies which business model does not fit to requirements of the newmality.

References

Deutsche Bundesbank 2020. *Monthly Report – May 2020. Deutsche Bundesbank*, Frankfurt am Main 2020.

Ferguson, *N.M 2020. Report 9: Impact of non-pharmaceutical interventions (NPIs) to reduce COVID-19 mortality and healthcare demand. Imperial College. London 2020.*

International Monetary Fund 2020. *World Economic Outlook April 2020*. Washington D.C. 2020.

Christian Buschmann, PhD, is Treasury Manager at a Frankfurt-based broker dealer, a subsidiary of one of Japan's largest banking groups. Before this he spent 11 years at a leading German Bank in several positions in Frankfurt am Main, London, and Luxembourg. He holds a diploma-degree in business administration from the Business and Information Technology School (BiTS) in Iserlohn and a MA and PhD from the Frankfurt School of Finance & Management. Since 2017 he is board member of the Allied European Financial Markets Associaton (AEFMA) and responsible for AEFMA's education programme. - cfc.buschmann@gmail.com.

Of Nemesis and Narcissus:
Lessons COVID may provide for enterprises – and ethics – of global health promotion and biosecurity

Diane DiEuliis, National Defense University, USA

Nikola B. Kohls, Coburg University of Applied Sciences, Germany

James Giordano, Georgetown University Medical Center, USA and Coburg University of Applied Sciences, Germany

Abstract

What will humanity learn from this crisis? The challenges posed by COVID-19 illustrate how gaps, weaknesses, and vulnerabilities in global biosecurity might become adversary opportunities, and exploited given the relative facility of new techniques of gene editing that could allow nation states or rogue actors to modify existing pathogens - like a coronavirus – or make other bioagents anew. The current crisis is a circumstance and period of change. What needs to change? What has changed based upon previous responses; what remains to be – and should be - changed? And will such change(s) be implemented, or will the hubris and superficial attractiveness of previously used methods seduce decisions and actions that lead to demise? COVID may provide a looking glass through which to view the past and present to gaze upon the relative successes and failures of national and worldwide postures of health promotion, public safety and biosecurity. But it may also serve as a pool of human sweat, blood, and tears in which we glimpse a reflection of humanity.

Key words

Learning, biosecurity, reflection

> *Nemesis is a goddess of ancient Greek mythology. She is described as the winged balancer of life; strictly impartial in distributing in due proportion to each that which is deserved, and enacting retribution against those who succumb to hubris and moral failure. Nemesis enacted such retribution on Narcissus for his vanity. After he rejected the advances of the nymph Echo, Nemesis lured him to a pool where he caught sight of his own reflection and fell in love with it, and could not bear to part from his own image, eventually leading to his own demise.*

The historian Joseph Campbell described myths as explanatory fictions that are intended to teach about aspects of life that bear important meaning to survival, flourishing, relationships, and their interaction. They offer lessons in benefits, burdens, and harms that may – and likely will – be encountered, and provide stories to illustrate human response, responsibility, successes, weaknesses, and failures. The COVID-19 pandemic is real, yet will be lyric in the tragic and epic aspects of manifest effect. What will humanity learn from this crisis? Looking ahead, there is increasing likelihood for both natural and man-made biothreats as humanity continues to disrupt global ecologies and develop emerging methods to modify biology. Such convergent human activity prompts question of whether societies – if not humanity at/large – is prepared to acknowledge and accept the responsibility to address the ethical challenges – and opportunities-instantiated by such 'progress'.

The challenges posed by COVID-19 illustrate how gaps, weaknesses, and vulnerabilities in global biosecurity might become adversary opportunities, and exploited given the relative facility of new techniques of gene editing that could allow nation states or rogue actors to modify existing pathogens - like a coronavirus – or make other bioagents anew. The current crisis should be regarded in its most literal sense: as a circumstance and period of change. But this prompts the questions: What needs to change? What has changed based upon previous responses; what remains to be – and should be - changed? And will such change(s) be implemented, or is the hubris and superficial attractiveness of previously used methods seduce decisions and actions that lead to demise?

To address these questions, our research group employs a process of Gap Identification, Analysis, and Compensation (GIAC), to detect and evaluate existing gaps in health promotions and biosecurity preparedness and response, so as to define tools and methods to bridge such gaps, and prevent their future occurrence. Evidently, COVID-19 presents a clear and present threat to nations' health public status and biosecurity in and across a number of different domains. To be sure, the biomedical threat impacts individuals' morbidity and mortality. The social and psychological effects – of individual and group sickness and death, as well as measures being implemented toward reducing their extent – impart social, economic and psychological disruptions across a range of scales and levels – from the personal to the populational.

This current situation may be seen as the horns of a bio-socioeconomic dilemma. On one side there is the need to address and maintain the best interests of those patients or currently infected, those on the road to recovery, those who are most serious, and those who may be vulnerable to infection in the future. On the other are desires – if not needs - to re-stabilize and mitigate economic loss - both nationally and internationally. In addressing these considerations and concerns it becomes important to differentiate what constitutes disruptive and destructive influences and effects. Indubitably, the effects of COVID-19 have been, and remain disruptive. This disruption induces ripple effects in and across a variety of sectors? Domains? and levels, which range from the cellular to the social. And while it is en vogue to utilize bellicose language to describe fighting this pandemic (and perhaps appropriately so), the disruptive and rippling effects are illustrative not of kinetic actions and results (such as those occurring in warfare), but rather of non-kinetic influences that can then rain disruptive effects in those domains and dimensions that lack preparedness and means of necessary and sufficient response.

To date, man-made threats have been well addressed by prior and present biological toxins, weapons (BTW) and chemical weapons (CW) conventions, and other signatory treaties. It may well be that the BTWC and CWC require re-visitation, review, and some revision. We argue that the current COVID-19 crisis prompts renewed and re-focused insight to the new vista of what constitutes health promotion in light of bio-risks, biothreats, and biohazards – both of natural origin and man-made design - which will require new stances of preparedness and response.

We opine that there is need for coordinated infrastructure and functions that engage adequate surveillance, communication of surveillance (with regard to qualification and quantification of burdens, viable risks and identified threats), and readiness. COVID-19 well-illustrates the "problem of novelty" as it affects an unprepared and uncoordinated system of biosecurity readiness, and response: it is a highly infectious biological agent with considerable – and somewhat ambiguous - variability in the morbidity, mortality, and factors contributory to the spread and severity of disease. The difficulties of addressing and dealing with these novelties have illuminated inherent gaps and weaknesses in various nations' systems of biosecurity preparedness and response.

As COVID has shown, risks and threats to biosecurity need not be man-made; climate change, coupled to the spread of human activities into faunal and floral ecologies make spillover effects of zoonotic disorders such as coronaviruses and ever more likely if not probable occurrences.

But the increasing possibility of natural events does not lessen the need to appreciate the growing risk and threat of man-made biological agents. To this end, our research group has been focusing upon biosecurity issues generated by the use and misuse of radical leveling and emerging biotechnologies. We have reported that misinformation and miscalculation about these risks and threats incur lack of readiness that can increase the pace of any disruptive influence, and extend the durability of effects of novel bio-techniques and tools in and across biomedical, socio-economic, political, and global positioning dimensions. Surely, these inadequacies in biosecurity, and are surely being recognized and noted by current and near-term global competitors (and potential adversaries).

If this provides a "description of the relative darkness", then the obvious query is how to "light a candle" – and keep it alight? There is merit in mobilizing a response that conjoins all the necessary levels of government - and social enterprise - that are required to maintain health promotions and biothreat suppression capabilities. Whole-of-government coordination, cooperation, and engagement is necessary, as evidenced by the response capabilities and effectiveness articulated in the aforementioned open societies. Yet, while necessary, whole-of-government activity alone does not – and cannot – afford the purchase to leverage the scale of services, resources, and human effort sufficient to mobilize an efficient, effective enterprise of biosecurity preparedness and response. To do this requires both whole-of-government and whole-of-nation approaches.

We have proposed that an effective whole-of-nation engagement would entail a four-thrust approach. The first thrust is focal to increasing awareness of existing and "on-the-horizon" biorisks and possible threats. Such awareness would mandate overview and deep surveillance to include identification and assessment of explicit and more tacit risk and threat factors and vectors. The second thrust entails translation of qualified risks into quantifiable prediction of threat. Such quantification requires modeling, gaming, and forecasting of threats and the impact and influence they make evoke in short-, intermediate-, and long-term. This allows evaluation of the resources that will be required for sustainable health promotion, and nimble readiness and responsiveness to identified threats. The third thrust is enterprise devoted to mitigating or counter the threat. Ultimately fourth thrust is dedicated to preventing, and decreasing or negating occurrence or effectiveness of (naturally-occurring and/or human-made) threats in the future, as an overarching goal in promoting and sustaining the health and safety of the polis. The four thrusts of this approach are not – and should not be – mutually exclusive.

In practice, the four thrust approach involves all of national resources, in a relatively seamless articulation of the so-called "triple helix", of government, (on national, regional and local and/or city levels), the research enterprise (of both public and private academia and foundations); and the commercial sector at a variety of scales. We propose that these entities be interactively and complementarily engaged in focus, scope and action(s). Thus, thrust one would facilitate thrust two via the conjoinment of academic institutions, research centers, and the informational resources to identify those risks that could become threats, and quantifying such threats and their influence, and potential effects. Moving from thrust two to three, quantification of threat is coupled to assessment and quantification of existing resources available and required to mitigate or counter influences and effects that would be rendered. Toward these goals, public health and safety systems and organizations, national laboratories, and industries are all brought to bear. Thrust three establishes a basis for the fourth: assessment of needs, and of existing and required resources, services and activities that will be essential to prevent some future event that threatens public health, safety and biosecurity. These third to fourth thrust efforts bring together whole-of-nation – communities in a coordinated effort to effect sustainable readiness and response.

But herein lies another dilemma. To what extent can and should these resources and services engage proactive efforts aimed at preparedness and response? Surveilling global ecologies (inclusive of populated environments) is evidently useful, if not arguably important to identify and assess health and biosecurity risks and threats. But what limits to surveillance should be defined, demarcated – and defended, to maintain the delicate balance of perspicuity, preparedness, (individual, and community) privacy, and commercial and national proprietary veiling? What system(s) of surveilling the surveillance can and need be developed and articulated to insure that "enough is enough; but not too much"; and what process and metrics will be used to delineate such distinctions? What will be identified as viable good, benefit, risk, burden, threat and harm? These constructs are nested in, and vested to meanings, ideologies, values, and needs; and arise from and reflect various communities' history, philosophies, ethics, and precepts and positions of power. There is a thin, and often ambiguous line between definitions of health, protection, and security, and what constitutes selection, separation, and subjugation.

The proverbial shield of health promotion, public safety and biosecurity also requires foresight to assess and predict risks and threats against which protection must be developed and rendered. Here too, we must ask, what agents and methods will be selected? Approaches such as gain-of-function research and investigations of possible bioagents and their respective antidotes are contributory to predictive preparedness and efficient response. Yet the dangers (of both possible biosafety accidents, as well as the potential dual-use of such studiers and their products) is evident and ominous. And, to reiterate, while current treaties and conventions may describe and constrain such activities, new developments in bioscience and technology enable skirting these treaties' restrictions, and there are no guarantees that nations will necessarily align with and/or ratify these conventions' precepts.

Perhaps then, COVID may provide a looking glass through which to view the past and present to gaze upon the relative successes and failures of national and worldwide postures of health promotion, public safety and biosecurity. But it may also serve as a pool of human sweat, blood, and tears in which we glimpse a reflection of humanity. What will we choose to see; and what will we learn from the explanatory story COVID affords? Will we succumb to hubris and vanity and remained affixed to some romanticized view of our own image? Or, will we take stock of our weaknesses as well as our strengths, in a more realistic view of both what we are, and what we may become through the power of science and technology, responsibility, and respect for a global community as an evolving story that we are capable of creating?

Acknowledgements

This work was supported in part by funding from the Henry Jackson Foundation (JG), and Leadership Initiatives (JG).

Disclaimer

The views and opinions provided in this essay do not necessarily reflect those of the United States government, Department of Defense, or those institutions and organizations that support the authors' work.

References

Campbell 1991. Campbell J. *The Power of the Myth*, NY: Random House.

DeFranco 2019. DeFranco JP, DiEuliis D, Bremseth LR, Snow JJ. Giordano J. 2019. Emerging technologies for disruptive effects in non-kinetic engagements. *HDIAC Currents* 6(2): 49-54.

DiEuliis 2017. DiEuliis D, Giordano J. Gene editing using CRISPR/Cas9: implications for dual-use and biosecurity. *Protein and Cell* 15: 1-2.

Gerstein 2017. Gerstein D, Giordano J. Re-thinking the Biological and Toxin Weapons Convention? *Health Security* 15(6): 1-4.

Gerstein 2020. Gerstein D, Giordano, J. How to re-open America. *CNN Opinions*, 3(27).

Giordano 2012. Giordano, J. Public health: History, theory and modern practices and challenges. In: Anheier K, Juergensmeyer M. (eds.) *Encyclopedia of Global Studies*. Fairfield CA: SAGE.

Giordano 2013. Giordano, J. Respice finem: Historicity, heuristics and guidance of science and technology on the 21st century world stage. *Synesis: A Journal of Science, Technology, Ethics and Policy* 4: E1-4.

Giordano, Benedikter 2012. Giordano J, Benedikter R. An early – and necessary – flight of the Owl of Minerva: Neuroscience, neurotechnology, human socio-cultural boundaries, and the importance of neuroethics. *Journal of Evolution and Technology* 22(1): 14-25.

Jesty 2012. Jesty J. Biotechnology: Who benefits; whom is harmed? In: Giordano J. (ed.) *Neurotechnology: Premises, Potential, and Problems*. Boca Raton: CRC Press, pp. 301-320.

Lanzilao 2013. Lanzilao E, Shook, J, Benedikter R, Giordano J. Advancing neuroscience on the 21st century world stage: The need for – and proposed structure of – an internationally relevant neuroethics. *Ethics in Biology, Engineering, and Med* 4(3): 211-229.

Shook 2014. Shook JR, Giordano J. A principled, cosmopolitan neuroethics: Considerations for international relevance. *Philosophy, Ethics, and Humanities in Medicine* 9 (1).

Shook 2017. Shook JR, Giordano J. Ethics transplants? Addressing the risks and benefits of guiding international biomedicine. *AJOB-Neuroscience* 8(4): 230-232.

Dr. **Diane DiEuliis** is a Senior Research fellow at National Defense University. Her research areas focus on emerging biological technologies, biodefense, and preparedness for bio-threats. Specific topic areas under this broad research portfolio include dual use life sciences research, synthetic biology, the US bioeconomy, disaster recovery, and behavioral, cognitive, and social science as it relates to important aspects of deterrence and preparedness. Dr. DiEuliis currently lectures in a variety of foundational professional military education courses across all the services.

James Giordano, Ph.D., is Professor in the Departments of Neurology and Biochemistry and Chief of the Neuroethics Studies Program of the Pellegrino Center for Clinical Bioethics, Georgetown University Medical Center, Washington DC, USA; Senior Research Fellow of the Project in Biosecurity, Technology, and Ethics, US Naval War College, Newport RI, USA; and Distinguished Visitingf Professor of Biotechnology, Health Promotions, and Ethics at the Coburg University for Applied Sciences, Coburg, GER; jg353@georgetown.edu.

Prof. Dr. **Niko Kohls** has over 20 years' experience in both research and business environments. He holds a diploma in psychology (1998) and a PhD (2004) from the University of Freiburg as well as habilitation thesis (Dr. habil. med.) in medical psychology from the University of Munich (2012). As a postdoc he has worked at the University Hospital Freiburg and at the University of Northampton in Great Britain, until he earned a Samueli-Rockefeller Scholar in 2007. From 2008 until 2014 Niko was responsible for co-directing and managing the Generation Research Program, a think tank of the University of Munich responsible for finding solutions for the dealing with the sociodemographic change. Since 2013 Niko is a professor for Health Sciences at the University of Applied Sciences Coburg, Germany with a special focus on health promotion. Niko's research is focussed on those aspects of states of consciousness including spirituality, mindfulness and inner coherence which are of particular relevance to the health promotion, neuroethics and organizational sciences.

The Coronavirus Pandemic
under Unfavourable Social Economic Conditions

Geni Maria Hoss, Faculdade EST, Brazil

Abstract

When the World Health Organization (WHO) classified the Coronavirus as a pandemic, rapid changes were already taking place in various countries. People in developing countries are affected and health workers are overburdened not only by the scientifically based safety measures to prevent and combat the pandemic, but also by the lack of health structures and unfavourable socio-economic conditions. Over and above observing security measures, solidarity and co-operation are required to meet the needs of people who have ended up in extreme poverty as a result of the pandemic. Important attitudes for a different future, too.

Key words

Coronavirus pandemic, social inequality, health system, solidarity, cooperation.

1. Health care during a pandemic

Also, in the case of a pandemic, the WHO has to deduce its task from Article 25 of the Universal Declaration of Human Rights, and, after analysing the complex global economic situation today, offer recommendations for its application to the health system of each country. Article 25 states:

"Everyone has the right to a standard of living adequate for the health and well-being of himself and of his family, including food, clothing, housing and medical care and necessary social services, and the right to security in the event of unemployment, sickness, disability, widowhood, old age or other lack of livelihood in circumstances beyond his control. [...]" (United Nations 1948)

In terms of this law directives for the primary health provision of all people were laid down in the Declaration of Alma-Ata 1978 (Kazakhastan), and re-confirmed forty years later after a Global Conference on Primary Health Care in Astana 2018 (Kazakhstan). Although many countries committed themselves to providing primary health care, there is still a huge lack in this field. The conferences drew attention to urgent social conditions and based themselves on a complex health policy. The Declaration of Alma-Ata states:

"The Conference strongly reaffirms that health, which is a state of complete physical, mental and social wellbeing, and not merely the absence of disease or infirmity, is a fundamental human right and that the attainment of the highest possible level of health is a most important world-wide social goal whose realization requires the action of many other social and economic sectors in addition to the health sector" (WHO 1978).

Such a concept presents many countries with a special challenge because of unfavourable conditions. The limitations caused by a lack of social justice, education, houses, healthy nutrition, sanitary provision, disease prevention, etc. come to a head in extraordinary situations such as epidemics and pandemics. Against this background we can expect very different effects of the coronavirus worldwide.

During a pandemic, in how far can the regulations and directives of the health system laid down at Alma-Ata or internal health politics, be applied in the countries? In this regard special mention must be made of equitable access to basic health care, equality (care according to regional standards and personal needs), integral care and treatment (preventative and clinical treatment and rehabilitation). In this instance we are dealing mainly with developing countries which have set up basic health structures, but where the public provision of health care and equipment is usually inadequate, and in many instances scrapped. In addition, the question arises here as to the extent to which the social deficit intensifies the provision of health care. What are the ethical questions that result from the lack or non-existence of medical technologies and medication?

When talking about developing countries we can say that people live in two worlds: an affluent country and also a country in which there are areas of extreme poverty. When a government fails, private initiatives take its place particularly in health care provision. We know that various demographic and social variables exercise an essential influence on health care provision. However, what is added by the coronavirus pandemic? Scientists are not yet able to answer all the questions, disregard of science, denial of the pandemic, conspiracy theories, and lack of trust in the government, fake news about the pandemic, which often gives rise to confusion among the people, widespread polarisation in politics, and as a result the lack of a uniting centre outside and above political ideologies, a lack of personnel in the hospitals and clinics.

We are justified in taking into consideration the complexity of health care provision in such adverse situations. Health care providers in general are not conversant with the rigid protective measures required by the pandemic, so that many of them become its victims. This negatively affects the psychological state of their colleagues. For doctors it is extremely difficult to come to ethical decisions when they are only presented with negative options. Not only have health professionals come into focus, but many ethical issues have been raised and, as a result, the whole of society has understood the health care dilemma, particularly in adverse conditions. Professionals need to be prepared to deal with a great ethic: how to make the right decisions in a chaos of health structures, lack of medical equipment, and where health professionals are constantly mentally and physically burdened?

The global action against a pandemic is also very complex. It is urgent to convince governments and citizens to follow the scientific evidence. Even though the Coronavirus baffles science in many ways, there is still general knowledge about how to deal with viruses in general, as well as knowledge gained in the last months, which is very important in supplying a suitable answer to the whole of society. Depending on the system of government, priorities and political leaders in the different countries, tensions often arise, because not all have a correct appreciation of the science and the global measures suggested by international organisations. The WHO guidelines cannot be applied by force, and we have to avoid interfering in the health care regulations of the individual countries, because this would offend against the remit of an international organisation. This raises the question: how to solve problems with a global impact without global involvement? When it comes to problems with a global impact on the health sector, this not only leads to international political tensions, but also to internal tensions in countries where political chaos already existed beforehand. Therefore, the WHO's guidelines are hardly, or are not applied in these countries. Local measures, especially where science is widely ignored, often have little or no effect. The necessary and urgent political unity to improve the joint commitment to solve the problem cannot be achieved overnight. Here, the lack of global leadership, including in humanitarian areas, is very evident. It is not enough to propose solutions, it is necessary to provide a kind of coordinating entity that helps to reconcile the global guidelines with every local reality, without violating the State's sovereignty. According to the Israeli philosopher Yuval Noah Harari (Harari 2020) the challenges of the Coronavirus are intensified by a lack of global leadership and trust between people. This can also lead to distrust regarding institutions that makes the adoption of global guidelines very difficult, which has a very negative effect in the event of a pandemic. Another aspect that can be highlighted here is the difficulty of gathering reliable information on the coronavirus pandemic, as reported in the

WHO Situation report 133:

"While steps are taken to ensure accuracy and reliability, all data are subject to continuous verification and change. Case detection, definitions, testing strategies, reporting practice, and lag times differ between countries/territories/areas. These factors, amongst others, influence the counts presented, with variable underestimation of true case and death counts, and variable delays to reflecting these data at global level" (WHO 2020).

These factors are repeated in particular in countries with political instability and with usual lack of articulation between the federal States and government entities in the area of public health, which depends on good data collection and interpretation. The result is incomplete information that undermines the credibility of the reports. Therefore, these countries are unable to inform the WHO correctly. In addition, incorrect information contributes negatively to decision-making and consequent actions, and may even compromise the rational use of scarce financial and human resources.

2. What the Coronavirus pandemic teaches us

The feeling of omnipotence, which was partly intensified by the new technologies, has been profoundly shaken. How helpless people suddenly are in the face of something unknown, because nothing can help us when we don't even know what to do. The way the virus has spread, as well as it terrible effects, show us in a cruel way that there is no dividing line between the various species. We must far more learn to share with one another the knowledge and respect for the specific qualities of each species. What Fritz Jahr, pastor and philosopher (1895-1953) noted applies here: "The sharp division between animals and human beings that was dominant from the beginning of European culture until the end of the 18th century, can no longer be maintained today" (Jahr 2013: 25). In actual fact this way of thinking has not been completely overcome even today. That is precisely why it is so important for human beings to understand their ethical responsibility in and for the whole world by distancing themselves from exercising absolute dominion over their relationship with other creatures, and instead approach them with respect. "When human beings declare their independence from reality and behave as the absolute ruler, the basis for their existence collapses automatically"(Pope Francis 2015). However human beings have to control how the various vital structures appear, and how a creature is related to the physical world around it and one another. This requires the contribution of science. The Mozambique biologist and author, Mia Couto, regrets the lack of knowledge about viruses in society as a whole:

"Viruses cannot be understood as the villains in history, or the rogues that are only studied for medical reasons. The scientific community questions whether these creatures are living organisms or inorganic particles. No matter, viruses are the great directors of the orchestra of life, the messengers and agents of exchange between the most varied genetic inheritances. They are not 'outside' or 'distant', they don't live in laboratories. They are where there is life, they are in us" (Couto 2020).

The unknown can lead to panic, and delay a measured and rapid reaction. It is not the first time that large numbers of people have died of epidemics (e.g. the so-called Spanish Flu pandemic of 1918). With regard to infectious diseases we may not forget that present-day technologies have made human mobility ever easier, and this promotes more rapid and more widespread infection. However, it remains an open question whether viruses wouldn't spread without these possibilities. The rhythm of their spread is a special challenge to the health care structures. Observing definite safety precautions is therefore important, because then the spread is retarded. In this way the health care systems of a country are not overtaxed so that they collapse. In addition, time is an important factor for science. Even though scientific knowledge today is far more advanced than in earlier pandemics, we may still not count upon a medical solution yet. Since the recommended measures exercise a huge effect on other areas of life, such as the economy, for example, or the employment market, they cannot be upheld for a longer period.

According to the information provided by the UN, many countries have noticed that domestic violence and the abuse of children, in all social classes, have increased greatly (cf. Mlambo-Ngcuka 2020). Can this be attributed only to the limitations of the housing situation and being thrown back onto one's own family? Of course, there is a complex spectrum of reasons for this situation. However, it is clear that in the multiplicity of lifestyles today, living together is no longer considered so important, and hence has to be learnt again.

At any rate, the situation that has developed as a result of the Coronavirus requires holistic and effective national measures, and the active responsibility of everyone for overcoming the pandemic as rapidly as possible, and for building up the areas impacted by it.

Not just me and those around me. "Whoever correctly carries out their moral duties towards themselves, will avoid harming many others" (Jahr 2013: 87). These words of Fritz Jahr, which he wrote in the context of a discussion of the Fifth Commandment "You shall not kill" (Ex 20,13), could also be a Golden Rule for the times of a pandemic. What matters here is not an egoistical attitude, but the realisation that everyone else and all creatures share in the same fate. Jahr asks: "What have been the practical effects of the ethical obligations of the Fifth Commandment for our own life? That we don't take our own lives, or that we don't shorten, damage or endanger it [...]" (Jahr 2013: 87). When we now talk about a pandemic, we are dealing in a special way with the effects of our personal attitudes on the collective. What matters, in the first place, is our own health as caring for the health of the whole of society. This often gives rise to tensions, because society today – particularly in the West – places great emphasis on private rights and personal freedom. Both of the highest values can give rise to the feeling that we live in a sort of "capsule" in which people experience that they are largely separated from the world around. When self-preservation is seen as an ethical duty, there is no limit between private and collective life. On the contrary, it makes us aware that they influence each other. It is obvious that the necessary safety precautions during the Corona pandemic have strongly encroached on our private lives, and again draw our attention to the social dimension, our collective lives. The core problem for many people is: What about my freedom? And my right to move around freely? To answer these questions we need to call upon social ethics:

"Social ethics rests upon the person and their intrinsic longing for freedom. It rejects two opinions that cannot be reconciled with freedom – Freedom is only a concession by society, which has the power to limit or suspend freedom. – Freedom is absolute and the human person is the lord of the universe" (Minnerath 2007: 35).

Where people place themselves and their wishes "above everything else", they remove themselves from their actual life in the world, i.e., they live together with others like themselves and with all other creatures. This offers them possibilities to develop themselves, but at the same time requires that they integrate themselves into society with its values and regulations for peaceful co-existence. Here one of the principles Pope Francis suggested in connection with social teaching for building up a people fits in:

The whole is greater than the part, but it is also greater than the sum of its parts. There is no need, then, to be overly obsessed with limited and particular questions. We constantly have to broaden our horizons and see the greater good which will benefit us all" (Pope Francis 2013).

We are not dealing here simply with a mass of people, but a global community in which every member is important and in which a greater sensitivity has to exist for the common good. Thus the security measures, when necessary and the only available means to protect ourselves from the pandemic, may not be seen as mere limitation of our freedom and private rights. The rapid spread of the Coronavirus, lack of knowledge and also unstable governments may have led to mistakes in determining the security measures, which may need to be modified. What is important is that people are open for such measures, and recognise that observing them is an act of self-preservation and serves the common good. Freedom is then not "I'll do what I want", but an affirmation that it is "good" for me and everyone even if only for a limited period. Just as our own good has an effect on the common good, so the common good has a role to play in the good of the individual person. The condition is that the knowledge on which these measures are based meets with our free acceptance, and avoids blind social obedience. Here, too, we can add: "Whoever protects themselves from harm, does good to their neighbours and their whole people" (Jahr 2013: 88).

3. Hope for a different future?

The possible changes for a future after the Coronavirus have to some extent already begun, because what happens and how it happens depends on how we react to the present challenges. Some things have changed because of the security measures that have ensured that many essential questions have been raised about our present lifestyle and attitude to life. These may differ worldwide depending on the political, economic and socio-cultural situation of each country. Undue pessimism or too much optimism has to be avoided. Faced with a surprisingly new situation for society in more and more countries, when even expert virologists were presented with more questions than they could answer, and when people's private and social lives were profoundly affected, we cannot suppose that it will not have consequences for the future. However, reactions to the quarantine already show that there is a desire to return to the "old" normal.

The economic consequences of the pandemic can also not be overcome overnight by waving a magic wand. All political and civic stakeholders have to act together. The challenge consists in bringing about such a project in societies marked by political polarisation and intolerance, which are more inclined to favour competition over co-operation. People in countries with a number of deficits in meeting basic needs are usually marked by solidarity and co-operation. For this reason, local solidarity organisations contribute towards mitigating the suffering of thousands of marginalised people. Yet just in these countries the policy makers are often involved in huge corruption scandals. If even in affluent countries the management of the pandemic has presented enormous challenges, what must it have meant for poor and developing countries, which are mostly marked by political instability? While people build up their solidarity organisations in order to help the poorest of the poor, there is a suspicion that during the pandemic the state is not using the augmented help to ensure a better future for its needy citizens, so that they can grow in their financial autonomy and live in decent conditions through their work and social integration. This is the background against which the UNO has raised the alarm, fearing that the current social inequalities and poverty will increase dramatically. The World Bank estimates that 60 million people worldwide could end up in extreme poverty (cf. Guterres 2020). Nevertheless, it is worth our while to highlight here what is good today and what gives hope for a better future.

Enjoy the break and live life creatively. An unplanned break in their social and working lives has challenged many people to re-discover themselves. The first days required a reorganisation of our private lives. Social customs and models of relationship required drastic modification. More time for the family, but how? More time on our own at home, but how do I cope with it? How do I cope with my inward self, because the time I otherwise lacked is now available for me to concern myself with my own life? Often people are overcome by profound sadness and depression. Many liberate themselves by learning to re-think and re-shape their lives. After the difficulties of the initial period, we may expect people to shape their lives differently by giving their own lives, their family and the ecology a greater value in their lives. Based on our present experiences, people will no longer see their private wishes and goals as an island, but as wholly integrated into the world around. They will concern themselves more with the unseen and its greater effects, and will have to consider their own position in relation to other created beings. Trust in science, whose research processes cannot be compared with the hectic pace of life today, will take on new significance: from scientism to a more balanced position of science in the life of the individual person and society. Countries in which politicians almost exclusively take their bearings from the economy have been particularly hard hit. A reorientation can be expected, which will be particularly promoted by civil agencies in society that will later be able to influence politics.

The ecology is grateful. Those who have attentively observed how the standstill of human activity has affected the ecology will understand better why the countryside needs a "Sabbath rest" from time to time. How could we interpret those words of the Bible to our present-day relationship to nature?

"The Lord said to Moses at Mount Sinai, "Speak to the Israelites and say to them: 'When you enter the land I am going to give you, the land itself must observe a sabbath to the Lord. For six years sow your fields, and for six years prune your vineyards and gather their crops. But in the seventh year the land is to have a year of sabbath rest, a sabbath to the Lord. Do not sow your fields or prune your vineyards. Do not reap what grows of itself or harvest the grapes of your untended vines. The land is to have a year of rest" (Lev 25, 1-5).

It is obvious that nature possesses a wonderful power of regeneration. It only needs the opportunity to do so, and to some extent this is now there. It would be naïve to suppose that without a very serious reason, such as the Coronavirus threat, people worldwide would go into quarantine again. However, we can expect that in the "new normal" with the Coronavirus – most likely there will be no "afterwards" – the pace of life will slow down and thus the earth will have more time to rest and recover.

A future with more co-operation and solidarity. The globalisation of the economy, mobility and communication has made a global network of many individual people and humanitarian organisations a reality. To what extent can the Corona pandemic provide an incentive so that co-operation and solidarity can increasingly prevail worldwide, but also locally, to benefit many people? The huge social inequalities have become far more visible, and through the collapse of the economy they will become even greater. In such unfavourable circumstances many people are taking creative initiatives to limit the negative effects on the people who are most endangered. These are often oriented to the future, because some of the measures taken today will contribute to a final solution. The involvement of social and financial agencies in extending health and social care structures for endangered people could offer examples for new models of public-private co-operation in the future.

In the sense of collectivity in developing countries, where social inequalities are blatant and with marked cultural differences, this time of pandemic is a real school for the future. It must be understood that these differences require actions appropriate to each reality. Solutions from a supervisor's perspective and which are often standardized may not have any effect. In Brazil, for example, because of the population density in slums, hotels were destined to welcome elderly people from these regions in order to facilitate the social distancing. However, this attempt to resolve the issue did not count on the fact that people are strongly bound to their homes and surroundings and feel unsafe to live, even if temporarily, in an environment that is not familiar to them. The same was observed among the indigenous people of the Amazon region. In the region, the exclusive hospitals for patients with coronavirus had to be equipped with hammocks since there was initial resistance to the hospitalization required, i.e. in hospital beds. These are challenges that turn this period into the school for the future. Dialog for specific localized actions is the first step to be taken rather than trying to get it right later on, which is why we need unity and engagement of all the players involved to be able to manage the pandemic.

Consolidation of network communication. Measures, such as closing borders, social distancing and quarantine could have caused some people stress. At the same time the distance between people was overcome by far more intensive networking. Many have only really discovered the internet and its possibilities for communication through the pandemic. Distance was experienced as a new way to be close. The extent of the digital integration achieved during the pandemic will surely set its stamp on a new mode of communication in the future, and in particular promote communication between the generations. People have learnt that physical distance can make personal closeness possible, and that worldwide networking does not have to bring about personal closeness if closer human relationships are lacking.

Work from home. The "home office" model, which is already a reality in many companies, was accelerated by the pandemic and has changed work relations in some areas. Some of these changes will certainly be consolidated as a new working model.

Considerations

The word "pandemic" indicates that we are dealing with an acute, global problem. The way it is dealt with varies depending on the possibilities of a country. When social conditions are unfavourable, fighting the Coronavirus is even more complex and requires more support by international organisations such as the WHO. The lack of global leadership and people's distrust regarding institutions and each other makes the implementation of security measures much more difficult.

In developing countries with significant political instability, however, not much can be expected in terms of major changes after the pandemic. The existing economic model, with all deficit, in large measure, should continue along its previous course. Despite citizens receiving more attention from the State during the pandemic, mainly in neoliberal countries, the economic recovery will occur according to the social urgencies of the population. Changes, despite being of little impact in relation to the size of the challenges, are expected from an organized society to the extent that the initiatives adopted are perpetuated, and the awareness of the citizens has aroused more to vindicate conditions that are more humane and supportive from political authorities to benefit the entire population.

The sharing of the experiences of health professionals who are constantly facing the border of life has certainly aroused greater empathy and understanding among the population, which may have a positive influence on working conditions and the recognition of the health professionals' services. In addition, there are also consequences for vocational training based on this experience. If the ethics of life is especially a daily dilemma in medicine, how much more are bioethical issues added in the case of a pandemic.

In conclusion, there are many new situations to overcome today and the hope of a different future to be promoted, even though many things will seem to go back to what they once were over time.

References

Couto   2020.   Couto,   Mia.   Notícias   Coronavírus   [URL: https://www.terra.com.br/noticias/coronavirus/mia-couto-o-virus-nao-pode-ser-o-vilao-da-historia,59daab636834a9cd510e2e766a449192y1qouhg9.html, visited Mai 15, 2020.]

Guterres 2020. Guterres, António. Global solidarity with Africa is an imperative. [URL: https://www.un.org/en/coronavirus/global-solidarity-africa-imperative, visited Mai 29, 2020.]

Jahr 1927. Jahr, F. Bio-Ethik. May, Arnd; Sass, Hans-Martin (Hg.). *Aufsätze zur Bioethik 1924-1948.* Münster: LIT-Verlag 2013 2nd Edition 25-31

Jahr 1934. Drei Studien zum 5. Gebot. Sass, H.M, May, A.T (Hg.). *Aufsätze zur Bioethik 1924-1948* Münster: LIT Verlag; 2013. pp. 85-93.

Mlambo-Ngcuka 2020. Mlambo-Ngcuka, P. Violence against women and girls: the shadow pandemic   [URL: https://www.unwomen.org/en/news/stories/2020/4/statement-ed-phumzile-violence-against-women-during-pandemic, visited Mai 29, 2020.]

Papst   Franziskus   2013.   Papst   Franziskus.   *Evangelii   Gaudium*   [URL: http://www.vatican.va/content/francesco/de/apost_exhortations/documents/papa-francesco_esortazione-ap_20131124_evangelii-gaudium.html, Mai 25, 2020.]

Papst   Franziskus   2015.   *Enzyklika   Laudato   Si*   [URL: http://www.vatican.va/content/francesco/de/encyclicals/documents/papa-francesco_20150524_enciclica-laudato-si.html, visitet Mai 26, 2020.]

UN   1948.   United   Nations.   *Allgemeine   Erklärung   der   Menschenrechte.* [URL: https://www.un.org/depts/german/menschenrechte/aemr.pdf, visited Mai 25, 2020.]

WHO   1978.   World   Health   Organization.   *Erklärung   von   Alma   Ata.*   [URL: http://www.euro.who.int/__data/assets/pdf_file/0017/132218/e93944G.pdf?ua=1,   visited Mai 25, 2020]

WHO   2020.   World   Health   Organization.   *COVID-19   Situation   Reports.*   [URL: https://www.who.int/emergencies/diseases/novel-coronavirus-2019/situation-reports, visited June 2, 2020.]

Yuval 2020. Yuval Noah Harari. In the Battle Against Coronavirus, Humanity Lacks Leadership.   [URL: https://time.com/5803225/yuval-noah-harari-coronavirus-humanity-leadership/, visited May 26, 2020]

Dr. **Geni Maria Hoss** holds a PhD in theology with a major in bioethics, from Faculdade EST, Brazil. She was professor of bioethics in the courses of human sciences. Currently is an independent scholar and is also active as guest lecturer and consultant in the area of bioethics, hospital humanization projects, health and spirituality, pastoral counseling and Christian Theology and environmental responsibility. E-Mail contact: geni.hoss@yahoo.com.br.

Post-Pandemic Business Pivot: 4 Trends to Watch

Sean Hull, Ashland University, USA

Abstract

History tells us that pandemics can - and usually do - have profound economic consequences, and there is no reason to believe that the current Coronavirus pandemic should be any different. It will not be business as usual when the dust settles. Businesses, no matter the size, need to accelerate to the future and there are some trends paving the way that might be worth watching.

Key words

Coronavirus, Pandemic, Economics, GDP, Income, Business, Proximity, Digital Technologies, Offline-to-online, Fourth Industrial Revolution, Exponential Organizations (ExOs), Low touch

1. The Black Death and Spanish Flu

The "Black Death" arrived on the shores of Italy in 1347 via ships, speculation goes from the east. The bubonic plague laid siege to Europe until 1353, when it petered out in western Russian.

In his book, *The End Is Always Near*, Dan Carlin cites:

"One chronicler, Agnolo di Tura, called the Fat, described the devastation: "Father abandoned child, wife husband, one brother another; for this illness seemed to strike through the breath and sight. And so they died. And none could be found to bury the dead for money or friendship."

Carlin goes on to say:

"We can't know how many people in all died. While estimates put the figure at 75 million, countless out-of-the-way farms and towns and even cities may not be included in the final toll. With the total population of western Europe at the time at a bit more than 150 million, this means that about half of the entire population of just that area was wiped out."

The clinical attack rate (CAR) and case fatality ratio (CFR) are standard measures. The CAR is an estimate of the number of individuals who are infected with the disease and the CFR expresses the percentage of infected individuals who die from the disease. Multiplying the CAR by the CFR provides the mortality rate for the population." If a CAR of 35% and CFR of 0.04% is moderate, and a CAR of 46% and CFR of 2.5% is severe, not sure how to classify a CFR close to 50%.

Almost six centuries later, the "Spanish Flu" arrived on the shores of the U.S. in 1918, also via ship. Adding insult to injury, World War I was still in full swing.

Again, Carlin citing this in his book:

"Four days after that Boston detachment (of returning soldiers) arrived, nineteen sailors in Philadelphia were hospitalized...Despite their immediate isolation and that of everyone with whom they had had contact, eighty-seven sailors were hospitalized the next day...two days later, six hundred more were hospitalized with this strange disease. The hospital ran out of empty beds, and hospital staff began falling ill."

Like the current Coronavirus pandemic, entire cities were shut down in the United States - with people staying home from work and school, masks becoming a common sight across the population - as the disease moved across the U.S.

In a paper titled *Economic Effects of the 1918 Influenza Pandemic*, (Thomas Garrett, 2007) cites a researcher:

"Spanish influenza moved across the United States in the same way as the pioneers had, for it followed their trails which had become railroads...the pandemic started along the axis from Massachusetts to Virginia...leaped the Appalachians...positioned along the inland waterways...it jumped clear across the plains and the Rockies to Los Angeles, San Francisco, and Seattle. Then, with secure bases on both coasts...took its time to seep into every niche and corner of America."

Per Marcus Keogh-Brown and others in *The Macroeconomic Costs of a Global*

Influenza Pandemic (2008): "The estimated death toll of the Spanish Flu ranged somewhere between 20 and 100 million people worldwide, with an estimated CFR of 2 to 2.5%."

The demographic damage of these pandemics is startling, but one can also not ignore the speed, scope and endurance (years) of these pandemics, with more damage occurring in subsequent "waves" of both.

And then there is the long(er) tail of economic damage that pandemics can induce.

2. Macroeconomic Consequences of Previous Pandemics

Hard economic data is scarce, if non-existent, for both, the Black Death and the Spanish Flu. Information comes from individual accounts and, in the case of the Spanish Flu, from print media (newspapers.) It should also be noted that, like the pandemics themselves, the economic effects were not uniform across countries.

The macroeconomic headline for the Black Death is the proverbial "tale of two cities."

Per David Routt in The Economic Impact of the Black Death (2008):

"The lion's share of the Black Death's effect was felt in the economy's agricultural sector, unsurprising in a society in which, except in the most urbanized regions, nine of ten people eked out a living from the soil."

Due to the demographic toll of the bubonic plague on the working (labor) class - i.e. severe reduction in supply - and other factors such as the availability of arable land, the English feudal law of desmende - land tenure - ceased to be viable for the landed gentry and manorialism died a slow death (Garrett, 2007.)

Commercial activity, primarily in urban areas where much of the working class was controlled by professional guilds, did not fare much better during the pandemic. The international conglomerates of the time ("super companies") struggled. Interestingly, though, one does see post-pandemic opportunity-taking by the entrepreneurs of the time, though these opportunities tended to be local and short term (thus reducing the downside risk.)

Again, Routt (2008):

"A fluctuating economy demanded adaptability and the most successful post-plague businessman not merely weathered bad times but located opportunities within adversity and exploited them. The post-plague entrepreneur's preference for short-term rather than long-term ventures, once believed a product of a gloomy despondency caused by the plague and exacerbated by endemic violence, decay of traditional institutions,

and nearly continuous warfare, is now viewed as a judicious desire to leave open entrepreneurial options, to manage risk effectively, and to take advantage of whatever better opportunity arose. The successful post-plague businessman observed markets closely and responded to them while exercising strict control over his concern, looking for greater efficiency, and trimming costs."

Fast forward almost 600 years to what might, surprisingly, be the macroeconomic headline of the day: The Spanish flu leaves almost no discernible mark on the aggregate US economy (Benmelech, 2020.)

Two pre-existing conditions might have contributed to the relative blunt impact of the Spanish Flu on the U.S. economy. One: "the influenza outbreak in the spring of 1918 occurred right after a downturn: the Dow Jones Industrial Average had actually declined 21.7% in 1917" (Benmelech, 2020.) Two: "When the pandemic unfolded, a significant share of the nation's resources at home and abroad were devoted to the war economy. Real government spending accounted for about 38% of GDP" (Benmelech, 2020.)

That said, on the ground it didn't feel so good, as illustrated by these actual newspaper clips of the day (Thomas Garrett, 2007):

Merchants in Little Rock say their business has declined 40 percent. Others estimate the decrease at 70 percent.

One department store, which has a business of $15,000 daily ($200,265 in 2006 dollars), is not doing more than half that.

Out of a total of about 400 men used in the transportation department of the Memphis Street Railway, 124 men were incapacitated yesterday. This curtailed service.

Fifty percent decrease in production reported by coal mine operators.

Although differences between the Black Plague and Spanish Flu abound on the economic front, two common themes might be a harbinger of what is to come (or already happening) with the current Coronavirus pandemic:

1. If not secular stagnation - i.e. negligible or no long-term growth - there was a period of tepid or contracted economic growth.

2. There were fundamental changes in, at least, some sectors of the economies, post-pandemic.

3. The Coronavirus Pandemic

The novel coronavirus (SARS-CoV-2) that causes the disease Coronavirus Disease 2019 (COVID-19) emerged late 2019 in the Chinese city of Wuhan. The virus was declared a pandemic on March 11, 2020, by the World Health Organization (WHO.) Lockdowns rolled across the globe as countries declared national emergencies, some more severe than others.

As of this writing, the virus has been reported on every continent except for Antarctica. Data is not definitive because of the relatively young age of the pandemic and differing reporting mechanisms, but, per Johns Hopkins Medicine (2020), there are over 11 million confirmed cases worldwide with over 530,000 related deaths. Per the U.S. Centers for Disease Control and Prevention (2020), the adjusted CFR rate for 82 countries, territories and areas is 4.24%.

On the economic front, Forbes (Klebnikov, 2020) reports:

The IMF forecast that global GDP will contract by 4.9% this year, a noticeable downgrade from its previous estimate in April when it projected GDP to shrink by 3%.

The IMF previously warned that the global economy was facing its worst financial crisis since the Great Depression—and now, despite some countries beginning to reopen, it says that the economic decline could be much worse.

But how does GDP play out for businesses (and making money)?

Rewind for some ECON 101:

1. The Gross Domestic Product (GDP) is the monetary value of all final goods and services produced within a geography within a given period of time.

2. It is important to discern between two types of "money": *income* (more liquid, like cash), which circulates through economies, and *wealth* (less liquid; assets like property) It is the income that makes economies go around (and move that GDP number.)

When income stops or slows circulating, one can get something like the Global Financial Crisis (GFC), aka as the Great Recession. From a U.S. Bureau of Labor Statistics (BLS) report (2014):

During the "Great Recession," which took place from late-2007 through mid-2009, the economy steeply contracted and nearly 8.7 million jobs were lost.6 Consumer spending experienced the most severe decline since World War II. Households cut spending, shed outstanding debt, and increased their rate of personal savings in response to reductions in income, wealth, confidence, and credit access. (BLS, 2014)

Cash is king, and, when the going gets tough, people and organizations tend to conserve, even hoard, it.

From an income generating perspective, the next 12 months will be tough.

4. Fast Forward to 2030

In August of 2001, one could walk up to the check-in counter of a commercial flight without so much as a ticket. That all changed, practically overnight, on September 11, 2001. History tells us that terrorist attacks, recessions, depressions - and pandemics - all can, and usually do, have sudden and profound consequences on business, be it an independent consultant, a local coffee shop or an international insurance company. There is no reason to believe that the current Coronavirus pandemic should be any different.

But what to do about it?

Skate to where the puck is going, not where it has been ~ Wayne Gretzky, former professional ice hockey player and coach

Before becoming the player that he was, Gretzky spent many years watching ice hockey games and plotting out the movement of pucks on paper. So much so that he was eventually able to predict exactly where the puck would be.

Here are some business trends, already in progress, worth watching:

Proximity as a platform: As the saying goes, all politics are local, and so it goes for business. There has always been a preference for horse trading within your community, what/wherever that might be, including online, and that will only be amplified by the pandemic. This has everything to do with attention and trust, and, as a report by the design firm Cake & Arrow states, "Trust lies close to home" (Cake & Arrow, 2020.).

Offline-to-online: Mary Meeker is a venture capitalist and well known for her annual Internet Trends Report, which many use as a reference for where tech is now and where it's going. She and her firm, Bond Capital, are out with a new 29-page report (Meeker et al., 2020) on how the coronavirus is shaping economic activity: "Many of these offline-to-online trends have been in place for a while," the report says. "COVID-19 just accelerated them."

Abundance through digital technologies: "The World Economic Forum has called the current period we are living in The Fourth Industrial Revolution, as digital technologies are now changing at a faster pace than ever due to their exponential nature." (Ismail, Palao, 2019) and Exponential Organizations (ExOs) are looking to tap into this environment of abundance to scale rapidly. Think buying a CD in the 80's v. streaming music now.

Low touch: Finally, per a global strategy and design firm (Board of Innovation, 2020), the post-Covid19 era will have a "low touch" economy shaped by new habits and regulations based on reduced close-contact interaction, which will disrupt how we eat, work, shop, exercise, manage our health, socialize, and spend our free time. Out of 511 epidemiologists asked, the majority do not expect to travel by airplane until next year (Sanger-Katz et al., 2020.)

History has also taught us that there will come a time when the economy picks up again, albeit different in some ways. The smart money will be on businesses that are ready: where (reiterating Mary Meeker) "COVID-19 just accelerated them" into 2030.

References

Carlin, D. (2019), *The End Is Always Near.* New York, NY: HarperCollins Publishing.

Garrett, T. (2007), "Economic Effects of the 1918 Influenza Pandemic", Federal Reserve Bank of St. Louis. Retrieved from https://www.stlouisfed.org/~/media/files/pdfs/community-development/research-reports/pandemic_flu_report.pdf

Keogh-Brown, M. et al. (2008), "The macroeconomic costs of a global influenza pandemic." Retrieved from https://www.gtap.agecon.purdue.edu/resources/download/3828.pdf

Routt, D. (2008), "The Economic Impact of the Black Death", University of Richmond. Retrieved from https://eh.net/encyclopedia/the-economic-impact-of-the-black-death/

Benmelech E. and Frydman C. (2020), "The 1918 influenza did not kill the US economy." Retrieved from https://voxeu.org/article/1918-influenza-did-not-kill-us-economy

Johns Hopkins Medicine (2020.) Retrieved from https://www.hopkinsguides.com/hopkins/view/Johns_Hopkins_ABX_Guide/540747/all/Coronavirus_COVID_19__SARS_CoV_2_

Centers for Disease Control and Prevention (2020.) Retrieved from https://wwwnc.cdc.gov/eid/article/26/6/20-0320-t1

Klebnikov, S. (2020), "IMF Slashes Global GDP Forecasts, Warning Of An Economic Crisis 'Like No Other". Retrieved from https://www.forbes.com/sites/sergeiklebnikov/2020/06/24/imf-slashes-global-gdp-forecasts-warning-of-an-economic-crisis-like-no-other/

Bureau of Labor Statistics (BLS) (2014), "Consumer spending and U.S. employment from the 2007–2009 recession through 2022." Retrieved from https://www.bls.gov/opub/mlr/2014/article/consumer-spending-and-us-employment-from-the-recession-through-2022.htm

Cake & Arrow (2020), "COVID-19 & the Gig Economy." Retrieved from http://go.cakeandarrow.com/covid-19-and-the-gig-economy

Meeker, M. et al. (2020), "Our New World." Retrieved from https://www.documentcloud.org/documents/6842117-Our-New-World.html#document/p1

Ismail, S and Palao, F. (2019), "Forget startups, ExOs (Exponential Organizations) are the new way to innovate." Retrieved from https://medium.com/openexo/forget-startups-exos-exponential-organizations-are-the-new-way-to-innovate-32305d628928

Board of Innovation (2020), "The Low Touch Economy is here to stay." Retrieved from https://www.boardofinnovation.com/low-touch-economy/

Sanger-Katz, M., et al. (2020), "When 511 Epidemiologists Expect to Fly, Hug and Do 18 Other Everyday Activities Again", New York Times. Retrieved from https://www.nytimes.com/interactive/2020/06/08/upshot/when-epidemiologists-will-do-everyday-things-coronavirus.html

Sean Hull is a technologist, problem solver and consultant with a 15+ year history of designing, planning and driving the delivery of strategic programs globally, primarily in the insurance domain. His track record includes work with Fortune 50 firms, Big Six Consulting, and not-for-profit organizations. Sean is a certified project manager and his academic qualifications include a Master of Business Administration (MBA) from Ashland University and a Bachelor of Arts (BA) in International Relations from the Ohio State University; sean.hull@gmail.com.

Strategies for the New World of Work

Paul Melot de Beauregard, Fernuniversität zu Hagen, Germany

Abstract

The corona pandemic is changing working conditions and the entire working life in a way never seen before. Some of the measures taken are very specific and are, therefore, likely to disappear soon again.[1] But others will remain, and mark the beginning of a new working life. If we look at the German market, these measures affect almost all areas regulated by labor and social security law. The following essay will describe some of the changes in the fields of work safety, social security law, and flexible working conditions, and give an initial assessment of related business strategies. The selection is only exemplary, and does not claim to be complete.[2]

Key words

Working conditions, Short-time work, Home Office, Remuneration, Health data

1. Assessment of the current situation

In international comparison, the German labor constitution is characterized by two main attributes: Firstly, there is a high level of employee protection, which goes hand in hand with a corresponding density of regulation. Secondly, the system can be described as rather static.

Both attributes have proven to be stabilizing in past crises and thus successful in economic terms. The combination of short-time work, protection against termination of employment and unemployment benefits in the financial crisis of 2008/2009 – admittedly in conjunction with other government incentive measures in the field of tax and subsidy law – has been able to secure jobs and promote the stability of the labor market.[3] The current challenges posed by the corona pandemic are not the same, however. The effects, as is already clear today, have a deeper impact on all social processes and thus also change the conditions under which day-to-day business operations are possible.

This reveals deficits: While the high stability of the employment relationship as a continuous obligation with a high level of protection has undeniably positive effects on the labor market, a lack of flexibility at the level of individual working conditions is often criticized. This lack of flexibility manifests itself, for example, in the legal hurdles to the introduction of short-time work, in the individual requirements for mobile and flexible work, or in the area of remuneration. Furthermore, in recent months it has become apparent that the German economy is not where it could be in terms of digitalization. Hopes are growing here that the experience of the Corona pandemic will lead to a digitalization push in all economic sectors. Finally, with regard to work safety, it can be said that Germany, compared internationally, already met the highest standards before the pandemic. However, the requirements that have now arisen as a result of Corona are specific and, therefore, can no longer be covered by the existing rules. In this context, employee data protection in particular is of crucial importance when introducing and implementing further protective and preventive measures.

---

[1] An example of this is the Act to facilitate access to social security and the use and protection of social service providers on the basis of the coronavirus SARS-CoV-2, Federal Law Gazette I 575, which came into force on March 28, 2020 and which provides for far-reaching authorizations of the legislator to extend the statutory maximum working hours, for details see *Löwisch*, BB 2020, 948 ff.

[2] For further "viral adjustments" in labor and social law, see for example *Fuhlrott/Fischer*, NZA 2020, 345 ff. The most comprehensive overview at present is probably provided by *Hohenstatt/Sittard* with their work "Arbeitsrecht in Zeiten von Corona", 1st ed., Munich, 2020.

[3] See *Wahlig/Geschke*, NZA 2010, 607 ff.

2. Work safety
    a) SARS-COV-2 work safety standards

Starting with the last topic mentioned, we can see that politics approached the business community in the most pragmatic, responsive, and low-threshold manner with regard to work safety. In addition to the general protection rules that must already be followed in working life, the Federal Ministry of Labor and Social Affairs (BMAS) provided companies with a flexible and at the same time in many respects detailed guideline by publishing the SARS-COV-2 occupational safety standards on 16 April 2020.[4] It should be noted that the work safety standards do not claim to be mandatory. It literally says: *"The responsibility for the implementation of necessary infection protection measures lies with the employer according to the result of the risk assessment"* (II. of the standards). However, the practical significance goes beyond that of a guide. The guidelines specify the employer's duty of care (cf. § 618 BGB[5]) and set a standard, which courts are likely to consult regularly in future proceedings. In this respect, companies will be well advised to comply with these standards.

    b) Health data

A particularly hot topic in the Corona Pandemic is the question of the permissibility of temperature measurements for employees. Such measures are just as important in terms of the safety of people at work, as they are controversial from a data protection point of view.

To begin with the implementation: Whether through contactless testing on the ear or thermal imaging, rapid on-site fever measurement has become a new, universally perceptible process during the corona pandemic. Airports require it for travelers, landlords of large office buildings require it at the entrance, and administrative agencies consider it before entering their premises. In most cases, these temperature measurements are accompanied by an explicit declaration of consent of the examined person. However, this leads to problems in terms of data protection law when the person concerned is in an employment relationship and is, therefore, an employee within the meaning of data protection law.

The opinions of the data protection authorities responsible for this vary from one federal state to another. For example, the data protection officer in Hesse already doubts the suitability of such measurements for work safety: "It should be noted that the mere fact that an increased body temperature is recorded does not automatically allow the conclusion to be drawn that corona disease is present. Conversely, an already existing corona disease does not necessarily have to be indicated by an increased body temperature."[6]

It is particularly important for companies to note that this ambiguity cannot be overcome by the employee's consent to the collection (or even further processing) of his or her health data. The Data Protection Commissioner of Hesse continues: "Obtaining a declaration of consent from employees to legitimize data processing operations that go further than those mentioned above is not permissible, as the voluntary nature required for this, i.e. the existence of a genuine choice, is lacking. The employee is in an economically dependent relationship with the employer or principal. If permission to perform work is made dependent on the disclosure of further personal (health) data, he or she must fear that this may lead to financial disadvantages

---

[4] https://www.bmas.de/SharedDocs/Downloads/DE/PDF-Schwerpunkte/sars-cov-2-arbeitsschutzstandard.pdf?__blob=publicationFile&v=1 (accessed on June 5, 2020).

[5] German Civil Code (Bürgerliches Gesetzbuch).

[6] https://www.datenschutz.rlp.de/de/themenfelder-themen/beschaeftigtendatenschutz-corona/ (accessed on June 5, 2020).

in the form of unpaid leave from work."[7]

If an employer nevertheless wishes to take temperature measurements, for example due to international compliance regulations, these should only be taken with the agreement of any existing works council, the company's data protection officer and the employees concerned. It is advisable to ensure that the design is as data protection-friendly as possible, which among other things prohibits the storage of data, reduces the perspective and scope (e.g. no sound) of the data collection as much as possible, and ensures that the personnel commissioned are specially trained and that the processing directory is updated.

3. Short-time work

German employment promotion law provides for the possibility for companies of all types and in all sectors to have the government step in with financial means, the so-called short-time work allowance, if working hours are reduced due to a considerable loss of workload (§§ 95 ff. SGB III[8]). This amounts – in the same amount as the unemployment benefit – to 60% of the net salary for the part of the work lost, or 67% of the net salary for employees with children, limited to the income threshold for the assessment of contributions. In these cases, the government also pays the social security contributions of the employees.

Already during the financial crisis, the provisions on short-time work made a significant contribution to relieving the labor market and to the rapid recovery of the German economy.[9] This is because, on the one hand, a company is relieved financially in the short term by the government covering its employees' costs. On the other hand, if the workload increases again, the employer can ramp up production or services with the experienced employees at short notice. This is a circumstance that is particularly important in static German labor law with its long planning horizons.

With the onset of the corona pandemic in mid-March 2020, companies in all sectors were able to make use of a tried and tested instrument for safeguarding jobs while at the same time conserving financial liquidity. Admittedly, the extent of the pandemic, and thus the burden on many companies, is now much greater than in 2008. Accordingly, the legislator has extended the provisions for short-time work at an unprecedented speed. For example, in the "Act on the temporary improvement of the regulations for short-time work compensation due to the crisis" of March 13, 2020[10], the German Federal Employment Agency (Agentur für Arbeit) has so far ordered the employer's social security contributions to be taken over during short-time work. Furthermore, employees are to receive an increased rate of 70% or 77% of net remuneration from the fourth month of short-time work and even 80% or 87% of net remuneration from the seventh month.[11]

Other facilitations made possible by the above-mentioned law are the reduction of the statutory quorum of those employees in the company, who must be affected by the loss of working hours (from 33% to only 10%), the extensive waiver of the accumulation of negative working time balances and the application of the law also to temporary workers.[12] These measures

---

[7] See fn. 5.

[8] German Social Security Code III (Sozialgesetzbuch III).

[9] *Wahlig/Geschke*, NZA 2010, 607 f.

[10] Official publication of the Bundestag 19/17893, 1.

[11] Social Protection Package II of May 14, 2020.

[12] (Retroactive) decision of the Federal Government by ordinance of March 23, 2020 on the basis of the aforementioned law. For further requirements of short-time work and their classification, see *Geulen/Vogt*, ArbRAktuell

were put into effect retroactively as of March 1, 2020 and are initially limited in time until December 31, 2020.

At the same time, collective agreements and works agreements as well as voluntary agreements at the level of the individual employee provide for so-called top-up contributions by the employer. Knowing that the job market was difficult from the companies' point of view before the onset of the Corona pandemic, and hoping that the consequences of the crisis will be overcome more quickly than previously predicted, most companies are still very interested in retaining their employees on the basis of further financial benefits.

What will remain of the extended short-time working allowance provisions? One deficit at the onset of the crisis was certainly the fact that many companies lacked collective agreements on the introduction of short-time work. The experiences of 2008 often did not lead to the conclusion that short-time work clauses should be introduced as standard in employment contracts. This is likely to change in the future. Where works councils exist, companies are well advised to enter into works agreements on short-time work for the future. Since short-time work is a case of mandatory co-determination, the works council must be involved.[13] Works councils, on the other hand, will use their right of co-determination to negotiate top-up amounts with the employer in such agreements and secure themselves a right of inspection and monitoring.

Where there is no works council, a short-time work clause should be included in the employment contract. Since these are general arrangements for the future, the employer will regularly want to waive the promise of an increase and will prefer to decide unilaterally in the event of a crisis.

4. Flexible working conditions
a) Voluntariness and discretion

Once working conditions have been agreed upon, they can only be changed again by means of a voluntary amendment to the contract by mutual agreement between the parties. The extension of the rules of the General Terms and Conditions of Business (§§ 305 ff. BGB) to employment contracts in 2002 has greatly restricted the use of reservation clauses by the employer. The Federal Labor Court in particular sets high standards for the effectiveness of such contractual provisions.[14]

Thereafter, the reservation of voluntariness must be mentioned again for each benefit. A blanket reservation clause in the employment contract could be too unspecific and, therefore, surprising. If an employer forgets to declare a benefit as voluntary and repeatedly provides the same benefit without such a reservation, the employee will develop a position of trust which will give him a claim based on so-called company practice.

If the employer promises the employee a variable remuneration for his performance, this cannot be made subject to the reservation clause. It must always be paid, even in the case of extraordinary termination (pro rata), since the courts assume that the purpose pursued with the variable remuneration – namely the incentive to perform – was achieved for the period until the employee left the company.

2020, 181 ff., on the extended possibilities of credit-free additional income in the case of short-time work *Klinkhammer/Mantel*, ArbRAktuell 2020, 213.

[13] See § 87 (1) No. 2 BetrVG (German Works Constitution Act).

[14] See for example BAG September 14, 2011 - 10 AZR 526/10, NZA 2012, 81 (reservation of voluntariness); August 3, 2016 - 10 AZR 710/14, NZA 2016, 1334 (reservation of discretion); on the whole *Lembke*, NJW 2010, 257 ff., 321 ff.

Even more difficult in practice are agreements on discretionary remuneration. If a reservation of the voluntary nature of a claim is intended to prevent it from arising, it must be assumed in the case of a discretionary reservation that a claim has already arisen and its fulfilment must now take place within the framework of a proper (i.e. reasonable) discretion (§ 305 (3) BGB). The exercise of this proper discretion is fully subject to review by the courts. The court, therefore, checks the timely setting of goals, their realistic achievability, the proper calculation of the degree of goal achievement, etc. Where this has not been properly implemented by the employer or even not at all, the employee's entitlement is quickly assumed to be 100%.[15]

A short-term deterioration in the business situation, such as that caused by the corona pandemic in many industries, shows in a special way how important it is to effectively agree variable remuneration. In future, employers will therefore pay even more attention than before to the effective and enforceable design of their bonus conditions.

b) Working from home and working hours

The experience gained with flexible working conditions during the Corona pandemic is certainly not limited to questions of remuneration. Rather, these have been on the agenda for some time and were only made particularly virulent by the crisis. What is new, however - at least in Germany - is the mass transfer of the workplace into the employee's home. Associated with this, working hours became much more flexible, from shift work to the almost complete mixing of private and working time.

Here too, German labor law is structured on a static and consensual basis. It is not possible for the employer to require the employee to work from home. The employer's right to issue instructions (§§ 611a BGB, 106 GewO) does not extend to the employee's private environment.[16] Conversely, the employee – for example in the case of health concerns – may not simply work from home.[17] A mutual agreement is always required.

The interests of both parties to the employment contract during the Corona pandemic were quite similar. Both employers and employees pursued the goal of social distancing, which was best achieved by working from home (where possible). Corresponding individual contractual agreements, including the provision of work equipment, the assumption of costs for electricity, telephone etc. as well as the special obligation for data protection were quickly drafted and concluded.[18] Often it became necessary to make improvements to these agreements in the first few weeks. With this experience, companies will in future have such work from home agreements in a more mature form ready for a crisis reaction. It should be noted that such agreements are to be entered into exclusively by employer and employee. Co-determination by the works council is not possible, as it would otherwise encroach on the employee's private sphere.[19]

Nevertheless, it is to be expected that current developments will accelerate further legislative measures to facilitate flexible working, including the possible introduction of an individual

---

[15] In detail *Lingemann/Pfister/Otte*, NZA 2015, 65.

[16] LAG Berlin-Brandenburg of November 14, 2018 - 17 Sa 562/18, BeckRS 2018, 34001. The situation is different for the special case of Corona according to *Krieger/Rudnik/Povedano Peramato*, NZA 2020, 473 (475 f.), who want to grant the employer an extended right of direction by way of exception.

[17] The situation may be different in the case of a considerable concrete danger. Here, especially in the case of risk groups, one can discuss a right to refuse performance under § 275 (3) BGB, cf. on this specifically in the context of the corona crisis *Dehmel/Hartmann*, BB 2020, 885 f. with reference to a first ruling of the ArbG Regensburg of March 19, 2020 - 6 GA 2/20 (n.v.) But this does not result in a right to work from home either, see LAG Rheinland-Pfalz of December 18, 2014 - 5 Sa 378/14, BeckRS 2015, 66249.

[18] *Halim/Wybitul*, DB Spezial 2020 No. 4, 6 ff.

[19] In detail *Krieger/Rudnik/Povedano Peramato*, NZA 2020, 473 (476 ff.).

right for employees to work from home. Echoes of this can already be found in the coalition agreement of March 12, 2018 between the CDU/CSU and SPD. Among other things it says here: "We want to promote and facilitate mobile work. We will create a legal framework for this. This will include a right of employees to obtain information from their employer about the reasons for the refusal to work from home and legal certainty for employees and employers in the dealing with privately used company technical equipment. The collective labor agreement partners should also reach agreements on mobile work."[20] If further legal measures were to be taken in this respect, these would have to be observed and included in the design of individual agreements.

In response to the contact restrictions imposed extensively during the Corona pandemic, it has proved helpful to have employees work in shifts - where not entirely or largely from home - in order to reduce contact between employees. Such shift schedules are subject to the mandatory co-determination of the works council.[21] In general, the works council is responsible for all issues relating to the distribution of working time. Working time accounts are also subject to the works council's co-determination. As already mentioned above in connection with short-time work, working time accounts are a thoroughly effective means of reducing positive time accounts during times of crisis without burdening the company's liquidity.

In addition, the corona pandemic has already led to an enormous digitalization of the working world. Data security plays a major role, especially when working outside the company's office. The increase in video and telephone conferences also makes corporate precautions against hackers and other cases of unwanted data leakage even more important. Here too, the adaptation and extension of existing agreements with works councils plays a major role.[22]

c) Infection Protection Act

In legal systems which, like the German legal system, are essentially characterized by norm enactments due to the Roman legal tradition, it can sometimes happen that one or the other norm is lost sight of or even forgotten. Such a circumstance can, fortunately, also be seen in the labor law provisions of the Infection Protection Act - specifically § 56 of the Infection Protection Act (IfSG).[23] The corona pandemic brought this back into view. § 56 IfSG regulates various cases:

First of all, it determines the employee's rights in the event of an officially ordered ban on work - for example, after returning from a risk area. § 56 (2) f. IfSG entitles the employee to six weeks' continued payment of wages, analogous to a case of illness under the Continued Remuneration Act. The risk is therefore initially allocated to the employer.[24] However, the employer can have the payment refunded by the responsible agency (§ 56 (5) and (12) IfSG). From the seventh week onwards, the employee can then – up to the income threshold for the assessment of contributions – receive compensation similar to the daily sickness benefit.

---

[20] Coalition agreement between CDU, CSU and SPD of March 12, 2018, lines 1822 ff., available at https://www.bundesregierung.de/resource/blob/656734/847984/5b8bc23590d4cb2892b31c987ad672b7/2018-03-14-koalitionsvertrag-data.pdf?download= (accessed on June 5, 2020).

[21] See § 87 (1) No. 2 BetrVG.

[22] See for example *Körner*, NZA 2019, 1389 ff.

[23] See in detail *Eufinger*, DB 2020, 1121 ff.: "§ 56 IfSG - Coronavirus SARS-CoV-2 und die Entdeckung einer Norm".

[24] The same applies in the event of loss of working hours if there is no other form of care for a child up to the age of 12. Here the new provision of § 56 (1a) IfSG also provides for a claim of the employee against the employer, see *Kleinschmidt*, DB 2020, 952 (955): "Der Arbeitgeber als Zahlstelle" (The employer as paying agent).

If, on the other hand, a business is shut down completely (§ 16 IfSG)[25], as is the case in the hospitality industry or in food production, the employer will also continue to have to pay the contractual remuneration. However, it is currently still unclear in which cases he can apply for a refund or - in application of the doctrine of business risk (§ 615 BGB) - will remain stuck on these costs. For such cases, it is recommended to examine an insurance solution (so-called business interruption insurance) even more closely in the future.

5. Assessment of the development

If one wants to classify the observations made, different perspectives are offered. It is obvious that in the future, employees will focus more on their own health and safety at work. The demand for flexible working, especially from home, is likely to have risen sharply.

The situation cannot yet be conclusively assessed under collective law. As far as can be seen, trade unions and works councils have been overrun by the latest developments. So far, they have been able to make a positive contribution, especially with regard to flexibility of work schedules. There will be further progress here in the foreseeable future.

However, the main focus must be on the issues arising for companies from these developments. The specific work tasks under labor law have already been identified. What is important, however, is that their implementation takes place by way of an overall crisis prevention orientation. The challenges facing companies have also already been mentioned many times.[26] A key word that is constantly recurring is "resilience", but also "load-bearing capacity" and even "failure safety". Future labor contract and collective law arrangements must fit in with this goal.

At the same time, questions are raised about work safety, insurance management and the cost-related deployment of staff on compliance issues that could lead to significant liability risks for those responsible. In the next pandemic, no one will be able to say they didn't know about it. In particular, within the framework of the Business Judgement Rule, board representatives will in future have to face questions about the crisis resistance of their organization.

Finally, opportunities arising from experience should be taken advantage of. For example, companies with business premises in expensive locations have already announced that they want to use work from home in the future to reduce costs.[27] Subsidies and liquidity-securing options expand the possibilities for economic activity. Whether or not opportunities can be seized in each case is sometimes a moral question beyond the law.[28]

6. Outlook

It is obvious that beyond the mentioned examples the Corona pandemic raises additional numerous questions of relevance for the future working live. What does it mean for the risk within a company in case that the supply chain is broken? What competitiveness do terms and

---

[25] On the fundamental permissibility of shutting down operations during the corona pandemic due to the constitutional obligation to protect life and physical integrity in accordance with Article 2 (2) of the Basic Law, see BVerfG of April 29, 2020 - 1 BvQ 47/20, BeckRS 2020, 7210.

[26] See for example statement of McKinsey of April 14, 2020: "The Future is not what it used to be: Thoughts on the shape of the next normal." https://www.mckinsey.com/featured-insights/leadership/the-future-is-not-what-it-used-to-be-thoughts-on-the-shape-of-the-next-normal (accessed on June 5, 2020).

[27] "Mehr Home-Office? Weniger Reisen-Was bleibt nach der Corona-Krise im Geschäftsalltag?" *Imwinkelried*, NZZ of May 7, 2020, https://www.nzz.ch/wirtschaft/mehr-home-office-weniger-reisen-was-bleibt-nach-der-corona-krise-im-geschaeftsalltag-ld.1555218 (accessed June 5, 2020).

[28] On the option of a "useful" breach of contract by managers in times of Corona, see *Bulgrin/Wolf*, AG 2020, 367 ff.

conditions require in case that the trade of products and services will be executed in an increasing way through multinationals via internet? What does home office mean for the safety of business secrets?

Seeing this amount of questions the topics covered above could only serve as examples. They did also not in any way fully present the regulatory measures during the corona pandemic. Nevertheless, it should have become clear that the framework conditions for employees have undergone a trial run over the past weeks and months, which has provided a number of lessons for companies, as well as works councils and employees. In view of the fact that similar or even worse pandemics, but also crises of a different nature, but comparable in their effects, could repeat themselves at any time in the future, the parties mentioned are well advised to prepare for the next eventuality in good time by making appropriate arrangements. What is needed now is the courage and consistency to learn the lessons and put them into practice.[29]

Paul Melot de Beauregard is a partner of the international law firm of Jones Day in Dusseldorf and honorary professor of Fern University Hagen (Germany). After finishing his studies at the universities in Munich and Wurzburg with the first state exam he earned his Ph.D. under Curt-Wolfgang Hergenröder at Wurzburg University with a thesis dealing with collective bargaining agreements. After that he earned the degree of an LL.M. (labour law) at the London School of Economics (UK). He advises and publishes in regard to all matters involving German and European employment law.

---

[29] The author thanks Ms. Melina Sonis for the translation of this article.

Home office in the pandemic: Curse or blessing?

Eva Dahlke, Independent Scholar, Germany

Peter Kegel, Independent Scholar, Germany

Abstract

Home office options have been discussed controversially in many companies. Currently, infection protection, lack of childcare, and the preservation of the business continuity often force to a mandatory home office. This national "workplace and communication trial" shows in detail opportunities and risks for the participants to work flexibly in terms of time and place. We refer to the basic principles of ethics beneficence, non-maleficence, autonomy, and justice to discuss the advantages and disadvantages for employers and employees. The drawn conclusions might offer opportunities for shaping the long-distance relationship during the pandemic and afterward.

Key words

Home office, flexibility, autonomy

Introduction

The physical presence in the workplace is often culturally anchored or determined by the work task. According to a survey performed in 2019, German companies of all sizes have offered their employees the opportunity to work on the move to about 25%. These were mostly hourly or daily models, which included home office as well as working in the context of customer contact on-site. Before the pandemic, employers cited a lack of suitability for the job, technical and data protection barriers, and personnel management aspects as arguments against the idea of a home office. On the part of the employees, there was both rejection and (unfulfilled) desire for home office models. Employees cited the preference of their superiors as a reason for not wanting to work in a home office due to the associated concern for their career, the lack of direct cooperation with colleagues on-site, but also the problematic distinction between professional and private life in the home environment (Grunau 2019). At the same time, the possibility of working in a home office was strategically placed in job advertisements to increase the attractiveness of the position for employees seeking this job option. Due to the rapidly rising COVID-19 cases in Germany at the beginning of March 2020, a shutdown, including the closure of schools and childcare facilities, restriction of the domestic economy, and closing of borders, took place within one week. The state-imposed contact reduction in combination with the frequent lack of childcare forced employers and employees to move to the home office in a disorderly manner within a short time to maintain the partial business continuity of companies and organizations. We will point out differences in pre-pandemic home office models, and possible deductions for workplace models of the future in the following concerning advantages, disadvantages, autonomy, and justice for those involved.

Beneficence

Generally, employers and employees unite the objective of maintaining at least partial business activity and, thus, also employment during and after the pandemic. This common starting position can be a strong motivator for the acceptance of this initially provisional workplace model. It can serve to overcome pre-pandemic obstacles and scepticism. The advance of trust in employees associated with a collaborative creative design of the new working conditions and fields of activity can lead to the recognition of empowerment and positive reinforcement of self-efficacy (Schwarzer and Jerusalem 2002). The experience of empowerment in adapting to changed conditions and thus, participation in the continued operation of the company can strengthen both self-esteem and a sense of belonging to the company. If there is also time flexibility in the home office, adaptation to individual work rhythms and thematic structuring can improve individual effectiveness. The content of the work can be in focus through the technical forms of communication via email, clouding, or video conferencing. External factors and possible role attributions, which may overlay or influence the (working) relationship in face-to-face work, may fade into the background. The elimination of commuting can relieve the mind as well as the environment and lead to a lower number of commuting accidents. According to a survey by a German health insurance company, 45% of the approx. 4 million insured persons surveyed worked outside their circle of residence, and over 10% of the insured persons worked more than 50 kilometers away from their residence (Steinmann et al. 2018). For part-time employees, the time saved may allow for a larger working time contingent. The elimination of long commuting distances can improve or fundamentally reconcile work and family life, especially in crises with limited care options. Flexibility in home office options, which allow time even outside of the previous working hours, e.g., at night or on weekends, may allow for further variations in care arrangements with partners.

Companies benefit from the newly created home office options in various ways, not only in maintaining their business activity during the pandemic. Outsourcing other areas to the home office may protect employees in functional areas that require on-site presence from contact with potential carriers. The home office can thus play its part in slowing down the spread of pathogens in the population. The pandemic may pose communication challenges to maintain or intensify contact with customers and suppliers. Communications strategies could involve reassigning other areas of work to employees. Flexibility in terms of location and, in some cases, time enables employees dependent on childcare to continue to work for the company. For managers, the work from the home office is essential to ensure continuous availability for coordinative tasks, especially during the pandemic. Ultimately, the home office can also be the previously unnoticed quieter workplace for conceptual, creative work due to the level of activity and communication within the company. Working in a familiar home environment can result in higher efficiency of the (overall) work performance. E.g. scheduling intermissions self-determinedly. The precondition is that individual factors (personality traits, characteristics of the home work such as equipment, ergonomic aspects, possibly existing disruptive factors) permit this.

Non-maleficence

The relocation of the workplace to the home environment results in technical and organizational challenges in the demarcation between work and private life. Tables that are not height-adjustable and chairs that are not very ergonomic must be independently compensated for by standing and walking breaks. Self-discipline during specific breaks and time management may be more difficult, especially in times of crisis-related anxiety and unattended children. The commute to work as a possible part of daily exercise, the lunch break, if possible, in the fresh air, and the unburdening way back home is no longer an option. The home environment can also lead to questionable differentiation between working hours and overtime, and the lack of spatial separation can promote sleep disorders (Sueddeutsche Zeitung). External indicators such as job appropriate clothing, labeling of the work area, or communication of the availability of time to roommates or family members can help with internal and external structuring. Finding a specific position between work and leisure time becomes more difficult as soon as other family members are involved, and several workplaces are used simultaneously, for example, for homeschooling. This balancing act becomes a challenge compared to when the home office was available while the partner or children were absent. The demarcation of the professional role when physically present in the family can be more difficult for female family members in particular, not only when children are young. Before the pandemic, surveys document the disproportion between the shares of unpaid work for both genders (Statistisches Bundesamt 2015). The challenge of combining home office and homeschooling is a particular one to exacerbate these already existing disparities. In the German-speaking world, this association is new for all those involved. The professional and content-related involvement of parents in the pedagogical work holds significant potential for conflict and requires professional understanding as well as time-intensive relationship work. Children need special attention due to the changed pandemic circumstances and their loss of social contacts. This situation can be incredibly stressful, especially for single parents during the pandemic due to the lack of childcare facilities. Besides, adults lack working hours as contact time with other adults. Social isolation can also be particularly significant for workers living alone.

Adapting to the new job situation during the pandemic, which may also put jobs at risk, is an additional burden for all concerned. At the same time, the pandemic leaves few options for personal stress management and compensation. Concerning illness at work, surveys before the pandemic showed that 75% of the employees surveyed had been present at work sick at least once a year, over 20% of them against medical advice. During a pandemic, both employers and employees generally demand and comply with early absence from work when symptoms of illness occur (Erbersdobler 2020). In the home office, however, these boundaries can become blurred. Hours of work, albeit perhaps with restrictions, instead of rest and recovery, are imaginable in the home environment. Due to their permanent involvement in strategic processes, especially during the pandemic and post-pandemic planning, executive staff tend to mix their professional and private lives and thus to work in specific situations, even beyond the contractually agreed working hours (Grunau 2019). Hence, the responsibility of managers is not only to maintain the department's productivity but also to protect themselves and their employees from excessive demands. Alienation of employees and a diminishing sense of belonging to the company can go hand in hand with work from home.

Autonomy

Working in a home office offers different degrees of freedom in the design, depending on the occupation. The temporal decoupling of attendance times to project agreements offers the possibility to adapt to the individual day and night rhythms of the employees or to the restrictions which are given by the cohabitation of several persons in one household. This degree of freedom within individual time management can often make it possible to continue working despite the obligation in childcare in the first place. Increasing their autonomy in shaping their roles requires trust in the loyalty and productivity of employees. This confidence may strengthen their sense of belonging and attachment to the company. The implementation may require a focus on the result of work rather than adhering to rigid time frames. However, even within fixed working hours, work from home can be structured individually. Freedom to organize the working environment beyond the boundaries of a company workplace can be beneficial to individual productivity and satisfaction (Foreman et al. 2017; Nittono et al. 2012). These degrees of freedom, actively used as an instrument of team leadership, can thus, despite increased individualization, strengthen cohesion and loyalty in and for the working group or team.

Justice

Certain activities cannot be executed in the home office, so working from the home office is already associated with a particular injustice, especially concerning employees on reduced working hours or dismissal. Often larger companies are more likely to outsource some of their activities to the home office due to the diversification of their work tasks. For some areas, such as sales and marketing, the transitions between mobile working and the home office are already fluid and do not represent a particular change. Even before the pandemic, managers were more often available privately for administrative and coordinating functions (Grunau 2019). Technical possibilities such as a separate quiet workroom with appropriate ergonomic equipment and environment are not available to every employee at home on an ad hoc basis. Making the private home environment visible within the framework of video conferences can emphasize social differences that are not visible in the neutral setting of uniform workplace design in companies. Besides, the location in the private sphere can reinforce the clichéd attribution of roles. The integration of childcare and home office is particularly dangerous for mothers of small children when returning to work. Due to the double burden, they can be considered for less demanding work tasks in a critical phase of their career. The primary stress factor for women is not the respective task, childcare, or professional commitment, but the change between these worlds several times a day. Other genders were not interviewed in the survey taken by the Federal Ministry for Family Affairs, Senior Citizens, Women, and Youth in 2010, but maybe affected similarly (BFSFJ 2010).

Conclusion

All participants may show increased stress levels as a result of the pandemic. Nevertheless, the basic assumption in business interactions with one another should be a fundamental trust in the integrity of all participants. In conjunction with untrained forms of interaction, respectful communication is especially important.

Before the pandemic, virtual leadership at a distance was not practiced extensively in many areas, so that uncertainty about communication can also be present at management levels (Universität Konstanz 2020). Continuous and constructive feedback is essential, mainly due to possible misunderstandings and the lack of regular analog contacts. It is necessary to practice an appreciative culture of discussion. Questions should be welcomed, and uncertainties addressed openly to avoid incorrect interpretations. There should be room for addressing the individual stress situation openly by employees and superiors should also raise this topic, even more so than in times of no crisis. Transparency regarding workload despite limited direct exchange requires structured planning of work steps and projects. The structuring of projects into subsections and the allocation of corresponding time frames can be a challenge for both managers and those carrying out the work. Communication hygiene should also include sound and regular feedback as part of an appreciative corporate culture.

In contrast to previous pandemic events, longer-term restrictions can be expected, so that a return to workplace normality is not yet foreseeable. This temporal dimension requires an accompanying exchange of information concerning the needs as they develop during the pandemic. Reevaluation and possible adaptation within the given possibilities can promote constructive cooperation and increasing appreciation and affection in physical, not social, and emotional distance. Companies whose business model was already based on digital exchange before the crisis can serve as role models for corporate culture outside the workplace. Companies invite employees to online after-work events for team building and offer participation in virtual sports programs. The challenge of mandatory absence from the workplace may improve internal communication and individual personal development to build on these newly acquired skills after the crisis (Grzanna 2020). Presence or absence as a mixed model between a home office and present work, coordinated according to individual needs, can also combine the advantages of both forms of work and compensate for the disadvantages. At the same time, the change of perspective can strengthen the empathic view and understanding of the respective work form.

References

BFSFJ 2010. Bundesministerium für Familie, Senioren, Frauen und Jugend: Beruflicher Wiedereinstieg nach der Familiengründung. Bedürfnisse, Erfahrungen, Barrieren. Hg. v. Bundesministerium für Familie, Senioren, Frauen und Jugend. Berlin. Online verfügbar unter https://www.bmfsfj.de/blob/93356/842fbc2a9c2172c460b7127e086bac35/beruflicher-wiedereinstieg-nach-der-familiengruendung-data.pdf.

Erbersdobler 2020. Erbersdobler, Julian: Wer hustet, wird jetzt schief angeschaut. In: Sueddeutsche Zeitung 2020, 19.05.2020. Online verfügbar unter https://www.sueddeutsche.de/karriere/job-arbeit-coronavirus-gesundheit-homeoffice-vorgesetzte-1.4907444?reduced=trueGut für den Arbeitnehmer (Arbeitsplatzsicherung, Betreuung + Arbeit, Flexibilität, Schutz).

Foreman et al. 2017. Foreman, Anne M.; Glenn, Margaret K.; Meade, B. Jean; Wirth, Oliver: Dogs in the Workplace: A Review of the Benefits and Potential Challenges. In: *International journal of environmental research and public health* 14 (5). DOI: 10.3390/ijerph14050498.

Grunau 2019. Grunau, Philipp: Mobile Arbeitsformen aus Sicht von Betrieben und Beschäftigten. Homeoffice bietet Vorteile, hat aber auch Tücken. Unter Mitarbeit von Kevin Ruf, Susanne Steffes und Stefanie Wolter. Hg. v. IAB-Kurzbericht. Institut für Arbeitsmarkt- und Berufsforschung. Nürnberg, Germany. Online verfügbar unter http://hdl.handle.net/10419/216702.

Grzanna 2020. Grzanna, Marcel. Kollegen, wo seid ihr? *Sueddeutsche Zeitung* 2020, 16.03.2020 (113), S. 59.

Nittono et al. 2012. Nittono, Hiroshi; Fukushima, Michiko; Yano, Akihiro; Moriya, Hiroki: The power of Kawaii: viewing cute images promotes a careful behavior and narrows attentional focus. *PloS one 7* (9), e46362. DOI: 10.1371/journal.pone.0046362.

Schwarzer et al. 2002. Schwarzer, Ralf; Jerusalem, Matthias (Hg.): Das Konzept der Selbstwirksamkeit. Selbstwirksamkeit und Motivationsprozesse in Bildungsinstitutionen. *Zeitschrift für Pädagogik* (44).

Statistisches Bundesamt 2015: Arbeitszeit von Frauen: ein Drittel Erwerbsarbeit, zwei Drittel unbezahlte Arbeit. Pressemitteilung Nr. 179. Wiesbaden (18.05.2015). Online verfügbar unter https://www.destatis.de/DE/Presse/Pressemitteilungen/Frueher/PD15_179_63931.html;jsessionid=A75DAB13E046CFBD0E1F408A58B8B1E8.internet8741, zuletzt geprüft am 07.06.2020.

Steinmann 2018. Steinmann, Susanne; Grobe, Thomas; Tendyck Hannah; Mess, Filip (2018): Mobilität in der Arbeitswelt. Datenanalyse und aktuelle Atudienlage 2018. Hamburg. Online verfügbar unter https://www.tk.de/resource/blob/2048574/98bacb6f0900b95f38e5b9feb723a096/gesundheitsreport--mobilitaet-in-der-arbeitswelt-data.pdf.

Sueddeutsche Zeitung: Schlaflos nach Feierabend. Ständige Erreichbarkeit macht krank. In: *Sueddeutsche Zeitung.* Online verfügbar unter https://www.sueddeutsche.de/karriere/staendige-erreichbarkeit-macht-krank-schlaflos-nach-feierabend-1.1028256.

Universität Konstanz 2020: Was das Arbeiten im Home Office mit uns macht. Universität Konstanz Kommunikation und Marketing (07.04.2020). Online verfügbar unter https://www.uni-konstanz.de/universitaet/aktuelles-und-medien/aktuelle-meldungen/aktuelles/was-das-arbeiten-im-home-office-mit-uns-macht/.

Dr. med. **Eva Dahlke**, physician in training to specialize in occupational medicine with a profound knowledge of emergency medicine and global assistance medicine. Postgraduate studies in medical ethics focusing on the interface between occupational medicine and ethics, primarily digital communication transformation concerning vulnerable groups.

Hans-Peter Kegel, born on 20.04.1981 in Homburg/Saar, works as a physician in the field of occupational, social and environmental medicine since 2009. His professional experience includes the planning, implementation and evaluation of scientific studies in the field of occupational, social and environmental medicine, working in student teaching and the training and further education of medical professionals, as well as providing occupational medical care for employees at schools in the state of Rhineland-Palatinate. Previously published contributions, including book contributions, range from topics of classical occupational medicine such as occupational toxicology to questions of future trends of occupational medicine with regard to new/digital media.

Declaration of War on Modern Civilization by the New Coronavirus is a Great Opportunity to Review it

Tsuyoshi Awaya, Okayama Shoka University, Japan

Abstract

The new coronavirus killed many people and pushed the world to the bottom of fear, but it is also trying to give lessons to humanity. Since the plague and the Spanish flu triggered, various changes including innovative changes, this is a chance. Now is the time to comprehensively review civilization, including its direction. The Corona Era should be the turning point for humanity and its civilization. The new coronavirus is testing mankind as a defective species that is not yet an endangered species but may face "extinction".

Key words

Coronavirus, Japan, man-made disaster, social impact, recovery

Introduction

The new coronavirus is raging. The lives of many people are being lost all over the world. I am also old and not other people's affairs a stranger at all. The new coronavirus kills many people and at the same time unveils the pathology of politics, economy, society and even modern civilization. This essay focuses on the relationship between such modern civilizations, and the new coronavirus and thus the corona disaster caused by it. It seems to be necessary because now we have noticed by the corona disaster that we have been relied upon how vulnerable political, economic and social systems, including the fragility of the health care infrastructure.

Some say that the new coronavirus is a warning for greedy humans. Some say it's a punishment for hubristic humanity. I think that the new coronavirus is a declaration of war against modern civilization, metaphorically speaking in a bit radical way. In other words, it is a challenge to humanity, the ruler of the earth. But at the same time, I also think that the new coronavirus gives us a chance to revisit its modern civilization, as we will see later. I think humanity should take advantage of this opportunity. In other words, humanity learns from "human enemies."

This essay is not a so-called scientific paper. In other words, this essay does not include a scientific argumentation. It was just a critique of a modern civilization that I wrote as soon as I was inspired by the corona disaster. Unfortunately or naturally, it is either mere lamentation or asking for the impossible.

1. The true value of modern civilization is being questioned

Currently, the new coronavirus shows the world as if it were poking a beehive. The world is always in contradiction and in chaos. The new coronavirus has dramatically increased those. The new coronavirus, as mentioned above, has made a ruthless declaration of war on our modern civilization. However, if we change our mindset, as a result, the new coronavirus and therefore corona disaster ironically give us a great opportunity to review modern civilization based on the human ego without a grand vision.

I am already tired of civilization that pursues only convenience and comfort. Economists will be furious if I radically say the modern civilization is an abnormal civilization that puts the economy ahead of all else with many wastes and contradictions. So, I will never say it again!

Now I think that the true value of modern civilization is being drastically questioned by the new coronavirus.

It is natural that various problems will occur if we continue to capture nature and plants and animals. In terms of corona disaster, civilization exactly caused it, as we will see later. Here again, that's why we need to review it.

Governments of some countries recommend just a small revision of everyday life. But it does not solve problems of modern civilization. First, the world needs to be aware of this.

2. Hotbed of Corona

The new coronavirus has spread to the world due to the global economy, which is an important factor supporting modern civilization. In that sense, the global economy, whether indirect or not, is one of the major causes of thecorona disaster. The price<cost> is too high. In different words and in short, it's the "hotbed" of the corona disaster. Of course, it goes without saying that the global economy brought about economic development in each country and region, and in turn, brought about a materially rich life for us. However, without fear of misunderstanding, I think that such an economic situation, and thus modern civilization, could be doubted.

Furthermore, an internationalized society based on the global economy is also a hotbed of corona disaster in the same sense. Of course, deforestation, urbanization with overcrowding<congested city>, and slums are part of the hotbed. It goes without saying that modern civilization depends too much on the global economy. "Local production for local consumption" is "a drop of water for a burnt stone".

It was exactly the human ego that created the hotbed of that corona disaster. To be exact, the human ego here is not only an individual ego but also an ego of an organization, a society, a nation, or the like. The root of this corona disaster is right here. Is corona disaster "divine justice" or "a taste of our own medicine?" The new coronavirus severely questions the human ego.

Considering the above, it would be no exaggeration to say that modern civilization itself is a hotbed of corona disaster.

3. Corona as a man-made disaster

corona disaster is not a natural disaster but a man-made disaster from a wide perspective. It does not mean that a particular act of a particular person in Wuhan is the origin. It is a man-made disaster in the sense that modern civilization itself produced corona disaster. Here the modern civilization has recreated nature, changed expression, destroyed it, exploited flora and fauna, left the contradiction of the human world aside, and further promoted the global economy.

4. The negative social impact of the new corona virus is immeasurable

The new coronavirus kills people. It's a mass murder. If it is a human, it means the crime of murder. In Japan, that would be the death penalty. corona disaster is like a calamity that jumped out of a Pandora's box. Originally, Japan suffered from earthquakes, tsunamis, heavy rains, typhoons, nuclear accidents, etc.

Murder is not the only crime of the new coronavirus. The negative social impact of the new coronavirus is immeasurable. The new coronavirus indirectly deprives people of their liberties and splits human, regional and national relations, etc., and fuels division of people, society and race through such countermeasures.

Furthermore, it also encouraged various types of discrimination, including racial discrimination and illness discrimination. However, it must be remembered that these are, despite the causation of the new coronavirus, ultimately based on one of the human habits of stupidity.

Especially, the socially vulnerable people such as poor people, immigrants and refugees are directly and indirectly be harmed due to the new coronavirus. Actually, they are being harmed. There is a word that "the hell is a matter of money.," I have made a word that "the life is a matter of money." The disparity creates the disparity. Economic disparities create life disparities, which are magnified by the corona disaster.

Also, I want to mention from a different perspective. The corona disaster accelerates the strengthening of national power because it has led to a dramatic increase in the dependence of the people on the nation in many countries. In other words, through the measures against the new coronavirus, indirectly the governments, either central or local, are increasingly strengthened. Of course, the so-called "blowing of administrative power", which has been pointed out before, will also be accelerated.

In addition, the corona disaster and its countermeasures may help the nation progress in a surveillance society. In the extreme, if all of these are taken together, it is possible to envisage a situation that could allow a significant tyranny of the nation. In addition, it can be easily assumed that corona disaster will accelerate the tension in the world.

5. Is Corona Disaster an Automatic Adjuster for Overpopulation?

The world population is increasing. A long time ago, in the Indian capital, Delhi, the air of the entire city was clouded white due to the exhaust gas of automobiles, causing a smoky smell. When I asked my friend, an Indian Supreme Court lawyer who came to pick me up when I arrived at Delhi International Airport, why the government left such air pollution that could cause lung cancer, he said: "The Indian Government think that there are too many people, so it is just OK." The world population has already exceeded 7.7 billion. Can the earth support it? Is the savior the new coronavirus? Is the new coronavirus an utomatic adjuster for Overpopulation?

In Japan, it has been a long time since the aging of society was pointed out. There is the flood of old people, including me. In addition, some of the questions are related to the harm of old people, that is so-called "harms from the old." Sometimes it is expressed by the words of "the runaway old". To the extreme, even "duty-to-die of the old" agitators have emerged. In other words, some celebrities have begun to argue that it is a problem that the old people will live long, and that the old people have an obligation to die early. What a sad claim! I feel sorry.

Corona's dead are mainly old people. Older people with chronic diseases are more likely to die. In the first place, there will almost never be an old person who has no chronic disease. If the troublesome old people, including me, disappear due to the new coronavirus, isn't the society as a whole happy with significant reductions in medical costs?

How about triage? Is it wasteful to use medical equipment for the old people who worked from morning till night, paid a lot of taxes and contributed to society because their lives left are short anyway? Though the arrival of a thought-provoking society, the corona disaster will encourage such triage thinking.

6. Turning disaster to advantage

Lockdowns and refraining from going out were taken as measures against the new coronavirus in cities all over the world. These inevitably led to a decrease in automobile operations and towns became quieter. In addition, exhaust gas was reduced and the air and sky were cleaned. The train stations and airports are also less crowded and comfortable.

Due to the new coronavirus, what used to be commonplace such as going out, traveling, talking with friends, eating and drinking, etc. has been no commonplace. When we lost it, we realized how grateful it was. That's a very good thing.

Other than those above, there are positive changes that are small on the surface but important in terms of meaning. corona disaster is transforming people's outlook on life <view of life> and values, even if only slightly. For example, people have begun to realize the importance of family, home and friends through various divisions as mentioned above.   I think it is not enough for people's outlook on life and values to change inevitably and automatically. Each of us needs to think corona disaster which is an unprecedented disaster is the opportunity to greatly change the outlook on life <view of life> and values. We need to consciously seek a big plus alpha. In other words, "doing" is more important than "becoming. It is not enough that the evil simply becomes good fortune. As the saying goes, we should "turn the evil into good fortune." Learning from the corona disaster, we should make Corona survivors lives happier, even if it is a little. Otherwise, the souls of many dead people will be not comforted.

7. What should we do as being triggered by corona disaster?

Needless to say, corona disaster is directly and indirectly a bad product of economic prosperity. In other words, it is a bad product of modern people being unaware of the abnormalities of modern society and even of modern civilization, or even blinding their eyes, therefore getting only benefits and living conveniently and comfortably. We are too stupid if we read the lesson.

Here, at the very least, it is necessary for us to change the way of thinking, overcoming the actual sadness of the fact that a large number of deaths are occurring all over the world. In other words, we need to turn a pinch into an opportunity. What kind of opportunity is that? As mentioned earlier, the new coronavirus and therefore corona disaster ironically give us a great opportunity to review modern civilization based on the human ego without a grand vision.

8. Economic V-shaped recovery?

So, what should we concretely do, being triggered by corona disaster? In Japan, it is often referred to as the "new everyday life of the Corona era" or the "new lifestyle." Der Kongreß tanzt. Words also dance hollowly. those contents are nothing but compassionate habits such as washing hands, gargling, avoiding a closed chamber, taking a social distance and promoting telework.

Suppose that they have suppressed the new coronavirus. Then, as if nothing had happened, as mentioned above, will we revisit our daily lives a little, and then return to the convenient, comfortable and wasteful civilization life we had before?

In many developed countries, governments say they will re-energize the economic activity that has fallen due to corona disaster. Japanese government loudly says, "Fighting and overcoming corona, and restoring the economy to a V-shape." Well, in itself, there may be no objection. Of course, there is no objection to industrial recovery. However, if the main part of the V-shaped recovery of the economy means to increase consumption, for example, to eat out at restaurants, to drink at taverns, to do sightseeing, etc. in order to drive the economy, a feeling of strangeness will be developed. Isn't it strange that the economy itself that only rotates on those assumptions? We have long abandoned the values of diligence, honesty, savings, and tolerance. Were these not universal values of humanity?

Now, the sharp in sales is declining at many tourist destinations all over the world and air pollution is decreasing as tourists are decreasing, indicating a calm aspect. Calm Kyoto as it used to be, Kathmandu where Everest can be seen... If the corona disaster is over, will a large number of foreign tourists come in Kyoto and it returns to noisy Kyoto? will Kyoto Station return to the place where hundreds of tourists line up at a taxi stand? I don't know who makes money, but have a simple question. "if you make money, is everything OK?"

9. Civilization as a desire satisfaction system

It has been a long time since the proposal of "reduced society" (http://shukusho.org/) was made, but no one listens to it. A modern civilization based on the market economy and technology, which runs with blinding eyes. Of course, that driving force is our insatiable desire. According to Hegel, civil society is a system of desires. I do not mean to be rude, but I'd like to say this. The civilization itself is, in the first place, a desire fulfillment system. In a bit more detail, it is a match-pump augmented reproduction and fulfillment system of desires that ignites and augments desires, then fills them out, then repeats. Unfortunately, it is our ego that nests at the center of that desire.

I think it is necessary to have a built-in desire auto-control system in the civilization as a desire satisfaction system. This is my claim from over 20 years ago ("Human Body Parts Business" 1999, Kodansha, Japan), but there is no sign that it will come true.

Human desires are very troublesome. It's difficult to treat. On the extension line of that desires are the competitive society and then the market economy. It goes without saying that the present time is a competitive society. The theory of enhancement and the theory of human remodeling, which are two of the themes of bioethics, have debates of a competitive society at their roots. Today's society is full of competition from small children and city salesmen to large politicians. A competitive society brings economic development and at the same time creates distressed human beings. In many developed countries, students are forced to take severe exams from childhood. Eventually, they will survive in a tough competitive society, become excellent bureaucrats and corporate warriors, and become the winners of life. They cannot afford to think of the weak and the losers of their lives. I have something to remember now. What a wonderful smile of small children in Southeast Asian slums who do not have to learn. However, there is no word of wealth in their future.

Originally, it is not limited to developed countries, but society as a whole is fully immersed in the principle of competition and the principle of market economy. The principle of competition does not make people happy. Those poison people's hearts. The principle of market economy brings about a materially rich society, but somehow or inevitably it gives a birth to money worshipers. In a society of market economy, sales are important even at university hospitals. Who made this kind of world?

In the first place, if economic development is enough to enrich rich people, then we do not need it at all. I'm fed up with politics, which are full of lies and cheats. Unfortunately, we are the dwellers of a world where justice is dying, and *where the ego is accepted*. Now, after a certain incident, the voice of "without peace without justice" is heard all over the world again. In the first place, according to Kant, if justice is destroyed, mankind does not need to live in this world. He also says it is important to overcome the ego. It is just a human being, he said.

Wonder if human beings are "non-discriminatory people". I wonder if, like at the time of the nuclear power plant accident, we forget corona disaster. Danger past, God forgotten.

10. Modern civilization without grand vision

We know immediately that the apple is round, but we do not immediately know that the earth is round. We can easily see criminal acts such as murder in front of us, but we do not easily notice the anomaly of civilization. If we go to the garbage disposal site, we can get a glimpse of the abnormalities of only modern consumer civilization.

I repeat the same arguments as above. The new coronavirus and therefore corona disaster gives us a great opportunity to review modern civilization based on the human ego without a grand vision, including reflections on individual life, and the state of politics, economy and society.

Change the point of view. The modern civilization suffers from "complex and progressive catastrophic syndrome" such as disparity, poverty, excessively competitive society, excessive consumption behavior and environmental pollution. This syndrome needs to be cured. And vaccine development is also important!

To begin with, civilization is made by humans. We can recreate it. I don't know if there is a post-corona world, but what is important is not that the world changes, but that we change the world. If we do not change, it will not change. It is not enough that the new coronavirus, and thus corona disaster automatically and inevitably move the times. We need to have the will to change.

11. Chance given by corona disaster

Corona disaster has specifically given us various "opportunities". I note some. Corona-infected people and their deaths are common in areas where vulnerable groups such as poor people, immigrants and refugees live. Now is the time to devote ourselves to helping the vulnerable. Rather, it must be done inevitably. Here are some things to remember. There are doctors and professors from poor countries participating in international bioethics congresses and conferences. They are wealthy people. There are somethings I can't always say to such people. "If you have time to discuss IT, robots, etc. in a comfortable meeting place, you had better manage the poor people who live on the street."

It is an opportunity to change our lives at a personal level. For that purpose, it is necessary to re-examine one's view of life and values. For example, now is a good time to change our lives into a slow life. It gradually transforms an energetic but noisy life into a relaxed and calm life.

People's outlook on life and values will probably change for the better, apart from their extent, due to corona disaster. But more than that, it's a chance to consciously re-question them, that is, to turn them into a good direction, with the Corona Era. Specifically, this is our chance to realize what is really important now.

Another point, the world is more and more forced to be divided. Maybe a dream story, but on the contrary, it can be said to be an opportunity for unity of humankind and solidarity in the world.

As described above, the new coronavirus offers mankind many opportunities. Saying is easy, doing is hard. So, only saying?

Conclusion

The new coronavirus killed many people and pushed the world to the bottom of fear, but it is also trying to give lessons to humanity. We need to remember that the plague and Spanish flu epidemics also triggered, at least indirectly, various changes including innovative changes.

We are swayed by the market economy, which is said to be more important than individual human lives, we are tossed about the modern civilization without a grand vision. We should have noticed the anomaly of modern civilization earlier. If so, corona disaster may not have occurred, or it may not have spread. But now it's no use worrying about it. Only the future can be changed.

I wonder if modern people still don't notice the size of the lost thing. Nostalgic to say, once there were clear air, pure water and beautiful starry sky in the world. We cannot make up for what we have lost.

Depending on how we look, I think the world is already crazy. Even if it isn't, it is better that we think so. When we are in the middle of something, we don't notice the anomaly. The new coronavirus says we need to be aware of the abnormality. The second "disastrous" is waiting for us, right there with a hand shin, counting from this time, I don't know if it's a virus or not.

Although I say it again and again, it is the time to say, but now is the time to comprehensively review civilization, including its direction. The Corona Era should be the turning point for humanity and its civilization. I am disappointed and desperate with many world leaders or men of powers, whether occasionally or always. Sometimes, no, they're often sly, cowardly, unreasonable, reckless, incompetent, insidious, and eager to have power. But, how to make use of the lessons of corona disaster under such leaders? It's a very difficult road. But without reviewing civilization, humanity's future will be disastrous.

Mankind must be a stupid group, but there is still hope. In the first place, it is not easy to judge which is worse, the new coronavirus that attaches to humans or the special virus that attaches to the earth, which name is a human. I'm also a member of the kind of a human who is overconfident and has a strong sense of self-esteem, so it would be biased if I judge. Aside from that, the new coronavirus is testing a mankind as a defective species that is not yet an endangered species but may be an "extinction-hoped" species. Whether or not corona disaster is a conspiracy or deliberate offense of the new Coronavirus, I hope we're not residents in extermination camps.

Tsuyoshi Awaya, B.Sc., LL.M., Ph.D., Professor of Bioethics and Medical Law, Faculty of Law, Okayama Shoka University, Okayama, Japan. (Professor Emeritus, Okayama University, Okayama, Japan). Specialization in Bioethics, Medical Law, Law and Sociology. Honors: 1. Testimony at the U.S. Congress on the Transplantation of Organs from Executed Prisoners in China, 1998, 2. Award for Promotion of Research from the Japan Association for Bioethics, 1996. *About 40 Books and Over 100 Academic Articles.* For many years, I have been conducting fact-finding surveys, legislative researches, etc. on organ transplantation in Asian countries.

Specifically, I have conducted various surveys on organ trafficking in India and the Philippines. I have also conducted various studies on excuted prisoners and Falun Gong transplants in China.I had testimony and a statement on the transplantation of organs from executed prisoners in China at the International Relations Committee and the Government Reform and Oversight Committee of the United States House of Representatives on June 4,1998.

Islam's Approach to Infectious Diseases through the Eyes of a Ninth Century Muslim Scholar

Tuba Erkoç Baydar, Assistant Professor at Ibn Haldun University, Turkey

Abstract

The religion of Islam does not only value the happiness of mankind in the life of the hereafter, but also in the life of this world. For this reason, it makes recommendations to human beings for them to pass the test of life in this world by setting out certain rules and prohibitions. Illness is one of the most serious tests that human beings face in the life of this world. Infectious diseases in particular have been a nightmare throughout human history. In this section, the approaches and recommendations that Islam adapted in the face of infectious diseases will be presented through the views of an important Muslim scholar who lived in the ninth century. The most important feature of this text is the fact that it includes references to the literature that precedes it and an all-encompassing evaluation of the subject at hand. It is also notable that Ibn Ḥajar al-ʿAsqalānī (d. 852/1449), who penned the work after having lost his three daughters to the plague, called the work Badhl al-maʿūn fī faḍl al-taʿūn, or the Benefits of the Plague.

Key words

Islam, infectious diseases, Ibn Ḥajar al-ʿAsqalānī

1. Introduction

Infectious diseases in human history have caused even greater destruction than wars and natural disasters. Throughout history, with the plague taking the lead, many infectious diseases such as tuberculosis, chickenpox, typhoid, flu, AIDS, and Ebola, have been a struggle for the human population. However, epidemic diseases are not only left behind on the pages of history. These diseases, which test humanity at certain intervals in world history, are still prevalent, as we see with COVID-19 in 2020.

Epidemics are critical events that not only signify death and survival but also change the culture, habits, values, and lives of societies. As historical experience shows us critical events and situations add momentum to history or help us overcome a significant threshold. Corona is just such an epidemic. In fact, with this epidemic, the world has made a rapid leap forward in preferring more virtual connections instead of physical ones. The COVID-19 pandemic, which has affected the lives of billions of people and caused thousands of people to die and face psycho-social and economic problems, is therefore an important issue that needs to be dealt with across many dimensions.

In order to contribute to the interdisciplinary analysis of the issue, this study will present an approach of Islam to epidemics. Given the fact that Islam wants people not only to be happy in the eternity, but also to live a happy and peaceful life in the world, it provides various recommendations for possible scenarios in the world. Moreover, according to Islam, a person should work not only for his/her own happiness, but also for the happiness of all living things, including the people, animals and plants around him/her. For this reason, important arrangements have been determined about what to do in case of diseases.

Since diseases is one of the leading phenomena which provide a powerful religious cognition, it is not surprising that Islam and Muslims have a great attention to issues related to diseases. In order to both express these regulations and present the approach of Islam, a work written by Ibn Ḥajar al-ʿAsqalānī (d.1449), one of the important scholars of the fourteenth century Islamic world, will be examined. Although Ibn Ḥajar's work is in a central position in this study, the views of other Islamic scholars will be consulted from time to time. However, this study will not go beyond the four Sunni sects. With comparative perspective, our methodology is to bring some central themes in the four Sunni sect literature on infectious diseases into clearer.

There are many stand-alone works written on infectious diseases in the Islamic world. Although some of these works are not extant, there are some that have survived until our present day and that provide important information (Ibn Ḥajar, 1991: 29-41). One of the works that has survived to this day is Ibn Ḥajar's *Badhl al-ma'ūn fī faḍl al-ta'ūn*, which is impressive in terms of its content and comprehensiveness. This work on the plague, as the French researcher Panzac puts it, is a collection of centuries of authority in its field (Panzac, 1997: 156). It was published by Ahmed Isam Abd al-Qadir al-Khatib in 1991 in Riyadh. The work, which is approximately four hundred and fifty pages, deals with the subject of epidemics in a very detailed way.

Ibn Ḥajar began to write his observations on the subject at a time when the plague epidemic had started to affect people intensely but then had come to a pause for unknown reasons. He completed his work after losing all of his three daughters to the plague epidemic. The author, who had personal experience in losing his daughters due to the plague and in the extent to which the epidemic affected people, is accepted as an authority in many fields such as hadith, *fiqh*, history, grammar, which makes this work even more valuable.

Ibn Ḥajar, who deals with the subject in a systematic way, mentions the topics he will address at the beginning of the text. He then mentions the verses on the subject and the hadiths. Ibn Ḥajar, who is known especially for his expertise in the field of hadith, also makes a detailed evaluation of the hadiths related to the subject in his work. First, he examines each person who narrates these hadiths one by one and provides a detailed analysis of their reliability by providing information about these individuals. He then evaluates the text of the hadiths and explains the parts that appear to be contradictory and conveys the views of the scholars to that end.

Ibn Ḥajar designed his work in five basic parts. In the first part, he explains how plague can turn into mercy, even though it is a torment sent to humanity. In the second part, he resolves the confusion caused by different terms used in epidemics and evaluates the theories put forward about the causes of the plague. In the third part, he talks about the situation of those who have the plague. This part provides important psychological support for those struggling with plague epidemics. Trying to answer any conceivable doubts and question marks, Ibn Ḥajar analyses human psychology. In the fourth part, referring to the quarantine issue, which is one of the most important issues in combating epidemic diseases, Ibn Ḥajar describes how to fight epidemic diseases based on the hadiths related to the subject. While describing these sections, Ibn Ḥajar, who gives examples from history, offers strong evidence to the reader by highlighting the practices of Islamic caliphs like 'Umar. In the fifth part, he describes, in detail, what to do when you catch epidemic diseases, precautions to be taken and rules to be followed. In the conclusion, Ibn Ḥajar summarizes his book by mentioning the plague epidemics that took place in Islamic geography.

2. Health Policy in Islam

Before moving on to Islam's approach to epidemics, it is necessary to describe its health policy more generally, because this policy is also effective in approaching epidemics. As Ibn Qayyim (d. 1350) stated, the health policy of Islam can be divided into three parts as preventive, therapeutic and health-maintaining. Arguing that all of these principles are included in the Qur'an, Ibn Qayyim said that a sick person should turn to alternatives instead of ablution with water (Qur'an 4/43), which is an example of preventive health; that a patient or a traveller should not fast, so as not to get sick (Qur'an 2/184), which is an example of maintaining health;

that there is healing for humans in honey" (Qur'an16/69), which is an example of the therapeutic side of these policies. Therapeutic and preventive health in particular are thought to be included in hadiths. The Prophet (pbuh) emphasized the value of health (al-Bukhārī 1991: 6412) and recommended quarantine for the plague and leprosy (al-Bukhārī 1991: 5707), promoted miswak (The miswak is a teeth cleaning twig) use, hand washing and cleaning in general – all of this is in line with the preventive medicine of our time.

According to Islam, it is essential to take precautions to prevent illness by knowing the value of health. However, when the disease starts, it is necessary to work toward treatment by making use of the data of medical science without despair. 1400 years ago, in the time of The Prophet, the idea that diseases occur due to the influence of evil spirits was rejected and treatment was encouraged based on various reasons. As a matter of fact, while many believed that the plague occurred due to the influence of evil spirits in medieval times, Ibn al-Khatib (d. 1375), one of the Islamic scholars, explained with scientific evidence that plague was an infectious disease and encouraged treatment (Tomar-Ubudī 2000: 75).

Since there are many hadiths about treatment, Islamic scholars have always encouraged treatment. The most frequently mentioned hadith about the treatment is the statement "Allah sent the healing of every disease" (al-Bukhārī 1991: 5678). With this promise, the Prophet (pbuh) encouraged Muslims to apply to medical science and to work on finding the cure of every disease by holding on to the belief that every disease has a cure. Moreover, besides encouraging the treatment of every disease, the fact that he personally sought out treatment and asked for health from Allah in his prayers (al-Bukhārī 1991: 5671). Also, al-Qarāfī's statement that, "The Prophet (pbuh) used medicine the most frequently among his contemporaries" (al-Qarāfī 1994: 307) shows how much he valued treatment. Moreover, The Prophet's wife Aisha talks about how frequently the Prophet consulted medicine. The Aisha stated that her knowledge on medicine was the result of the frequent visits he received from doctors. (al-Haythamī 1991: 388).

The treatment approach in the Islamic world is two-dimensional. The first dimension is to apply to physical means such as treatment from the doctors; while the second dimension is more spiritual, such as praying to Allah and hoping for a full recovery. Islam addresses both physiological and transcendental factors. Along with this physiological aspect of man, transcendental characteristics make him a meeting point between material and spiritual realms. For this reason, in case of illness, as in every case, both physical reasons and praying to the creator and trusting Him are important for a full recovery. As a matter of fact, the Hanafī scholars who accepted the legitimacy of treatment emphasized the importance of intention when seeking treatment by saying that if the healing is not thought to come from Allah, it will impact the legitimacy of the treatment (al-Fatawa 1973: 354). This attitude is evident both in the approach of Islam to calamities in general as well as being evident in the approach towards epidemics.

3. The Approach of Islam to Diseases and Calamities

Diseases are a part of life. As emphasized in the Qur'an and hadiths (al-Bukhārī 1999: 6487), and by the Islamic scholars, the problems in the world are all a part of the test. For example, Al-Zamakhsharī (d. 538/1144), one of the *tafsīr* scholars, clearly states that misfortunes were sent to test people (Al-Zamakhsharī 1947: 232-33). On the other hand, theologians who have important views on the meaning of misfortunes such as illness, describe the misfortunes as lessons, exams and signs for both those exposed and those around them (al-Māturīdī 2003: 351-458).

According to Sarrāj al-Tūsī (d. 988), one of the most important Sufī scholars, there are three kinds of troubles and misfortunes: trouble and calamities are either punishment for sins, purification of sins, or a means of spiritual elevation (Sarrāj al-Tusī 1996: 362). In addition, diseases bring the beloved servant of Allah closer to Him, serve as a reminder of God's purpose in sending the servant to the world, erase his sins, raise his position and are a response to the mistakes he made in the world (Qadi ʿAbd al-Jabbār 2013: 286). People's patience, sincerity, violations in their beliefs and devotion to Allah are tried through misfortunes. Therefore, as it is stated in the story of Prophet Job, there is a wisdom in the pain and suffering sent by Allah, and if one does not rebel against them, it is stated that one will face reward in eternity and that one's sins will be forgiven (al-Nīshāpurī 1990: 350). Like the verses, the ʿulama are united in saying that the troubles in the world will be atonement for sins (Âlûsī nd: 152). For example, the founder of the Māturīdī school, Imam al-Māturīdī, stated that "the end of those who pass the test will be eternal salvation will turn into mercy for those who pass the test" (al-Māturīdī 2009: 505), and many theologians said that the misfortunes in the world will have the reward of eternal blessing (al-Juwaynī 1992: 247; al-Ghazālī 2008: 287). For this reason, according to Islam, the fact that illnesses that happen to people on Earth are seen as purely bad results in an incorrect evaluation of this issue. As a matter of fact, we are reminded in the Holy Qur'an that something should not be evaluated as good or bad merely by consideration of its apparent results (Quran 2/216).

One of the most important points which Islam recommends while being tested with a calamity is tawakkul. *Tawakkul*, which means trusting and leaning on Allah, is counted as a qualification of believers in the Quran (Quran 8/2) and is praised by the Prophet (pbuh). The Prophet said, "If a Muslim comes across an illness, Allah will shed his mistakes and sins as the leaves of the tree fall at the time of autumn." (al-Bukhārī 1999: 5660). In addition, in other hadiths, the Prophet stated that the disease which comes across the believer will increase his spiritual degree and cause the forgiveness of his sins. However, showing trust does not mean being patient with the disease and waiting for his reward from Allah while not seeking treatment for his illness. Allah, Who creates the cause-effect relations in worldly life, is the creator of both causes and consequences. Nevertheless, Allah condemns anyone who wants to give up without applying to the possible means He has prepared and says, "They are like anyone who opens their two hands towards the water for it to come to their mouths. Whereas (unless he takes the water to his mouth) water is not going to enter his mouth. " (Quran 13/14.).

Epidemic Terms and Historical Background

In the literature in the Islamic world, the words wabā' and *tā ʿūn* are most often used to refer to epidemics. According to Ibn Manzūr (d. 1311), the word *wabā'* is derived from the Arabic letters "wāw, bā', yā'" and is an umbrella concept that denotes all infectious diseases. *Tā ʿūn* is a kind of *wabā'*. (Ibn Manzūr nd: 198). Ibn Sīnā (d. 1037), whose medical works were accepted as a reference in the Western and Eastern world of science for hundreds of years, states that because tā ʿūn was common in the towns were infectious diseases often occurred, they called tā ʿūn, wabā' in those areas while this term doesn't comply with the meaning of the actual term. (Ibn Ḥajar 1991: 99) Ibn Ḥajar gives a detailed analysis of the word of *tā ʿūn* and the *wabā'* and conveys the views of scholars on the subject, drawing attention to the difference between *tā ʿūn* and *wabā'* and explaining that every *tā ʿūn* is included in the term *wabā'*. Ibn Hajar takes on the view which is based on the distinction made by the linguists and physicians, who state that not every *wabā'* can be counted as a *tā ʿūn* (Ibn Ḥajar 1991: 102-104).

Throughout the history, we see that Muslim communities fight against many epidemic diseases. The biggest epidemic in the history of Islam was during the time of the second caliph of the Caliphate of the *khulafā' al-rāshidūn*, 'Umar. This plague epidemic, which caused many important companions of The Prophet to be martyred, caused the death of approximately 25 thousand people (Ibn Ḥajar 1991: 362). Apart from that, it is known that the plague was seen in many Muslim cities such as Egypt, Shiraz, Basra, Turkestan, Iraq, and, later, Bursa and Istanbul, and caused serious deaths (Varlik 2011: 175). Many companions, scholars and leaders died in epidemics in the Islamic world. As a matter of fact, Mu'ādh Ibn Jabal (d. 639), who was among the companions who were promised heaven in eternity; the Prophet's step-son, Hind b. Hāla (d. 656); Mughīra b. Shu'ba (d. 670); Abu Naṣr Tāj al-Dīn al-Subkī (d. 1370); the three daughters of Ibn Ḥajar, whom we are discussing in this article; and many scientists and statesmen in the Ottoman period died due to infectious diseases.

4. Precautions against Infectious Diseases and Quarantine

Infectious diseases raise many socio-economic and psychological problems. Therefore, serious measures should be taken against epidemic diseases and they should be prevented as much as possible. It is possible to summarize the measures adopted and recommended by Islam in line with health policy, in three main categories: preventive health, treatment and prayer. While preventive health precautions are recommended to be taken in order not to catch the disease, treatment is recommended after catching the disease, and prayer, both before and after catching the disease.

In Islam, preventive measures are part of the daily rituals of Muslims. It is emphasized that health is a great blessing in the religion of Islam, and, through the duties, it imposes on believers; it includes measures that provide health and protection. Cleanliness is a constant requirement of faith in Islam according to the words of the Prophet (Muslim 2000: 534). Muslims who need to pray five times a day wash their hands, face, arms and feet before these prayers, paying attention to dental cleaning, and to the cleanliness of their clothes and the cleanliness of the place of prayer for their worship to be valid. This also reduces the risk of the spread of the disease.

When it comes to epidemics, important measure is to prevent the spread of the disease. One of the most effective ways to do this is quarantine. Shortly after the establishment of a quarantine organization and the implementation of new health regulations in the middle of the nineteenth century, plague outbreaks in Anatolia, Egypt and the Eastern Mediterranean were greatly reduced (Varlik 2011: 176). Today, also it has been decided that the most effective way to fight Coronavirus is to prevent the spread of epidemic disease. Wuhan was considered the place where COVID-19 started, and if a strict quarantine were applied from the very first moment, we would not have to struggle with the Coronavirus in many parts of the world. This experience has again shown how vital quarantine is against infectious diseases.

Quarantine (*quarantenadan*), which is an Italian word in origin, is defined as "keeping travellers under surveillance for a period of forty days" (Sariyildiz 2001: 463). The understanding of quarantine in Islam is twofold: for a sick person not to leave from where s/he is located, and for a healthy person to keep away from the region where the disease is located. This determination was made based on Qur'anic verses and hadiths. It is clearly stated in the Qur'an that no one should jeopardize even her/his own life (Qur'an. 2/195). Based on this verse, it is said that no one should enter the region where the disease is located. The source that provides more detailed information on quarantine is hadiths. The Prophet (pbuh) said, "If you hear that there is a plague, do not enter there. If it occurs in your location, do not leave" (al-Bukhārī 1999: 5729) and these words summarize the way quarantine is implemented. In another hadith, it is seen that he mentions the importance of staying away from a person with leprosy through a metaphorical expression involving the image of escaping from a lion (al-Bukhārī 1999: 5707).

The recommendations of the Prophet (pbuh) on quarantine were also implemented by the Companions after his death. When the second caliph 'Umar arrived in the town of Sargh while on a journey to Damascus to inspect the army in the Syrian region, he was informed that there was a plague in Damascus. After consulting with the Companions, he decided that they would turn back, and even though there were objections accusing 'Umar of trying to flee from the decree of Allah, 'Umar did not change his decision, saying that that they would be fleeing from the decree of Allah to the other decree of Allah (i.e., whether they went on to Damascus or not, that would be the decree of Allah). Then, when a latecomer said that the Prophet (pbuh) made a recommendation not to enter a region where disease was located, he realized that he had made the right decision and praised Allah (al-Bukhārī 1999: 5729). This behaviour of 'Umar is an important example for Muslim scholars and political leaders, since 'Umar held both political authority and religious authority. As can be seen in the example of 'Umar, not entering the region where the disease is located reflects the quarantine understanding in Islam.

Just as one should not travel to a region where there is an outbreak of an infectious disease, one should not leave that place if one is in it. Indeed, the words of the Prophet forbade anyone to travel to a region with the plague, and forbade anyone to leave that area. Al-Jaṣṣāṣ, one of the important Ḥanafī scholars, mentions this hadith and other evidences, saying that it is not right to try to escape from the disease. Al-Jaṣṣāṣ conveys the hadiths coming from the Prophet and argues that in a situation where infectious disease occurs, that area should not be left or visited (al-Jaṣṣāṣ 1996: 165). Many Islamic scholars like al-Jaṣṣāṣ also warn that one should not leave the quarantine area. As a matter of fact, according to the report of al-Zarkashī, from the fourteenth century Shafi'ī scholars, Taqī al-Dīn b. Daqīq thinks that escaping from the city where infectious disease started is prohibited, and it should be prohibited to enter that area. Because entering that town means putting your own life in danger with your own hands, which is prohibited in the Qur'an (Ibn Ḥajar 1991: 305).

One of the influential Shafi'ī scholars Taj al-Dīn al-Subkī says that leaving a region where there is the plague is *harām* according to the Shafi'ī school. According to him, the prohibition of leaving the area with plague becomes certain when paired with the intention of escaping from Allah's predestination. The uncertain situation is to leave the plague area for the purpose of treatment. Ibn Khuzayma thinks that escaping from the plague is a great sin. According to him, Allah will punish the person who is in such a position (Ibn Ḥajar 1991: 275).

According to Ibn Ḥajar, there is important wisdom in the command of the Prophet regarding quarantine. However, it is not always possible to grasp this wisdom. Although the causes are not fully understood, the important thing is obedience to the order. The behaviour that man must fulfil is submission to the command of Allah (Ibn Ḥajar 1991: 302). Ibn Ḥajar gives a long speech about being able to leave the area where infectious disease occurs. To this end, he deals with the views and evidence of many scholars, many questions about quarantine, the understanding of trust and fate, and the relation of interest and the wisdom of the quarantine (Ibn Ḥajar 1991: 274-306).

According to some of the scholars, this disease affects everyone in the region where plague is seen. For this reason, it is not beneficial for any person to flee from the place where the plague occurs. To escape from illness and not to escape from it are equal. Likewise, it can be considered otherwise (Ibn Ḥajar 1991: 302). In addition, if people escape from this area, people who cannot escape from there will experience the sadness of this. Moreover, when they die due to this disease, there will be no one to shroud them and put them in a grave. Therefore, one should not leave the region where the epidemic is located (Ibn Ḥajar 1991: 303). Some scholars have said that one of the wisdoms of this prohibition is to prevent people from trusting means other than relying on God and trusting them (Ibn Ḥajar 1991: 304). On this subject, Ibn ʿAbd al-Barr al-Subkī, one of the Shafiʿī scholars, makes an important comment. According to him, the prohibition of leaving the plague area is for faith, and the prohibition of entering the plague area is to protect the *nafs* (Ibn Ḥajar 1991: 303). Similarly, one of the important Hanafī scholars, al-Sarakhsī (d. 1090) drew attention to this with the following statements: "As long as the person has the belief that everything happens by the decree of Allah, there is no trouble in entering the place of the plague or leaving it. However, it is *makrūh* for the person to believe that he will not catch the disease by not going where the plague is, or that he will get rid of it by leaving the infectious place. In order to protect his faith, one should not enter or leave the plague." (al-Sarakhsī 1993: 166). As seen in these examples, many scholars of Islam evaluate the issue in faith framework.

According to Ibn Ḥajar, as can be seen from the letters of the second caliph ʿUmar to ʿUbayda b. Jarrāḥ, there are some exceptions for not being allowed to leave a plague city. One of these exceptions is to go elsewhere for treatment. Likewise, it is possible to leave a city in order to return to one's original homeland (Ibn Ḥajar 1991: 273). In the second half of the sixteenth century, the contagiousness of the disease had increased so *fatwas* were given related to the response of going from a place where the epidemic was seen to a place with clean air. For example, Taşköprüzade Ahmed Efendi expresses this explicitly in the treatises he penned. Abu Suud Efendi also has fatwas on the matter. In response to the question of whether there is a permit to escape from *taʿūna* (the plague), he made a fatwa to the end that it would be permissible to take refuge in the favour of the Creator (Duzdag 1983: 182). Especially those who play important roles in the fight against the epidemic, such as healthcare professionals, should not leave this region. In fact, he ruled out the punishment of grave for those who did not escape and did his duty (Duzdag 1983: 182). Muslim scholars also see escaping from the quarantine zone as a weakness. In fact, in this regard, the Prophet said, "Escaping from where the disease originated is like escaping from the war. Patience and staying there are like the ones who persevere in the war" (Ibn Ḥajar 1991: 280). The fact that the Prophet likened running away in case of an epidemic disease to leaving those around one alone in the face of war in this hadith shows the importance of the issue.

There are also some well-known facilities for patients in the Islamic religion. Islam is the religion of convenience. The Prophet said, "Make things easy for the people, and do not make it difficult for them, and make them calm (with glad tidings) and do not repulse them (al-Bukhārī 1999: 6125). For this reason, facilitating the lives of Muslims when an epidemic occurs, is also considered important by Islamic scholars. *In case of necessity, some amenities have been determined in order to protect people's lives, property, honour, mind and religion in Islam.* For example, in a situation where fasting is harmful to health, one is asked to postpone fasting and help the poor instead. In this context, some measures may be taken to prevent the spread of epidemics. For example, Muslims may be asked to worship individually in their homes instead of coming together. Indeed, ʿAbdullah b. ʿAbbās, after reciting the Islamic testimony of faith on a rainy day, had asked the caller of Muslims to the mosque to say, "Complete your prayers in your home" instead of "come to prayer". For those who criticized him, he stated that he had seen it this way from the Prophet (Muslim 2000: 1604). In addition, when it is possible that the Prophet forbade those who eat garlic to come to the mosque due to the smell (Muslim, 2000: 1248), going to the mosque due to a life-threatening virus can easily be forbidden.

When illnesses occur, it is an evident responsibility of the administrators of that society to take any precautions that prevent these diseases, especially that of quarantine, to prevent the disease from spreading to more people. Indeed, in the Umayyad period, Caliph Walīd I. (d. 715) allocated an allowance for those suffering from leprosy and quarantined them to prevent them from interfering with the society by taking over all of their care and expenses (al-Tabarī 1967:437). Any actions that endanger one's own health and that of others must be avoided and the rules set by the competent authority to prevent epidemics must be followed. Every Muslim is expected to comply with rules like wearing a mask, paying attention to social distance, isolation, and controlled social life and curfew. It is the responsibility of an infected person to act cautiously and avoid transmitting this disease to another. That is why the Prophet describes the Muslim as the person at whose hands and words other Muslims do not suffer. Therefore, Muslims have responsibilities towards their environment. Every Muslim should fulfil their duty to protect their family and their environment.

5. What to Do with Those Who Have Infectious Diseases

According to Islam, the first thing to do after catching the disease is to increase the psychological immunity. Even in the worst case, without psychological rebellion or breaking down, one can relax by considering the good tidings of Allah. Indeed, the approach of scholars and companions in Islamic history is a great example at this point. Although Ibn Ḥajar lost his three daughters, he gave his work the title: *the Virtues of the Plague* and said that the disease was a mercy sent to the people. The governor of Damascus, to whom it was proposed that he become a caliph after the Prophet but who did not want it, was ʿUbayda b. Jarrāḥ and he said that when the plague came out, it was a mercy sent by God. When he died of plague, Muʿādh Ibn Jabal became the new governor. His first two sons and then he himself passed away due to plague. He said that his condition when he died was the most beautiful he could ever want in the world (Ibn Ḥajar 1991: 268).

As stated before, human beings are of two dimensions, material and spiritual. They should feed these two aspects in case of epidemic. People should protect their body by taking material precautions, and protect their spiritual aspect against diseases with spiritual measures. For this reason, besides the measures mentioned above, such as cleaning and quarantine, it is necessary to rely on Allah and to pray to Allah with patience. According to Imam Shafi'ī, one of the four great Imams, the best thing to cure plague is to remember Allah, because remembrance removes punishment. For example, if the forgiveness of Yūnus (pbuh) were not related to his constant and patient prayers, he would have stayed in the belly until the apocalypse (Ibn Ḥajar 1991: 317).

In addition, according to Islam, one is encouraged to pray for himself, as well as for others. The Prophet said, "Muslims are like a single body in loving each other, pitying each other, and protecting each other. When one organ of that body is disturbed, all of the other organs feel discomfort." Because of this statement, Islamic scholars have also encouraged those who live in a region where there is no plague to pray for those in a region where the disease is present (Ibn Ḥajar 1991: 317).

Finally, according to some Islamic scholars, seeing the disease as an opportunity for forgiveness for sins from Allah makes it controversial to pray for the elimination of diseases. This is not a common opinion, although there are those who do not welcome praying to get rid of the plague because of Allah's mercy. Ibn Ḥajar criticizes those in this view and provides various evidences (Ibn Ḥajar 1991: 319). The fact that the disease is written in God's decree does not prevent prayer, because Allah Almighty ordered us to pray. Moreover, leaving the prayer means leaving a righteous deed. The attitude of the Muslim against the plague is that he knows that it is a trial sent by Allah, and patience and prayer without leaving the region where the disease is occurring is required. As the second caliph ʿUmar said, the existence of the disease is destiny, and salvation from the disease through prayer is destiny. In addition, measures to be taken against the disease have been determined in destiny.

6. The Status of Those Who Die from Epidemic Diseases

The condition of those who die in epidemics is one of the important issues discussed in literature. While illnesses are sometimes sent to people as a mercy, sometimes it is a misfortune. On this question, Ibn Ḥajar says that such illnesses were sent to people when they were dismissed and disrupted by the prophets sent to them (Ibn Ḥajar 1991: 82). However, epidemic diseases in Islamic thought are generally considered a mercy based on the words of the Prophet. The Prophet gives glad tidings to those who died because of the epidemic, saying that death from the plague is a martyrdom for every Muslim (al-Bukhārī 1999: 5732). In addition, in another hadith: "Certainly, Allah made the plague martyrdom for believers. Wherever the plague appears, and a believer who is there patiently endures, thinking that this plague comes across those whom Allah appreciates, and doesn't leave where he is located, Allah will bestow upon him the reward of a Martyr." (al-Bukhārī 1999: 5734). What is meant by being patient here is that he does not give himself over to sorrow, but surrenders himself, and does not rebel, as he is pleased with God's decree and fate. As stated in the hadiths, for those who die from epidemic diseases to be counted as martyrs, they must rely on Allah and show patience.). It is stated in the hadith that this disease is rendered as a means of mercy for the Muslims and this mercy will be manifested as martyrdom for those who comply with the conditions. Likewise, Ibn Ḥajar said that no one should leave the region where he is to receive martyrdom and that this calamity was given by Allah and that it will disappear only with His wish. (Ibn Ḥajar 1991: 199-203).

Finally, Ibn Ḥajar makes an interesting comment based on the statements in the hadith about infectious diseases. According to him, it is possible for not only for those who died from the epidemic disease, but also for everyone who died during the time of an epidemic disease to be regarded as a martyr. In the hadith the word 'epidemic' is used with the preposition "*fī*". In the Arabic language, this preposition means both reason and time. When we take the letter "*fī*" in the hadith as time the meaning of the hadith comes to the meaning that everyone who dies not only because of the epidemic disease, but who died in the time of the epidemic is considered a martyr. Reminding us that Allah's mercy is great, Ibn Ḥajar says that if Allah wishes, He can give martyrdom to everyone who died in that period (Ibn Ḥajar 1991: 200).

7. Conclusion

The complex psychology and somatic physiology of human beings must be dealt with in case of epidemic diseases, as in every issue. Therefore, Islam adopts a two-way approach to combating epidemic diseases. The first is to strengthen spiritual immunity. When spiritual immunity is strong, even if someone is plagued by spiritual viruses such as sadness, grief, anxiety attacks, these will be eliminated by spiritual immunity. Spiritual antibodies produced by the body's past sorrow, grief and exams will strengthen the immune system, just as it occurs in the physical plane. Strengthening spiritual immunity is as important as strengthening material immunity. As a matter of fact, socio-economic and psychological problems that people experience during this process will open the door to a psychological pandemic after the COVID-19 outbreak. In order to avoid such a pandemic, spiritual immunity needs to be strengthened. In this context, the issues recommended by Islam are very important. The praise of those who do not complain about the disease and show patience both in the world and in the hereafter provides an important motivation. In addition, seeing those who died due to the epidemic as martyrs is an important glad tiding for both the relatives of the deceased and those who struggle against this disease.

However, spiritual behaviours such as praying and patience in the face of epidemic diseases in Islamic thought are not enough in the struggle. Material measures must also be taken. The most important order of Islam in the face of epidemics is maintaining quarantine. As is pointed out in other hadiths related to the subject, entering and exiting the region where an epidemic disease is seen is prohibited. This is a complete quarantine and it is meant to maintain tightly. Based on the words of the Prophet, Islamic scholars regarded quarantine as a religious order. It was said that a person who did not pay attention to quarantine and who left the city was sinful, or who caused someone to die by bringing him to the city should pay a fine.

Some measures, such as quarantine, must be taken by the state and the people must comply. It is important to take some precautionary measures. However, some criteria have been developed to ensure that these requirements are objective and do not open doors to abuse. The most important of these criteria is that the reason for why something is good is genuine, inherent, does not conflict with any other concerns and is suitable for the spirit of Islam. It is necessary to pay attention to these criteria so that the measures taken within the scope of responding to Coronavirus does not violate the rights of the people.

References

al-Bukhārī 1999. Abū 'Abd Allāh Muḥammad ibn Ismā'īl ibn Ibrāhīm Ibn al-Mughīrah ibn Bardizbah al-Ju'fī. Ṣaḥīḥ al-Bukhārī: al-Jāmi' al-Musnad al-Sahīh al-Mukhtaṣar min umūr Rasūl Allāh wa sunnanihi wa ayyāmihi. Riyadh: Dār al-Salām Press 1999.

al-Fetāwā al-Hindiyye 1973. ed. Burhanpurlu Sheyh Nizam, Sheyh Vecîh al-Dīn, Sheyh Jalal al-Dīn Muhammad, Qadī Muhammed Hüseyin, Molla Hamid, Diyarbakır: al-Maktaba al-Islamıyyah 1973.

al-Ghazālī 2008. Abū Hamid Muhammad b. Muhammad. Ihya al-Ulum al-Dīn. Cario: al-Maktaba al-Tavfekiyye 2008 I.

al-Haythamī 1991. Nur al-Dīn 'Ali ibn Abi Bakr ibn Sulayman Abū Hasan al-Haythamī, Majma' al-Zawa'id wa Manba' al-Fawa'id, Beirut: Dār al-Fikr 1991 III/388.

al-Jaṣṣāṣ 1996. Abū Bakr Aḥmad ibn 'Alī al-Rāzī. Aḥkām al-Qur'ān. Beirut: Dār al-Kutub al-'Ilmiyya 1996 II.

al-Juwaynī 1992. Imam al-Haramayn., Kitâb al-Irshād, ed. Esad Temim, Beirut: Müessese al-Kutub as-Sakāfiyya 1992 257.

al-Māturīdī 2003. Abū Manṣūr Muḥammad b. Muḥammad b. Maḥmūd al-Samarḳandī. Kitāb al-Tawhid. Puplished by Muhammad Aruji. Ankara: TDV Press 2003 351-458.

al-Māturīdī 2009. Abū Manṣūr Muḥammad b. Muḥammad b. Maḥmūd al-Samarḳandī. Tawilât al-Qur'ân. ed. Muhammad Masum Vanlıoğlu, Istanbul: Mizan Press 2009 II.

al-Qarāfī 1994. Shihāb al-Dīn Abū Abbās Aḥmad ibn Abi 'l-'Alā' Idrīs ibn 'Abd al-Raḥmān. al-Dhakhīrah. Puplished by Muhammad Hubze, Beirut: Dār al-Garb al-Islami 1994.

al-Sarakhsī 1982. Muhammad b. Ahmad b. Abi Sahl Abū Bakr, al-Mabsût. Istanbul: Çağrı

Press, 1982 X.

al-Ṭabarī 1967. Abū Jaʿfar Muḥammad ibn Jarīr ibn Yazid, Tarikh al-Rusul wa al-Muluk (History of the Prophets and Kings). Puplished by Muhammad Abu Fadl Ebrahim, Egypt: Dār al-Mearif 1968 VI.

al-Taftāzānī 1998. Saʾad al-Dīn Masud Ibn Umar Ibn Abd Allah. al-Talvīh ilā Kashfi Haqāiq al-Tanqīh. thk. Muhammed Adnan, Beirut: Dār al-Erkam b. Abū Erkam 1998 I.

Âlūsī nd. Shihab al-dīn Maḥamud b. ,Abd Allah al-Alusī al-Baghdadī. Ruh al-Ma'anı fī Tafsir al-Qur'an. Beirut: Dār al-Ihya at-Turās al-Arabī, t.y. V.

al-Zamahsharī 1947. Abū al-Qasım Jarallah Mahmud b. Omar b. Mohammed. al-Kashshaf ,an Haqa'iq al-Tanzil. Beirut: Dār al-Marife 1947 I /232-233.

al-Nīshāpurī 1990. Abū Abd-Allah Muhammad ibn Abd-Allah al-Hakim an-Nīshāpurī. Al-Mustadrak ,alâ al-Sahîhayn. Puplished by Mustafa Abd al-Qadir Ata, Beirut: Dār al-Kutub al-Ilmiyyah 1990 IV/350.

Düzdağ 1983. M. Ertuğrul. Sheikh al-Islām Ebussuud Efendi Fetvaları Işığında 16. Asır Türk Hayatı. Istanbul 1983 154-182.

Ibn Ḥajar 1991. Ahmad b. Ali Ibn Ḥajar al-Askalānī. Badhl al-maʿūn fī faḍl al-taʿūn. Published by Abd al-Qadir al Khatip, Riyadh: Dār al-Asıma Press 1991 1nd edition.

Ibn Manzūr nd. Jamal al-Dīn Muhammad b. Mukarram Lisān al-Arab. Beirut: np nd, 1nd edition.

Ibn Qayyim 1981. Shams al-Dīn Abū 'Abdullah Muhammad Ibn Abū Bakr Ibn al-Qayyim al-Jawziyyah. Zad al-Maʿad. Puplished by Shuayb Arnaut, Abd al-Qadir Arnaut, Beirut: Muesset al-Risala 1981 2nd edition IV 6-8.

Kandemir 2005. M. Yasar. Muaz. In Encyclopedia of Islam, Istanbul: TDV Press XXX/338-339.

Muslim 2000. Abū al-Ḥusayn 'Asākir ad-Dīn Muslim ibn al-Ḥajjāj ibn Muslim ibn Ward ibn Kawshādh al-Qushayrī an-Naysābūrī. Ṣaḥīḥ Muslim: al-Musnadu al-Sahihu bi Naklil Adli. Riyadh: Dār al-Salām Press 2000.

Panzac 1997. Daniel. Osmanlı İmparatorluğu'nda Veba. translate Serap Yılmaz, Istanbul: Tarih Vakfı Yurt Press 1997.

QadiʿAbd al-Jabbar 2013. Ibn Ahmad Ibn 'Abd al-Jabbar al-Hamadanī. Mu'tezile'nin Beş İlkesi. translated by İlyas Çelebi, Istanbul: Türkiye Yazma Eserler Kurumu Başkanlığı Press 2013 II/ 286.

Sarıyıldız 2001. Gülderen. "Karantina". In Encyclopedia of Islam, Ankara: TDV Press XXIV/ 463-465.

Sarrāj al-Tusī 1996. Abū Nasr Abdullah b. Ali al-Sarrāj. Kitab al-Luma fi al-Tasawwuf. translated by Hasan Kâmil Yılmaz, İstanbul: Altınoluk Press 1996.

Tomar-Ubūdī 2000. Cengiz-Casim. Ibn al-Hatīb Lisān ad-Dīn. In Encyclopedia of Islam, Istanbul: TDV Press 2000 XXI/74-76.

Unat 1975. Ekrem Kadri. Bulasıcı Hastalıklarla Savas ve İslam Dini. Istanbul: Fatih Press 1975.

Varlık 2011. Nükhet, Tāun. In Encyclopedia of Islam, Istanbul: TDV Press 2011 XL /175-177.

Tuba Erkoç Baydar is Assistant Professor with Ibn Haldun University. She was born in Bitlis, graduated from Uludag University Faculty of Theology with minor in Social Sciences in 2009. She completed her master's degree at the Faculty of Theology at Istanbul University in 2011 with her thesis, "Command and Prohibition in Abû Ishâq Al-Shîrâzî's Legal Thought". In 2011, her doctorate studies started at Marmara University in the field of Islamic Law and she continued to work as research assistant at the same department. In 2017, she gained the title of doctor with the thesis of "Euthanasia and Withholding Treatment: an Islamic Legal Analysis". Tuba Erkoc Baydar was born in a scholarly family and began her studies at an early age under her family. Her madrasah education continued at Bursa and at Istanbul. Meanwhile, she completed ISAM's AYP program. She has been in France, Syria and Jordan for educational purposes and in 2014, she stayed for a year at United States at Georgetown University Kennedy Institute of Ethics for conducting research and participating several courses. Tuba Erkoç Baydar is currently working as an assistant professor at Ibn Haldun University. Her special interests are Shafii law, methodology of Islamic Law, family law, bioethics, medical ethics, euthanasia, withholding and withdrawing of treatment and end of life. Tuba Erkoç Baydar is also the chair of the EDEP foundation. She is married and mother of one child and speaks Arabic, English, Ottoman Turkish, Persian and Kurdish languages.

How Can God Let this Happen?
A Theological Reflection on the Pandemic

Martin Eberle, Wuppertal-Bethel Church University, Germany

abstract
Abstract

The corona pandemic is shattering confidence in the natural environment. If several world religions, and with them about half of the world's population, call this natural environment, God's good creation, how is it possible that there is so much physical evil? Formulated from a religious perspective: How can God allow suffering and catastrophes? What does Judeo-Christian biblical tradition, understood as an important part of the cultural memory of humanity, say about this? Does this tradition make sense in conversation with contemporary scientific and philosophical positions? Can cultural memory also provide insights as to how we can act sensibly and responsibly in the face of the challenges of a pandemic?

Key words

Bible, theology, philosophy, cosmology, creation, God, suffering, theodicy, anthropic principle, Martin Luther, ethics

1. The anthropic principle, or: for whom is the world created?

The modern differentiation of the sciences has gone hand in hand with restricting the object of investigation to comprehensible and repeatable experiments, that are intersubjective. Since God and theology are located outside the field of experimentation, religion has become an historical and sociological field of research. The formerly theistic world view has been replaced by the naturalistic world view. Against this background, religious traditions have become part of the cultural heritage, which is historically interesting, but only serves to a very limited extent, to explain the world.

A few years ago, however, the Berlin philosopher Holm Tetens made an interesting plea for belief in God[1] - and he did so in confrontation with precisely this so-called naturalistic world view, which has either suspended the question of God or excluded it from the horizon of science.

Tetens, as a critically thinking philosopher, approaches the idea of God with the help of logic. He comes to the quite surprising conclusion that theistic arguments for the assumption of the idea of God are far more reasonable than naturalistic assumptions that reject the idea of God.

At this point, we will first discuss a concept that he includes in his argument, that is interesting from a theological point of view.

This is the concept of "the anthropic principle", which has gone from physics into cosmology, becoming an important basic assumption about the world. The anthropic principle describes the astonishing fact that the whole universe in all its parts seems to be in exactly the right condition for a human being to emerge as an intelligent observer, indeed, that the universe seems to be as it is for the sake of the human being. (Tetens 2017:42).

With the anthropic principle, therefore, a thought has now been formulated that builds a bridge between scientific and theological thinking.

From a biblical-theological point of view, the concept of a Creator God, whose will and work, is the source of the world and mankind, can be particularly relevant here. (Tetens

---

[1] Tetens 2017. Tetens, Holm. Gott denken. Ein Versuch über rationale Theologie (Think God. An experiment in rational theology). Stuttgart: Reclam 2017 6th edition.

2017:43)

Biblical texts look at the created world with open wonder. In Psalm 104, the psalmist praises this Creator God with the words

v24: *O Lord, how manifold are your works!*

In wisdom, you have made them all; the earth is full of your creatures. (NRSV)

This does not mean, however, that everything is created only for the disposal of the human being. The psalmist also mentions creatures that do not exist for human's sake, but have their own realms on earth:

You make darkness, and it is night,

when all the animals of the forest come creeping out.

The young lions roar for their prey,

seeking their food from God.

When the sun rises, they withdraw

and lie down in their dens.

People go out to their work

and to their labor until the evening.

...

Yonder is the sea, great and wide,

creeping things innumerable are there,

living things both small and great.

There go the ships,

and Leviathan that you formed to sport in it.

(verses 20-23, 25-26, NRSV)

The mention of the mythical creature called Leviathan could tempt us to regard the biblical tradition as a reminder of past world views that have no relevance today. But the Bible demythologizes and historicizes ancient cosmology.[2] The world is God's well-ordered creation.

It could also be chaotic, disorderly and hostile to life, but the punch line of the Bible is that God has tamed chaos. The world as God's creation is both a living and creative space for humanity, with the challenge to use this creative power in the right way.[3]

In a central text of biblical cosmology and anthropology, the ambivalent characteristic of humanity is exemplarily addressed. The first biblical creation narrative in Genesis 1 states:

Be fruitful and multiply, and fill the earth and subdue it." (v.28 NRSV)

The terms used reflect the reality of human empowerment of the world since the Neolithic era. The self-reflecting human being sits at the head of the creatures. The biblical narrative still passes on the insight that the dominium terrae included dominion but not killing. But, according

---

[2]　Anderson 2011. Bernhard W. Anderson, Interpreter's Dictionary vol 1, 726; quoted after: Plaut, Gunther W. Die Tora in jüdischer Auslegung. Vol. 1: Bereschit/Genesis, Gütersloh: Gütersloher Verlagshaus 2011, 80.

[3]　Marti 2004. Marti, Kurt: The Psalms. Approximations. Stuttgart: Radius-Verlag 317, with reference to Ebach, Jürgen: Creation in the Hebrew Bible. In: Ecological Theology. Perspektiven zur Orientierung, ed. by Günter Altner, Stuttgart 1989.

to the Bible's creation narrative, this did not prevent the emergence of violence.[4] From a biblical perspective, violence is inseparable from the world populated by humans.[5] Humankind, however, has taken this freedom to exercise violence, without God having wanted this. Humankind's mandate to rule is in the context of its being made in God's image. It can therefore only be interpreted as "reign of peace without the 'right over life and death'".[6]

Thus, also the second biblical story of creation assigns to man the role of the gardener:

The Lord God took the man and put him in the Garden of Eden to till it and keep it. (Genesis 2: 15 NRSV)

So the anthropocentric world view does not correspond to the biblical tradition. According to biblical testimony, God created the world to glorify God. However for this, humanity is not absolutely necessary.

Psalm 19 states:

The heavens are telling the glory of God;

and the firmament proclaims his handiwork.

Day to day pours forth speech,

and night to night declares knowledge.

There is no speech, nor are there words;

their voice is not heard;

yet their voice goes out through all the earth,

and their words to the end of the world. (verses 2-4; NRSV)

In the theocentric worldview of the Bible, the human being is thus not master of everything but part of the community of creation, created and called by God to act as God's partner in the world (Moltmann 1993:44f).

2. Theodicy as a way to maintain trust in God

God gave the world autonomy. It includes not only free will, which enables the human being to bring death and destruction upon other people and nature. The own weight that God gives to the world is also shown in the laws of nature. does not abolish the independence of the world. But that would be the case if God were to constantly intervene with miracles in the fate of the world.

Becoming and passing are basic characteristics of the created world. So it is also a basic characteristic of the human being to be limited and finite. Only in this way - as a material being, i.e. in physical existence - can man be a subject and enter into a relationship with others. (Tetens 2017:30ff)

The theologian Wolf Krötke therefore points out that a world without suffering is only

---

[4] Crüsemann 1997. Crüsemann, Frank: Die Tora. Theologie und Sozialgeschichte des alttestamentlichen Gesetzes. [The Torah. Theology and Social History of the Old Testament Law.] Gütersloh, Chr. Kaiser/Gütersloher Verlagshaus 1997, 2nd ed., 339.

[5] Even the violence among animals - to eat and be eaten - is, according to biblical interpretation, a sign of the imperfect world.

[6] Moltmann 1993. Moltmann, Jürgen. God in Creation, Gütersloh: Chr. Kaiser/Gütersloher Verlagshaus 1993, 4th ed., 44th ed.

conceivable by surrendering our independence and is thus tantamount to human self-negation.[7]

However, the physical existence of man inevitably brings with it the experience of suffering and pain. While it can just about be endured when a person dies " in a good old age, an old man and full of years"[8], the suffering of others and one's own illness often leads to the question: Why?

Why me and why now? Why do nurses and doctors fall ill and die from coronavirus while they are helping other people? Why does indescribable suffering always hit "innocent" people, while criminals are spared?

The answer to these questions was discussed in the 18th century under the question of God's justification (theodicy). The German universal scholar Gottfried Wilhelm Leibniz dealt comprehensively with the theodicy question in 1710. In the end he postulates that God did not create a perfect world, but the "best of all possible worlds". But only a few decades later, this argument also proved to be fragile. After an earthquake off Lisbon on November 1, 1755, a tsunami and subsequent fires devastated the city; tens of thousands died. The tragic event soon had a considerable influence on European philosophy and literature.[9]

The COVID 19 pandemic seems to raise the theodicy question again on the microbiological level: how can God allow a deadly virus to infect mankind and kill hundreds of thousands?

The answer to the theodicy question is relatively easy to understand, as long as it refers to moral evils, that is, what is called "an evil deed". Paradigmatically, the Holocaust stands for this. Why does God allow people to do such incredibly horrible things to others? The best known answer to this question is called "free-will-defence". She argues that God has endowed humankind with a free will. In comparison with the alternative - the non-freedom of human beings, that is to say, a puppet existence - this is preferable - despite the possibility that human beings make destructive decisions.[10] That God must therefore allow moral evils does not mean, however, that God wants them. (Tetens 2017:64).

But what about the physical evils?

The theodicy question is based on a theistic image of God, which ascribes to God qualities that are contradicted by experienced suffering. At the same time it testifies to an anthropocentric understanding of man and the world, which judges everything created from a utility point of view. This in turn is undoubtedly due more to wishful thinking than to life experience.

For Tetens, physical evils are a basic condition of being human. They simply follow from the fact that man is a finite being, that is, mortal. "Insofar as dying and death are connected with physical and psychological suffering, physical evils must occur in the empirical world, i.e. evils that are not the responsibility of human beings but that occur naturally according to general natural laws. (Tetens 2017:72) With this, it is first of all stated, that a world without suffering and pain is not conceivable. They are as much a part of life as death. Of course, this does not

---

[7]   Krötke 2019. Krötke, Wolf: Der gute Gott und das Leiden der Geschöpfe. Ist Gott verantwortlich für Leid und Gewalt? [The Good God and the Suffering of Creatures. Is God responsible for suffering and violence?] 8. [URL https://wolf-kroetke.de/news-ansicht-1-
1.html?tx_ttnews%5Btt_news%5D=305&cHash=e013eb478f2669d6422adee496a1c1b6, visited April 2020]. Cf. also Krötke, Wolf: Gottes Klarheiten [God's Clarities]. Tübingen: Mohr Siebeck 2001, 230-245.

[8]   Genesis 25:8 (NRSV) on the death of Moses; cf. Job 42:17.

[9]   This is the case with Johann Wolfgang Goethe, for example, who reports on it in retrospect in his memoirs: Goethe. Dichtung und Wahrheit (Poetry and truth). 1st book. [URL https://www.projekt-gutenberg.org/goethe/dichwah1/dichwah1.html, visited April 2020]

[10]   Polkinghorne 2011. Polkinghorne, John: Science and Religion in Quest of Truth, London: SPCK 2011, 81.

explain the suffering that goes beyond what is bearable. One might think of infirmity, as well as of extraordinary events that we experience as catastrophes.

The physicist and theologian John Polkinghorne goes a step further here. He also sees - analogous to the "free-will-defence" - the possibility of a "free-process-defence". Natural processes are interwoven processes in which it is simply impossible to separate the good from the bad. "At the heart of the free process defence lies the conviction that the desease and disaster present in nature is not gratitious, something that a creator who was a bit more competent or a bit less callous could easily have remedied, but it is the inescapable consequence of the nature of a freely fertile world. (Polkinghorne 2011:82.) As an example he also refers to tsunamis - they are the result of earthquakes that are possible due to tectonic plate shifting. If God had provided the earth with a solid crust, how would minerals from the earth's interior come to the surface to renew its fertility?

Creation is thus interpreted as God's self-limitation. At the same time, evolution is understood as God's mode of action.

Nevertheless, Tetens finds consolation in the possibility that man, despite all this, trusts in God and acts accordingly: in practising charity or "radical solidarity" as a reaction to the physical and moral evils in the world. Following the concepts of Alfred North Whitehead's philosophy of process, he formulates: "God waits for the participation of man in the success of creation and answers it with radically emergent innovations with which he 'can and will still let good things arise from the most evil'" (Tetens 2017:77 - in inclusion of a quotation from Dietrich Bonhoeffer)

In this way the reflection of theodicy becomes almost the possibility to maintain trust in God. Anthropocentrism is overcome in favour of a humble attitude, which nevertheless does not lapse into resignation. It goes hand in hand with the distancing from the human tendency to self-deification, which often manifests itself in the "illusory belief in human self-redemption" (Tetens 2017:76). Even an optimism of progress that overestimates human possibilities does not do justice to the reality of the extent of the world's suffering. (Tetens 2017:79)

3. God as the addressee of the cry for help and salvation

Unfortunately, our physical existence does not only allow us sensual pleasure and the experience of joy and happiness. It is also accompanied by illness and pain. Natural processes beyond human control are suffered and sometimes catastrophically experienced. In such moments, prayer is the way to express the unbearable, the terrible, and at the same time the hope of staying alive, nourished by the hope that the horror will end. The Bible gives many examples of how to put into words the struggle with suffering. One of them is mentioned here as an example:

They are verses from the Temple Consecration Prayer of King Solomon. According to the Biblical tradition, this was spoken at the consecration of the first temple of the people of Israel for the biblical God:

37 "If there is famine in the land, if there is plague, blight, mildew, locust, or caterpillar; if their enemy besieges them in any of their cities; whatever plague, whatever sickness there is; 38 whatever prayer, whatever plea there is from any individual or from all your people Israel, ... 39 then hear in heaven your dwelling place, forgive, act ...

41 "Likewise when a foreigner, who is not of your people Israel, comes from a distant land because of your name 42—for they shall hear of your great name, your mighty hand, and your outstretched arm—when a foreigner comes and prays toward this house, 43then hear in heaven your dwelling place, and do according to all that the foreigner calls to you ... (Verses 37-39.41-43; NRSV)

The prayer cited here as an example shows the view - quite fundamental for the Bible - that God is approachable and that it can be expected that he will listen to the requests of people - not just the requests of his people Israel, but of all people who turn to him. His power is so great that nothing can resist him.

By turning to God, God is present in the life of man: as an addressee of lamentation and petition and as a reason for hope.

But this is only one side. The Bible does not only report God's presence as humanity's hope. It also shows enough examples where prayers remain unheard.

The Old Testament book of Job, for example, tells of inexplicable suffering that befalls a good person. When Job loses his possessions, he says: *"the Lord gave, and the Lord has taken away; blessed be the name of the Lord"* (Job 1:21; NRSV). When he himself becomes terminally ill, he finally accuses God - without first receiving an answer.

The Gospels, in turn, tell of Jesus, the Son of God, praying to God in the Garden of Gethsemane: *"My Father, if it is possible, let this cup pass from me; yet not what I want but what you want."* (Matthew 26:39; NRSV) Jesus' way finally leads to the cross, where he says words from Psalm 22: *"My God, my God, why have you forsaken me?"* (Matthew 27:46) God's own Son, says the New Testament, suffered pain and died a death by torture.

Finally, at the heart of the Christian faith is not the message that God answers all prayers, not even in the face of blatant injustice and senseless suffering. Thus the New Testament does not see God's assistance and his redemptive action happening precisely in passing by suffering, but in suffering and through suffering. With it the specific perspective of the Christian tradition comes into view. Where the suffering of God in Jesus Christ is taken as the starting point, the question changes fundamentally.

4. The basic existential situation of man and God's presence in suffering

Finiteness is a basic condition of human life. Suffering and death are inevitable. God expects man to exist independently, to make his own decisions - but also to lead a finite life connected with suffering and death. The decisive question is now: how can we bear this imposition?

Christian theology emphasizes that God has revealed himself in Jesus Christ. Thus the life and suffering of Jesus becomes at the same time a statement about God, who does not remain in the position of the spectator, but takes part in the suffering of the world and its creatures. God affirms the existential situation of man, which could only be made free of suffering by surrendering creaturely existence. But God expresses solidarity with man in his physical existence. The cross as the place of Jesus' execution becomes the symbol of the compassionate God.

Suffering is thereby neither condoned nor belittled. It appears as a component of the human condition, which in some respects is to be simply accepted.

But in enduring suffering man does not have to feel abandoned by God. The apostle Paul, for example, sees the whole natural creation and man as a community of suffering that longs for redemption - united by God's Spirit.

19 For the creation waits with eager longing for the revealing of the children of God; 20 for the creation was subjected to futility, not of its own will but by the will of the one who subjected it, in hope 21 that the creation itself will be set free from its bondage to decay and will obtain the freedom of the glory of the children of God. 22 We know that the whole creation has been groaning in labor pains until now; 23 and not only the creation, but we ourselves, who have the first fruits of the Spirit, groan inwardly while we wait for adoption, the redemption of our bodies. 24 For in hope we were saved. Now hope that is seen is not hope. For who hopes for what is seen? 25 But if we hope for what we do not see, we wait for it with patience.

26 Likewise the Spirit helps us in our weakness; for we do not know how to pray as we ought, but that very Spirit intercedes with sighs too deep for words. (Romans Ch. 8, verses 19-26; NRSV)

Here we can see that the Bible recognizes transitoriness as an existential fact. As a cause and expression of suffering it is a torment and cause for complaint. But God does not leave man alone in it. By the power of his Spirit, God participates in the groaning of creatures about the suffering sides of creaturehood. In his Spirit God is present in the world and works in it. The help he gives is essentially the power of hope. It creates patience and helps to bear suffering. When Paul writes: the Spirit himself intercedes for us with inexpressible groaning, he is expressing that God shares suffering in solidarity with humanity and aims to overcome it.

Paul can speak from his own experience, for he was plagued by a persistent suffering. He repeatedly asked God to free him from his disease. But God's answer Paul found is

"My grace is sufficient for you, for my power is made perfect in weakness." (2 Corinthians 12:9; NRSV)

5. Suffering should not only be endured, it should be reduced and overcome

The biblical tradition, however, is not limited to stating suffering and discussing ways in which life is possible despite all this. Nor does it hope only for an otherworldly overcoming of suffering. Its goal is the reduction of suffering and its overcoming in this world. To this end, it changes the perspective from passive suffering to the possibilities of man to actively deal with the evil he has experienced. If God shows solidarity with the suffering people, then people should do the same. Within the Christian tradition this is succinctly demonstrated in Jesus' so-called speech of the Last Judgment in the Gospel of Matthew. Jesus calls for merciful and solidary action wherever we encounter a person in physical distress. At the end Jesus says the famous sentence: *"Whatever you did for one of the least of these brothers and sisters of mine, you did for me."* (Matthew 25:40; NIV)

That the demanded solidarity cannot be limited to members of one's own group, but includes all people, is again clearly expressed in Jesus' parable of the Good Samaritan (Luke 10:25-37): the mercy demanded by God is universal. Every person is "neighbour".

The transgression of the group ethos common to Judeo-Christian thinking is not the decisive point here, but rather the view that human beings are challenged and able to reduce suffering. As God's partner, they are enabled and challenged to stand by their fellow human beings: in jointly bearing what cannot be changed, and in striving to reduce and prevent suffering as much as possible. The well-being of the fellow human being thus becomes the point of reference for action.

From a theological point of view, knowledge of the natural and social sciences is an important prerequisite for being able to practice this solidarity especially where there are more complex contexts involved or realities that are not intuitively accessible to us. In the horizon of biblical theology, the further development of the possibility of opening up the world through the sciences is part of the human being's ability to act as God's partner in the world.

6. Martin Luther's advice on how to behave in an epidemic

A historical example from Germany shows how this can be achieved in concrete terms. When the plague raged in 1527, the Wittenberg reformer Martin Luther discussed the question of how a Christian should act in such a situation. In a letter to a pastor in Breslau he writes:[11] *"Therefore I shall ask God mercifully to protect us. Then I shall fumigate, help purify the air, administer medicine, and take it. I shall avoid places and persons where my presence is not needed in order not to become contaminated and thus perchance infect and pollute others, and so cause their death as a result of my negligence."* (Luther 1527) With this he pleads for social distancing.

With regard to medical questions, he relies on experts instead of his own wishes and convictions. Taking the question of how plague victims are to be buried as an example, he says: *"I leave it to the doctors of medicine and others with greater experience than mine in such matters to decide whether it is dangerous to maintain cemeteries within the city limits. I do not know and do not claim to understand whether vapors and mists arise out of graves to pollute the air. If this were so my previously stated warnings constitute ample reason to locate cemeteries outside the city. As we have learned, all of us have the responsibility of warding off this poison to the best of our ability."* (Luther 1527)

Overall, Luther's attitude is oriented towards the welfare of his fellows. Emergency aid for the sick and poor is also required during the epidemic. *"If my neighbor needs me, however, I shall not avoid place or person but will go freely, as stated above. See, this is such a God-fearing faith because it is neither brash nor foolhardy and does not tempt God."* (Luther 1527)

Here it is good to see how the possibility of opening up the world with reason and reducing suffering in it develops into a moral imperative. For the one who earnestly hopes and asks for the overcoming of suffering, but does not himself contribute to it, deceives himself, his fellow human beings and God.

Far too often God is accused of the physical and moral evils in the world, instead of asking about one's own responsibility. The Bible calls this attitude "sin".[12]

Instead, man is called upon to become aware of his responsibility for the world.

7. Ethical conclusions

a. Recognizing creaturely boundaries

From an ethical point of view, the first question to be asked is the responsibility of the human being. What can be expected of him?

The answer will initially be: the human being is capable of radical solidarity (charity). In view of the suffering and the striving to overcome it, precisely this solidarity is demanded of humans. At the same time, the limits of human action must be recognized. It consists first of all in the fact that we will never be able to put an end to suffering. Neither physical nor moral evil can be banished from this world for good. We must therefore warn against not only moral but

---

[11] Whether One May Flee From A Deadly Plague. Martin Luther, Luther's Works, Vol. 43: Devotional Writings II, ed. Jaroslav Jan Pelikan, Hilton C. Oswald, and Helmut T. Lehmann, vol. 43 (Philadelphia: Fortress Press, 1999), 119–38.

[12] "An appeal to God's power ... which veils human guilt, only becomes more and more entangled in it, and is just such an expression of the refusal of a humane behaviour." [Translation: ME] - Krötke 2019:10.

also technical-civilisational immoderation and hubris. There is no self-redemption, no end to suffering in the world attainable.

The recognition of human limits also includes the insight into the entanglement of man in culpable contexts. Christianity would define this as being in sin. As finite human beings, we are sometimes involved in the world's evil and suffering as perpetrators, sometimes as victims. This also means that we ourselves are confronted with our own guilt and failure to the best of our knowledge and belief. This becomes most obvious in TRIAGE and other dilemma situations. Here we as human beings are dependent on comfort and forgiveness. (Tetens 2017:74f; Krötke 2019:10f)

b. Responsibility for consequences

Conversely, it can be observed how man steals from the responsibility for the consequences of his actions. This is often justified by ambiguous research results or complex contexts. Take the corona pandemic as an example: The SARS-CoV 2 virus is probably a zoonosis - an infection that spreads from animals to humans. A possible reason for the increasing number of zoonoses in recent decades is the reduction in biodiversity due to human intervention in existing ecosystems. Regardless of unhygienic slaughter and market conditions that played a role in the spread of the virus, it appears to be a physical evil for which humans themselves are partly responsible. In view of the corona crisis and the large number of serious and fatal cases of disease, to ask why God allows this to happen would be tantamount, in this sense, to man's self-disempowerment and flight from responsibility.

Nevertheless, impact assessment is always limited by our limited knowledge. And, of course, many different interests flow into decisions on action - even when power imbalances are excluded, conflicts of interest thus exist, leading to decisions that are sometimes risky. However, complexities and contingencies are no licence for indifference towards possible consequences of action. From an ethical perspective "caution" then becomes a guiding principle that can also be qualified from a theological point of view as the equivalent of God's action on man.[13]

c. Freedom and self-restraint

Even if the actions of finite man cannot be anything other than fallible, the question must be asked how freedom can be lived responsibly. With the so-called Golden Rule and the commandment to love one's neighbour the biblical tradition passes on the guiding idea of an ethics of reciprocity. It is also found in many other religious traditions and can rightly be considered part of the cultural memory of humanity.

Golden Rule (Matthew 7:12; NRSV):

"In everything do to others as you would have them do to you; for this is the law and the prophets.

Charity commandment (Matthew 22:39; NRSV):

"You shall love your neighbor as yourself."

Both sentences go beyond strategic reciprocity. They aim at mutual consideration and the

---

[13] "By forgetting that suffering is also part of humanity, people owe each other the prudence that corresponds to the prudence with which God acts on us". [Translation: ME] Krötke 2001:241.

priority of the other person's well-being, independent of selfish calculations of benefit.[14]

The connection between freedom and self-restraint in Martin Luther's work also follows this line.[15] The possibility of reducing suffering through restrictions on freedom then appears to be preferable to the freedom to be allowed to expose oneself to the risk of infection.

d. Ethos Formation

It is of course debatable to what extent the restriction is to be imposed from outside, i.e. freedom is to be restricted by the state. At this point, we should consider in more detail the legitimacy of the state's exercise of power, its responsibility and its limits, especially under the condition of a democratically ordered delegation of power. It is however plausible that voluntary self-restriction is desirable, since it can serve the fellow human being independently of state-ordered measures. So how can it be possible for people in crisis situations to voluntarily find a way to act calmly, considerately and in solidarity?

The formation of an appropriate ethos plays an important role here. It can be understood as practice in behaviour patterns that happen intuitively and not only as a result of critical reflection. From the perspective of Christian ethics, it is a matter of practising an ethos of charity that has strong situational features, but is also oriented towards norms and rules.[16] The formation of such an ethos can be understood to be the starting point of a task to make well-founded and humane decisions in crises - even when guilt and failure cannot be avoided.

e. Prevent suffering, reduce suffering

In view of the hundreds of thousands of cases of suffering as exemplified by a pandemic, we must take care of one another - not only to assess the risks for ourselves, but also for others, globally speaking: for the totality of human beings, as far as that is possible. Using the example of wearing face masks and social distancing: all this is not only about self-protection, but also about the protection of others.

In the face of suffering from suffering - keyword theodicy - precaution comes to the fore as a task. Just as it is simply dishonest to reproach God when a house built in a flood zone is flooded, so it is necessary to take precautionary measures, for example by expanding medical capacities.

When humanity as a whole is faced with a humanitarian challenge - which, from the point of view of charity, is the case even in a regional crisis - worldwide cooperation in the development, production and distribution of vaccines and medicines will be advisable.

The goal of all efforts must be to prevent suffering and reduce suffering. Where this succeeds - and it can only succeed to a limited extent - we humans live according to the possibilities that are intrinsically given to us. However, this also includes taking into account the fundamental nature of human existence - relationship. In a pandemic, this is pushed into the background when social distancing leads to old and sick people being kept from social contacts and,

---

[14] Cf. the discussion in Ulrich 1998: 59-62. Ulrich, Peter: Integrative Wirtschaftsethik [Integrative Economic Ethics]. Bern. Stuttgart. Vienna: Haupt 1998, 2nd ed.

[15] Luther, Martin: Von der Freiheit eines Christenmenschen [On the freedom of a Christian]. Gütersloh: Chr. Kaiser/Gütersloher Verlagshaus 1995.

[16] Fischer 2002. Fischer, Johannes: Theologische Ethik. Grundwissen und Orientierung. Stuttgart. Berlin. Köln: Kohlhammer 2002, 160ff.

in extreme cases, to lonely suffering or dying. On the other hand, in recognition of the creative limits of the human being, the challenge of accepting death as part of life and accompanying people in it becomes apparent. In the Christian perspective, precisely this is a "relative testimony of [God's] power that cannot be limited by death". (Krötke 2001:245)

References

Anderson 2011. Bernhard W. Anderson, Interpreter's Dictionary vol 1, 726

Crüsemann 1997. Crüsemann, Frank: Die Tora. Theologie und Sozialgeschichte des alttestamentlichen Gesetzes. [The Torah. Theology and Social History of the Old Testament Law.] Gütersloh, Chr. Kaiser/Gütersloher Verlagshaus 1997, 2nd ed.

Ebach 1989. Ebach, Jürgen: Creation in the Hebrew Bible. In: Ecological Theology. Perspektiven zur Orientierung, ed. by Günter Altner, Stuttgart 1989.

Fischer 2002. Fischer, Johannes: Theologische Ethik. Grundwissen und Orientierung. Stuttgart. Berlin. Köln: Kohlhammer 2002, 160ff.

Genesis 25:8 (NRSV)

Goethe. Dichtung und Wahrheit (Poetry and truth). 1st book. [URL https://www.projekt-gutenberg.org/goethe/dichwah1/dichwah1.html, visited April 2020]

Job 42:17.

Krötke 2001. Krötke, Wolf: Gottes Klarheiten [God's Clarities]. Tübingen: Mohr Siebeck 2001, 230-245.

Krötke 2019. Krötke, Wolf: Der gute Gott und das Leiden der Geschöpfe. Ist Gott verantwortlich für Leid und Gewalt? [The Good God and the Suffering of Creatures. Is God responsible for suffering and violence?] 8. [URL https://wolf-kroetke.de/news-ansicht-1-1.html?tx_ttnews%5Btt_news%5D=305&cHash=e013eb478f2669d6422adee496a1c1b6, visited April 2020]

Luther 1999. Martin Luther, Whether One May Flee From A Deadly Plague. *Luther's Works*, Vol. 43: Devotional Writings II, ed. Jaroslav Jan Pelikan, Hilton C. Oswald, and Helmut T. Lehmann, vol. 43 (Philadelphia: Fortress Press, 1999)

Luther, Martin: Von der Freiheit eines Christenmenschen [On the freedom of a Christian]. Gütersloh: Chr. Kaiser/Gütersloher Verlagshaus 1995.

Marti 2004. Marti, Kurt: The Psalms. Approximations. Stuttgart: Radius-Verlag

Moltmann 1993. Moltmann, Jürgen. God in Creation, Gütersloh: Chr. Kaiser/Gütersloher Verlagshaus 1993, 4th ed., 44th ed.

Plaut 2011. Plaut, Gunther W. Die Tora in jüdischer Auslegung. Vol. 1: Bereschit/Genesis, Gütersloh: Gütersloher Verlagshaus 2011

Polkinghorne 2011. Polkinghorne, John: Science and Religion in Quest of Truth, London: SPCK 2011

Tetens 2017. Tetens, Holm. Gott denken. Ein Versuch über rationale Theologie (Think God. An experiment in rational theology). Stuttgart: Reclam 2017 6th edition.

Ulrich 1998. Ulrich, Peter: Integrative Wirtschaftsethik [Integrative Economic Ethics]. Bern. Stuttgart. Vienna: Haupt 1998, 2nd ed.

Dr. theol. **Martin Eberle** studied Protestant Theology in Heidelberg, Leipzig, Berlin, Bielefeld and Madurai (India). With an interdisciplinary work on the topic "Understanding Economic Ethics. Max Weber's Studies on Ancient Judaism from a theological-ethical perspective" he received his doctorate from the Kirchliche Hochschule Wuppertal/Bethel (Germany). He is the pastor of the German Lutheran Church Washington, D.C.

Beyond Pandemics: the Reorganization of Powers and the New Face of Society

Christian Byk, Court of Appeals, France

Abstract

Epidemics have often been a means for states to assert their power, while the globalization of trade and colonial expansion have made international cooperation necessary. With the emergence of new globalized actors (GAFAM), not only are pandemics at stake in a redistribution of power but they are also marked by the integration of emergency policies into the policy of social control.

Keywords

pandemics, states, power, society, freedom

Epidemics have long been an opportunity for states to assert their power because quarantine, to be effective, requires strong power. Health policy during an epidemic still remains largely dependent on the action of States, which have an extensive administrative and health system. The role played by organizations such as the World Health Organization (WHO) is now added to the action of States (I).

However, these two dimensions are insufficient today in a "globalized" world if one does not take into account the other powers, which exist at this level. And, faced with the pandemic, each power is in search of the assertion of its sovereignty, either in the field which is strictly its own (this is the example of trade law and the measures adopted to fight against pandemics in international trade), or to conquer new areas as do the GAFAM (II).

I The decline of national sovereignty and distrust of international organizations

A States on the front line: a jump before the decline?

Epidemics can be an opportunity for a state to consolidate its power - such as Italy and the COVID-19 pandemic[1] - but they can also endanger its economy and its power. The United States and China may well find themselves in this situation because the former struggles to maintain its "leadership" when the latter does everything to snatch it away[2].

1) A start based on a policy rejecting the traditional logic of epidemic management

The epidemic being the abnormal propagation of a natural disease, and not a divine punishment, "the management of care and medicines is a challenge for sovereignty: it is necessary both to respond urgently by the distribution of adapted products and anticipate by building up

---

[1] Jean-Pierre Darnis, La crise du COVID-19, les leçons du cas italien. Note de la FRS n°07/2020, 23 mars 2020, https://www.frstrategie.org/publications/notes/crise-covid-19-lecons-cas-italien-2020.

[2] Institut Montaigne, François Godement, La guerre commerciale Chine – Etats-Unis : quelles conséquences ? https://www.institutmontaigne.org/blog/la-guerre-commerciale-chine-etats-unis-quelles-consequences; Jean Dominique Seval, La Chine pourrait s'imposer comme la première puissance mondiale dès la fin de l'épidémie, Le Monde, 11 avril 2020, https://www.lemonde.fr/idees/article/2020/04/11/la-chine-pourrait-s-imposer-comme-la-premiere-puissance-mondiale-des-la-fin-de-l-epidemie_6036349_3232.html. Laurence Nardon, COVID-19 : la fin du leadership américain ? Chroniques américaines, Institut français des relations internationales, 14avril 2020, https://www.ifri.org/sites/default/files/atoms/files/nardon_leadership_covid_2020-2.pdf.

stocks "[3].

But, when the State fails in this anticipation, what can it do?

In this regard, Italy's situation with the COVID-19 pandemic, which affected it from the first quarter of 2020, is a good example.

The idea of fostering the development of collective immunity and allowing economic activity to continue was rejected, unlike the United Kingdom, inspired by a liberal tradition. On the contrary, it is the will to protect the population as much as possible which has been affirmed, even if that means restricting public freedoms.

Thus, "... by establishing general containment and by choosing to suspend all non-essential activities ..., Italy has demonstrated the capacity of a democratic state to take radical measures to combat the epidemic"[4]. It has in fact served as a model for other European countries[5].

The Italian ethical choice, which one can think that it also integrates the place that Catholicism preserves in the country, did not stop the epidemic but, will have, at least, avoid (narrowly) to endanger the system health and the lives of many people.

By comparison, the situation in other countries appears more chaotic.

2) Situations of chaos, both ideological and organizational

a) The two chaos: USA, Brazil

➤ United States

In the United States, chaos is primarily ideological in nature and affects both the federal government and its relationship with the States. At the federal level, the chaos resides in the presidential objective which is, in the logic of the slogan "Make America great again", to safeguard the economic power of the country. If the plan (April 16, 2020) to restart the United States[6] is apparently cautious, the president has nevertheless expressed his wish that the "healthy" states restart before May 1st.

This attitude does not facilitate relations with States, whose governors are responsible for lifting or not the containment. Indeed, the president openly supported those who denounced the

---

[3] Florence Bretelle-Establet et Frédéric Keck, Les épidémies entre « Occident » et « Orient », *Extrême-Orient Extrême-Occident* [En ligne], 37 | 2014, para.27, http://journals.openedition.org/extremeorient/327.

[4] Institut Montaigne, Les Etats face au coronavirus : l'archétype italien, 20 avril 2020, https://www.institutmontaigne.org/blog/les-etats-face-au-coronavirus-larchetype-italien.

[5] Gary P. Pisano, Raffaella Sadun, Michele Zanini, Lessons from Italy's Response to Coronavirus, Harvard Business Review, https://hbr.org/2020/03/lessons-from-italys-response-to-coronavirus.

[6] Huffington Post, Le plan de Trump face au coronavirus pour rouvrir les États-Unis, 17 avril 2020, https://www.huffingtonpost.fr/entry/le-plan-de-trump-face-au-coronavirus-pour-rouvrir-les-etats-unis_fr_5e98da5cc5b6ead1400a1b32. Département d'État des États-Unis, Bureau de la porte-parole, Publication du plan d'action du gouvernement des États-Unis pour soutenir la réponse internationale face au COVID-19 , fiche d'information, 16 avril 2020, https://fr.usembassy.gov/fr/publication-du-plan-daction-du-gouvernement-des-etats-unis-pour-soutenir-la-reponse-internationale-face-au-covid-19/.

containment measures as an attack on American freedom and democracy[7].

> ➤ This context is also that of Brazil[8].

In both countries, the gravity of the situation is also linked to deficiencies in the health system, which leaves many people on the path, due to lack of resources.

b) China and the hidden chaos of the effects of the pandemic

If China has succeeded in demonstrating its organizational capacities in the face of an initial health "chaos", it is only thanks to its ideological rigidity and the lack of transparency as to the origin and the real effects of the pandemic and as regards the number of sick people and deaths[9].

B Emergence and role of international organizations

The transport revolution, industrialization and the development of free trade increased in the 19th century the speed of proliferation of epidemics and led to the establishment of health cooperation between States in the form of international conferences[10]. Experts develop standards there, which are based on three essential ideas: the protection of European powers against epidemics, the preservation of trade and that of colonization [11].

1) International organizations

a) From the International Office of Public Hygiene to the World Health Organization

-It was not until **the beginning of the 20th century**[12] that a first organization appeared, the International Office of Public Hygiene[13]. At the end of the First World War, during which several important epidemics (Spanish flu, typhus…) raged, was created in 1923, the Office of Hygiene

---

[7] AFP, Encouragées par Donald Trump, les manifestations anti-confinement se multiplient aux Etats-Unis, Le Monde, 19 avril 2020, https://www.lemonde.fr/international/article/2020/04/19/etats-unis-encouragees-par-trump-les-manifestations-anti-confinement-se-multiplient_6037052_3210.html.

[8] Achim Lipold, Le Brésil face au coronavirus: autoritarisme et politique de déni, RFI, 11 mai 2020, http://www.rfi.fr/fr/am%C3%A9riques/20200511-le-br%C3%A9sil-face-coronavirus-autoritarisme-et-politique-d%C3%A9.

[9] Olivier Meuwly, Le Coronavirus et la Chine. Le révélateur d'un système, Le Temps, 9 avril 2020, https://blogs.letemps.ch/olivier-meuwly/2020/04/09/le-coronavirus-et-la-chine-le-revelateur-dun-systeme/
Simone Pieranni, Le Coronavirus change tout : préparez-vous à la nouvelle hégémonie chinoise, Le Grand Continent, Cartographier le coronavirus, L'Observatoire géo-politique du COVID-19, https://legrandcontinent.eu/fr/2020/03/12/coronavirus-chine-surveillance/.

[10] Neville Mariott Goodman, International Health Organizations and their Work, Editions J. and A. Churchill, 1952, Londres, p. 77.

[11] Mark Harrison, Disease, Diplomacy and International Commerce: the Origins of International Sanitary Regulation in the Nineteenth Century, Journal of Global History, 2006-1, p. 197-217.

[12] Anne Rasmussen, Tournant, inflexions, ruptures : le moment internationaliste , Mil neuf cent. Revue d'histoire intellectuelle, n° 19, 2001, p. 30 ; Sylvia Chiffoleau, Genèse de la santé publique internationale. De la peste d'Orient à l'OMS, Presses universitaires de Rennes, Rennes, 2012.

[13] Créé en 1907, la mission de l'OIHP est principalement le suivi des règles de quarantaine dans les ports ; il sera intégré à l'OMS en 1947 : OIHP, Vingt-cinq ans d'activité de l'Office international d'hygiène publique, Paris, 1933.

of the League of Nations[14], to which succeeded in 1947 the World Health Organization.

Benefiting from a competence extended to all questions relating to health, the WHO had to face, from the end of the 1980s, a management crisis, which seriously affected its image and its credibility[15]. The rise of new epidemics was a good indicator of this situation. Indeed, the "governance" reforms undertaken from the end of the 1990s destabilized the Organization[16] while making it more dependent vis-à-vis certain states (the United States, China) and private interests (foundations, pharmaceutical industry)[17].

-**Under such influences, its action has been reoriented** towards the short term and emergency situations arising from the emergence of new pandemics, neglecting recurrent pandemics so that this reorientation seems to have benefited certain pharmaceutical companies[18]. To this observation is added the manifestation of the economic and political interests of certain States, major contributors to the budget. Is it the risk of criticism of this dependence, or the fact of not wanting to create panic, that led the WHO to wait until March 11, 2020 to declare the pandemic alert concerning COVID-19? Unless the State, from whose territory the virus came out to spread around the world, put pressure on?[19]

b) The European Union: a "supporting competence"

➤ Remember that **the EU can only intervene in the health field on the basis of subsidiarity and solidarity**[20]. Indeed, if Article 168 of the Treaty on the Functioning of the EU recognizes the legitimacy of the Union to fight against the great scourges as well as the surveillance of serious cross-border threats to health[21], the text specifies that it is about fostering cooperation and coordination while respecting the responsibility of States [22]. It is in this context that in 2016 the Commission presented a strategic plan targeting epidemics

---

[14] Céline Paillette, De l'Organisation d'hygiène de la SDN à l'OMS. Mondialisation et régionalisme européen dans le domaine de la santé, 1919-1954, *Bulletin de l'Institut Pierre Renouvin*, 2010/2, n° 32, pp. 193-198, https://www.cairn.info/revue-bulletin-de-l-institut-pierre-renouvin1-2010-2-page-193.htm.

[15] Chloé Maurel, L'OMS et la gestion des crises et catastrophes sanitaires mondiales : perspectives pour une réforme, Chantiers politiques, 5 mars 2011, https://www.nonfiction.fr/article-4323-loms-et-la-gestion-des-crises-et-catastrophes-sanitaires-mondiales-perspectives-pour-une-reforme.htm. L'OMS, une histoire entre combat contre les maladies et luttes d'influence, The Conversation, 30 mars 2020, https://theconversation.com/loms-une-histoire-entre-combat-contre-les-maladies-et-luttes-dinfluence-134597.

[16] Nicole Scholz, L'Organisation mondiale de la santé au cœur de sa réforme, Service de recherche du Parlement européen, oct. 2015, https://www.europarl.europa.eu/RegData/etudes/BRIE/2015/571307/EPRS_BRI%282015%29571307_FR.pdf.

[17] Christophe de Brouwer, L'OMS: organisme scientifique ou bureaucratie politique comme les autres? Contrepoints, 10 avril 2020, https://www.contrepoints.org/2020/04/10/368721-loms-organisme-scientifique-ou-bureaucratie-politique-comme-les-autres; Jean-Loup Motchane, Quand l'OMS épouse la cause des firmes pharmaceutiques, Le Monde diplomatique, juillet 2002, https://www.monde-diplomatique.fr/2002/07/MOTCHANE/9250.

[18] Chloé Maurel, Ce que les crises épidémiques révèlent des dérives de l'OMS, The Conversation, 20 mars 2020, https://theconversation.com/ce-que-les-crises-epidemiques-revelent-des-derives-de-loms-133639.

[19] Marieke Louis, L'OMS dans le maelstrom du covid-19, entretien avec Auriane Guilbaud, Collège de France, la vie des idées, 1 avril 2020, https://laviedesidees.fr/L-OMS-dans-le-maelstrom-du-covid-19.html.

[20] Marco Inglese, L'Union Européenne et la santé, thèse, Universités de Strasbourg et de Bologne, 2014, https://tel.archives-ouvertes.fr/tel-01148538/document.

[21] Art.168 1 alinéa 2 TFUE, consolidated edition, 9 mai 2008, JOUE, C115/47, https://eur-lex.europa.eu/resource.html?uri=cellar:88f94461-564b-4b75-aef7-c957de8e339d.0010.01/DOC_3&format=PDF.

[22] CourtJEU, Royaume-Uni c. Commission, C-180/96, Rec. 1998 p. I-02265.

and took, at the end of January 2020, with regard to Covid -19, several initiatives, notably support for research and support for State savings. However, the limited nature of the latter once again caused public disappointment.

Indeed, the Union's credibility can only suffer from the lack of concretization of the essential principle which gives meaning to the Union, solidarity and, as pointed out by J. Delors, there is a risk that "the lack of solidarity puts Europe in mortal danger". This is why, once the pandemic has been brought under control, the essential question will have to be asked: "Can the European Union and the member States come together to build health sovereignty together?"[23].

➢ Thus, the arrival of "new epidemics" (AIDS, H5N1, SARS, Ebola, COVID-19), has put the responsiveness of international organizations to the test due to the difficulties in assessing the effects of these viruses and the importance political issues. Bringing the member states together in an organization of a specific legal nature, community and union, the European Union has not, it seems, been more successful in this direction.

Is then the emergence of new sovereignties in the health field only the result of this feverishness of international organizations or is it the sign that the actors of these new sovereignties are becoming the real holders of legitimacy and power to act in this area?

2) The emergence new sovereignties

a) Awakening of nationalisms, attempt to reconstitute the Empires (China, Russia, Turkey…), disappointment vis-à-vis Europe, all these elements combine to announce **that the 21st century is the century of return to the idea of sovereignty** (Thierry Charles, The new perspectives of sovereignty, L'Harmattan, Paris, 2015). But, beyond the maintenance of the old forms of sovereignty, it is new sovereignties which appear and which invest in the field of health   technosciences.
But what do we mean when we speak of new sovereignties? In fact, it is a question of realizing that actors other than States and infra or supra-state entities, assume a power of full authority in certain fields, which thus constitute cross-border areas governed by common rules, at least in part, independent of the States.

b) From "lex mercatoria" to "lex numerica"

For centuries, international trade law has been an example of an autonomous space, which establishes and controls rules and customs without the need for State power to guarantee control and sanction.[24]

---

[23] Paul Hudson, directeur général de Sanofi, L'Europe doit construire sa souveraineté sanitaire Les Echos, 28 mars 2020,   https://www.lesechos.fr/idees-debats/cercle/opinion-leurope-doit-construire-sa-souverainete-sanitaire-1189846.

[24] Berthold Goldman, Frontières du droit et « lex mercatoria », Archives de philosophie du droit, 1964, pp. 177-192 ; Alain Pellet, La *lex mercatoria*, »tiers ordre juridique ? Remarques ingénues d'un internationaliste de droit public *in* Mélanges en l'honneur de Philipe Kahn, Souveraineté étatique et marchés internationaux à la fin du XXème siècle, Litec, Paris, 2000, pp.53-74, http://pellet.actu.com/wp-content/uploads/2016/02/PELLET-2000-Lex-mercatoria-tiers-ordre-juridique.pdf; Agnès Lejbowicz, III. La « lex mercatoria », dans Philosophie du droit international. L'impossible capture de l'humanité, sous la direction de Agnès Leibowitz, Presses Universitaires de France, « Fondements de la politique », Paris, 1999, pp. 77-129, https://www.cairn.info/philosophie-du-droit-international--9782130497219-page-77.htm.

More recently, it has been joined by science and technology[25], such as digital technology, the uses of which are difficult to control in a limited geographical area[26]. But, there is something new in this independence of the normative system. The "old model of sovereignty" of merchants was limited to the framework of their international trade and, even more, to a targeted activity (maritime transport of goods, for example) or a specific product (cotton, wheat, precious metals ...). However, today, there is a will and capacity, financial and technological, of the big digital companies (those that we call the GAFAM) to project beyond their "core business" and economic power[27]. Motivated by an objective of human enhancement, both ideological, technological and consumerist, they get ready to invest in areas of activity likely to give them a power of control over all that is still within the jurisdiction of States (health, scientific research, education, the military, exploration of space, humanitarian action, dispute resolution, etc.) but also what is intended to stay outside (information, privacy, art and culture...). From enhanced humanity to the digital administration of the World, would the path be open to the irresistible "siliconization"[28] of the World?[29]

Certainly, these hegemonic powers have not yet acquired all the traditional elements of sovereignty, such as in matters of money, justice or ethical bodies. But, on the other hand, they already escape ordinary taxation[30] and, by their influence, are the subject of quasi-diplomatic recognition[31].

In contrast to the chain of actors, who aim to go beyond the concept of the state, we find the partisans of "individual sovereignty"[32]. Very present in the United States with the rise of bioethics (the principle of autonomy), they show great activism as a reminder that only individual freedom constitutes the fundamental value of society[33].

Does not the multiplicity of actors, their nature and the objectives of their action condemn them to reveal their ineffectiveness and lose their legitimacy? This is why, failing to believe in

---

[25] Christian Byk, Le droit international de la « bioéthique » : « jus gentium » ou « lex mercatoria » », JDI, vol. 4, 1997, pp. 913-944.

[26] Since the 2000's, it exists an embryonic sset of international texts: Commission nationale française pour l'UNESCO, Liste des initiatives et normes internationales concernant l'intelligence artificielle, https://unesco.delegfrance.org/Intelligence-Artificielle-Liste-des-initiatives-et-normes-internationales-3405.

[27] Jacques Fontanel, Natalia Sushcheva, La puissance des GAFAM : réalités, apports et dangers. Annuaire français de relations internationales, Paris : La Documentation française, 2019, XX. hal- 02196915, http://hal.univ-grenoble-alpes.fr/hal-02196915/document.

[28] The word derives from the « Silicon Valley », a place in California where are located the headquarters of Google, Apple and Facebook, those of Amazon and Microsoft are in the State of Washington.

[29] Eric Sadin, L'Humanité Augmentée. L'administration numérique du monde, Ed. L'échappée, 2013 ; La Silicolonisation du monde. L'irrésistible expansion du libéralisme numérique, Ed. L'échappée, 2016.

[30] J. Fontanel, Paradis fiscaux, pays « filous », La fuite organisée des impôts vers les pays complices, L'Harmattan, Paris, 2016 ; Nikos Smyrnaios, L'effet GAFAM : stratégies et logiques de l'oligopole de l'internet, Communication & langages, 2016/2, n°188, pp. 61-83, https://www.cairn.info/revue-communication-et-langages1-2016-2-page-61.htm.

[31] Alexis Feertchack, Le Danemark aura un ambassadeur dans la Silicon Valley, Figaro Vox , 8 mars 2017, https://www.lefigaro.fr/secteur/high-tech/2017/02/01/32001-20170201ARTFIG00116-le-danemark-aura-un-ambassadeur-dans-la-silicon-valley.php; Marc Rameaux, Les GAFA élevés au rang de puissance diplomatique ou la tyrannie des géants du Web, Figaro Vox, 2 fév.2017, https://www.lefigaro.fr/vox/monde/2017/02/02/31002-20170202ARTFIG00113-les-gafa-eleves-au-rang-de-puissance-diplomatiqueou-la-tyrannie-des-geants-du-web.php.

[32] Jean-Gabriel Ganascia, Eric Germain, Claude Kirchner, La souveraineté à l'ère du numérique, rapport, 27 mai 2018, CERNA, p.12, https://www.allistene.fr/files/2018/05/55160_AvisSouverainete-CERNA-2018-05-27.pdf.

[33] Op.cit. note (7), para.3.

collective action, some see in individual freedom the only dynamic that can give man some hope of escaping pandemics, which remind him of his vulnerability. They therefore adopt the rule that one could neither want nor be able to protect life by coercive policies without making it totally unlivable by the programmed death of social relations and the economy. This begs the question: should the idea that the authority implied in the measures to be taken to fight the pandemic be aimed at helping us to live in emergency or to preserve our freedoms? Unless the balance between these two objectives leads to define our political future as the enjoyment of freedom in a permanent framework of emergency governance?

II The emergence of a new social ontology

The COVID-19 pandemic acts as a catalyst for social change. It makes us aware of what was still for many a vague impression.

We had, in fact, already flipped into another world that the strength of the measures taken to fight the pandemic reveals to us. These are first justified by urgency. However, we hypothesize that the emergency already rhythms our social life enough to accustom us to it. We have entered a society and an economy of urgency and immediacy and we have already admitted that it is in this context that our freedoms will be exercised

A Contingency emergency...

The state of emergency has a history and a practice, which demonstrate that it is a temporarily necessary legal framework.

1) A legal framework with a history

a) The state of emergency allows the government, in a situation of imminent danger, to take measures to combat this situation, by freeing itself from ordinary law rules and procedures, including in the area of fundamental rights and freedoms. **Borrowed from the Roman Republic,** it is a disputed "remedy"[34]. Some point to the risk of dictatorship . The others recall with Rousseau that in the event of danger, "it is evident that the first intention of the people is that the State does not perish"[35].

b) Under French law[36], the state of emergency results from the act of 3 April 1955[37] adopted in the context of the events in Algeria. Implemented three times during this period, it was also applied overseas during the 1980s, then in 2005, during riots in the suburbs, and between November 14, 2015 and November 1 2017 following the attacks committed by "Islamic State".

"Declared by decree taken in the Council of Ministers, (it) confers on the civil authorities

---

[34] Dominique Albertini, L'état d'urgence, une histoire d'exceptions, Libération (9 avril 2020).

[35] *J-J Rousseau,* Du contrat social/Édition 1762/Livre IV/Chapitre 6 : la dictature, Marc Michel Rey, 1762 (p. 283-290).

[36] (36)   Olivier Beaud, Cécile Guérin-Bargues, L'état d'urgence ,Une étude constitutionnelle, historique et critique , 2ème édit, LGDJ, Paris,2018.

[37] Légifrance, loi n° 55-385 du 3 avril 1955 relative à l'état d'urgence, version consolidée au 15 mai 2020, https://www.legifrance.gouv.fr/affichTexte.do?cidTexte=JORFTEXT000000695350.

... exceptional police powers but ..., beyond twelve days, the extension of the state of emergency can only be authorized by law[38].

2) A temporary legal framework

a) Based on the model of the 1955 act, the state of health emergency was provisionally introduced, during the COVID-19 pandemic, in the public health code[39] until 21 April 2021 by the law of March 23, 2020[40]. The same law provided for the entry into force of the state of health emergency for a period of two from March 24, 2020, a date extended until July 10 by the law of May 11, 2020[41].

b) It takes up, in fact, the criterion of "health catastrophe endangering, by its nature and gravity, the health of the population"[42]. The measures provided for in article L.3131-15 of the public health code "are strictly proportionate to the health risks incurred and appropriate to the circumstances of time and place (and that) they are immediately put to an end when they are no longer necessary"[43]. In any event, they "cease to have effect at the same time as the state of health emergency ends"[44].

However, the number of these measures, which affect many aspects of the exercise of freedoms, including freedom of movement and respect for private life, raise questions about their relevance.

B Fears of the state of emergency

They relate to the extent of restrictions on public freedoms and their limited control, but also to the gradual integration of the concept of urgency into ordinary law.

1) The health emergency: broad powers and little control

a) Article L3131-15 of the Public Health Code provides for ten categories of measures limiting individual freedom (freedom of movement, placement in solitary confinement), collective freedoms (prohibition of assemblies and therefore limitation of freedom of political and religious expression) and also freedom of trade and industry (requisitions, general administrative closings). However, "The state of emergency does not ... give the state a blank check"[45]. Indeed, our most basic values and rights cannot be restricted such as dignity, the right to life and

---

[38] Sénat,   Étude   de   législation   comparée   n° 156   -   janvier   2006   -   L'état   d'urgence, https://www.senat.fr/lc/lc156/lc156_mono.html.

[39] Art.L3131-12 to 20 of the French Public Health Code (PHC).

[40] Loi n° 2020-290 du 23 mars 2020 d'urgence pour faire face à l'épidémie de covid-19, JORF n°0072 du 24 mars 2020.

[41] Loi du n° 2020-546 du 11 mai 2020 prorogeant l'état d'urgence sanitaire et complétant ses dispositions, 9 mai 2020, JORF n° 116 du 12 mai 2020.

[42] Art.L3131-12 PHC.

[43] Art. L3131-15 PHC, last paragraph.

[44] Art.L3131-14 PHC.

[45] Catherine Le Bris, La sauvegarde des libertés en temps de « guerre » contre le coronavirus, The Conversation, 27 mars   2020,   https://theconversation.com/la-sauvegarde-des-libertes-en-temps-de-guerre-contre-le-coronavirus-134913.

the prohibition of inhuman and degrading treatment.

b) In fact, some nuances must be made: the dignity of the deceased and their families has been affected by the end-of-life and bereavement conditions that have been imposed on them. Likewise, the priority of care given to patients with COVID-19 has deprived access to care for other patients. If health surveys to find people in contact with infected people are essential, is a mobile app project to locate these people really useful?[46].

As for the control by a judge, the variety and the limited number of cases hardly allow to say that it plays an essential role to ensure the control of the measures taken in application of the state of emergency[47].

Finally, with regard to parliamentary control, contrary to the provisions of the 1955 law, which provided for Parliament to intervene after a period of 12 days, the law relating to health emergencies provides that Parliament will only decide on its extension a month after his proclamation!

2) The lasting emergency

The health crisis caused by the COVID-19 pandemic reveals another phenomenon, the gradual integration of health emergency measures into our common law.

a) Emergency integrated into ordinary law

The National Consultative Commission on Human Rights declared itself "worried ... about a tendency to justify by the urgency of administrative acts and practices which, objectively, do not fall under it and which affect legal certainty[48]. The CNCDH also denounced the extension over time, beyond the end of the state of health emergency, and in other areas of the measures that the law of March 23, 2020 authorizes. It considers that "the law of March 23 leads to a concentration in the hands of the Executive of the power to restrict the rights and freedoms that the Republic has never known in peacetime"[49].

Would legal certainty have given way to legal flexibility, that is to say, the need for the law

---

[46] CNIL, Délibération n° 2020-046 du 24 avril 2020 portant avis sur un projet d'application mobile dénommée « StopCovid » ; https://www.cnil.fr/sites/default/files/atoms/files/deliberation_du_24_avril_2020_portant_avis_sur_un_projet_dapplication_mobile_stopcovid.pdf; CNCDH, *Avis sur le suivi numérique des personnes,* 28 avr. 2020, https://www.cncdh.fr/sites/default/files/avis_2020_-_3_-_200424_avis_suivi_numerique_des_personnes.pdf; Nathalie Devillier, Backtracking: comment concilier surveillance du COVID-19 et respect des libertés? The Conversation, 26 mars 2020, https://theconversation.com/backtracking-comment-concilier-surveillance-du-covid-19-et-respect-des-libertes-134843; Amnesty International déclaration publique conjointe, « Déclaration : Le recours aux technologies de surveillance numérique pour combattre la pandémie doit se faire dans le respect des droits humains », 2 avr. 2020. Cette déclaration a été signée par une centaine de groupe de la société civile, 2 avril 2020, https://www.amnesty.org/fr/documents/pol30/2081/2020/fr/.

[47] Hélène Christodoulou, L'État de droit déstabilisé par l'état d'urgence sanitaire : menaces et encadrements, Observatoire de la justice pénale, 13 mai 2020, https://www.justicepenale.net/post/l-%C3%A9tat-de-droit-d%C3%A9stabilis%C3%A9-par-l-%C3%A9tat-d-urgence-sanitaire-menaces-et-encadrements.

[48] CNCDH avis sur l'état d'urgence et l'état de droit, 28 avril 2020, 020,https://www.cncdh.fr/sites/default/files/avis_2020_-_2_-_200424_avis_etat_durgence_sanitaire_et_etat_de_droit.pdf.

[49] Commission nationale consultative des droits de l'homme , avis sur l'état d'urgence et l'état de droit, 28 avril 2020, IIIème partie de l'avis, https://www.cncdh.fr/sites/default/files/avis_2020_-_2_-_200424_avis_etat_durgence_sanitaire_et_etat_de_droit.pdf.

and lawyers to adapt to a society that lives at the pace of urgency and immediacy?

b) From the state of emergency to the society of emergency

1 ° **Many authors and human rights bodies denounce this excitement of the law.** Already in 2017, the law strengthening the fight against terrorism introduced into ordinary law, until December 31, 2020, administrative house arrest, search as well as border controls; these measures can be taken exclusively in the prevention of terrorism but outside a state of emergency[50].

Agreeing with this observation, the lawyer Raphaël Kempf affirmed that "the continuous erosion of individual freedoms observed since September 11, 2001 knows, in France, a brutal acceleration with the confinement of the population and the state of health emergency". He asked the question: "In the absence of checks and balances, will fundamental rights succumb to a virus?"[51]

2°. If we must be right, we must nonetheless rejoice that these critics help to realize **the insufficiency of theoretical analyzes of the state of emergency** [52]. Thus, in view of the time that punctuates society, urgency has imposed itself as a sign of modernity. "We have moved from the concept of rhythm (ages of life, rhythm of the seasons) to the concept of measurement: time is broken up in moments at the heart of which human beings disperse while accessing the feeling of multiplication and power ... The "emergency cult" testifies to a desire to control time in its most immediate dimension. What place then for a time that is seeking ... "[53]. And to conclude," with the advent of the reign of urgency ... it is not the thickness of time that re-emerges, it is its violence"[54].

Conclusion

Let the State survive trough urgency and by the mean of urgency would necessarily diminish our liberties. The state of emergency, by becoming our ordinary state, may allow us to survive a pandemic but it will also help us to forget what it is to live.

In order to combat this drift, we must analyze the question of urgency "from a broad and synthetic perspective ... embracing a series of diverse grounds ... (medicine, economy, justice, environment, politics, culture, etc.), but also drawing on many theoretical fields (philosophy,

[50] Loi n° 2017-1510 renforçant la sécurité intérieure et la lutte contre le terrorisme, rapport de Marc-Philippe Daubresse fait au nom de la mission de contrôle et de suivi de la loi renforçant la sécurité intérieure et la lutte contre le terrorisme, 26 fév.2020, https://www.senat.fr/fileadmin/Fichiers/Images/redaction_multimedia/2020/2020-Documents_pdf/20200226_Rapport_Senat_SILT.pdf.

[51] Raphaël Kempf, Et le gouvernement décida de confiner les libertés, Le Monde diplomatique, mai 2020, https://www.monde-diplomatique.fr/2020/05/KEMPF/61747.

[52] Véronique Champeil-Desplats, Histoire de lumières françaises : l'état d'urgence ou comment l'exception se fond dans le droit commun sans révision constitutionnelle, Revue interdisciplinaire d'études juridiques, 2017/2, volume 79, pp. 205-227, https://www.cairn.info/revue-interdisciplinaire-d-etudes-juridiques-2017-2-page-205.htm.

[53] Nicole Aubert, Le culte de l'urgence: la société malade du temps, Edition: Flammarion, Paris 2003, http://files.caferuis8.webnode.fr/200000046-ed960ef88b/n-3%20le%20culte%20de%20l-urgence%20correction.pdf.

[54] Nicole Aubert, L'urgence, symptôme de l'hypermodernité : de la quête de sens à la recherche de sensations, Communication et organisation, 29 | 2006 : Figures de l'urgence et ommunication, pp.11-21, https://journals.openedition.org/communicationorganisation/3365?lang=en.

sociology, psychology, economics, etc.)"[55].

References

AFP 2020. AFP, Encouragées par Donald Trump, les manifestations anti-confinement se multiplient aux Etats-Unis, Le Monde, 19 avril 2020, https://www.lemonde.fr/international/article/2020/04/19/etats-unis-encouragees-par-trump-les-manifestations-anti-confinement-se-multiplient_6037052_3210.html.

AI 2020. Amnesty International déclaration publique conjointe, « Déclaration : Le recours aux technologies de surveillance numérique pour combattre la pandémie doit se faire dans le respect des droits humains », 2 avr. 2020, https://www.amnesty.org/fr/documents/pol30/2081/2020/fr/.

Albertini 2020. Dominique Albertini, L'état d'urgence, une histoire d'exceptions, Libération (9 avril 2020).

Aubert 2003. Nicole Aubert, Le culte de l'urgence: la société malade du temps, Edition: Flammarion, Paris 2003, http://files.caferuis8.webnode.fr/200000046-ed960ef88b/n-3%20le%20culte%20de%20l-urgence%20correction.pdf.

Aubert 2006. Nicole Aubert, L'urgence, symptôme de l'hypermodernité : de la quête de sens à la recherche de sensations, Communication et organisation, 29 | 2006 : Figures de l'urgence et ommunication, pp.11-21, https://journals.openedition.org/communicationorganisation/3365?lang=en.

Beaud 2018. Olivier Beaud, Cécile Guérin-Bargues, L'état d'urgence ,Une étude constitutionnelle, historique et critique , 2ème édit, LGDJ, Paris,2018.

Bretelle-Establet et al. 2014. Florence Bretelle-Establet et Frédéric Keck, Les épidémies entre « Occident » et « Orient », *Extrême-Orient Extrême-Occident* [En ligne], 37 | 2014, para.27, http://journals.openedition.org/extremeorient/327.

Brouwer 2020. Christophe de Brouwer, L'OMS: organisme scientifique ou bureaucratie politique comme les autres? Contrepoints, 10 avril 2020, https://www.contrepoints.org/2020/04/10/368721-loms-organisme-scientifique-ou-bureaucratie-politique-comme-les-autres

Byk 1997. Christian Byk, Le droit international de la « bioéthique » : « jus gentium » ou « lex mercatoria » », JDI, vol. 4, 1997, pp. 913-944.

Champeil-Desplats 2017. Véronique Champeil-Desplats, Histoire de lumières françaises : l'état d'urgence ou comment l'exception se fond dans le droit commun sans révision constitutionnelle, Revue interdisciplinaire d'études juridiques, 2017/2, volume 79, pp. 205-227, https://www.cairn.info/revue-interdisciplinaire-d-etudes-juridiques-2017-2-page-205.htm.

---

[55] Jérôme Thomas, Christophe Bouton, *Le temps de l'urgence*, Lormont, Le Bord de l'eau, séries: Diagnostics , 2013, https://journals.openedition.org/lectures/11761.

Chiffoleau 2012. Sylvia Chiffoleau, Genèse de la santé publique internationale. De la peste d'Orient à l'OMS, Presses universitaires de Rennes, Rennes, 2012.

Christodoulou 2020. Hélène Christodoulou, L'État de droit déstabilisé par l'état d'urgence sanitaire : menaces et encadrements, Observatoire de la justice pénale, 13 mai 2020, https://www.justicepenale.net/post/l-%C3%A9tat-de-droit-d%C3%A9stabilis%C3%A9-par-l-%C3%A9tat-d-urgence-sanitaire-menaces-et-encadrements.

Conversation 2020. L'OMS, une histoire entre combat contre les maladies et luttes d'influence, The Conversation, 30 mars 2020, https://theconversation.com/loms-une-histoire-entre-combat-contre-les-maladies-et-luttes-dinfluence-134597.

Darnis 2020. Jean-Pierre Darnis, La crise du COVID-19, les leçons du cas italien. Note de la FRS n°07/2020, 23 mars 2020, https://www.frstrategie.org/publications/notes/crise-covid-19-lecons-cas-italien-2020

DEEU 2020. Département d'État des États-Unis, Bureau de la porte-parole, Publication du plan d'action du gouvernement des États-Unis pour soutenir la réponse internationale face au COVID-19, fiche d'information, 16 avril 2020, https://fr.usembassy.gov/fr/publication-du-plan-daction-du-gouvernement-des-etats-unis-pour-soutenir-la-reponse-internationale-face-au-covid-19/.

Devillier 2020. Nathalie Devillier, Backtracking: comment concilier surveillance du COVID-19 et respect des libertés? The Conversation, 26 mars 2020, https://theconversation.com/backtracking-comment-concilier-surveillance-du-covid-19-et-respect-des-libertes-134843

Feertchack 2017. Alexis Feertchack, Le Danemark aura un ambassadeur dans la Silicon Valley, Figaro Vox , 8 mars 2017, https://www.lefigaro.fr/secteur/high-tech/2017/02/01/32001-20170201ARTFIG00116-le-danemark-aura-un-ambassadeur-dans-la-silicon-valley.php; Marc Rameaux, Les GAFA élevés au rang de puissance diplomatique ou la tyrannie des géants du Web, Figaro Vox, 2 fév.2017, https://www.lefigaro.fr/vox/monde/2017/02/02/31002-20170202ARTFIG00113-les-gafa-eleves-au-rang-de-puissance-diplomatiqueou-la-tyrannie-des-geants-du-web.php.

Fontanel 2016. J. Fontanel, Paradis fiscaux, pays « filous », La fuite organisée des impôts vers les pays complices, L'Harmattan, Paris, 2016

Fontanel 2019. Jacques Fontanel, Natalia Sushcheva, La puissance des GAFAM : réalités, apports et dangers. Annuaire français de relations internationales, Paris : La Documentation française, 2019, XX. hal- 02196915, http://hal.univ-grenoble-alpes.fr/hal-02196915/document.

Ganascia 2018. Jean-Gabriel Ganascia, Eric Germain, Claude Kirchner, La souveraineté à l'ère du numérique, rapport, 27 mai 2018, CERNA, p.12, https://www.allistene.fr/files/2018/05/55160_AvisSouverainete-CERNA-2018-05-27.pdf.

Godement 2020. Institut Montaigne, François Godement, La guerre commerciale Chine – Etats-Unis : quelles conséquences ? https://www.institutmontaigne.org/blog/la-guerre-commerciale-chine-etats-unis-quelles-consequences

Goldman 1964. Berthold Goldman, Frontières du droit et « lex mercatoria », Archives de philosophie du droit, 1964, pp. 177-192

Goodman 1952. Neville Mariott Goodman, International Health Organizations and their Work, Editions J. and A. Churchill, 1952, Londres, p. 77.

Harrison 2006. Mark Harrison, Disease, Diplomacy and International Commerce: the Origins of International Sanitary Regulation in the Nineteenth Century, Journal of Global History, 2006-1, p. 197-217.

Hudson 2020. Paul Hudson, directeur général de Sanofi, L'Europe doit construire sa souveraineté sanitaire Les Echos, 28 mars 2020, https://www.lesechos.fr/idees-debats/cercle/opinion-leurope-doit-construire-sa-souverainete-sanitaire-1189846.

Huffington Post 2020. Huffington Post, Le plan de Trump face au coronavirus pour rouvrir les États-Unis, 17 avril 2020, https://www.huffingtonpost.fr/entry/le-plan-de-trump-face-au-coronavirus-pour-rouvrir-les-etats-unis_fr_5e98da5cc5b6ead1400a1b32

Inglese 2014. Marco Inglese, L'Union Européenne et la santé, thèse, Universités de Strasbourg et de Bologne, 2014, https://tel.archives-ouvertes.fr/tel-01148538/document.

Institut Montaigne 2020. Institut Montaigne, Les Etats face au coronavirus : l'archétype italien, 20 avril 2020, https://www.institutmontaigne.org/blog/les-etats-face-au-coronavirus-larchetype-italien.

Kempf 2020. Raphaël Kempf, Et le gouvernement décida de confiner les libertés, Le Monde diplomatique, mai 2020, https://www.monde-diplomatique.fr/2020/05/KEMPF/61747.

Le Bris 2020. Catherine Le Bris, La sauvegarde des libertés en temps de « guerre » contre le coronavirus, The Conversation, 27 mars 2020, https://theconversation.com/la-sauvegarde-des-libertes-en-temps-de-guerre-contre-le-coronavirus-134913.

Lejbowicz 1999. Agnès Lejbowicz, III. La « lex mercatoria », dans Philosophie du droit international. L'impossible capture de l'humanité, sous la direction de Agnès Leibowitz, Presses Universitaires de France, « Fondements de la politique », Paris, 1999, pp. 77-129, https://www.cairn.info/philosophie-du-droit-international--9782130497219-page-77.htm.

Lipold 2020. Achim Lipold, Le Brésil face au coronavirus: autoritarisme et politique de déni, RFI, 11 mai 2020, http://www.rfi.fr/fr/am%C3%A9riques/20200511-le-br%C3%A9sil-face-coronavirus-autoritarisme-et-politique-d%C3%A9.

Louis 2020. Marieke Louis, L'OMS dans le maelstrom du covid-19, entretien avec Auriane Guilbaud, Collège de France, la vie des idées, 1 avril 2020, https://laviedesidees.fr/L-OMS-dans-le-maelstrom-du-covid-19.html.

Maurel 2011. Chloé Maurel, L'OMS et la gestion des crises et catastrophes sanitaires mondiales : perspectives pour une réforme, Chantiers politiques, 5 mars 2011, https://www.nonfiction.fr/article-4323-loms-et-la-gestion-des-crises-et-catastrophes-sanitaires-mondiales-perspectives-pour-une-reforme.htm.

Maurel 2020. Chloé Maurel, Ce que les crises épidémiques révèlent des dérives de l'OMS, The Conversation, 20 mars 2020, https://theconversation.com/ce-que-les-crises-epidemiques-revelent-des-derives-de-loms-133639.

Meuwly 2020. Olivier Meuwly, Le Coronavirus et la Chine. Le révélateur d'un système, Le Temps, 9 avril 2020, https://blogs.letemps.ch/olivier-meuwly/2020/04/09/le-coronavirus-et-la-chine-le-revelateur-dun-systeme/
Simone Pieranni, Le Coronavirus change tout : préparez-vous à la nouvelle hégémonie chinoise, Le Grand Continent, Cartographier le coronavirus, L'Observatoire géo-politique du COVID-19, https://legrandcontinent.eu/fr/2020/03/12/coronavirus-chine-surveillance/.

Motchane 2002. Jean-Loup Motchane, Quand l'OMS épouse la cause des firmes pharmaceutiques, Le Monde diplomatique, juillet 2002, https://www.monde-diplomatique.fr/2002/07/MOTCHANE/9250.

Nardon 2020. Laurence Nardon, COVID-19 : la fin du leadership américain ? Chroniques américaines, Institut français des relations internationales, 14avril 2020, https://www.ifri.org/sites/default/files/atoms/files/nardon_leadership_covid_2020-2.pdf.

OIHP 1933. OIHP, Vingt-cinq ans d'activité de l'Office international d'hygiène publique, Paris, 1933.

Paillette 2010. Céline Paillette, De l'Organisation d'hygiène de la SDN à l'OMS. Mondialisation et régionalisme européen dans le domaine de la santé, 1919-1954, *Bulletin de l'Institut Pierre Renouvin*, 2010/2, n° 32, pp. 193-198, https://www.cairn.info/revue-bulletin-de-l-institut-pierre-renouvin1-2010-2-page-193.htm.

Pellet 2000. Alain Pellet, La *lex mercatoria*, »tiers ordre juridique ? Remarques ingénues d'un internationaliste de droit public *in* Mélanges en l'honneur de Philipe Kahn, Souveraineté étatique et marchés internationaux à la fin du XXème siècle, Litec, Paris, 2000, pp.53-74, http://pellet.actu.com/wp-content/uploads/2016/02/PELLET-2000-Lex-mercatoria-tiers-ordre-juridique.pdf

Pisano 2020. Gary P. Pisano, Raffaella Sadun, Michele Zanini, Lessons from Italy's Response to Coronavirus, Harvard Business Review, https://hbr.org/2020/03/lessons-from-italys-response-to-coronavirus.

Rasmussen 2001. Anne Rasmussen, Tournant, inflexions, ruptures : le moment internationaliste , Mil neuf cent. Revue d'histoire intellectuelle, n° 19, 2001, p. 30

Rousseau 1762. J-J Rousseau, Du contrat social/Édition 1762/Livre IV/Chapitre 6 : la dictature, Marc Michel Rey, 1762 (p. 283-290).

Sadin 2013. Eric Sadin, L'Humanité Augmentée. L'administration numérique du monde, *Ed. L'échappée, 2013*

Sadin 2016. Eric Sadin, La Silicolonisation du monde. L'irrésistible expansion du libéralisme numérique, *Ed. L'échappée, 2016.*

Scholz 2015. Nicole Scholz, L'Organisation mondiale de la santé au cœur de sa réforme, Service de recherche du Parlement européen, oct. 2015, https://www.europarl.europa.eu/RegData/etudes/BRIE/2015/571307/EPRS_BRI%282015%29571307_FR.pdf.

Seval 2020. Jean Dominique Seval, La Chine pourrait s'imposer comme la première puissance mondiale dès la fin de l'épidémie, Le Monde, 11 avril 2020, https://www.lemonde.fr/idees/article/2020/04/11/la-chine-pourrait-s-imposer-comme-la-premiere-puissance-mondiale-des-la-fin-de-l-epidemie_6036349_3232.html

Smyrnaios 2016. Nikos Smyrnaios, L'effet GAFAM : stratégies et logiques de l'oligopole de l'internet, Communication & langages, 2016/2, n°188, pp. 61-83, https://www.cairn.info/revue-communication-et-langages1-2016-2-page-61.htm

Thomas et al. 2013. Jérôme Thomas, Christophe Bouton, *Le temps de l'urgence*, Lormont, Le Bord de l'eau, séries: Diagnostics , 2013, https://journals.openedition.org/lectures/11761.

Christian Byk, judge at the Court of Appeal, Paris, Secretary General of the International Association of Law, Ethics and Science and Chairman of the Intergovernmental Bioethics Committee of UNESCO (2017-2019).

The Syndemic Perspective
and the Need for Health Hermeneutics

Fernando Lolas, University of Chile and Central University of Chile, Chile

Abstract

This contribution emphasizes a *syndemic perspective* considering synergistic interactions of viral pandemics with other conditions, pathological or not, in creating societal disease-states or disorders. It proposes that causal thinking, aimed at explaining occurrences, needs to be complemented by a hermeneutic approach, related to understanding, comprehending and interpreting through an integral view. In order to constitute a complement to the usual scientific outlook a transdisciplinary approach is needed, avoiding the hegemony of one method over others and relying on *Erlebnis* of stakeholders and their narratives. The aim is to aid in *setting priorities* for goal-directed action in accordance with value orientations of the communities and justifying decisions on the basis both of their consequences and personal convictions. This involves examining and harmonizing different discourses. The clash between *common good* and *individual advantage* can thus be approached from the perspective of both *evidence-based* and *value-based* considerations, stressing the dialogical structure of ethical judgement and decision-making.

Key words

Syndemic Perspective, Health Hermeneutics, Value

Since it was proposed, the neologism syndemics[1] has enjoyed wide acceptance. It has served to emphasize the co-occurrence of pathological conditions at a population level, describing interactions among entities such as hunger, obesity, viral infection, and other conditions defined for the clinical setting and redefined for use at the community level[2]. Whereas in clinical thinking terms such as co-morbidity or dual pathology are employed for the coexistence of nosological entities, the interaction of these conditions at the group or community level generates new challenges. So-called "social determinants of health" are important for defining public policy but causal thinking poses the question of the intermediate links between those "determinants" and the "final common pathways" of disease-states. Isolating factors and cancelling out confounding influences lead to endless piecemeal research, where new influences, dangerous or protective, are discovered or rediscovered.

Conceptualizations such as the bio-psycho-social model[3], apparently useful at the individual level, end up in a juxtaposition of methodological data-generating tools. In medicine, this has meant a predominance of analytical methodologies derived from the hard sciences; the approach has not essentially modified clinical practice and social healthcare. Its impact on the design of institutions is reflected in the addition of specialty treatments without changing usual practices.

Traditional scientific method multiplies causal attributions if pure experimental or quasi-experimental observational designs are employed. This applies both to the biological and the social scientific foundations of scientific medicine; the prestige of science and rigorous experimentation is deemed essential for sound conclusions.

The isolation of causal influences is a complex process that begins with the definition of

---

[1] Singer, Merrill. (2009). *Introduction to syndemics : a critical systems approach to public and community health.* Jossey-Bass. ISBN 978-0-470-48298-8. OCLC 428819497.

[2] Singer M Bulled N Ostrach O Mendenhall ESyndemics and the biosocial conception of health.Lancet. 2017; 389: 941-950

[3] Engel, G L The need for a new medical model: a challenge for biomedicine. Science (1977) 196:129-136.

entities. Miettinen proposes the neologism "etiogenesis"[4] implying first the "genesis", the creation of the entity, and then the cause, that what leads to the entity. Diseases are not givens, are constructs. After formed they enter into the culture of the profession and into lay people talk, with different meanings and connotations. Specialized jargon characterizes the division of labour and the fragmentations of knowledge.

Community problems present themselves as riddles for experts and lay people. There are complex webs of meaning along with emotional reactions to threat, death, and disability. Political authorities impose restrictions on individual liberties in order to control the spread of the disease and to manage resources for coping with emergencies. Reactions vary widely, from fake news disseminated by interested parties to prejudices related to affected people and fight for scarce resources.

Health hermeneutics

Knowledge is not simply information. It is organized information. As important as the facts is the architecture or order imposed on them for organizing the information into understandable concepts. To know is to participate in a community of meanings embedded in culture.

There is no knowledge without active *mimesis* or reconstruction of the context in which the information was created. This includes the valoric milieu, the prejudices of those affected by the information and the unavoidable interests associated with every form of knowledge since knowledge- as organized information- is always knowledge *for something and for someone.*

The narratives associated with the pandemics vary according to the perspective from which the phenomena are analyzed. A *hermeneutic approach* aims at reconstructing meaning from the vantage point of multiple observers. Beyond analysis and causal thinking it strives at considering the impact of context on the way events and facts are understood and interpreted. Essentially, in the case of a societal phenomenon, it presupposes interpretating *dialogical interactions of conflicting narratives.*

Health hermeneutics for syndemic times does not imply change in data gathering processes or in causal inferences. It suggests a *change in data interpretation*, placing emphasis on *narratives* from different perpectives and viewpoints. The *meta-narrative* arising from multiple sources, properly interpreted, provides useful clues for reconfiguring dilemmas and problems from a more inclusive standpoint. The advantage lies in considering at the outset the valoric structure of judgment as one context embedded in narratives. Essentially, this should be used for an *appropriate priority-setting strategy*, an end in itself.

Four perspectives should be considered: organizations, disciplines, culture, history. These influence individual observers determining tone and contents of narratives. The relativ weight of these influences varies from group to group and from discourse to discourse. Priorities may vary widely within a society, depending upon experience, tradition, perceived need, social position, and moral considerations.

During a pandemic, not only a virus threatens human welfare. Poverty, hunger, social disruption, psychological suffering are part of the process. The interpretation must take all those points of view into consideration. The interpretation should center on a *metanarrative*, composed by the partial renditions of the phenomenon. Where the economist sees a problem, the epidemiologist sees another facet, and the mental health expert places other priorities in front.

---

[4] Miettinen, O.S. (2015) *Medicine as a scholarly field: An introduction.* Springer International Publishing Swizterland.

The "real" problem depends on the power of the narrative for defining it. Despite agreement that the pandemia is a health problem, no one would deny that it is also an economic one. Why is the standard argument oriented toward the vague notion "life is first"? The habit of ethical thinking obliges people to put welfare of humans first. But the other arguments are as forceful as the health one, since people may die from starvation or develop grave psychological disturbance due to measures taken to combat viral epidemics.

The syndemia notion suggests *Horizontverschmelzung*, a fusion of horizons expressed as narratives from different voices. The *first person* voice of those who are affected, either by a disease-state or any of its consequences, including those derived from preventive measures. The *second person* voice reflects the impact on relational activities brought about by the pandemics. Finally, the *third person* voice expresses the causal thinking of scientific discourse, apparently neutral and objective.

Which is then the real problem? What is health, social health, under these considerations? Evidently health cannot reside solely in eliminating the virus, for a totally undernourished or impoverished community will not enjoy it. It cannot consist in ignoring the real threat of infection. The real health is an aggregate of narratives that escapes a comprehensive definition. H.G. Gadamer uses the term *Verborgenheit*[5] for referring to individual health, something hidden and difficult to explain with numbers, an enigma. The same holds true for *societal well-being*. Health is harmony, everything working in accord. Healthy communities live in silence and peace, everything seems to be where it should be, there is a feeling of plenitude and tranquil strength. It cannot be expressed solely from the medical, the economic, the political, and the social point of view. It is a *metanarrative* with many voices that need to be understood as a whole by an interpreter provided with sensibility and understanding, trying to unravel the meaning of situations. The productive use of prejudice is of the essence of the hermeneutic enterprise. It helps enter the cycle of interpretation-application where the meaning of the "text" is put to work under real circumstances. To analyze, to comprehend, to interpret is to apply what has been learned (knowledge) in a prudent way (phronesis) to restore the state of plenitude, that hidden dimension of well being we call health at the community level.

This position may add complexity to the "paradigmatic instability" of medicine as a social practice. For medicine, as a science of actions and not of objects[6], derives its power from lacking an epistemological status in its own right, but by being "applied" biochemistry, physiology, sociology, and politics. The famous Virchow expression "medicine is a social science" opposed the standard thinking of his time. Medicine as politics of the body was similar to politics as the medicine of society.

Politicians refer to this integration as "intersectorial thinking": Health problems are approached from one specialized, closed, perspective, to which economic and social discoursed are added. Multidisciplinary or interdisciplinary thinking are *stressed,* juxtaposing rationalities but ignoring that an interpretive stance is needed working on a transdisciplinary basis, that is, from a multiperspectivistic approach from the outset.

Facing this problem at the individual level, we reinterpreted the psychiatric case not as personal disease history but as a *multinarrative* derived from the discourses of patients, relatives,

---

[5] Gadamer, H.G. (1993) *Über die Verborgenheit der Gesund*heit. Suhrkamp, Frankfurt a.M.

[6] Lolas, F. Theoretical medicine: a proposal for reconceptualizing medicine as a science of actions. *The Journal of Medicine and Philosophy* 21: 659-670, 1996.

relevant others, and physicians[7]. The "case" was not an indidivual sick person but a *complex multilayered narrative,* composed by different speakers with different aims and different rhetorics[8]. The task was to achieve a total picture, beyond particular narratives: The suggestion then as now is to approach the challenge from a *narrative/hermeneutic* position considered as the ppropraite context for bioethical thinking[9].

Ethical implications: Priority-setting, evidence-based and value-based decisions

A distinction should be made between axiological norms and thetic norms. The first derive either from a deontological or a teleological perspective and are supposedly binding. The second consider the contrast between group common good and personal advantage and modulate what is perceived as a duty to the community, as horizontal or vertical solidarity, as reciprocity and as benevolence or non maleficence. The isolation of different principles for action is an artifact, virtue is a general stance and it is incorporated into judgements and actions in an imperceptible way.

It is important to stress that many narratives are involved in syndemic approaches, the first, the second and third person narratives place different priorities on the construction of the "plot". They seem to be referring to different events and occurrences, making dialogue difficult. They are different "*axiological narratives*": each one places emphasis on one aspect or factor ignoring or diminishing the importance of others. They are *value-laden narratives,* manifesting choices on the importance each discourse gives to different aspects. The economist attributes importance to economic factors, the politician tries to influence public opinion and obtain power, and so on.

The lesson is that a metaethical discourse is needed. Not to impose a particular worldview or set of rules but to harmonize and interpret the metanarrative established considering all the voices involved.

The basic information is the same as in other investigative endeavours. What is different is the approach to data and information and the type of knowledge sought. It is not simply one more type of information and a further method. The hermeneutic approach is, more that a *method,* a *modus,* other form creating realities and apprehending meaning.

The aim of ethical reasoning is to understand the reasons behind decisions and to justify them with good theories. Each societal "*order*" (the scientific, the medical, the religious, the political,etc.,.) is characterized by a *scale of priorities.* What is important in one discourse may not be relevant in others. The idea of an order is exactly that: a scale or gradient of importance for different actions or occurrences. A clash between the economic and the medical order is evident in decisions regarding the syndemic. Different and contradictory discourses are difficult to harmonize; both are relevant for life. The hegemony is dictated by power. Those who have power and authority can impose their priorities. No discussion on ethics is possible without reference to power relations within a given society. The dialogical/hermeneutic approach based on

---

[7]   Lolas, F., Valdebenito, C. Hacia una reconstrucción técnico-axiográfica del caso en psiquiatría: una nota bioética. *Revista de Neuro-Psiquiatría* (Lima) 67 (3-4):182-187, 2004. -   Lolas, F., Valdebenito, C. La inter-textualidad en la construcción del caso psiquiátrico. *Revista de Psiquiatría Clínica* (Santiago) 41(1): 27-31, 2004.

[8]   Lolas, F. L'éventail des pratiques en psychiatrie: intégration des processus complémentaires de narration. *L'Evolution Psychiatrique* (Paris) 82(2):18-23, 2017.

[9]   Lolas, F. The hermeneutical dimension of the bioethical enterprise.Notes on the dialogical/narrative foundations of bioethics. Acta Bioethica (Santiago) 24(2):153-159, 2018.

narratives tries to achieve a wider consensus on priority-setting because narration is argument[10]. This does not mean setting the priorities as such in detail but to devise methods for considering the feelings and dispositions of stakeholders in a comprehensive form.

The tension between common good and individual preferences may find, if not resolution or elimination, at least a compromise. Also, the distintion between technical foundation and moral justification is better appreciated. Value-based decisions are thus harmonized with evidence- based ones.

Concluding remarks

A pandemic threat presents essentially two challenges. The need for sound causal inference in scientific terms, on the one hand, an an appropriate ethical response on the other.

In a syndemic perspective the disruption caused by the etiological factor virus is one element in a complex web. The disorder also includes perceptions, alterations in personal relations, economic and social problems plus diversity due to cultural imprint.

It is difficult to isolate the relative importance of each factor for the final condition.

In the sphere of ethical judgement the identification of core values and the assessment of principles and guidelines are best served by a hermeneutic approach based on the narratives of the different stakeholders involved. It is not a suggestion for producing more or more reliable data but a method – or better, *modus-* for restructuring and organizing information in order to prioritize actions and decisions. Since many interests are relevant, each one associated with a different discourse and interest ("orders") the predominance of one rationality over others may determine the final outcome. For instance, in some countries the pressure for not interrupting economic activity may be as strong, or even stronger, than the measures of isolation and confinement indicated by the public health rationality.

The fusion of these two perspectives – causal scientific inference and narrative/hermeneutic understanding of the "case" at hand- allows for a treatment of decisions that do not necessarily overlap. The epistemology of causal thinking is not enough for an adequate priority-setting, even if it involves horizontal and vertical integration of disciplines. The wider picture is gained through methods for organizing the totality of experiences and data in comprehensive texts composed by the perceptions, discourses, and actions of social actors. Priority-setting, a challenge in itself, may then result in different outcomes in different societies after the predominant core values and the relevant ethical justifications, axiological and thetic, are uncovered by an appropriate "reading".

This is health hermeneutics.

References

Engel 1977. Engel, GL Die Notwendigkeit eines neuen medizinischen Modells: eine Herausforderung für die Biomedizin. Science (1977) 196:129-136

Gadamer 1993. Gadamer, HG *Über die Verborgenheit der Gesundheit.* Suhrkamp, Frankfurt aM

Lolas 1996. Lolas, F. Theoretische Medizin: Ein Vorschlag zur Rekonzeptualisierung der Medizin als Handlungswissenschaft. *The Journal of Medicine and Philosophy* 21 : 659-670,

---

[10] Olmos P, editor (2017) *Narration as argument.*Springer International Publishing

1996.

Lolas 2017. Lolas, F. L'éventail des pratiques en psychiatrie: Integration des Processus Complémentaires de Narration. *L'Evolution Psychiatrique* (Paris) 82 (2): 18-23, 2017.

Lolas 2018. Lolas, F. Die hermeneutische Dimension des bioethischen Unternehmens. Anmerkungen zu den dialogischen / narrativen Grundlagen der Bioethik. *Acta Bioethica* (Santiago) 24 (2): 153-159, 2018.

Lolas et al. 2004a. Lolas, F., Valdebenito, C. Hacia und die Rekonstruktion des Falles und der Psiquiatrie: una nota bioética. *Revista de Neuro-Psiquiatría* (Lima) 67 (3-4): 182-187, 2004

Lolas et al. 2004b. F. Lolas, C. Valdebenito. *Revista de Psiquiatría* C línica (Santiago) 41 (1): 27-31, 2004.

Miettinen 2015. Miettinen, OS *Medizin als wissenschaftliches Gebiet: Eine Einführung* . Springer International Publishing Schweiz

Olmos 2017. Olmos P, Herausgeber *Erzählung als Argument*. Springer International Publishing

Singer 2009. Singer, Merrill. Einführung in die Syndemie : Ein kritischer Systemansatz für die öffentliche und kommunale Gesundheit . Jossey-Bass. ISBN 978-0-470-4 8298-8. OCLC 428819497.

Singer et al. 2017. Singer M Bulled N Ostrach O Mendenhall ESyndemics und das biosoziale Konzept der Gesundheit.Lancet. 2017; 389: 941-950

Fernando Lolas, is Medical Doctor both at the University of Chile as well as the Central University of Chile.

Between Ego(centr)ism and Cooperation:
Would People become Moraly Disengaged
or More Altruistic after the COVID-19 pandemic?

Ana Fritzhand, University "Ss. Cyril and Methodius", North Macedonia

Dejan Donev, University "Ss. Cyril and Methodius", North Macedonia

Abstract

The world is facing great health challenge since COVID-19 pandemic was declared. However, it is not only immense health issue, but also psychological, bioethical, economical, and political one. There are many unanswered questions. Among them is how this pandemic will affect people's mental health and their moral behavior? In this paper, the authors are focusing on the dilemma whether people will become more morally disengaged, or more altruistic after the pandemic is over. Hence, the knowledge from ethics and psychology is integrated, having in mind that people have potential for being both good and bad in their actions towards others.

Key words

egocentrism, egoism, cooperation, moral disengagement, altruism, bioethics

1. Introduction

COVID-19 pandemic is the most popular daily issue since the day it was declared by WHO. It raises unique ethical dilemmas because it is not only immense health issue, but also psychological, bioethical, economical, and political one. Thus, it makes demands on society from all domains of life, worldwide. According to Regilme Jr. (2020), although only twenty years of the 21st century have passed, the world already faced three grand crises. The first one is related to the 9/11 terrorist attacks in the USA. The second happened in 2007-2008 and was related to the global financial crisis that was considered the worst economic crisis since 1930s. Finally, the third one is still happening and is called "COVID-19" pandemic. This newest crisis has also accelerated the emergence of an epistemic crisis that became obvious in delegitimation and pervasive doubt of/in professional expertise, scientific knowledge as well as the reliability and legitimacy of established institutions, including public health institutions.

Following this, there are many open questions regarding various aspects of social and personal functioning that are important, especially from the bioethical standpoint. Concepts like "social distancing", "the new reality/normality", "isolation", "lockdown" etc., are already common in the media. As Khoo and Lantos (2020:1) point out, everybody are facing restriction on freedom of movement and must deal with it the best they can. But, how the application of these concepts relates to everyday quality of peoples' life? It is almost sure that this pandemic will affect and is already affecting the mental health of individuals. However, there is still no final answer on how it will affect people's mental health and their moral behavior on short and long-term basis? Finally, although everybody speak of "new normality" and that "the life will never be the same", what it is really going to look like when this is all over?

2. Moral Disengagement vs. Altruism

There is an increasing interest among psychologists, both researchers and practitioners, about the concept of moral disengagement. Albert Bandura (2016), the author of this concept, points out that in order to understand morality and moral behavior as a whole, it is necessary to be able to explain not only what motivates people to behave morally, but also why in certain circumstances people behave passively, inhumanly and/or violently, but still have a positive opinion of themselves. Theories of morality are usually directed towards the inhibitory aspect of moral agency, which is manifested in one's ability to refrain from inhumane behavior. However, there is also a proactive form of moral agency. It is recognized in compassion for the suffering of others or in efforts to improve their well-being, often to one's own detriment.

In the past, moral development theories have focused on the adoption of moral standards and the development of moral reasoning as prerequisites for moral behavior. However, it is quite clear today that these concepts are not the most important factors leading to individual's moral behavior. Moral disengagement is one of the arguments that underpin this view. This is because selective activation and disengagement from self-sanctioning, enables different actions by individuals with the same moral standards. This is observed in certain situations where moral disengagement is manifested by individuals who otherwise show compassion in other areas of their lives. Moral disengagement is closely linked to the self-regulation mechanisms that need to be activated first. Therefore, some individuals can be both cruel and humane towards different people at the same time, depending on whom they include and exclude from their category of humanity (Bandura, 2016).

According to Khoo and Lantos (2020:2), there are evidence of increased domestic violence and alcohol abuse during the quarantine period, where children are mostly vulnerable due to their lack of power. Travel restrictions and the lockdowns of schools, universities and work places are main factors for emerging feelings of loneliness, boredom, confusion, anger, frustration, as well as continuous feeling of being inadequately informed. Some or all of these are reflected in peoples' actions and can result in various forms of unadapt or dysfunctional reasoning and behavior. However, having in mind the global focus on the at-risk populations, the fear for the safety of others, i.e *altruistic fear* (Warr & Ellison, 2000; as cited in Sloan et al., 2020:3), has also become apparent. This type of fear is perceived in those individuals who fear for their families, friends and members of the close community of getting the virus, instead of feeling frightened exclusively for their own health.

As Jeronimus (2020) points out, COVID-19 pandemic already entered every aspect of peoples' lives and accelerated societal transformations. Although this pandemic affects individuals to a different level, depending on various factors (ex. age, gender, socioeconomic status, culture, personality, resilience etc.), it is more than obvious that at least secondary stress is present among majority of people. There is also change in values, politics and resources in the countries, especially those mostly affected by the virus. Furthermore, the number of lockdowns and prolonged social isolation is closely linked to financial and mental health issues. It also influences the way people organize their social networks, which can lead to the need of readjustment at the individual and social level as well. In this sense, when analyzing different cohorts it becomes obvious that youth and emerging adults are facing the challenge of maturing faster than their peers from previous generations. As for the others, it is plausible to experience increased level of introversion, uncertainty, and become more risk-aversive. Thus, the COVID-19 pandemic influence the individual's complex set of feelings, thoughts, behaviors, values, goals, and perspectives on the world.

During these circumstances caused by COVID-19 pandemic, altruism matters more than ever, because it is necessary for overcoming the outbreak. When discussing altruism, authors usually refer to the moral practice of concern for the happiness of others. It appears as a virtue in many cultures and is central to a various religions worldwide (Jenkins, 2020). However, if there is no sufficient motive, means and opportunity, altruism will not occur. It always requires the ability to assess and influence others' welfare. Altruism can also be undermined by fostering any seemingly incompatible beliefs. Therefore, it should be promoted as something common, attractive and expected (Farsides, 2007). In this sense, the *effective altruism* movement grounded in practical ethics and Socratic philosophy, is showing to be of significant importance. According to Singer (2015), effective altruism is based on the idea that individual should do the most good he/she can. Looking at the two poles of the continuum, there is one pole which involves living the minimally acceptable ethical life that underline using a substantial part of the spare resources to make the world a better place for all people. On the other pole stands fully ethical life, according to which, individual should do the most good he/she can. When trying to summarize the characteristics of the effective altruism, one should be listing several important things. First, effective altruism is directed toward making a difference to the world, for example, by providing incentives for charities to demonstrate their effectiveness. Second, it gives the meaning in one's life, since by doing what is good and right, one feels good about him/herself in the same time. Third, effective altruism revoke the question that connects the psychological and philosophical perspective of whether people are driven by their inner feelings and desires, or the reason has the substantial role in determining the way a person live his/her life?

3. Methodology

For the purpose of this paper, authors reviewed relevant literature and conducted data analyses of the articles in scientific journals as well as the latest news in popular texts, blogs and opinions in the media. Discursive analysis, comparative analysis and an interpretive text analysis were also made, in order to gain insight into the power of discourse in constituting practice.

The main research question is whether the COVID-19 pandemic will produce more ego(centr)ism and moral disengagement, or would people become more cooperative and altruistic over time, especially after this whole state of pandemic is over?

Consequently, the following hypothesis is formulated, stating that: Individual characteristics such as personality, personal values and emotional maturity would be more relevant to moral behavior of people, than the context of pandemic itself.

4. Would people become egocentric or cooperative after COVID-19: What does evidence show?

The lasting implications of the pandemic are still yet to come, but meanwhile, there is wide place for doing bioethical research. It is evident that moral distress, conflicts and mixed sentiments that affect everybody in different extent, are much related to the present global circumstances. In this sense, the fear and uncertainty are probably the two most frequent emotions among many individuals. In psychology, fear is understood as an adaptive response of the organism when danger is perceived. In other words, it is functional because it motivates the individual to engage in protective behavior. It is quite expected for people to experience such feelings, especially when witnessing shocking pictures of severely ill patients in the hospitals, knowing that many of them would probably die of this virus. Then, there are news on the media about lockdowns and quarantines that sometimes last for several days, so again, mentioned feelings appear understandable. In many countries around the globe, media register similar behavior of people in stores – people panickly buying products in huge amounts in order to satisfy the basic need for security and survival (at least in their heads) when the time of the lockdown comes.

In psychology, it is well known that people have natural tendency towards altruism, especially when it comes to the members of their own group. Even small personal sacrifices, such as donation to charities are also counted as altruism. However, altruism could also be enhanced to its extremes, such as risking one's own life and wealth for helping complete strangers – there are examples of this during wars and during this pandemic, where health workers risk their own health and lives on daily basis, while helping severely ill patients (Savulescu & Wilkinson, 2020). According to Schaffner (2020), research show that crises generally bring out the best in people. Author refers to data from hundreds of case studies run by the University of Delaware's Disaster Research Centre, which indicate that when faced with disasters, the vast majority of individuals help one another, by engaging in altruistic and pro-social activities, such as volunteering, sharing goods and services, and even acts that may expose them to risk.

However, Nettle (2020), reports the recent data from studying the intuitive theories of human nature to adversity, together with his colleague Saxe, which are more pessimistic than optimistic. Namely, they asked participants about hypothetical societies where various events happen during epidemic and received bad predictions, such as that people would become more selfish and less moral; less cooperative and more nepotistic; less rule-bound and more likely to generate conflict. Participants also expressed greater perceived need for strong leadership and policing, as well as severe punishment for those who are not following the rules in such times. Furthermore, when asked about the response of their fellow citizens to the current real pandemic, participants also strongly predicted that other people will behave selfishly, compare to low or variable possibility of them behaving cooperatively. As Nettle points out, the participants are perceiving this pandemic as leading slightly more to conflict and distrust, than to solidarity. These findings could be explained by a perceived social threat, but also by a systematic gaps between the intuitive theories of behavior and the actual behavior of people in real-life situations.

There were many opportunities in the last couple of months for authors to search for the evidence of peoples' moral behavior. Whether it is the store, the hospital, at work, the waiting line in the bank or the post office, or even at home, some people stressed by the uncertainty (because that is what COVID-19 is called – "an invisible enemy"), could manifest egoistic or egocentric behavior, while others could be highly empathetic and altruistic. The former could be perceived, for example, when people panickly buy the last few products left on the shelves, fistfights over toilet paper, profiteering and thinking only on themselves (Schaffner, 2020), or when people refuse to follow the safety rules for social distancing, or when someone refuse to donate blood plasma to save someone else's life.

On the other side, there are individuals who are giving donations to hospitals or to poor citizens, the young and healthy ones who shop for the elderly, women sewing face masks for free, musicians playing concerts outside to keep the positive spirit of the people (Schaffner, 2020), the organizations that provide their data bases of books, journals, arts, and software for free to the public (ex. museums, software companies, publishing companies etc.). Then again, there are those on the "first line of fire" – the healthcare workers, doctors and nurses, who are risking their own lives while trying everything they can to save the lives of others. They are facing their own moral dilemmas, balancing between available resources and their own conscience, sometimes forced by limited number of beds and respiratory machines to decide who is going to live, and who to die.

In the beginning of the pandemic, one of the most frequently heard phrase from the officials in many countries, was to keep "social distance" in order to prevent the spread of the COVID-19 disease. Then, after some time it has been reformulated into "physical distancing" as more appropriate phrase, since "social distancing" can imply a sense of staying away from the social connections so people could stop communicating with one another (Gudi, 2020). As

Hensley (2020) explains, social distancing refers to a distance across social boundaries. Thus, it can lead one to think about social distancing as minding only one's own health. Yet, it could also be truth that it is something people need to do to protect others. With such interpretation, social distancing leads to social responsibility and solidarity as ethical virtues (Vergin, 2020), that does not depend exclusively on feelings, but on a deeper sense of commitment to a higher, more noble cause than individual's self. The virtue of solidarity also includes a commitment to social justice, which is another very important bioethical issue in this time of pandemic (Vaughan Brakman, 2020). Following this, some philosophers and medical ethicists place social distancing as a moral imperative. According to Howard (as cited in Litvack, 2020), promoting health and saving lives is a morally good goal for society. Having in mind this, as well as considering research data which clearly show that social distancing contributes to halt the spread of the virus, it is logical to support the judgment that it is morally wrong not to practice social distancing.

However, everyday evidence show that not everyone is following this advice. Not everyone is keeping required physical distance in public. Not everyone is being empathic, altruistic and helping. As stated previously, there are many examples around the world of people behaving selfishly in the stores or elsewhere, fighting, profiteering and so on. So, it is obvious that people tend to advance their own interests at the expense of others. In many countries during May this year (ex. Germany, Britain, Poland, Belgium, Italy, USA, Australia, South Africa, Brazil)[1], many people protested against the lockdowns. Why is this the case when Covid–19 is one of the 10 greatest pandemics in history of humanity[2]? There could be many answers to this. According to Howard (as cited in Litvack, 2020), poor logical reasoning of individuals demonstrated in the tendency to seek out or only listen to information that confirms what they already believe, could be one possible explanation of such behavior. The author also points out that many times practice show that people could be very self-interested and could display egoistic thinking which leads their actions afterwards. Hence, there are many examples of people refuse to stop partying, going out in cafeterias and restaurants, or gathering with friends in large groups, because they are not willing to give up the things they enjoy. In psychology, it is called *self-serving bias* present to various extent in every individual (Prentice, 2020). As an example of this, recently several new clusters of COVID-19 patients in North Macedonia appeared, provoked by weddings, birthday parties, home celebrations, religious gatherings and so on, which contribute significantly to the emergence of the second pick of the disease in the country.[3]

5. Conclusion

Plagues were not uncommon during history. There were plagues in the ancient world too, such as the one in Athens in 430 BC, similar to COVID-19 in its behavior, symptoms, and ef-

---

[1] https://www.reuters.com/news/picture/anti-lockdown-protests-around-the-world-idUSRTX7H61S.

[2] http://earth5r.org/covid-19-coronavirus-and-other-pandemics.

[3] https://www.dw.com/mk/%D0%BE%D0%B4-%D0%BA%D1%80%D1%88%D1%82%D0%B5%D0%B2%D0%BA%D0%B8-%D0%BD%D0%B0-%D1%81%D0%B2%D0%B0%D0%B4%D0%B1%D0%B8-%D1%81%D0%B5-%D1%88%D0%B8%D1%80%D0%B0%D1%82-%D0%BA%D0%BB%D0%B0%D1%81%D1%82%D0%B5%D1%80%D0%B8%D1%82%D0%B5-%D0%BD%D0%B0-%D0%BA%D0%BE%D1%80%D0%BE%D0%BD%D0%B0%D0%B2%D0%B8%D1%80%D1%83%D1%81%D0%BE%D1%82/a-53779962. https://360stepeni.mk/sobiraneto-vo-grupi-sozdade-novi-klasteri-na-kovid-19-vo-tetovo/. https://www.slobodnaevropa.mk/a/30665470.html. https://24.mk/details/nov-klaster-vo-okhrid-gosti-na-semejna-veselba-za-novorodenche-zarazeni-so-kovid-19.

fects. Although the culture and the way of living in that time were very different in many aspects compared to the present, the Epicurus teachings could also be applied today. In other words, people should try to be as calm and positive as possible, be thankful for what they have, review the way they have been living their lives, reassess their priorities and values and be focused more on their moral well-being, than on the material prosperity in order to achieve the peace of mind and true happiness (Smith, 2020).

Yet, having in mind some examples mentioned previously, an inevitable question arises: are some people too selfish to change their behavior? As Prentice (2020) advises, the modern science of moral decision making should be followed in looking for the answer. Relating this to the effective altruism explained before and the question of whether people are driven by their inner feelings and desires, or the reason has the substantial role in determining the way a person live his/her life, it seems that the former is obviously the case in many actions of some people during this pandemic. Therefore, now, more than ever is important to build "moral imagination" and a sense of shared identity so individuals could act more cooperatively. The fact is that human beings are not born to live as individual and separated atoms from others and the societies. The diseases like COVID-19 reminds every person of the importance of interdependence and interconnectedness (Khan, 2020), because if everyone look only after oneself, the humanity would lose chance to survive.

There is much goodness in the world, but there is also selfish and egoistic side of individuals and groups. Moral disengagement is closely linked to the self-regulation mechanisms of individual that need to be activated first. Thus, we should bear in mind, as Bandura (2016) points out, that some individuals can be both cruel and humane towards different people at the same time, or as Staub (2003) would say, people could both be good and bad. Hence, what is most important in the end, is that in even most extreme circumstances, how people would react highly depends on who they are, on their personality and values, on their emotional maturity. Some people would easily behave selfishly or aggressively, while others would be willing to die while saving the life of another, sometimes even a complete stranger. Thus, whether this "new normality/reality" after the COVID-19 pandemic will be optimistic and altruistic, or egoistic and morally disengaged, depends mostly on those who construct it – on us, the people.

References

Bandura 2016. Bandura, A. Moral Disengagement: How People Do Harm and Live with Themselves. New York: Worth Publishers 2016

Farsides 2007. Farsides, T. The Psychology of Altruism. The Psychologist, 20, 8, 474-477 [URL: https://thepsychologist.bps.org.uk/volume-20/edition-8/psychology-altruism visited June 1, 2020.]

Gudi 2020. Gudi, S. K. Language Matters: Is it Social or Physical Distancing to be followed during the COVID-19 Pandemic? Plos Blogs. Your Say. [URL: https://yoursay.plos.org/2020/05/29/language-matters-is-it-social-or-physical-distancing-to-be-followed-during-the-covid-19-pandemic visited June 1, 2020.]

Hensley 2020. Hensley, L. Social distancing is out, physical distancing is in — here's how to do it. Global News [URL: https://globalnews.ca/news/6717166/what-is-physical-distancing visited April 23, 2020.]

Jenkins 2020. Jenkins, M. Humanity, Above All: Facing COVID-19 with Altruism, Compassion and Empathy. Social Space [URL: https://socialspacemag.org/humanity-above-all-facing-covid-19-with-altruism-compassion-and-empathy visited June 1, 2020.]

Jeronimus 2020. Jeronimus, B.F. (2020). Personality and the Coronavirus COVID-19 Pandemic. University of Groningen Press (pre-print)

Khan 2020. Khan, M. R. How crisis awakens altruism in humanity. International Centre for Climate Change & Development (ICCCAD) [URL: http://www.icccad.net/dr-mizan-r-khan-articles/how-crisis-awakens-altruism-in-humanity visited April 23, 2020.]

Khoo & Lantos 2020. Khoo, E. J. & Lantos J. D. Lessons learned from the COVID-19 pandemic. Acta Paediatrica. Nurturing the Child. 1-3 DOI: 10.1111/apa.15307 [URL: https://onlinelibrary.wiley.com/doi/10.1111/apa.15307 visited April 23, 2020.]

Kluger 2020. Kluger, J. The Moral Dilemma of Coronavirus Quarantines. New Your Times: IDEAS COVID-19. [URL: https://time.com/5800379/coronavirus-quarantine-morality visited March 13, 2020.]

Litvack 2020. Litvack, E. Social Distancing as a Moral Dilemma: Notes From a Medical Ethicist. The University of Arizona. [URL:https://uanews.arizona.edu/story/social-distancing-moral-dilemma-notes-medical-ethicist visited May 15, 2020.]

Nettle 2020. Nettle, D. Are people selfish or cooperative in the time of COVID-19? Personal blog [URL: https://www.danielnettle.org.uk/2020/03/25/are-people-selfish-or-cooperative-in-the-time-of-covid-19 visited June 1, 2020.]

Prentice 2020. Prentice, R. More of Us Need to Think About Morality in the Time of COVID-19. University of Texas at Austin. Texas Perspectives. [URL: https://news.utexas.edu/2020/04/08/more-of-us-need-to-think-about-morality-in-the-time-of-covid-19 visited May 15, 2020.]

Regilme Jr. 2020. Regilme Jr., S. S. F. (June, 12, 2020). Opinion – COVID-19: Human Dignity Under Siege Amidst Multiple Crises. E-International Relations [URL: https://www.e-ir.info/2020/06/12/opinion-covid-19-human-dignity-under-siege-amidst-multiple-crises visited June 15, 2020.]

Savulescu & Wilkinson 2020. Savulescu, J. & Wilkinson. D. Extreme altruism in a pandemic. Journal of Medical Ethics blog [URL: https://blogs.bmj.com/medical-ethics/2020/04/23/extreme-altruism-in-a-pandemic visited April 23, 2020.]

Schaffner 2020. Schaffner. A. K. (Apr 10, 2020). The Power of Altruism: Why it matters even more in times of crisis. Psychology Today. [URL: https://www.psychologytoday.com/intl/blog/the-art-self-improvement/202004/the-power-altruism visited April 23, 2020.]

Silva 2020. Silva, V. Motivation, agency and morality in the coronavirus crisis. Social Policy Association blog. [URL: http://www.social-policy.org.uk/spa-blog/motivation-agency-and-morality-in-the-coronavirus-crisis visited June 15, 2020.]

Singer 2015. Singer, P. The Logic of Effective Altruism. Boston Review. A Political and Literary Forum. [URL: http://bostonreview.net/forum/peter-singer-logic-effective-altruism visited May 15, 2020.]

Sloan et al. 2020. Sloan, M. M., Haner, M., Graham, A., Cullen, F. T., Pickett, J. T., & Jonson, C. L. Pandemic Emotions: The Extent, Correlates, and Mental Health Consequences of Personal and Altruistic Fear of COVID-19. 1-47 Working Paper, University of South Florida.

Smith 2020. Smith, M. F. Confronting COVID-19 with Help from Ancient Philosophy. *The*

Shetland Times, p.16 in the paper "Ancient Plagues Displayed Similar Symptoms". [URL: http://www.martinfergusonsmith.com/COVID-19%20AND%20EPICUREAN%20PHILOSOPHY.pdf visited April 23, 2020.]

Staub 2003. Staub, E. The Psychology of Good and Evil: Why Children, Adults and Groups Help and Harm Others. Cambridge: Cambridge University Press

Vaughan Brakman 2020. Vaughan Brakman S. Social distancing isn't a personal choice. It's an ethical duty. VOX [URL: https://www.vox.com/future-perfect/2020/4/9/21213425/ coronavirus-covid-19-social-distancing-solidarity-ethics visited April 23, 2020.]

Vergin 2020. Vergin, J. Solidarity: How the coronavirus makes us more willing to help. DW Science [URL: https://www.dw.com/en/solidarity-how-the-coronavirus-makes-us-more-willing-to-help/a-52968633 visited April 23, 2020.]

Media websites

1. https://www.reuters.com/news/picture/anti-lockdown-protests-around-the-world-idUSRTX7H61S

2. http://earth5r.org/covid-19-coronavirus-and-other-pandemics

3. https://bit.ly/3lUtD51 (original: https://www.dw.com/mk/..........)

4. https://360stepeni.mk/sobiraneto-vo-grupi-sozdade-novi-klasteri-na-kovid-19-vo-tetovo/

5. https://www.slobodnaevropa.mk/a/30665470.html

6. https://24.mk/details/nov-klaster-vo-okhrid-gosti-na-semejna-veselba-za-novorodenche-zarazeni-so-kovid-19

Ana Fritzhand. Born in Skopje, North Macedonia, in 1978. She completed her studies in psychology at the Faculty of Philosophy, Ss. Cyril and Methodius University in Skopje in 2001. She received master degree from the same University in 2007, and doctoral degree in May 2010, both in psychology. The key research interests of prof. Fritzhand are in Developmental psychology, Moral psychology, and the Psychology of peace and conflict. During her professional career she has published numerous scientific papers, participated in a number of referent international scientific conferences and congresses, as well as in national and regional scientific research projects. Prof. Fritzhand is currently the head of the Department of Psychology at the Faculty of Philosophy in Skopje and Vice President of the Chamber of Psychologists of North Macedonia. E-mail contact: anaf@fzf.ukim.edu.mk.

Dejan Donev. Born in Skopje, North Macedonia, in 1976. He completed his studies in philosophy at the Faculty of Philosophy, Ss. Cyril and Methodius University in Skopje in 1999. He received master degree from the same University in 2005, and doctoral degree in June 2008, both in philosophy. The key research interests of prof. Donev are in Ethics, History of Ethics, especially Bioethics, Ecological Ethics and Animal Ethics. During his professional career he has published numerous scientific papers, participated in a number of referent international scientific conferences and congresses, as well as in national and regional scientific research projects. Prof. Donev is working on the Department of Philosophy at the Faculty of Philosophy, University "Sts.Cyril and Methodius", in Skopje, N. Macedonia and currently is the Head of the Center for integrative bioethics at the same faculty. E-mail contact: donevdejan@fzf.ukim.edu.mk.

Statement on individual autonomy and
social responsibility within a public health emergency

World Emergency COVID19 Pandemic Ethics (WeCope) Committee

18 July 2020

As an independent, multidisciplinary and cross-cultural committee, comprised of experts from cultures and nations across the world, we offer the following recommendations on the concepts of individual autonomy and social responsibility in the context of the COVID-19 pandemic.[1]

Introduction

Since the advent of modern Western bioethics, 'autonomy', generally defined as capacity to make informed decisions in relation to oneself, has developed as an axial ethical principle. Autonomy implies an obligation to respect. Autonomy soon became hegemonic in some contexts and thus underestimates other relevant ethical principles in our shared human existence, with great loss to our common morality.

One of the neglected ethical principles was responsibility, which is generally defined as the obligation to answer for one's own actions and omissions. Specifically, social responsibility is the obligation to contribute to the welfare of a pluralist society. However, 'responsibility' has often been viewed from a narrow legal perspective, as 'accountability', as being the direct cause of an effect, acknowledging authorship, and being subject to the penalty stipulated by law. 'Responsibility' has a broader, moral meaning as the capacity to answer for what has been done, and also for what, while having the power to do it, was not done and what ought to be. For the purpose of this statement, "responsibility' is a function of moral agency and not a legal or political construct.

Individual 'autonomy' and social 'responsibility' have been too frequently perceived as opposed concepts and realities, as if being responsible would somehow restrain the exercise of autonomy, or as if autonomous individuals would somehow dismiss their social responsibility. This is what is still happening today, in the context of the pandemic in some parts of the United States of America, for example, regarding the use of masks, with a current strong movement against their use in the name of individual autonomy, totally discarding the whole notion of responsibility.

However, this has not been the common understanding of 'autonomy' and 'responsibility' outside modern Anglo-American bioethics. At the turn of the 20th century to the 21st century, as bioethics asserted itself globally, there was a broader reconceptualization of autonomy and a parallel strengthening of its relationship with other ethical principles, namely that of responsibility, such as is already stated in article 5 of the *Universal Declaration of Bioethics and Human Rights* (2005):

"Autonomy and individual responsibility: The autonomy of persons to make decisions, while taking responsibility for those decisions and respecting the autonomy of others, is to be respected."

The awareness that autonomy requires a proportional assumption of responsibility was thus

---

[1] The chair of this WeCope Subcommittee is *Maria do Céu Patrão Neves*, PhD., Universidade dos Açores, Portugal (Email: m.patrao.neves@gmail.com). The following persons made written contributions to this Statement: *Aldrin Quintero, Darryl Macer, Dhastagir Sultan Sheriff, Fabrino Atanásio, Hasan Erbay, Kala Perkins, Lakshmi Vyas, Manuel Lozano, Marlon Lofredo, Mireille D'Astous, Raffaele Mantegazza, Rogelio P. Bayod, Şükran Sevimli, Suma Jayachandran and Nader Ghotbi.* This Statement draws on ideas and literature from many sources, and benefited through comments from other persons as well. Selected academic references are provided in background papers. https://www.eubios.info/world_emergency_covid19_pandemic_ethics_committee.

globally recognized by all countries.

The current COVID-19 pandemic has confronted each individual with their own autonomous behavior and their own obligations towards society, aware that each person can affect the well-being of the community. Indeed, this pandemic, to which there is no proven effective treatment and where the control of the infection depends on individual behavior, has dictated the valoriza-tion of the community's interest to the detriment of the individual's, voluntarily or legally, also encouraging to reframe the concepts of 'autonomy' and 'responsibility' and their relationship, within a global context of public health emergency.

1. The concepts: from a classic definition to a global understanding

Broadly, 'autonomy' is the capacity and the right to make choices by yourself towards yourself; and 'responsibility' is the duty and the obligation to acknowledge agency or to be accountable for the consequences. The individual is the direct cause of something (effect), by their own deci-sions or actions, and thus becomes accountable for the consequences. However, this is a legal, narrow, definition; the moral, broader definition is that the recognition that the exercise of autonomy is always contextualized (and not abstract) and that responsibility also falls on what was not done but what could and should have been done.

Beyond the more general and formal definition of 'autonomy' and 'responsibility', developed by different professionals and scholars, it is important to recognize that the notions these concepts convey can also be expressed by other words in different cultures.

In communities where these concepts are not common, the same idea may be present in other terms, and it is important to have this sensitivity to recognize those terms and how when they are culturally embedded also express the notions of 'autonomy' and 'responsibility'. The con-cepts of 'autonomy' and 'responsibility' can and should also be recognized in daily practice.

Recalling the example of facial masks, it is known that they have long been common in several Asian countries but were less used outside Asia. Today, it is recognized that the widespread use of masks creates two barriers to the risk of infection and therefore their use is highly recom-mended from a public health point of view.[2] In many countries where masks were not available, people started to produced them, with cultural meaningful colors and drawings, using their own resources and creativity for a common purpose.

A broad view on autonomy and responsibility allows, in the current pandemic situation and in the diversity of geo-cultural contexts in which it spreads, to engage people towards a greater awareness, both of what they can freely do and what they need responsibly to do.

Recommendation 1: *The concepts of autonomy and of responsibility should be considered in their broad moral meaning (and not in a narrow legal meaning), and in the cultural context to understand the different ways they can be expressed and the specific meaning they can ac-quire. In the current pandemic individual autonomy must be balanced with social responsibil-ity to control the spread of the infection.*

2. The context: from theoretical requirements to everyday practice

The definition of 'autonomy' and 'responsibility' as moral obligations to be acknowledged by the self and respected by others is not enough for their true and effective compliance.

Formal principles require material conditions to be fulfilled. These material conditions can in-clude political (e.g. a dictatorship weakens both, the autonomy and responsibility of citizens

---

[2] Statement of the World Emergency COVID19 Pandemic Ethics (WeCope) Committee, *Wearing Masks and Face Covers as Social Responsibility during COVID-19 pandemic* (23 April 2020).

who are expected to obey given rules), economic (e.g. low income people have to be totally focused in their survival and are not really free to make choices beyond their most basic needs), social (e.g. within some cultural and religious environments, people are constraint to follow what is traditionally established for them), educational (low level of education and/or lack of a critical mind narrow the range of choices and the awareness of responsibility) requirements. These different contexts influence the exercise of autonomy and responsibility. Also urban, rural, or tribal communities have different internal dynamics.

'Autonomy' is not only about making decisions freely about oneself, feeling empowered, and being self-confident; but also being free from fears that limit one's decision, such as violence or hunger. 'Responsibility' is not just responding from one's own decisions and actions; but also being cooperative with others, supportive at least among those close to you (a smile, listening, a prayer, are gestures of kindness available to all). Both attitudes admit different levels of performance.

In the context of a pandemic, it is important to adopt behaviors that are expected from each person as a contribution to the common good, and, above all, to urgently provide the adequate and necessary means for the exercise of both autonomy and responsibility. SARS CoV-2 can infect everyone, but not everyone is equally exposed, nor does everyone have the same conditions to protect themselves. The pandemic has worsened inequalities, further compromising the autonomy and responsibility of the most disadvantaged, in this crisis as in the future.

Recommendation 2: *The exercise of autonomy and of responsibility require some basic political, economic, social, and educational conditions to be truly and effectively developed. Otherwise, people can neither be recognized as autonomous, nor can they be held morally responsible. In the current pandemic, basic conditions for the exercise of autonomy and responsibility should be assured.*

3. The balances: from a single pattern to a diversity of dynamics

The current pandemic has revealed what was already a (underground) reality, hidden by the banner of hegemonic individualistic autonomy: individual autonomy is only ethically legitimate when exercised responsibly; likewise, responsibility can only be assumed if grounded in autonomy. Individual autonomy without responsibility lacks awareness and converts freedom into libertinism; social responsibility without autonomy can lead to violence and tyranny. Therefore, 'autonomy' and 'responsibility' are complimentary, insofar as they reinforce each other, and also interdependent, insofar as they need each other to both develop fully.

Indeed, communities are not built by a summation of single individuals. Communities are straightened nets of relationships where each part, each person evolves and defines itself by the relationships it keeps with different people and institutions. The whole is greater than the parts, the community is greater than the individuals.

The recognition of the other is the premise for self-recognition, and it is by participating in different collective works for the common good that individuals fulfill themselves.

Relationships redefine the persons.

Therefore, the responsible exercise of autonomy does not diminish personal autonomy, but recognizes that each human being is constituted in his interaction with his community. There are many gratifying examples such as volunteering, giving blood donations, food banks, animal shelter, helping old aged people, and supporting public causes like environmental protection, reducing child labor, recycling of wastes, and so on.

In the context of the pandemic, there has been many moving examples of persons who sacrifice themselves to help others: health professionals working far beyond their hours to take care of the patients; young people who satisfy some of the basic needs of elderly and others who are confined; or ordinary citizens who distribute food for those who have lost their jobs.

Recommendation 3: *Autonomy and responsibility should not be viewed separately. They are complementary concepts, and interdependent realities, so their respective exercise is reciprocally enhanced. The current pandemic has confirmed that true autonomy is always responsible and responsibility is only effective with consideration of autonomy.*

4. The interdependencies: a responsible autonomy

The recognition that both individual autonomy and social responsibility towards the community are inalienable and mutually reinforcing ethical requirements, leads to the imperative of assuming responsible autonomy in all circumstances, including the most demanding as in exceptional pandemic situations.

In the context of the SARS-CoV-2 pandemic, the balance between autonomy and responsibility was put to the test from the beginning and at four main levels: isolation of patients, quarantine for suspects, population lockdown and social distancing. Each of these different levels imposed some sort of limitation to the individual's freedom of movements, always according to the needs of the wellbeing of the community, thus viewed as a personal contribution to the common good. The pandemic will eventually contribute to a greater awareness of the human condition of community and also global interdependence and thus to the deepening of our sense of belonging and duty towards society.

Recommendation 4:

The exercise of responsible autonomy requires that each and every one recognizes the impact that one's choices can have in the community to which one belongs and to which one has duties. The current pandemic stresses the importance of responsible autonomy for everyone's life and wellbeing, as interdependent beings.

5. The citizens' obligations developing a socially responsible individual autonomy

Each person is also a citizen benefiting from the goods society provides and contributing to common good. Therefore, each person before acting, should check if his/her decision were to be adopted by all, would it contribute to a peaceful coexistence. Indeed, morality of individual decisions and actions depend on the possibility to become universal. This requirement applies directly to the current pandemic and addresses each of the following question: if my autonomous decisions and actions ought to be followed by all my fellow's citizens would my community be safer, healthier, and better than before? This is a question that each and every person is able to answer; and if they do it honestly, and act accordingly, then we would most certainly build a better world for humanity.

Different circumstances, such as the SARS-CoV-2 pandemic, require different contributions. In this context there are key ethical principles and critical procedures that should be observed:

- rejecting a narrow and limiting self-centered attitude, acknowledging that no one lives alone;

- embracing an integrated vision of oneself, as belonging to a community and coexisting with other people, as well as being inhabitants of a shared world with other beings;

- adopting a global view of the world in recognition of the network of interdependencies in which we all live;

- requiring high-quality public consultation, with the capacity to identify misinformation, and promote interdisciplinary approaches;

- understanding that the current pandemic situation requires a more altruistic, cooperative and solidarity attitude;

- recognizing that strengthening equality, that is, equal opportunities to all, is a moral challenge that will benefit each and every one.

Recommendation 5: *Moral legitimacy of individual autonomous decisions depends on their universal potential to be adopted by all. Therefore, they ought to be altruistic, cooperative, and helping to strengthen solidarity and equality. These general requirements for moral behavior become even more important in exceptionally vulnerable and demanding situations such as the current pandemic.*

6. The states' obligations promoting a socially responsible individual autonomy

States have the power and the duty to intervene in order to promote citizens' social responsibility, while protecting their individual autonomy, namely through the establishment of norms to protect public health, the supervision of their compliance and the penalty for non-compliance. Therefore, states should also balance the citizens' right to autonomy and the citizens' capacity to social responsibility when adopting public health measures, respecting individual human rights, evaluating economic and social conditions of the population to actively participate in public policies and also to comply with public health rules, and enhancing social justice. Each political decision should thus check, previously to become a rule, if there had been an opportunity to listen to all citizens, would it be reasonable to expect their agreement.

In this context there are key ethical principles and critical procedures that should be observed:

WeCope Statement on Autonomy and Responsibility within a public health emergency (18 July 2020)

6

- respect for human rights (for the three first generations of Human Rights) as the common morality worldwide;

- accuracy, taking well-informed decisions, relying on the best scientific knowledge and evidence;

- proportionality when limiting, provisionally, individual rights on behalf of the common good;

- equity or fairness in distributing burdens and benefits;

- truthfulness on the presentation of facts and doubts, probabilities and predictions;

- transparency over the definition of criteria and their implementation;

- open communication fostering a broad dialogue and enhancing a pluralistic debate;

- accountability for the decisions taken and the actions implemented.

Recommendation 6: *The moral legitimacy of political decisions depends on their consensual acceptance. Therefore, they ought to respect human rights, be accurate, proportionate, fair, truthful, transparent, inclusive, accountable. These general requirements for an ethical public policy become even more important in exceptional situations as the current pandemic, where some human rights can be provisionally limited on behalf of the common good.*

7. The international community's obligations to enhance globally responsible cooperation

States have the responsibility to work together, to cooperate and act solitarily, mostly when facing global problems, as a pandemic. This pandemic affects all human beings in the world. Although every person can be infected, the living conditions of any person may make others susceptible to infection, severe harms, and less likely to receive medical care, and to benefit from economic assistance, and less resourceful to overcome the crisis, etc. Therefore, international solidarity, at the medical, economic and social levels can contribute to the access of all people to a basic package of emergency help. Moreover, the huge endeavor to create a vaccine against the coronavirus and a safe and efficient treatment for COVID-19 can only be accomplished in a reasonable time frame through international cooperation, at the scientific level.

Recommendation 7: *Sovereign states have the obligation to cooperate with one another, at all possible levels, to contribute to global justice. In the current pandemic, all states should cooperate to the extent of their capabilities, in finding a drug or vaccine against COVID-19, and these therapies, once discovered, should be accessible to all who need them.*

Members, World Emergency COVID19 Pandemic Ethics (WeCope) Committee

Dr. Thalia Arawi (Lebanon)
Dr. Mouna Ben Azaiz (Tunisia)
Dr. Lian Bighorse (San Carlos Apache Nation, USA)
Dr. Andrew Bosworth (Canada)
Dr. Rhyddhi Chakraborty (India, UK)
Mr. Anthony Mark Cutter (U.K.)
Dr. Mireille D'Astous (Canada)
Dr. Ayoub Abu Dayyeh (Jordan)
Dr. Nilza Maria Diniz (Brazil)
Dr. Hasan Erbay (Turkey)
Prof. Nader Ghotbi (Japan)
Prof. Abhik Gupta (India)
Prof. Soraj Hongladarom (Thailand)
Prof. Miwako Hosoda (Japan)
Prof. Dena Hsin-Chen Hsin (Taiwan)
Dr. Anower Hussain (Bangladesh)
Prof. Bang-Ook Jun (Republic of Korea)
Prof. Hassan Kaya (South Africa)
Dr. Sumaira Khowaja-Punjwani (Pakistan)
Prof. Julian Kinderlerer (South Africa)
Dr. Lana Al-Shareeda Le Blanc (Iraq)
Prof. Marlon Lofredo (the Philippines)
Dr. Manuel Lozano Rodríguez (Spain)
Prof. Darryl Macer (New Zealand)
Prof. Raffaele Mantegazza (Italy)
Dr. Aziza Menouni (Morocco)
Dr. Endreya Marie McCabe (Delaware Nation, USA)
Prof. Erick Valdés Meza (Chile, USA)
Dr. Ravichandran Moorthy (Malaysia)
Prof. Firuza Nasyrova (Tajikistan)
Dr. Suma Parahakaran (Malaysia)
Prof. Maria do Céu Patrão Neves (Portugal)
Prof. Deborah Kala Perkins (USA)
Prof. Osama Rajkhan (Saudi Arabia)

Ms. Carmela Roybal (Tewa Nation, USA)
Prof. Mariodoss Selvanayagam (India)
Prof. Mihaela Serbulea (Romania)
Dr. Jasdev Rai Singh (England)
Dr. Raquel R. Smith (USA)
Prof. Takao Takahashi (Japan)
Dr. Ananya Tritipthumrongchok (Thailand)
Dr. Lakshmi Vyas (UK)
Prof. Yanguang Wang (China)
Prof. John Weckert (Australia)
Dr. Anke Weisheit (Uganda)

Inquiries to: Prof. Darryl Macer, Chair, WeCope Committee; Email: darryl@eubios.info, Tel. +1-949-439-9307

Martin Woesler, Hans-Martin Sass (Eds.)

Medicine and Ethics in Times of Corona

ISBN: 978-3-643-91320-3

Reihe: Ethik in der Praxis / Practical Ethics - Studien / Studies , Bd. / vol. 47

Albert Camus in La Peste (1947) describes how a plague of 1849 affects and kills not only people but changes and kills also societies, values, technologies, businesses. The global Corona pandemic of 2019/2020 has not come to an end and a vaccine is still under development in fall 2020. Countries set aside civil and basic human rights. The pandemic brought about triage, changes in employment, social contacts, and schooling. Families and friends cannot get together, visiting the sick, nor attending funeral. This pestilence is clearly a cultural, economic and political disease. What impact does the pandemic have on our global networks of commerce and communication? How do and will different countries respond? Leaders in medical and sociological research, in politics, religion, and consulting have different solutions. Martin Woesler (Changsha and Witten/Herdecke) and Hans-Martin Sass (Washington DC) have collected 40 diverse, sometimes controversial answers from over 24 countries.

Professor Martin Woesler lives and works in Bochum/Germany and Changsha/China; Professor Hans-Martin Sass lives in Reston VA and works in Washington DC and Bochum/Germany.

Ethik in der Praxis/Practical Ethics
Studien/Studies
hrsg. von Ilhan Ilkilic (Universität Istanbul), Arnd T. May (Erfurt), Amir Muzur (Universität Rijeka), Hans-Martin Sass (Universität Bochum/Georgetown University Washington), Martin Woesler (Universität Witten/Herdecke)

Die Reihe ETHIK IN DER PRAXIS setzt sich in interdisziplinären *Studien,* in kontroversen *Diskursen* und in der Bereitstellung von *Materialien* mit der Validierung und Integration ethischer Prinzipien und Tugenden im beruflichen Alltag auseinander. Fragen der Abschätzung von Wertfolgen und von Technologiefolgen sind zunehmend Gegenstand gesellschaftlicher Auseinandersetzung und akademischer Analyse, nachfolgend auch der politischen und verordnenden Steuerung im nationalen und transnationalen Rahmen. Insbesondere Forschung und Praxis der sich im globalen Maßstab rasant entwickelnden Technologien von Kommunikation, Molekulargenetik und Biomedizin werden international Gegenstand interdisziplinärer Güterabschätzung.

Die Reihe ETHIK IN DER PRAXIS/PRACTICAL ETHICS in ihren drei Abteilungen STUDIEN, KONTROVERSEN und MATERIALIEN, gegründet und herausgegeben von Hans-Martin Sass (Institut für Philosophie, Ruhr-Universität, Bochum, und Kennedy Institute of Ethics, Georgetown University, Washington DC), wird seit 2018 von einem erweiterten Editorial board ediert.

Hermes A. Kick
Border Situations – Crises – Postcritical Creativity
Karl Jaspers and Processdynamic Perspectives
For none of the central survival problems of mankind, which include the increase of the world population, limited resources, transcultural communication problems and information overload, convincing solution concepts exist so far. The areas of tension mentioned are taken up in this volume and placed in the context of overstrain and rebellion of the individual and society. They are the impetus for philosophical thinking and for the conceptualization of the process-dynamic approach as a survival strategy that leads to practical philosophy. Overcoming the borderline situation shows "what man actually is and can become" (Karl Jaspers). Using numerous examples from the fields of psychotherapy, artistic and political action, this book shows that historical and phenomenological analysis needs to be complemented by a process-dynamic approach.
Bd. 46, 2020, 218 S., 39,90 €, br., ISBN 978-3-643-91287-9

Sybille Fritsch-Oppermann (Hg.)
Technik für das Leben?
Interkulturelle Hermeneutik und Ethik der Wissenschaft
Bd. 45, 2022, ca. 240 S., ca. 39,90 €, br., ISBN 978-3-643-14556-7

Arnd T. May; Barbara Seehase
Advance Care Planning (ACP) in der Eingliederungshilfe
Grundlagen und Praxis zur gesundheitlichen Versorgungsplanung (SGB V §132 g)
Bd. 44, 2020, ca. 120 S., ca. 39,00 €, br., ISBN 978-3-643-14292-4

Iva Rinčić; Amir Muzur
Fritz Jahr and the Emergence of European Bioethics
The book presents the results of a long research into the life and work of the German theologian and teacher Fritz Jahr (1895 – 1953) from Halle an der Saale, who was the first to use the term "bioethics", as early as 1926. It is a revised history of bioethics with an overview of all 22 of Jahr's known published papers. The analysis follows the diffusion after 1997 of the discovery of Fritz Jahr worldwide and particularly the contribution of Croatian bioethicists to it.
Bd. 43, 2019, 154 S., 34,90 €, br., ISBN 978-3-643-91134-6

LIT Verlag Berlin – Münster – Wien – Zürich – London
Auslieferung Deutschland / Österreich / Schweiz: siehe Impressumsseite

...nčić; Amir Muzur
...n Rensselaer Potter and His Place in the History of Bioethics
Van Rensselaer Potter (1911 – 2001), the biochemist-oncologist of University of Wisconsin-Madison, was long been related to the invention of the term "bioethics". Even today, knowing that the German theologian Fritz Jahr (1895 – 1953) is to be credited for this invention, Potter's ideas do not lose on their importance, primarily for his opposition to a bioethics narrowed down onto biomedical issues. The book represents the first monograph on Potter's life and work worldwide, telling a fascinating story about a concerned top scientist and humanist.
Bd. 42, 2019, 126 S., 29,90 €, br., ISBN 978-3-643-91133-9

Tatjana Grützmann
Interkulturelle Kompetenz in der klinisch-ethischen Praxis
Kultursensible Ansätze zum Umgang mit interkulturellen Situationen in der Klinischen Ethikberatung
Bd. 41, 2016, 244 S., 34,90 €, br., ISBN 978-3-643-13489-9

Hans-Martin Sass
Cultures in Bioethics
Bd. 40, 2016, 260 S., 39,90 €, br., ISBN 978-3-643-90755-4

Simone Horstmann
Ethik der Normalität
Zur Evolution moralischer Semantik in der Moderne
Bd. 39, 2016, 268 S., 34,90 €, br., ISBN 978-3-643-13146-1

Amir Muzur; Hans-Martin Sass (Eds.)
Fritz Jahr and the Foundations of Global Bioethics
The Future of Integrative Bioethics
Bd. 37, 2012, 400 S., 49,90 €, gb., ISBN 978-3-643-90112-5

Ralf Jox; Katja Kühlmeyer; Georg Marckmann; Eric Racine (Eds.)
Vegetative State – A Paradigmatic Problem of Modern Society
Ethical, legal, social and medical perspectives on chronic disorders of consciousness
Bd. 36, 2012, 216 S., 34,90 €, br., ISBN 978-3-643-90097-5

Georg Bollig
Palliative Care für alte und demente Menschen lernen und lehren
Bd. 35, 2010, 128 S., 19,90 €, br., ISBN 978-3-643-90058-6

Jochen Vollmann; Jan Schildmann (Hg.)
Empirische Medizinethik
Konzepte, Methoden und Ergebnisse
Bd. 34, 2011, 304 S., 29,90 €, br., ISBN 978-3-643-10763-3

Johannes Huber
Totipotenz – überfordertes Kriterium der Schutzwürdigkeit?
Eine naturphilosophische Untersuchung zu den biologischen Grundlagen eines normativ gewordenen Begriffs. Geleitwort Prof. em. Dr. med. Dr. rer. nat. Henning M. Beier
Bd. 33, 2009, 200 S., 24,90 €, br., ISBN 978-3-8258-1998-9

LIT Verlag Berlin – Münster – Wien – Zürich – London
Auslieferung Deutschland / Österreich / Schweiz: siehe Impressumsseite

Acta Bioethica Supplementa
Estudios transdisciplinarios – Transdisciplinary Studies -'Etudes transdisciplinaires

edited by Prof. Dr. Fernando Lolas Stepke (Universidad de Chile)

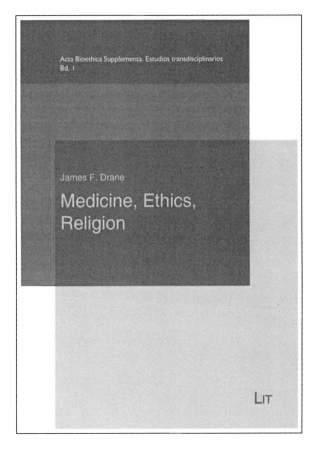

James F. Drane
Medicine, Ethics and Religion
A Christian Bioethics and A Philosophy of Life. Preface: Fernando Lolas Stepke
Medicine, Ethics, Religion addresses three topics that inevitably will be confronted at some level in every human life. Academic understanding of all three fields provides background for entering the field of medicine.
Understanding of Bioethics is part of every contemporary student's higher education. The discipline is presented as an important background understanding of contemporary culture for students. This textbook is required reading for an entry-level course in bioethics or for an introductory philosophy course with a focus on medicine. It may also help readers to understand their own lives, adding e religious dimension to the practice of medicine.
The doctor-patient relationship, an analysis of contemporary culture, the impact of technology on human life and the interfaces between medical practice, bioethics, and religion are core themes of this volume.
Bd. 1, 2018, 174 S., 34,90 €, br., ISBN 978-3-643-91015-8

LIT Verlag Berlin – Münster – Wien – Zürich – London
Auslieferung Deutschland / Österreich / Schweiz: siehe Impressumsseite

LIT aktuell

Hans-Martin Sass
Health and Happiness of Political Bodies
Environment, Business, Bio-Politics
In 1926, the German pastor Fritz Jahr in Halle coined the term 'Bioethik' and defined a 'Bio-Ethical Imperative: Respect every living being as an end in itself and treat it, if possible, as such'. Bioethics since then has grown from medical ethics and social and political strategies to multidisciplinary and integrated disciplines of research and consulting. In 2020, reflecting and mediating the interactive and integrated ecosystems and interactive networks in biology, society, business, technology and communication, I submit a wider integrated biocultural, corporate and political 'Bio-Cultural Imperative: Support direct human inter-action and common-sense as an end in itself and use hardware and software tools only in stabilizing healthy and happy cultures in the bodies of ecologies, corporations and politics'.
In 1969 a human walked on the moon, in 1989 the Berlin Wall fell down, in 2001 the World Trade Center in New York fell down, in 2020 a global Corona pandemic fell down on people and communities. Biological, political and corporate bodies change, and we change with them and in them: 'tempora mutantur et nos mutamur in illis'.
(Hans Martin Sass, preface)
Bd. 15, 2020, 88 S., 24,90 €, br., ISBN 978-3-643-91305-0

LIT Verlag Berlin – Münster – Wien – Zürich – London
Auslieferung Deutschland / Österreich / Schweiz: siehe Impressumsseite